AF770129

STATISTICAL METHODS FOR BIOMEDICAL RESEARCH

STATISTICAL METHODS FOR BIOMEDICAL RESEARCH

Editor

Jiqian Fang

Sun Yat-sen University, China

Associate Editors

Yuantao Hao • Chuanhua Yu

Yanbo Zhang • Jing Gu • Tianhe Xu

World Scientific

EW JERSEY • LONDON • SINGAPORE • BEIJING • SHANGHAI • HONG KONG • TAIPEI • CHENNAI • TOKYO

Published by

World Scientific Publishing Co. Pte. Ltd.
5 Toh Tuck Link, Singapore 596224
USA office: 27 Warren Street, Suite 401-402, Hackensack, NJ 07601
UK office: 57 Shelton Street, Covent Garden, London WC2H 9HE

British Library Cataloguing-in-Publication Data
A catalogue record for this book is available from the British Library.

STATISTICAL METHODS FOR BIOMEDICAL RESEARCH

Copyright © 2021 by World Scientific Publishing Co. Pte. Ltd.

All rights reserved. This book, or parts thereof, may not be reproduced in any form or by any means, electronic or mechanical, including photocopying, recording or any information storage and retrieval system now known or to be invented, without written permission from the publisher.

For photocopying of material in this volume, please pay a copying fee through the Copyright Clearance Center, Inc., 222 Rosewood Drive, Danvers, MA 01923, USA. In this case permission to photocopy is not required from the publisher.

ISBN 978-981-122-886-5 (hardcover)
ISBN 978-981-122-887-2 (ebook for institutions)
ISBN 978-981-122-888-9 (ebook for individuals)

For any available supplementary material, please visit
https://www.worldscientific.com/worldscibooks/10.1142/12060#t=suppl

Typeset by Stallion Press
Email: enquiries@stallionpress.com

PREFACE

This book is an English version of the second edition of the Chinese textbook titled 《生物医学研究中的统计学方法》 for postgraduate students in the bio-medical field.

Over the course of the last 10 years, the first edition of the book has accompanied the growth of tens of thousands of postgraduate students and has been viewed fondly by their advisors. In particular, the advisors have paid much more attention on statistics courses than before, as they expect their students to have solid knowledge in basic statistics and be able to blend statistical thinking into research. In addition, they have requested that we teach more about the rule and art in statistical design, for both interventional study and observational study, as well as the multivariate analyses that are necessary to clarify complex relationships. It is delightful that while facing big data, some of the postgraduate students have been self-learning the statistical models and methods not covered by our first edition to enhance their thesis writing.

Encouraged by such a trend, the authors of the original textbook have tried to reform statistics courses. Based on the practice of more than 10 institutions, we would suggest 4 short courses for postgraduates in Bio-medical field: BASIC STATISTICS (compulsory), STUDY DESIGN AND IMPLEMENT (selective 1), FREQUENTLY USED POWERFUL STATISTICAL METHODS (selective 2), and INTRODUCTION TO ADVANCED STATISTICAL METHODS (seminar). The second edition is prepared just for these courses.

Part I of this book is for the compulsory course of BASIC STATISTICS and includes nine chapters from statistical description, parameter estimation, and hypothesis testing to simple correlation and regression. In total, it needs 27 class hours for theory and practice, respectively. The concepts and logic of parameter estimation and hypothesis testing as well as the methods for univariate analyses and their prerequisites are expected to be mastered. Additionally, Part I teaches the primary operation of statistical software to allow students to be able to solve simple practical problems. Beyond the knowledge delivered, this part emphasizes cultivating statistical attainments, which might be useful to the students later in their careers.

Part II is for the selective course of STUDY DESIGN AND IMPLEMENT and includes eight chapters from sampling survey, interventional study, observational study, diagnosis study, and missing data to article writing. In total, it needs 24 class hours for theory and practice, respectively. Students are required to understand the rule of statistical design and actively apply the methods and skills being taught into their research.

Part III is for the selective course of FREQUENTLY USED POWERFUL STATISTICAL METHODS and includes seven chapters, from complex analyses of variance and variety of regressions to classical multivariate analyses. In total, it needs 21 class hours for theory and practice, respectively. This part emphasizes the selection of appropriate methods and implementation by statistical software, so intensive practice and discussion are necessary. Instead of a final exam, an essay might be required for each student to search for and analyze a set of existing data in one's own field.

Part IV is for the seminar course of INTRODUCTION TO ADVANCED STATISTICAL METHODS and includes eight chapters from meta analysis, time series, item response theory, structure equation model, multilevel model, bioinformatics and genetic statistics to data mining. In total, it needs 24 class hours for theory and practice, respectively. Rather than requiring an exam, trying new methodology is encouraged for this part. In fact, for students who are not major in statistics, it is enough to just know the idea and function of the new tools and how to apply them. Similar to eating at a restaurant, one should be able to read the menu, order dishes, and know how to enjoy the dishes after they are cooked by professionals.

Following the style of the first edition, the main body of each chapter is followed by five extra sections: Report Writing, Case Discrimination, Computer Experiments, Frequently Asked Questions & Summary, and Practice & Think.

Moreover, there are 3 appendices attached. Appendix A includes Introductions to SPSS, Excel and R, respectively. Appendix B includes all the programs, data, and printouts for Computer Experiments and the reference answers for Case Discrimination as well as Practice & Think. Appendix C includes the Statistical Tables.

As the reserve team for academic research, the postgraduate students should be cultivated with fine statistical attainments. Coming from more than 10 universities, the authors would like to devote this book to the postgraduate students in bio-medical field and sincerely hope to see them growing and prospering academically.

Jiqian Fang
December 2019, Guangzhou

CONTENTS

CHAPTER 0

INTRODUCTION

What is statistics? As defined in *Webster's Third New International Dictionary* (1961), statistics is "A science dealing with the collection, analysis, interpretation, and presentation of masses of numerical data." According to the *Dictionary of Epidemiology*, 4th ed. (John M. Last, 2000), statistics is "The science and art of collecting, summarizing, and analyzing data that are subject to random variation."

Since data and variation are ubiquitous, statistics exists in all aspects of human life. With the rapid advancement of technology and the increasing popularity of computers, statistics is becoming more and more important. In order to summarize experiences, obtain information, explore the unknown, and make precise decisions, almost all kinds of science and technology need the help of statistics. British statistician Francis Galton (1822–1911) once said "[Statistics are] the only tools by which an opening can be cut through the formidable thicket of difficulties that bars the path of those who pursue the science of man."

What is medical statistics? Medical statistics is a discipline that creates and applies statistical knowledge and methods for medicine and life sciences. In the catalog of discipline category, it is both a branch of statistics and a branch of medicine, an interdisciplinary subject combining statistics and medicine.

0.1. Why study statistics?

Looking back into history, it is not difficult to find that statistics is closely related to medicine, genetics, eugenics, and biology. Pierre

CA Louis (1787–1872), the founder of evidence-based medicine, had applied statistics to medical research long ago. In order to evaluate the popular bloodletting therapy at that time, 52 patients with severe typhoid fever were divided into two groups: 39 cases were treated through bloodletting, with an average survival time of 25.5 days; 13 cases were not given the treatment with an average survival time of 28 days; thus, the bloodletting therapy was deemed an ineffective treatment for typhoid fever. In view of the controversy over lithotripsy, Louis counted the fatality rate of patients who received traditional surgery ($1237/5715 = 21.6\%$) and compared it to that of patients who received lithotripsy ($6/257 = 2.3\%$), and determined that lithotripsy was superior to traditional surgery. After that, Karl Pearson (1857–1936) laid the foundations of biostatistics through research on eugenics and heredity and named them Biometrics. Ronald A. Fisher (1890–1962) is recognized as the founder of modern statistical science and also is hailed as the greatest biologist since Darwin.

Nowadays, medical statistics has become an invaluable tool for medical research. In order to test the effectiveness and safety of new drugs, countries around the world have laws that require researchers to conduct strict clinical trials and consider possible issues in the statistical analysis plan. Outstanding medical journals have published a variety of statistical guidelines, and have been inviting statistical experts to review manuscripts so that the medical research reports would only be published if the statistical requirements were met. Research groups who apply for research funds are encouraged to include strong statistical members . . . and so on. Because the importance of medical statistics has become a consensus, undergraduate and postgraduate students who major in clinical medicine, nursing, laboratory, rehabilitation, radiology, public health, and others, all should study medical statistics.

0.1.1. *Discovering the regularity behind uncertain phenomena*

Children born to the same parents (even twins) have different heights, weights, and personalities. Students taught by the same teacher in the same classroom have different test scores. Differences are common phenomena in nature. The differences among comparable objects are called variation. Variation makes the results of observational or experimental study uncertain, behind which statistics discovers the regularity. For example, a researcher found that the attendance rates of nurses are different in the department of psychiatry and the department of obstetrics and gynecology. Are attendance rates really different between the two departments? There are two possibilities: one is that the attendance rates of two departments are the same, and the observed difference is only an accidental phenomenon; the other is that the observed difference is not accidental and the attendance rate of psychiatric nurses is indeed lower than that of obstetrics and gynecology nurses. Which one is the actual regularity? This question can be answered by statistical inference.

0.1.2. *Considering problems in research with statistical thinking*

The main content of the section "results" in the articles of medical journals are often the results of statistical analysis. It is very important to critically understand and treat these results.

0.1.2.1. *Is the "positive" result really positive?*

For example, if a group of patients with colds was treated with a drug with a cure rate of 90% for 1 week, can we say that the anti-cold drug is effective? The therapeutic effect seems effective only in terms of cure rate, but the high self-healing rate of bad cold should also be taken into account. Is the cure rate of 90% due to the anti-cold drug or the self-healing caused by autoimmune function? Answering this question involves the establishment of a control group. If the objects were randomly divided into two groups; one group using the anti-cold drug and another group not using it, then when and only when the difference of cure rates between the two groups is statistically significant, it can be said that the anti-cold drug had a therapeutic effect. If otherwise (not statistically significant), the "positive" result would be doubtful.

0.1.2.2. *Is the "negative" result really negative?*

Seventy-one papers published in famous medical journals such as *Lancet*, *JAMA*, and *N Engl J Med* were analyzed for their negative results. It was found that 62 of them (93%) might be false-negative due to an insufficient sample size. Back to the example above, even if the drug was found to be indeed effective, the difference between the two groups might not be observed if the sample size was small and large variation within groups existed, causing a false negative result.

0.2. Biomedical research and data are inseparable

0.2.1. *Common data sources*

0.2.1.1. *Experimental records*

Experimental records, which are the main data source of biomedical research, include laboratory records and clinical trial records. For example, in a pharmacological experiment of a new drug where the experimental animals are allocated to different dose groups, the reaction of animals is observed, and median effective dose or median lethal dose is calculated; detailed records of the medication and condition changes of observed patients are taken to evaluate the efficacy of new drugs. In the long-term follow-up of clinical trials, the accumulated data are more valuable. The statistical methods for design and analysis of such interventional studies are relatively mature.

0.2.1.2. *Field investigation records*

When the required data are not available from the regular records, a field investigation can be performed to collect data. For example, in order to understand the prevalence of diabetes in an area, it is necessary to conduct a field survey. Hospital records can't meet the needs of this study because some patients with diabetes are not hospitalized, some not even diagnosed. Statistical methods for the design and analysis of such observational studies are also relatively mature.

0.2.1.3. *Electronic documents kept routinely*

Generally, various kinds of business organizations have routinely kept electronic documents. For example, a hospital's medical record information system preserves the inpatient's medical records; the medical insurance department maintains the patient's reimbursement data; and the physical examination department keeps reports of the general population. Researchers can obtain relevant information from these data resources according to their research interests. For example, in order to study the therapeutic effect on a disease over many years, the primary medical record databases of inpatients can be used to analyze the cure rate, the incidence of complications, and days of hospitalization.

Data contained in routinely kept electronic documents are relatively reliable of that full utilization will save time, labor, and money for research. Such kind of data can serve a wide range of research projects though since they are not initially designed to be used for one specific topic, researchers need to rely on more statistical methods to answer their specific questions.

0.2.1.4. *Widespread big data*

Widespread big data are also important resources for conducting biomedical research using statistical methods. (E.g., the census data every 10 years, China Health Statistics Yearbook, the national health service survey reports, etc.) In addition, there are publicly published reports, commercial databases, special research literature, and Internet data. The fourth part of this book helps in mining and analysis of such big data.

0.2.2. *Example*

In order to study whether days of hospitalization, delivery method and pregnancy outcome are related to age, height, weight, occupation, and level of education, an obstetrician has collected a total of 1402 pregnant women in a hospital from 2004 to 2005 using routinely kept primary medical records (Full data see data0-1.xls in Appendix B Computer Experiment). After ranking by hospitalization number, the data of the top 10 women are shown in Table 0.1.

Table 0.1 Data of the top 10 pregnant women

Hospitalization number	Age (y)	Height (cm)	Weight (kg)	Days of hospitalization (d)	Occupation	Level of education	Delivery method	Pregnancy outcome
20040001	25	162	76.0	9	others	middle school	natural childbirth	others
20040002	32	153	60.0	7	others	primary school	caesarean section	full term
20040003	28	158	64.0	10	others	middle school	natural childbirth	full term
20040004	29	162	68.0	8	worker	university	caesarean section	full term
20040005	27	158	68.0	6	farmer	primary school	natural childbirth	others
20040006	39	158	66.5	8	worker	middle school	caesarean section	others
20040007	23	162	68.0	11	others	primary school	caesarean section	others
20040008	20	162	70.5	4	manager	university	natural childbirth	full term
20040009	27	160	71.5	3	others	middle school	natural childbirth	others
20040010	22	162	70.0	7	worker	university	caesarean section	full term

Table 0.2 The categories of some categorical variables

Variable	Category
Occupation	worker, farmer, manager, intellectual, business service, others
Level of education	illiteracy, primary school, middle school, university, and above
Delivery method	natural childbirth, threatened preterm birth, accouche, caesarean section
Pregnancy outcome	full term, others

The category of variables such as occupation, level of education, delivery method, and pregnancy outcome are shown in Table 0.2.

The raw data are generally arranged according to the format of Table 0.1, with the variable name as the header. Each row represents the data of an individual (basic analysis unit). The first column shows the identification numbers of the individuals, and the other columns represent the observed records of the variables. The format like Table 0.1 can be considered "standard format," a format that has been widely adopted by various international standard statistical software for data analysis.

0.2.3. *Type of variables*

Usually "data" consist of the individuals' observed values of several variables. Here "individual" refers to the basic unit of research: each patient in the database of medical records, each animal in the animal experiment, and so on. A variable is a quantity that reflects an individual's characteristics or attributes. In Table 0.1, the hospitalization number, age (y), height (cm), weight (kg), occupation, level of education, days of hospitalization (d), delivery method, and pregnancy outcome are variables. Different individuals may have different values, causing variation, but otherwise, they are called constants. For example, in a study on pregnant women, "gender" is not a variable but a constant. The variables involved in statistics are random variables indeed, which can be categorized two types: quantitative variables and qualitative variables.

0.2.3.1. *Quantitative variable*

Quantitative variables are also called numerical variables, which are most common in statistical analysis. Depending on whether there are "gaps" among possible values, the quantitative variables are classified as continuous variables or discrete variables. The former can take any value in a certain interval without any "gaps," such as age (y), height (cm), weight (kg). Meanwhile, the latter can't take any value, there are "gaps" among the values, such as number of family members, number of pulse beat and many more.

0.2.3.2. *Qualitative variable*

Qualitative variables are also called categorical variables. Depending on whether there is order, rank, or size among the possible categories, qualitative variables are further divided into ordinal variables and nominal variables. The former is such as the level of education (illiteracy, primary school, middle school, university, and above) and the severity of illness (mild, moderate, and severe). The latter has no order, rank, or size among the possible categories, such as occupation, delivery method, and pregnancy outcome in Table 0.2, etc. Both ordinal variables and nominal variables can be classified as binary variables (such as gender for male or female, test scores for passing or failing, patient's survival or death) and polynomial classification variables (the "values" of occupation can be worker, farmer, manager, intellectual, business service, or others, the "values" of blood type can be A, B, AB, or O).

0.2.4. *Conversion and coding of variables*

0.2.4.1. *Transforming quantitative variables into qualitative variables*

Depending on the needs of study, sometimes quantitative variables can be converted into qualitative variables. For example, the actual measured blood pressure is a quantitative variable. Clinically, the diastolic blood pressure $<$ 80 mmHg is defined as normal blood pressure, 80–90 mmHg is pre-hypertension, 90–100 mmHg is stage I hypertension, and 100 mmHg or more is stage II hypertension. The quantitative variable of blood pressure is converted into an ordinal variable on this account. If the individuals are classified as normal or abnormal according to whether their diastolic pressures are higher than 90 mmHg, the quantitative variable of blood pressure is converted into a binary variable.

However, qualitative variables can no longer be converted into quantitative variables, in fact, quantitative data should be collected as much as possible during the data collection phase, as quantitative data contain more information than qualitative data.

0.2.4.2. *Digital encoding of qualitative variables*

In order to perform statistical analysis, the qualitative variables often need to be digitized. Digital encoding is an important skill. The binary variable can be encoded as 0 and 1. For example, a male is represented by sex = 0 and a female is represented by sex = 1; thus, the variable sex can also be referred to as the indicator variable of females. Usually, 1 indicates the category of interest, and 0 indicates the category of less interest. If the value "full term" is more interesting in variable "outcome," then we can define the indicator variable of "full term" by pregnancy outcome = 1 for full term, and pregnancy outcome = 0.

For nominal variables, any codes can be entered for the computer to recognize their classification. Each code or number serves only as a name or identifier, without the meaning of numeric values. However, in multivariate analysis, the coding of a dummy variable is needed in order to put nominal variables into the mathematical model. For example, if occupation is classified into six categories: workers, farmers, managers, intellectuals, business services, and others, then 5 dummy variables (1 less than the total number of categories) can be defined and recorded as J_1, J_2, J_3, J_4, J_5, respectively. The coding method is shown in Table 0.3.

If an individual's occupation is farmer, the values of J_1, J_2, J_3, J_4, J_5 are 0, 1, 0, 0, 0, 0; if an individual's occupation is intellectual, the values of J_1, J_2, J_3, J_4, J_5 are 0, 0, 0, 1, 0; if an individual's occupation is others, the values of J_1, J_2, J_3, J_4, J_5 are

Table 0.3 The coding method of dummy variables

	Labels of dummy variable				
Occupation (J)	J_1	J_2	J_3	J_4	J_5
Worker	1	0	0	0	0
Farmer	0	1	0	0	0
Manager	0	0	1	0	0
Intellectual	0	0	0	1	0
Business service	0	0	0	0	1
Others	0	0	0	0	0

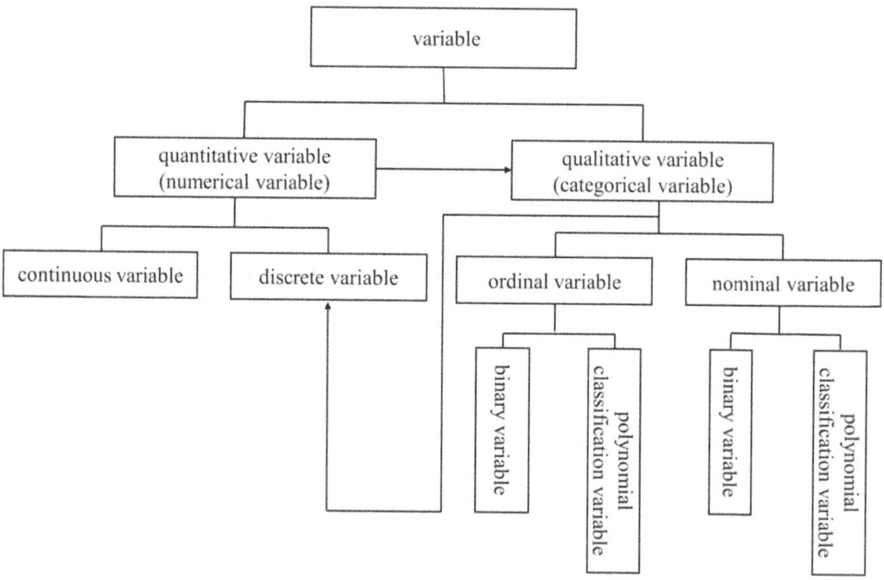

Figure 0.1 Variable types of statistical data

0, 0, 0, 0, 0. In this way, these 5 dummy variables are indicator variables of workers, farmers, managers, intellectuals, business services taking "others" as reference. Given the number of categories, most statistical software can automatically generate dummy variables similar to the above, as long as the variable is a categorical one.

Ordinal variables can be encoded as $1, 2, 3$, in order from smallest to largest. The corresponding scores can also be given according to the actual situation. For example, "level of education" can be coded as $1, 2, 3, 4$ corresponding to illiteracy, primary school, middle school, university and above, respectively; or it can also be coded as 0, 6, 12, 16 according to the years of study.

The types and transformations of variables can be summarized as Figure 0.1.

0.3. Common basic concepts

0.3.1. *Homogeneity and variation*

Individuals with the same attributes are called homogeneous. However, even if the individuals are homogeneous, there may be differences among them, which are called variations. For example, the height, weight, and other characteristics of twins can be considered homogeneous, but there must be variation within twins on a homogeneous basis. Variation is the basis of statistical research, without which there is no need for statistics. Statistics is the science and art dealing with variation within data.

0.3.2. *Population and sample*

The homogeneous subjects to be studied for certain research purposes as a whole constitute a population. The population is usually very large. For example, if the research purpose is whether the water quality of East Lake in Wuhan is polluted, the population is the water of entire East Lake. If the research purpose is to estimate the white blood cell count of normal adults in an area, the population is all the white blood cells of normal adults in the area. There are two kinds of population, finite population and infinite population.

We will not extract the water of the entire East Lake to study its water quality, nor will we extract all the blood of normal adults in an area to study their white blood cell counts, but we will extract a portion of individuals from the population for study. The subjects that are extracted from the population constitute a sample. Random sampling allows each individual in the population to have the same opportunity to be selected as a member of the sample, helping to ensure the reliability and representativeness of the sample.

In general, if the number of individuals in a sample is much smaller than the total number of individuals in the population (e.g., the total number of individuals in the population is 10,000 and the number of individuals in the sample is 450, the number of individuals in the sample is less than 5% of that in the populations), then the population can be approximately regarded as an infinite population.

0.3.3. *Parameter and statistic*

The quantity describing the statistical characteristic of a population is called a parameter. Once the population is determined, the parameters are the constants that define it. Parameters such as mean, standard deviation, and probability of population are denoted by Greek letters μ, σ, and π, respectively.

The quantity describing the statistical characteristic of a sample is called a statistic. Statistics are obtained from a sample. The variation of individuals makes the samples different, causing variation among the values of statistics that are based on the differing samples. Therefore, it can be concluded that a statistic is also a random variable that changes around the population parameter. Sample statistics such as mean, standard deviation, and probability of sample, are commonly expressed in English letters, and are denoted by $\bar{X}, S$, and P, respectively.

0.3.4. *Error*

Error refers to the difference between the measured value and the true value. Generally there are two types of error, random error and systematic error. Random error is limited by the precision of measurement. The actual measured values obtained by repeated measurements are often different, but fluctuate around a certain value in an undirected way, which is subject to random error (Figure 0.2). Due to the existence of variation, random error is inevitable. However, it can be reduced by increasing the number of repeated measurements

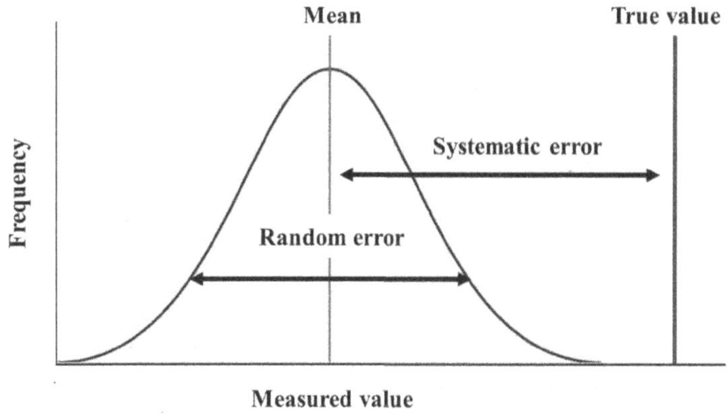

Figure 0.2 The diagram of error

(in other words, increasing the sample size) and calculating the average value.

Another type of error is systematic error, also called bias. It is the difference between the actually measured value and the true value (Figure 0.2). In theory, systematic error runs through the whole research process, usually caused by the lack of calibration of instruments and some bias in subjectivity, but can be avoided if the above problems can be overcome. Accuracy is usually used to describe the proximity between measured values and true values.

In addition, there is a gross error, which is caused by accidental mistakes of researchers during the experiment like instrumental failure, mistakes in records, wrong decimal points, wrong units, etc. Gross error is not included in the error analysis, and must be eradicated from the study.

0.3.5. *Random event*

Given a research purpose and certain conditions, the observation or experiment of a random phenomenon (uncertainty phenomenon) is called a random trial. The outcome of a random trial, which is called a random event or simply an event, is uncertain beforehand. Contrary to random events, there are certain events and impossible events, which are out of the focus of statistics.

0.3.6. *Probability and frequency*

A measure of the likelihood of occurrence of an event is called probability. It is generally represented by the capital letter P, with values ranging from 0 to 1. The probability of a certain event is 1, the probability of an impossible event is 0, and the probability of a random event is $0 < P < 1$.

When the probability of a random event $P \leq 0.05$ (5%) or $P \leq 0.01$ (1%), it is commonly called a small probability event. Since the probability of an event is small, it is unlikely to occur in one round of sampling. In practice, people often treat "unlikely" as "impossible"; thus, whenever a small probability event occurs in once of sampling, people can't help but ask "What's the matter? That's a coincidence. Is there something wrong?" Statistics is based on such thinking in order to perform statistical inference.

In real life, the population probability of random event is often unknown, and the actual sample frequency of the event is often used to estimate the population probability. If under the same conditions, n trials are repeated independently, and event A occurs f times, the frequency of event A is f/n.

The relationship between sample frequency and population probability is as follows: the frequency always fluctuates randomly around the probability; when the sample size n is larger, the range of fluctuation will be smaller, and the sample frequency is closer to the population probability.

0.4. Statistical work throughout the entire process of biomedical research

Statistical work in medical research includes research design, data collection, data sorting, statistical analysis, and report writing.

0.4.1. *Research design*

Before engaging in disease investigation, clinical trials, laboratory tests, and other research works, research design should be completed. Whether the intervention is applied to the research subjects or not, the research can be classified as either experimental study or observational study. Experimental studies, including animal experiments and clinical trials (research subjects of the latter are human), require interventions on the subjects; the corresponding design is called experimental design. The experimental design should follow four basic principles: randomization, control, replication, and balance. Observational studies, on the other hand, do not impose any intervention measures on the research subjects, and data are obtained mainly through field investigations. Before the investigation, it is necessary to make a careful plan for the research purpose, subjects, content, method, progress, expected results, and so on, which is called a survey design.

Statistical work must begin with research design. Fisher, the pioneer of statistics, has repeatedly emphasized in his work that collaboration between statisticians and scientific researchers should begin at the design stage, not during data processing. In his words, "To consult the statistician after an experiment is finished is often merely to ask him to conduct a post mortem examination. He can perhaps say what the experiment died of." The second part of this book will focus on the methods and art of research design.

0.4.2. *Data collection*

Earlier, the main sources of data were introduced. Whether they are experimental data, field investigation data, or routinely kept electronic documents, data collection should adhere to three principles: accuracy, completeness, and timeliness. To this end, data collecting personnel should have high enthusiasm, a strong sense of responsibility, and have received uniform and strict training.

0.4.3. *Data sorting*

Data sorting, also known as data cleaning, aims to sort the raw data through systematization and organization for further statistical analysis.

Sorting or cleaning includes the inspection, verification, and correction of the raw data, as well as preprocessing the data. For a quantitative variable, the maximum value, minimum value, and mean can be calculated to check whether these values are in conflict with reality. For example, if you find that the maximum age is over 150 or there is a negative value of age, you will need to check whether the raw data are recorded incorrectly or the computer input is incorrect. For a qualitative variable, the frequency distribution of the categories can be calculated. If there is a category that does not match the actual situation, it should be checked and corrected.

Systematization and organization refer to reasonable grouping and rational summarization of the raw data for further analysis according to research purpose.

0.4.4. *Statistical analysis*

Statistical analysis is the core component of statistics, mainly including statistical description and statistical inference.

Statistical description includes the calculation of mean, frequency and indicators for their variation (such as standard deviation and coefficient of variation), and the production of statistical tables and charts.

Statistical inference is the process by which the sample data are used to estimate or understand its corresponding population, such as through confidence interval and hypothesis testing.

In addition to the first 2 parts, the third part of this book will introduce popular multivariate analysis, including multiple linear regression, logistic regression, the Cox's model, etc. The fourth part will introduce useful modern statistical models and methods, including the structural equation model, the multi-level model, item response theory, and statistical methods and data mining techniques in bioinformatics, genetic research, etc. Usually, the calculation is very heavy, so we will help readers applying these advanced and complex methods to their own studies with the statistical software SPSS, EXCEL and R package.

0.5. Report writing

In the era of computers, most tasks of statistical analysis can be completed by technology. It is increasingly important to correctly comprehend the statistical thoughts and output results of statistical software, and make appropriate interpretations and expressions in the scientific papers. Previous textbooks have not emphasized this statistical step enough, resulting in frequent statistical errors in professional journals.

In the scientific report, it is generally necessary to clearly point out the statistical design and analysis methods, the statistical software used, the estimated values of statistics and the corresponding probabilities, and make a reasonable explanation of statistical analysis results combined with the professional knowledge of various disciplines. For training, Report Writing is focused in each chapter.

The following paragraph is a brief summary and description of the data in Section 0.2.2:

In order to study the risk factors of delivery method and pregnancy outcome, the medical records from routinely kept hospital records were used. The population was the whole pregnancy women and the sample consisted of 1402 pregnant women in a hospital within 2 years from 2004 to 2005. Age (y), height (cm), weight (kg), days of hospitalization are quantitative variables which include 3 continuous variables (age, height, and weight) and a discrete variable (days of hospitalization); occupation, level of education, delivery method and pregnancy outcome are qualitative variables which include a binary variable (pregnancy outcome), 2 nominal variables (occupation and delivery method), and 1 ordinal variable (level of education).

0.6. Case discrimination

Case 0.1 To study the physical and mental health status of college students and its influencing factors, a researcher investigated the students (3-year program) in a vocational-technical college. Sixty science students, 38 engineering students, 19 literature students, and 46 medical students were selected, and the general health status, anxiety and depression status of each student were collected by questionnaires. The conclusion of this study was: "The physical and mental health of college students is not optimistic, academic problems, employment pressure, poor physical condition, poor interpersonal communication and inadequate social support are the main influencing factors." Is the conclusion reasonable? Why? How should we improve it?

Case 0.2 Two drugs were tested as treatments for a certain disease. Of the 5 patients who were treated with drug A, 4 improved, and of the 50 patients who were treated with drug B, 36 improved. Hence a researcher concluded that drug A is better than drug B. Is this conclusion reasonable? Why? How should we improve it?

Case 0.3 In order to investigate the monitoring indicators of early renal tubular damage in hypertensive patients, 74 cases of hypertensive patients found negative for both urinary routine test and protein qualitative test and normal for both of serum creatinine and urea nitrogen were selected as the case group. The group included 43 males and 31 females with an average age of 61 years (40–73 years). According to the course of hypertension, the patients were divided into three subgroups: subgroup I included patients with hypertension less than 10 years, subgroup II included patients with hypertension for 10–20 years, and subgroup III included patients with hypertension for more than 20 years. Another 53 healthy workers were selected as the control group. The values of four quantitative indicators including urinary RBP, mALB, β_2-MG, and NAG were observed in two groups. The conclusion was that urine RBP, mALB, β_2-MG, and NAG were sensitive indicators for early glomeruli and renal tubules damage in hypertensive patients. What is wrong with this design? What is the correct way to do it?

Case 0.4 There were 1200 persons in an army, of which 120 persons (114 males and 6 females) suffered from a disease in a certain period. After statistical analysis, a health worker said that the incidence rates of the disease between male and female were significantly different (male $114/120 = 95\%$ and female $6/120 = 5\%$), and thus concluded that males were prone to this disease. What do you think of this conclusion? If the conclusion is wrong, then what is the type of error? What is the correct way to do it?

0.7. Computer experiments

Experiment 0.1 Opening an Excel file with SPSS Assuming that the data file data0-1.xls is stored in the "D:\data\" subdirectory, learn how SPSS opens the file.

Experiment 0.2 Automatically recoding data with SPSS SPSS has a variety of coding methods for qualitative variables. This experiment learns simple automatic recode.

Because SPSS sometimes does not display the names of the character variables (such as Analysis ——> Compare Means ——> One-way ANOVA), regression analysis also needs variable digitization, so it is necessary to code variables. SPSS has a variety of coding methods, and this experiment only introduces relatively simple automatic recode.

0.8. Frequently asked questions and summary

0.8.1. *Frequently asked questions*

1. Is study population and target population the same thing?

They're not the same thing. The study population is also called the sampling population or sampling frame, and the target population is the population of homogeneous research objects determined according to the research purpose. Although sometimes they can be consistent, when the study population does not fully cover the target population, they are inconsistent. For example, suppose one wants to study the growth curve of children in the country, and has sampled from a few local elementary schools of 10 cities in the country. In this case, the target population is the children of the country, but the study population is the local students in the 10 cities.

2. Is red blood cell count a continuous variable or a discrete variable?

Red blood cell count is a discrete variable because there are "gaps" among the values of the red blood cell count. However, because the values are relatively large and the "gaps" among these values are relatively small, it is often regarded as a continuous variable in practice.

3. Are the conclusions drawn from different coding methods the same?

As mentioned above, "level of education" is assumed to be an ordinal variable, and can be coded as 1, 2, 3, 4 according to illiteracy, primary school, middle school, university and above, or 0, 6, 12, 16 according to the years of schooling. The conclusions of statistical analysis obtained from different codes are generally consistent, but some statistics obtained may be different (see the frequently asked question in Chapter 20).

0.8.2. *Summary*

1. Statistics is a discipline related to research design and data analysis, which is known as a science that collects data from specific circumstance and extracts information and knowledge from the data.
2. The methods of statistical analysis are selected according to the purpose of analysis, the attributes of data and the type of outcome (effect) variables. There are two kinds of variables, quantitative and qualitative variables. Qualitative variables are also called categorical variables. According to whether order exists among categories, qualitative variables can be classified as ordinal variables and nominal variables. Quantitative variables can be classified as discrete variables and continuous variables, while qualitative variables can only be discrete variables after encoding.
3. The basic concepts of random event and random variable, homogeneity and variation, population and sample, parameter and statistic, random error and bias, frequency and probability, etc. will frequently appear in the following chapters. Readers will need to deepen their understanding of them.
4. Statistical work runs through the entire process of medical research, including research design, data collection, data sorting, analysis, and report writing. It should be noticed that statistics is not simply limited to "data analysis."

Think and Practice

I. Best Choice

1. The basic unit of medical research is ( ).
   A. Sample B. All objects C. Influencing factor D. Individual E. Population
2. The purpose of sampling from a population is ( ).
   A. Studying sample statistics B. Inferring population parameters from sample statistics C. Studying typical cases D. Studying population statistics E. Calculating statistical indicators
3. Parameter as a term refers to ( ).
   A. The number of participating individuals B. The quantity describing the statistical characteristic of a population C. The quantity describing the statistical characteristic of a sample D. The sum of samples E. The number of involved variables
4. Which of the following is a nominal variable ( ).
   A. White blood cell count B. Days of hospitalization C. Number of outpatients and emergency patients D. The classification of patient's condition E. ABO blood type
5. Which of the following is incorrect about the term of random error? ( ).
   A. Limited by the precision of measurement B. Non-directional C. Also called bias D. Inevitable E. Can be reduced by increasing the sample size

II. Interpretation of Terms

1. Random variable
2. Homogeneity and variation
3. Population and sample
4. Parameter and statistic
5. Error
6. Random event
7. Frequency and probability

III. Questions

1. What are the differences and connections between biostatistics and other branch of statistics?
2. There are 50 boys in each of Class A and Class B. Ten boys were selected from each of the two classes to measure their heights, and average values were calculated respectively. If the average height of Class A is higher than that of Class B, can we infer that the average height of boys in Class A is higher than that of Class B? Why?
3. In order to study the height and weight of 100,000 normally developed 7-year-old boys in a region, 200 are randomly selected from them to measure their height and weight. Please answer the following questions.
   (1) What is the population in the study?
   (2) What is the meaning of population mean of height in this study?
   (3) What is the meaning of population mean of weight in this study?
   (4) What is the relationship between the population mean and population in this study?
   (5) What is the sample in the study?

Jiqian Fang, Chuanhua Yu, Fang Shi

Part I

Basic Concepts and Methods

CHAPTER 1

STATISTICAL DESCRIPTION

Statistical analysis includes statistical descriptions and statistical inferences. For statistical description of the collected data, statistical charts, tables or statistical measures can be chosen.

1.1. Statistical description of quantitative data

1.1.1. *Frequency table of quantitative data*

(1) Frequency table and frequency histogram

In order to study the distribution of quantitative data, enough individuals need to be drawn randomly from the population. Through further sorting, the frequency distribution table is constructed, which is called frequency table for short.

Example 1.1. The weights (kg) of 1402 parturient mothers observed by an obstetrician are as follows (see data file data1-1.xls or data1-1.sav for complete data).

76.0	60.0	64.0	68.0	68.0	66.5	68.0	70.5	71.5	70.0	57.0	68.0	65.5	58.0
63.0	65.0	71.5	74.0	56.5	64.0	60.0	64.5	68.0	65.0	68.0	65.0	63.0	62.0
	...												
59.5	62.0	76.5	61.0	75.0	56.0	73.0	69.0	53.5	65.0	60.0	69.0	65.0	66.0
72.0	55.0												

Through the following steps, a frequency table (Table 1.1) is obtained. In the table, the first column divides the data into several

Table 1.1 Frequency table for weight (kg) of 1402 parturient mothers

Interval (1)	Mid-value (2)	Counts (3)	Frequency f_i (%) (4)	Cumulative frequency (%) (5)
48~	50	6	0.4	0.4
52~	54	54	3.8	4.2
56~	58	162	11.6	15.8
60~	62	293	20.9	36.7
64~	66	359	25.6	62.3
68~	70	298	21.3	83.6
72~	74	140	10.0	93.6
76~	78	70	5.0	98.6
80~	82	17	1.2	99.8
84~88	86	3	0.2	100.0
Total	—	1402	100.0	—

intervals (usually 10–15 groups). The first interval should include the minimum value, and the last interval should include the maximum value. It is customary to set each interval as half-open with left closing and right opening, such as the first interval [48, 52). The mid-value in column 2 is the representative value for each interval, which is actually the average of the upper limit and the lower limit of this interval. Columns 3 and 4 are counts and frequency, count is the number of individuals falling within each group, frequency is the proportion of a count in the total number of individuals, also known as the relative frequency or constituents. Column 5 is the cumulative frequency.

If the horizontal axis is the weight and the vertical axis is the frequency density of each group (the ratio of frequency to length of interval, where the frequency is the fourth column of Table 1.1, the length of interval is 4 kg), the data in Table 1.1 can be drawn as frequency histogram (Figure 1.1).

As can be seen from Figure 1.1, the bar locating in the middle of the chart is the highest (the peak locates at center). Either left or

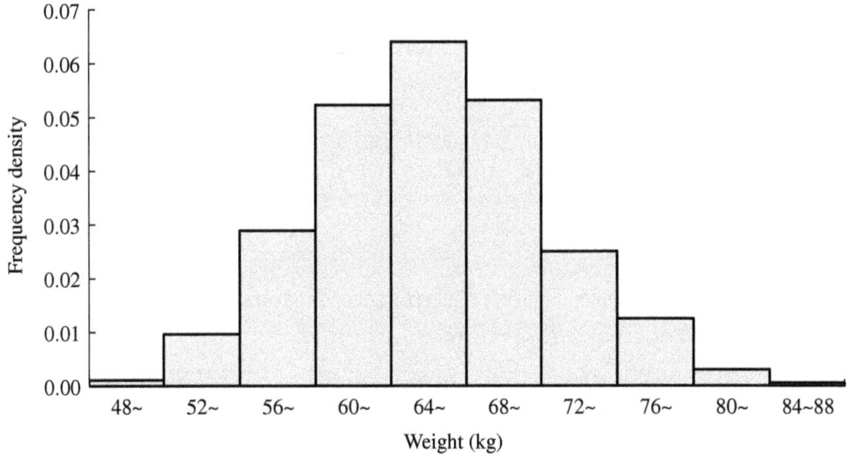

Figure 1.1 Frequency distribution for weight (kg) of 1402 parturient mothers

right parts decline almost symmetrically. The area of each of bars is the frequency of the corresponding interval, the sum of the frequencies of all the intervals is the sum of the areas of the corresponding bars, and the sum of the whole histogram area is 1.

(2) Two characteristics of the frequency distribution

Two important characteristics of frequency distribution can be seen from the frequency table and frequency distribution histogram: central tendency and tendency of dispersion. As can be seen from Table 1.1, the weight of 1402 parturient mothers varies from high to low, but it obeys a certain distribution rule: (1) The weights closer to the central part tend to have higher frequency, which is called central tendency; (2) The majority of individual values do not coincide with average completely. Instead, they deviate from average in varying degrees, which is the tendency of dispersion. Central tendency and tendency of dispersion are two important perspectives of frequency distribution, they can comprehensively summarize the information contained in quantitative data.

1.1.2. *Statistical description measures of quantitative data*

Quantitative data are described by statistical measures in two aspects: central tendency (i.e., average) and tendency of dispersion (i.e., severity of variation).

1.1.2.1. *Central tendency*

(1) Arithmetic mean is also simplified as mean. The population mean is represented by Greek letters μ and the sample mean is represented by $\overline{X}$. The mean reflects the quantitative average of observations following a symmetric distribution. The formula is

$$\overline{X} = \frac{X_1 + X_2 + \cdots + X_n}{n} = \frac{\sum X}{n} \tag{1-1}$$

(2) Median, M. The median is the observation value that ranks in the middle of a group of observations. Arrange the observations from minimum to maximum, the one locates in the middle is the median.

In statistics, percentile is a commonly used parameter of location, expressed as P_x (read as the x-th percentile). P_x divides all observations in the population (or sample) into two parts, with x % of observations smaller than it, and the remained (100-x) % of observations larger than it. According to this, P_{50} is the median, that is, the median is a special percentile.

(3) Geometric mean, G. Some data in medical research, such as antibody titer, bacterial count, etc. are all larger than 0. Their frequency distribution is obviously asymmetric. However, logarithm transformation to observed values may approximately lead to a symmetrical distribution. For this data, the geometric mean can be used to describe its average level.

The formula is to extract an n-th root to the product of n observed values $X_1, X_2, X_3 \ldots, X_n$.

$$G = \sqrt[n]{X_1 \cdot X_2 \cdot X_3, \ldots, X_n} \tag{1-2}$$

Or displayed in logarithmic form

$$G = \lg^{-1}\left(\frac{\lg X_1 + \lg X_2 + \lg X_3 + \cdots + \lg X_n}{n}\right) = \lg^{-1}\left(\frac{\sum \lg X}{n}\right) \tag{1-3}$$

In the formula, $\lg^{-1}$ represents the antilog based on 10, and each observation value $X > 0$ is required. If there are any negative numbers, a positive number is added to each observation value before hand.

Example 1.2. Serum antibody titers of 5 people were 1:2, 1:4, 1:8, 1:16, 1:32. Please calculate the average titer.

In this example, the reciprocal values of the titers are statistically described as 2, 4, 8, 16, 32.

Severely dominated by the maximum value, its arithmetic mean is 12.4, which does not represent the average of these five observations. Their geometric mean is

$$G = \sqrt[5]{2 \times 4 \times 8 \times 16 \times 32} = 8$$

or $\lg G = \frac{\lg 2 + \lg 4 + \lg 8 + \lg 16 + \lg 32}{5} = 0.903$

$$G = \lg^{-1} 0.903 = 8$$

Therefore, the average antibody titer is 1:8.

1.1.2.2. *Tendency of dispersion*

(1) Standard deviation It is used to measure the variability of quantitative variables.

$X - \mu$ is the measurement of deviation from mean, which is the difference between the observed value and the population mean. The average of $X - \mu$ cannot be used to show the variability of individuals in the population, because summation of $X - \mu$ is 0. In practice, we use average of $(X - \mu)^2$ to summarize the deviation for the individuals in the population, as it treats the variation same if two observations have an equal absolute value of $X - \mu$. The average of $(X - \mu)^2$ is named population variance, denoted as σ^2.

The dimension of the variance is the square of the dimension of the original data. In order to express variability by the original dimension, we calculate the square root of the population variance. It is called the population standard deviation σ. The larger the standard deviation, the greater the variation among individuals.

In practice, it is often impossible to calculate the population means μ and only the sample mean $\overline{X}$ can be applied to replace μ. If is found that when $\overline{X}$ is used instead of μ, the variability of individual deviation from $\overline{X}$ in the sample is smaller than the degree of deviation from μ, so that the average value of the squared deviation also tends to be small. British statistician W.S. Gosset proposed using $n - 1$ instead of n to calculate the average level of the square of the deviation in the sample, that is, the sample variance

$$S^2 = \frac{\sum (X - \overline{X})^2}{n-1} \tag{1-4}$$

The arithmetic root of the above formula is the sample standard deviation, where $n-1$ is called the degree of freedom. In this example, $S = 6.07$ kg can be obtained from SPSS based on the original data.

The degree of freedom is a statistical term, the meaning of which is the number of random variables that can be "freely" valued; in this case, $\overline{X}$ is used as a given condition, resulting in only $n - 1$ of the observations being arbitrarily valued. The summarized variability in the sample should use denominator $n - 1$.

(2) Range (R) is the difference between the maximum and minimum values of a set of observations, which may roughly reflect the variability of observed values.

When range is used, the explanation of the variability is simple and clear, so it is widely used, such as to evaluate the incubation period of the disease. But the disadvantages are (1) only the information provided by the maximum and minimum values is used. It fails to summarize the variability of other individuals in the sample. (2) Due to the influence of sampling error, the calculated results of range tends to be unstable. (3) When the sample size increases, the possibility of drawing more extreme observations also increases, resulting in a wider range. Therefore, it is not appropriate to compare two ranges when they are obtained by very different sample sizes.

(3) Inter-quartile range Quartiles (Q) are also two special percentiles. Including P_{25} and P_{75}. There are one-fourth of all observations smaller than P_{25}, which is called lower quartile, and sometimes it is denoted as Q_L; there are one-fourth of all observations larger than P_{75}, which is called upper quartile, and sometimes it is denoted as Q_U. The inter-quartile range is the difference $Q_U - Q_L$, covering half of all observations. The wider the range, the higher the degree of variation; on the contrary, the smaller the degree of variation. For example, in a study on incubation period of poisoning by salmonella in food, $P_{25} = 15.3$ h, $P_{75} = 36.1$ h, and the inter-quartile range is $Q_U - Q_L = 36.1 - 15.3 = 20.8$ h. This value reflects the degree of variability in the latency of this type of disease caused by salmonella poisoning in food. In many circumstances, we prefer to provide the exact locations of Q_L and Q_U instead of inter-quartile range for description. It shows the range that the middle half of the individuals cover. In this example, the inter-quartile range could be reported directly $(Q_L, Q_U) = (15.3, 36.1)$ h.

(4) Coefficient of variation (CV) is the ratio of the standard deviation to the mean, expressed as a percentage. The formula for calculating the CV based on sample information is

$$\text{CV} = \frac{S}{\overline{X}} \times 100\% \tag{1-5}$$

The standard deviation, inter-quartile range, and range are all dimensional indicators, and the dimensions are the same as the original observations. The CV is a relative value and it has no dimension. It is often used to: (1) Compare the degree of variation between variables with different dimensions. (2) Compare the degree of variation between variables with the same dimension but a severe difference in the scale, for example, $\times 10^3 p$ mol/L vs. $10^6 p$ mol/L.

1.2. Statistical description of qualitative data

Like quantitative data, qualitative data can also be described by frequency table, and some popularly used parameters to show the relative level can be applied for statistical description.

1.2.1. *Description of categorical data — frequency and frequency distribution*

(1) Description of the binary variable — frequency

When there are only two possible outcomes, a relative frequency is often used to describe the regularity of the outcome. Two possible outcomes in medical research are common, such as positive and negative in skin test results, survive and death of living status, etc. At this time, researchers often focus on one of the outcomes (referred to as positive events in this study). For example, the study on survival status may focus on the frequency of death, and the study of disease status may focus on the frequency of illness.

Example 1.3. An obstetrician recorded the pregnancy status of 1402 parturient mothers, resulting in 1148 full-term births. If the positive event of interest to investigator is full-term production, the full-term production frequency can be calculated as 1148/1402 = 81.9%.

Generally, in a specific study, the positive event of interest needs to be defined first, and then the frequency of the positive event is calculated as follows, which is referred to as the positive rate.

$$\text{Positive rate} = \frac{\begin{array}{c}\text{Number of individuals who actually have a}\\ \text{positive event in the observed persons}\end{array}}{\begin{array}{c}\text{Total number of observed individuals who}\\ \text{may have a positive event}\end{array}} \times K \tag{1-6}$$

Among them, the numerator is part of the denominator. K is the proportional base, usually taken as 100%, 1000‰, 10,000/10,000 and 100,000/100,000, etc. It is customary to ensure that the calculated result contains 1 or 2 integers. For example, we use 7.5×10^{-6} to show the prevalence rate instead of 0.0075%, which means that more than 7 out of every 1,000,000 people suffer from a certain disease. The essence of the positive rate is relative frequency, which is an estimation to the probability of occurrence of a positive event in the population.

Sometimes researchers are not only concerned with the relative frequency of full-term production (81.9%), but also the relative frequency of premature production $(1402 - 1148)/1402 = 18.1\%$. Here the sum of these two relative frequencies must be 100%. Once one of them is known, another is fixed. Thus, the binary categorical variable requires only one relative frequency that is sufficient to describe the distribution characteristics of outcome.

(2) Description of multi-classification data — frequency distribution

When observations have more than two possible forms of outcome, distribution of frequencies is often used to describe distribution characteristics of outcome.

Example 1.4. An obstetrician recorded the occupations of 1402 parturient mothers. The results are listed in column 2 of Table 1.2. Calculate the frequency distribution of various occupations in column 3.

Table 1.2 Frequency distribution of a survey on the occupations of parturient mothers

Occupation	Count	Relative frequency (%)
Physical labor	208	14.8
Farmer	102	7.3
Intellectual labor	206	14.7
Manager	141	10.1
Service trade	208	14.8
Other	537	38.3
Total	1402	100.0

1.2.2. *Description of person-time data — intensity*

In epidemiological follow-ups, the lengths of time that individuals stay in the cohort vary. The sum of person-time is commonly used to represent the total amount of observations. For example, if a person is observed for half a year, the total amount he contributes is 0.5 years $\times$ 1 person $=$ 0.5 person years; the other 2 people are observed for 1 year respectively, and the total amount of their contribution is 1 year $\times$ 2 persons $=$ 2 person years.

Example 1.5. A hospital had A and B surgery treatments for the same disease, and 100 patients were randomly selected to evaluate the recurrence rate. The lengths of time after surgery are different, and the final follow-up of patients who have not relapsed is January 1, 2018. In order to save space in this book, only a part of data is given in Tables 1.3 to illustrate the statistical description.

If we neglect the characteristics of person-time data and calculate by formula (1.6), we will mistakenly conclude that the recurrence rates of the two operations are the same, both of which are 1/3. The correct way is to first calculate person-years observed for each patient without recurrence after operations. See the last column in

Table 1.3 Comparison of recurrence rates between two operations (shorted data)

Operations	Completion date of surgery	Recurrence	Person-years of observations
A	January 1, 2002	Recurrence on January 1, 2017	15.0
	July 1, 2003	No recurrence	14.5
	January 1, 2008	No recurrence	10.0
	Total	—	39.5
B	January 1, 2006	Recurrence on January 1, 2007	1.0
	January 1, 2016	No recurrence	2.0
	July 1, 2016	No recurrence	1.5
	Total	—	4.5

Table 1.3, and then divide the number of recurrences by the person-years observed as the intensity of the positive event of recurrence. The general formula is

$$\text{Person-Time positive rate} = \frac{\text{Positive numbers}}{\text{Summation of person} - \text{Time for individuals under a negative state}} \times K \quad (1\text{-}7)$$

Here, the numerator is the number of positive individuals, and the de-nominator is the sum of observed person-time under a negative state. The choice of the proportional base is the same as (1-6).

The data of Table 1.3 were substituted into formula (1.7). Operation A: $1/39.5 \times 100\% = 2.53\%/\text{year}$, Operation B: $1/4.5 \times 100\% = 22.22\%/\text{year}$, which indicated that the average recurrence rate was 2.53% in the patients receiving operation A and 22.22% in the patients receiving operation B. The two schemes had different intensity of positive events. Here, the discussed positive event is recurrence, the unit of time is year, so it is called recurrence rate of person year.

1.2.3. *A compound parameter — ratio*

We sometimes use the ratio of two associated variables A and B as a parameter to describe the state of affairs.

$$\text{Relative ratio} = \frac{A}{B} \quad (1\text{-}8)$$

Among them, A and B themselves can be absolute or relative numbers; the dimensions of A and B can be different or the same.

If the dimensions of A and B are different, the relative ratio is a parameter with dimensions. For example, the number of doctors per 1000 community people and the number of beds per 1000 community people reflect the allocation of health resources. If the dimensions of A and B are the same, the relative ratio is a dimensionless parameter, for example, the gender ratio in demography. Another example is ratio of the incidence rate in the exposed group to the unexposed group, it actually is the relative risk (RR) commonly used in epidemiology.

1.2.4. *Issues in the application of parameters for relative level*

(1) Clear definition is needed. The calculation of parameters for relative level is the ratio of the two elements of the observation. According to the characteristics of these two elements, it can be known which type of parameter that the ratio belongs to. However, some terms used in practice cannot literally correspond with the type of parameter. For example, abortion rate = number of abortions in the year/number of women within childbearing age in the same year × 100%. The term itself seems to be a rate. However, according to the elements in the formula, it is easily found as a ratio. Therefore, when discussing the type of relative frequency, it is necessary to know the definition of both the numerator and the denominator.

(2) When estimating the parameter of relative level, the denominator should not be too small. Generally speaking, when enough observations are obtained, the calculated result of the parameter of relative level is relatively stable and can correctly reflect the actual situation. For example, 100 patients accept regimen A, and 60 cases are effective; 5 patients accept regimen B, and 3 cases are effective. The efficient rates of these two regimens are both 60%. However, the calculation for regimen B is based on a smaller sample size, and the sampling error is large. It cannot guarantee that the efficient rate is close enough to the actual level of efficiency. In practice, when sample size is small, it is suggested to report the absolute number directly. For example, the efficiency of regimen B is reported as "3/5 cases are effective."

(3) If several relative frequencies are calculated by different sample sizes, their average level cannot be directly estimated by the arithmetic mean of them. In 1.5, the observation of person-years for regimen A and regimen B are quite different, the average

recurrence rate cannot be calculated with $(2.53\% \pm 22.22\%)/2 = 12.38\%$. The correct approach is to pool the numerator and the denominator separately, that is, $(1 + 1)/(39.5 + 4.5) = 4.55\%$.

(4) When comparing relative levels, we need to pay attentions to the comparability. Multi factors are involved in the observations for us to estimate parameters of relative levels. Except for the concerned exposure factors, all the other factors should have same or similar influential strengths.

1.3. Statistical table and statistical chart

Statistical tables and statistical charts are important statistical tools for describing the information contained in the data. In scientific research reports, the results of statistical analysis are often listed in a table, called a statistical table. The statistical chart is supposed to visually present the quantitative relationship of the affairs in study. There are different patterns of charts — by the location of points, the trend of curves, the height of bars, or the size of the area. Statistical tables and statistical charts have their own advantages in revealing the information contained in the data. The former is accurate and quantitative, and the latter is intuitive. However, in academic journals, in order to save space, the results given by statistical tables should not be repeated with statistical charts, or vice versa.

1.3.1. *Statistics tables*

(1) The structure of a statistical table. As an ordinary format, each statistical table should have a title to introduce the main idea of the table. There are horizontal headings to indicate the meaning of horizontal digits, and vertical headings to indicate the meaning of vertical digits. If necessary, the horizontal (vertical) headings can be further defined, as shown in Table 1.3. The horizontal items "regimen A, B" are subdivided into 100 patients (for saving space, only 3 of them are listed). Tables contain digits, lines, and sometimes follow a description or annotation with a font that is different from the main part.

As to the contents, each table has a subjective part and a predicative part. The subjective part is the object to be explained, such as the "occupation" in Table 1.2, usually locates at the left side of the table. And the predicative part is used to explain the characteristics of the subject, such as the columns after the "occupation" in Table 1.2, generally listed on the right side of the table.

(2) Types of statistical tables. Statistical tables are divided into simple tables and combinative tables. The data in simple table is grouped by a single feature, as shown in Table 1.2, divided into 6 groups by occupation. Combinative table combines two or more features to group the data. Table 1.4 combines occupations with hospital days to analyze the cesarean section rate of women in different occupations and hospital days.

(3) Principles and general requirements for the application of statistical tables. One of the principles is that the table should be concise and have clear aims. Only one topic should be included in a table to make readers understood easily. The second principle is that the subject and the predicate are distinct and relationship among the digits is logically displayed. The position of the subject and predicate

Table 1.4 An obstetrician investigates the cesarean section rate of maternal in different occupations and different hospital days

	Hospital stay ≤7 days			Hospital stay >7 days		
Occupation	Observed numbers	Cesarean section	Cesarean section rate (%)	Observed numbers	Cesarean section	Cesarean section rate (%)
Worker	169	57	33.7	39	26	66.7
Farmer	75	25	33.3	27	17	63.0
Intellectuals	148	41	27.7	58	35	60.3
Manager	119	32	26.9	22	10	45.5
Service	168	37	22.0	40	24	60.0
Other	425	102	24.0	112	71	63.4
Total	1104	294	26.6	298	183	61.4

should be accurate. Arrangement of the headings and their further subdivisions should satisfy professional considerations. The general requirements are:

① Title. Summarizes the contents in the table and locates at the top of the table.
② Headings. The text should be concise. If there are any dimensions for the digits, the dimensions need to be given after headings.
③ Lines. We use as few as possible lines in table. Except for the top line, the bottom line, the horizontal lines below the vertical headings and above the total, the rest should be omitted as much as possible. Vertical lines and diagonal lines should not be used.
④ Digits. Arabic numerals should be used in the table. The decimals of the same measurements should be consistent. The digits should be vertical aligned by the decimal dots. There should be no blank in the table, and the content that has not been observed can be represented by "..."; the content that does not exist can be represented by "—". When the observed result is "0", the digit "0" cannot be omitted.
⑤ Annotations. If there are any required annotations or descriptions in the table, we marked the digits with "*" or other symbols, and the corresponded explanations are written below the table.

The above requirements are general for all statistical reports. Different academic journals sometimes give their own special regulations and please refer to their requirements (guidelines) if necessary.

1.3.2. *Statistical chart*

The popularly used statistical charts in medical scientific reports include bar charts, percent bar charts, pie charts, line charts, scatter plots, box plots, heat maps, etc. The basic requirements for statistical charts are:

① Choose the appropriate chart according to the properties of the data and the purposes of the research.

② Arrange the title at the bottom of the graph. The title may summarize the contents in the table.

③ The comparison of different affairs in the same chart should be distinguished by different patterns or colors. The legends should be provided in appropriate positions (usually on the right side of the chart, the bottom of the chart, or the upper right blank area of the chart).

④ If coordinate axes are used in the statistical charts (such as bar charts, line charts), the orientation of the horizontal axis should be rightwards, and the orientation of the vertical axis should be upwards. Both axes have their headlines. When the coordinate axes represent quantitative data, the origin, dimension, and appropriate scales should be marked. When the coordinate axes represent qualitative data, the notations of groups should be given. For the sake of aesthetics, it is suggested to draw the statistical chart with height: width = 5:7 (approximate to golden ratio).

Different statistical charts have their own applications and special considerations of drawing, which are explained as follows:

(1) Bar chart The heights of the equal-width bars represent the values of the measurements in different compared groups. Bar charts include single bar charts (only a unique grouping factor) and multiple bar charts (at least two grouping factors, as shown in Figure 1.2, such as the categories of bacteria and the types of antibiotics). The scale of the axis which indicates the heights of the bars (usually the vertical axis) must start from 0. Otherwise, it may lead to distorting the comparisons among the groups.

(2) Percent bar chart Percent bar charts are used to represent frequencies of various categories in frequency distribution data. For example, the total lengths of the two bars in Figure 1.3 both equal 100%, and the lengths of the stacked bars correspond to the frequencies of different categories, respectively.

(3) Pie chart The application of pie chart and the arrangement of slices are similar as percent bar charts. The area of a slice (or

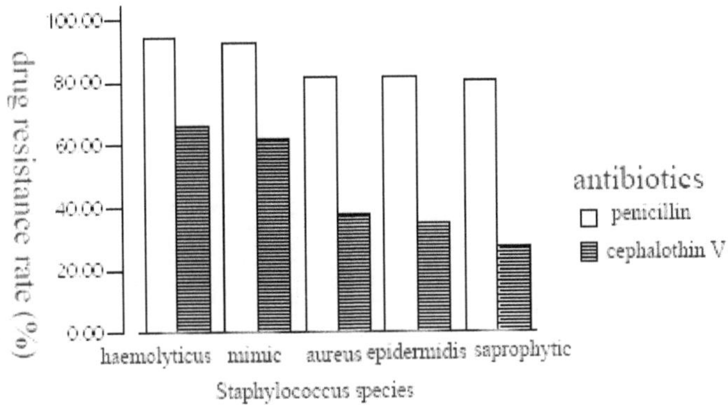

Figure 1.2 Drug resistance rates of five kinds of staphylococcus applying in two kinds of antibiotics in a children's hospital

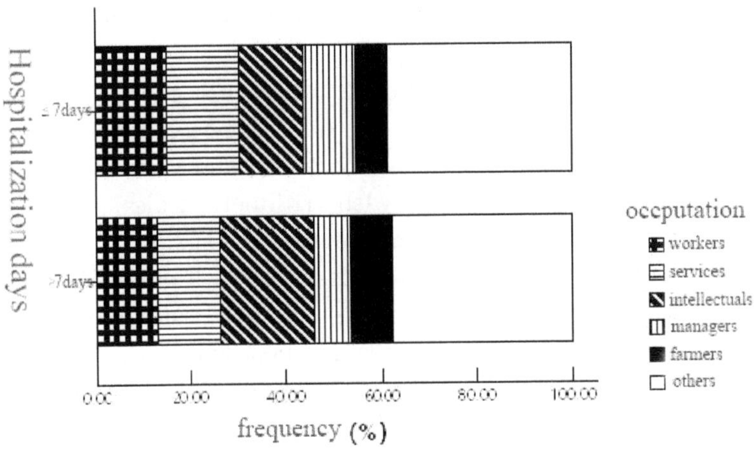

Figure 1.3 The frequency distribution of occupations for parturient mothers with different hospitalization days during prenatal period

its central angle) corresponds to the frequency of each category, while the area of the whole pie (or the central angle 360°) represents 100%. The first slice starts from the position of the clock at 12 o'clock. If there are no special professional considerations, it is usually arranged clockwise from the largest slice to the smallest slice.

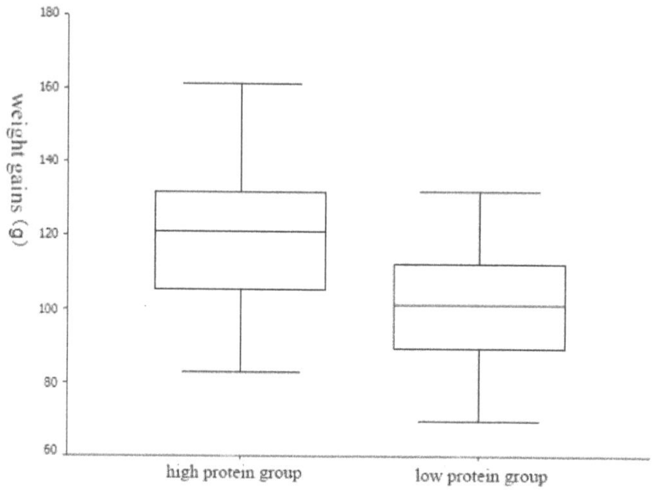

Figure 1.4 Weight gains in rats fed by two diets with different protein amount

(4) Line chart The rise or decline of a line in a coordinate system indicates changes of affairs over time or evolving levels along with an ordinal variable. The horizontal and vertical axes of an ordinary line chart are both with arithmetic scales.
(5) Box plot It is used to compare the average level and variation between several groups of data. As in Figure 1.4, for each group of data, its minimum, Q_L, M, Q_U, and maximum are presented. M represents its average position, both the range of minimum~maximum and the range of $Q_L \sim Q_U$ can illustrate the variation of data.

1.4. Repot writing

For the statistical description of quantitative data, the following contents are often required to be reported:

(1) Definition of the population or sample according to the purpose of the study.
(2) Pattern of data distribution.
(3) Choose appropriate statistical measurements to describe the average level and the degree of variation.

Table 1.5 Descriptive statistics for weight (kg) of 1402 parturient mothers

Variable (unit)	N (sample size)	Minimum	Maximum	Mean	Standard deviation
Weight (kg)	1402	48.0	87.0	65.66	6.07

(4) For a good illustration, sometimes statistical tables or charts are required.
(5) Give necessary professional explanations.

The following report is the analysis results of the body weight (kg) of 1402 parturient mothers in Example 1.1.

Data in Example 1.1 was collected from parturient mothers, according to which the frequency table (Table 1.1) and histogram (Figure 1.1) were obtained. It showed that the weights of the parturient mothers followed a symmetric distribution. Arithmetic mean and standard deviation were suggested for statistical description.

Based on the data of 1402 parturient mothers, the range of weight was 48.0~87.0 (kg), the mean ± standard deviation was 65.66 ± 6.07 (kg) (Table 1.5).

1.5. Case discrimination

Case 1.1 In this case, the doctor observed the hospital days of 1402 parturient mothers as shown in Table 1.6, and he found that the average hospital days were 6.6 days. Please comment on this result.

The average hospital days can be calculated.

$\bar{X} = 2 \times 0.0563 + 4 \times 0.2254 + \cdots + 24 \times 0.0014 + 26 \times 0.0021 = 6.6$ (days)

Case 1.2 Someone compiled a statistical table. What improvements are needed in your opinion? (Table 1.7)

Case 1.3 Someone drew the following statistical chart. What do you think needs to be improved?

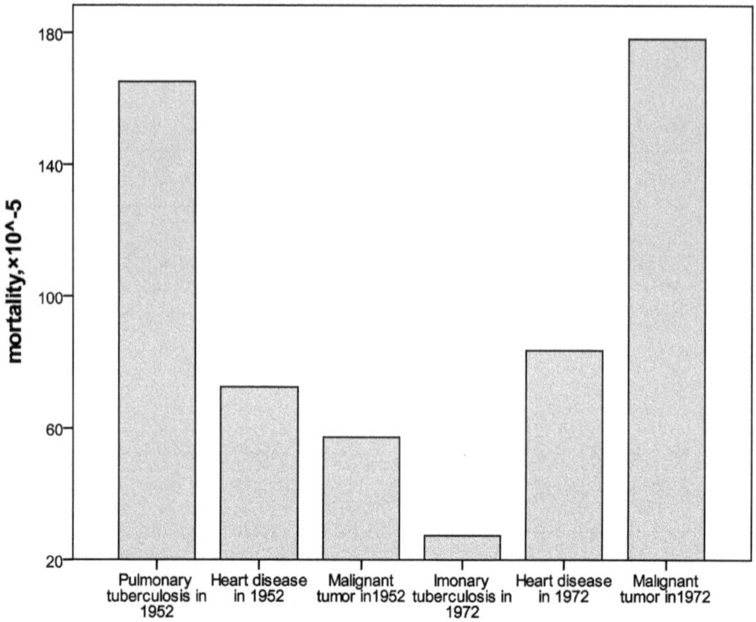

Table 1.6 Hospital days during delivery period of 1402 parturient mothers

Interval (1)	Mid value (2)	Number (3)	Relative frequency % (4)
1∼	2	79	5.63
3∼	4	316	22.54
5∼	6	559	39.87
7∼	8	243	17.33
9∼	10	89	6.35
11∼	12	57	4.07
13∼	14	23	1.64
15∼	16	19	1.36
17∼	18	9	0.64
19∼	20	1	0.07
21∼	22	2	0.14
23∼	24	2	0.14
25∼	26	3	0.21
Total	—	1402	1

Table 1.7 Mortality of various types of malignant tumors in Jilin city from 1976 to 1979

Diseases \ A	0~	15~	35~	55~	75~
Gastric cancer	None	1.13/100,000	19.92/100,000	150/100,000	313.4/100,000
Esophageal cancer	None	0.1/100,000	2.18/100,000	35.20/100,000	73.56/100,000
Live cancer	0.34/100,000	1.64/100,000	25.30/100,000	97.51/100,000	134.33/100,000
Lung cancer	None	0.41/100,000	20.21/100,000	125.10/100,000	137.53/100,000

Table 1.8 Comparison of fatality rates of a disease between two hospitals in 2000

	Hospital A			Hospital B		
Severity of disease	Number of discharged patients	Number of death	Case fatality rate (%)	Number of discharged patients	Number of death	Case fatality rate (%)
Mild	100	8	8.0	650	65	10.0
Moderate	300	36	12.0	250	40	16.0
Heavy	600	90	15.0	100	18	18.0
Total	1000	134	13.4	1000	123	12.3

Case 1.4 The case fatality rate was used to compare the treatment levels of a certain disease in two hospitals, and the results were shown in Table 1.8. From the combined case fatality rate, it was concluded that the treatment level of hospital B was better than that of hospital A. Please comment on this conclusion.

1.6. Computer experiments

Experiment 1.1 Statistical description of quantitative data

Draw a histogram of the data in Example 1.1. Based on the raw data, calculate the arithmetic mean, standard deviation, median and inter-quartile range, etc.

Experiment 1.2 Statistical description of qualitative data

According to the requirements of Example 1.4, illustrate the frequency distribution of occupations.

Experiment 1.3 Draw percent bar chart

According to data file data1-2.sav, group the individuals as hospital days $\leq$7 days and >7 days, and then draw a percent bar chart as Figure 1.3.

Experiment 1.4 The relationship between mean and median from different distributions of variables

Using data1-3.sav, this experiment illustrates the calculation of statistics from frequency table. For data with both symmetric distribution and asymmetric distribution, the relationship between medians and means are shown.

1.7. Frequently asked questions and summary

1.7.1. *Frequently asked questions*

1. To give a statistical description with proper statistics, distribution of variables is assumed. In actual situation, how do we know the distribution of the variables?

In general, the distribution of variables can be obtained by retrieving literatures. For example, in literatures, data of weight and vital capacity of adults follow symmetric distribution, while selenium in hair of adults follow positive skewness distribution. Then, we can follow the literatures when dealing with adults' weight, vital capacity and the selenium in hair, especially when the data of the references are based on large sample sizes.

Sometimes the distribution of some certain medical measurements cannot be found in published literatures while we are academically interested in it. Then, by large enough samples, we can use statistical analysis software such as SPSS, to perform hypothesis test. You may move to Chapter 2 in this book to get some further knowledge about distribution.

2. Why do we use semi-logarithmic line chart instead of general line chart, when displaying the rate of change?

When displaying the trends over time with a general line chart, the vertical position only indicates the value at the corresponding time.

For example, if a variable changes as "10 → 100 → 1000", in step 1, the variable increases by 90, and in step 2, it increases by 900. It is obvious that the magnitude of change in step 2 is larger than that in step 1. However, when it comes to the rate of change, we can see that in step 1, the variable multiplies 10 and in step 2, it multiplies 10 as well. In these two steps, the variable has the same rate of change. A general line chart can easily display the increment, but fails to display the rate of change.

So, we use semi-logarithmic line chart, in which the vertical axis uses the logarithmic scale. After transformation, the change"10 → 100 → 1000"is now"1 → 2 → 3". In this way, the chart reveals clearly that same rate of change happen in the 2 steps.

1.7.2. *Summary*

1. The data collected with some certain purpose of study contain abundant information. The purpose of statistical description is displaying broadly the main information, with proper methods (making statistical table, drawing statistical chart, or calculating statistics).
2. Pinpoint types of variables, and make statistical description with different statistics.

   (1) Quantitative variable: we can use arithmetic mean, geometric mean, or median to describe the average level, according to the patterns of distribution. As to describe the variation, we can use range, standard deviation, variance, inter-quartile range, or CV (Table 1.9).
   (2) Qualitative variable: we can use frequency, frequency distribution, intensity, and ratio to describe the qualitative data based on properties of data and purposes of study (Table 1.10).
   (3) It is necessary to use statistical tables and charts in high-quality reports and we need ensure that they are appropriate for the data and to support the main purpose of the study (Table 1.11).

Table 1.9 Statistical description of quantitative variable

Statistical description	Statistics	Meanings	Circumstances
Average Level	Arithmetic mean	Average of individuals	Symmetric distribution
	Geometric mean	Average multiples	Symmetric distribution after logarithmic transformation
	Median	A value cut the individuals into two parts with half of the cases smaller than it	① Asymmetric distribution; ② Semi-quantitative data; ③ Values beyond any ends; ④ Uncertain distribution
Variation	Range	The difference between maximum and minimum	Any distribution
	Standard deviation (variance)	Quantify average deviations from mean	Symmetric distribution
	Inter-quartile range	P_{75}–P_{25}	① Asymmetric distribution; ② Semi-quantitative data; ③ Values beyond any ends; ④ Uncertain distribution
	Coefficient of variation	Standard deviation/Mean	① The variations of two variables with different dimensions; ② variables with same dimension but a severe difference in the scale

Table 1.10 Statistical description of qualitative variable

Statistics	Formula	Application
Frequency	n/N	Estimated probability for an event
Frequency distribution	$n_1/N, n_2/N, \ldots, n_k/N$	Estimated probabilities for all events
Intensity	Positive cases/ total person time	Relative frequency per unit of time
Ratio	A/B	Any quantity over another

Table 1.11 The applications and instructions of graphs

Graphs	Applications	Instructions
Bar chart	Comparisons between groups	Heights of bars are determined by amount in each category
Histogram	Frequency distribution of quantitative variable	Area of rectangle represents the relative frequency
Percent bar chart	Frequency distribution	The height of each stacked part in a bar represents the relative frequency
Pie chart	Frequency distribution	Slices of a pie show proportions
Line chart	display trends over time of quantitative variable	The arithmetic scales are used for both vertical and horizontal axes
Box plot	Display distribution of quantitative variable	Use box and line to describe Q, M, and R
Heat map	The change of quantitative variable	The colored elements in two- or three-dimensional space are used to show the values or average values

Think and Practice

I. Questions for Reflection

1. What statistics should be chosen when making statistical description to quantitative variables?

2. Give an example to show the differences and associations between frequency and frequency distribution.
3. What should be noticed when analyzing relative levels?
4. What are the frequently used graphs in statistics? What are the different circumstances for the applications of different types of graphs?

II. Questions on Calculation

1. In a survey, the total cholesterol (mg/dL) of 100 healthy male adults between 40 and 50 years of age was tested. The data is as follows:

227	190	224	259	225	238	180	193	214	195	213	193	209	172	244
199	155	208	203	199	253	181	196	224	210	220	255	257	216	249
235	220	190	203	197	149	175	236	202	209	174	184	174	185	167
235	167	210	171	248	201	266	189	222	199	197	214	199	198	230
246	209	202	186	217	206	200	203	197	161	247	138	186	156	195
163	273	178	190	207	259	186	194	246	172	234	232	189	172	235
207	208	231	234	226	174	199	278	277	181					

Questions:

(1) Please work out a frequency table, a histogram, and then discuss the distribution pattern.

(2) With the result of (1), choose proper statistics to describe the average level and variation of the data.

(3) Calculate P_{25}, P_{75}, and P_{95}.

2. After 3 courses of treatment in 120 patients with micro-filaremia, the antibody titers measured by indirect fluorescent antibody test (IFAT) were as follows. Please calculate the average level of antibody titer.

antibody titer	1:5	1:10	1:20	1:40	1:80	1:160	1:320
case	5	16	27	34	22	13	3

Table 1.12 The incidence and the mortality of hemorrhagic fever within 6 years

Year	Newly found case	Death case
1975	32	4
1976	56	5
1977	162	12
1978	241	13
1979	330	10
1980	274	5

3. The data of the incidence and the mortality of hemorrhagic fever from the year 1975 to 1980 are collected as follows. Here, we assume the population sizes remain unchanged during these 6 years (Table 1.12).

Questions:

(1) What is the trend of incidence rate along with years?
(2) What is the trend of case fatality rate along with years?
(3) What kind of chart should be applied to display the analysis results above?
(4) Comment on the evaluation results about the effectiveness for preventing and controlling hemorrhagic fever.

Jinxin Zhang

CHAPTER 2

PROBABILITY DISTRIBUTION

In Chapter 1, the univariate description is introduced using frequency distribution table and histogram. However, it is just about the description of the sample distribution. Due to variation among individuals, even if two samples are taken from the same population, the frequency distribution of the samples will be different. A very important further objective is to describe the population distribution. In this chapter, we introduce several population distributions commonly used in biomedical research, including the normal distribution of continuous random variable, the binomial distribution, and Poisson distribution of discrete random variable.

2.1. Normal distribution

2.1.1. *Basic concept*

What is the way to know the population probability distribution of a continuous random variable? In fact, the frequency density histogram introduced in Chapter 1 approximates the distribution of a variable. When the sample size is larger and the class interval width is smaller, the continuous probability distribution of the population can be obtained.

The above process can be illustrated by the example of weight distribution of expectant mothers in Table 1.1. The bars of Figure 2.1 are the frequency density histogram corresponding to Table 1.1.

Connecting the midpoints at the top of each bar in order to get a polyline (frequency density polyline, see Figure 2.1). When the

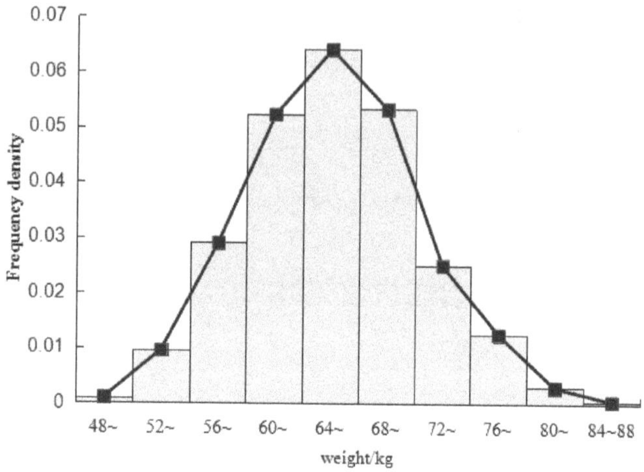

Figure 2.1 Weight frequency density graph

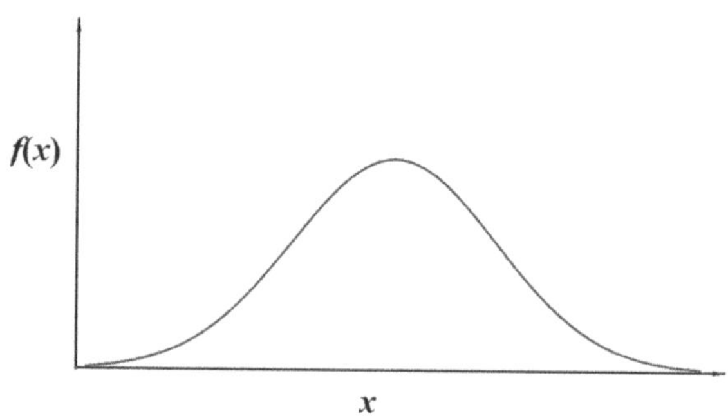

Figure 2.2 Diagram of probability density curve

sample size n is larger and larger, the frequency of each sub-interval is more stable and closer to the corresponding probability. If the number of sub-intervals increases and the length of each sub-interval is reduced, then the polyline will be close to a smooth curve with a "bell shape," which is higher in middle, lower on two sides, and basically symmetric. When n and the number of sub-intervals tend to infinity, and the length of each sub-interval tends to 0, the polyline will tend to a smooth curve, which is called the probability density curve (see Figure 2.2).

If the probability density function of a continuous random variable X can be expressed as

$$f(x) = \frac{1}{\sigma\sqrt{2\pi}} e^{-\frac{(x-\mu)^2}{2\sigma^2}}, \quad -\infty < x < +\infty \tag{2-1}$$

Then we say the random variable X follows a normal distribution and denoted by $X \sim N(\mu, \sigma^2)$, where μ is population mean and σ^2 is population variance.

The normal distribution was firstly discovered when the German mathematician C.F. Gauss studied the error theory. It is also called Gaussian distribution.

According to the above analysis, the body weight approximately follows a normal distribution. The data in Table 1.1 can be used to calculate the frequency or approximate probability (i.e., the corresponding area) of body weight taking value in any interval, for example

$$P(Weight < 64\text{kg}) \approx 0.0043 + 0.0385 + 0.1155 + 0.2090 = 0.3673$$

is the sum of the area of the bars where the body weight falls in the four sub-intervals of $48\text{kg} \leq weight < 52\text{kg}, 52\text{kg} \leq weitht < 56\text{kg}, 56\text{kg} \leq weitht < 60\text{kg}$ and $60\text{kg} \leq weight < 64\text{kg}$. In theory, it approximates to the corresponding area under the probability density curve, which is the cumulative probability.

In general, if the continuous random variable $X \sim N(\mu, \sigma^2)$, its probability density function can be set as $f(x)$ in Formula (2-1), then the cumulative probability of the value falling in the interval $(-\infty, x)$ equals to the integral of $f(x)$ from $-\infty$ to x, denoted as $F(x)$, that is,

$$F(x) = P(X < x) = \frac{1}{\sigma\sqrt{2\pi}} \int_{-\infty}^{x} e^{-\frac{(t-\mu)^2}{2\sigma^2}} dt \tag{2-2}$$

where $F(x)$ is called the distribution function of $N(\mu, \sigma^2)$. Its value represents the probability of the variable falling in the interval, corresponding to the area of the shadow under the probability density curve (often called the left tail area), as shown in Figure 2.3.

The distribution function $F(x)$ can be used to calculate the probability that the variable takes value in any interval $[a, b)$ as shown in

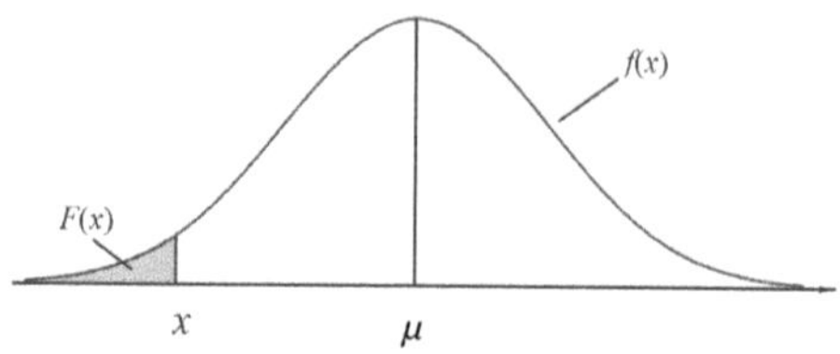

Figure 2.3 Probability density function and distribution function of normal distribution

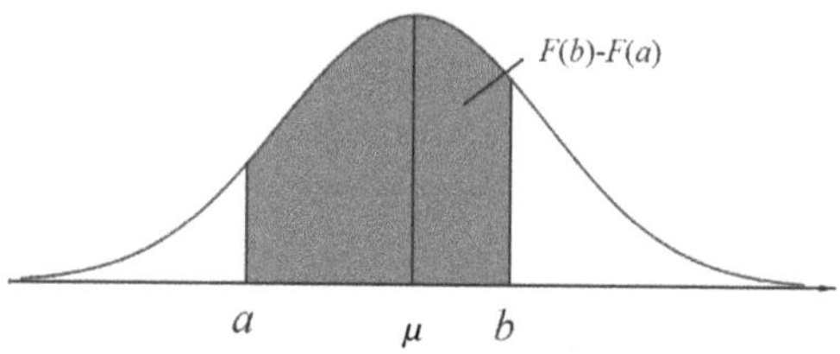

Figure 2.4 The probability of a normal distribution

the shaded part of Figure 2.4,

$$P(a \leq X < b) = F(b) - F(a) \tag{2-3}$$

As a special case, when $b = +\infty$,

$$P(X \geq a) = 1 - P(X < a) = 1 - F(a) \tag{2-4}$$

2.1.2. *Characteristics of normal distribution*

As can be seen from Equation (2-1) and Figure 2.3, the normal distribution has the following important characteristics.

(1) The normal distribution is unimodal and symmetric, with the axis of symmetry at $x = \mu$.
(2) The normal distribution $N(\mu, \sigma^2)$ has two parameters, namely the position parameter μ and the shape parameter (or variation parameter) σ. The position parameter represents the position of the peak of the probability density curve. When σ is fixed and μ is increased, the curve moves to the right along the X-axis, otherwise, the curve moves to the left along the X-axis, as shown

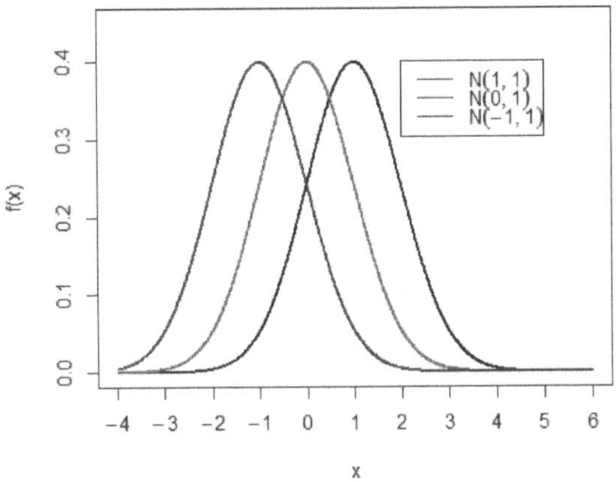

Figure 2.5 Curve of normal distribution probability density under different μ

in Figure 2.5. The shape parameter σ represents the degree of deviation of the variable X. When μ is fixed, the larger σ is, the more values of X disperse, and the curve is more "chunky," the smaller σ is, the more values of X concentrate around μ, and the curve will be "thinner and taller," as shown in Figure 2.6.

(3) The probability density function $f(x)$ maximizes at $x = \mu$, and $f(\mu) = \frac{1}{\sigma\sqrt{2\pi}}$.

2.1.3. *Standard normal distribution*

When the mean μ and variance σ^2 of the normal distribution are known, according to the formulas (2-2), (2-3), and (2-4), the probability that the value of the normal variable falls into any interval can be calculated. It all comes down to calculate the area under the probability density curve of normal distribution, or the distribution function values at the endpoints. However, it is difficult to calculate any random variable X following general normal distribution into Z,

$$Z = \frac{X - \mu}{\sigma} \tag{2-5}$$

It can be proved that the new random variable Z after the transformation of Equation (2-5) follows a normal distribution of mean

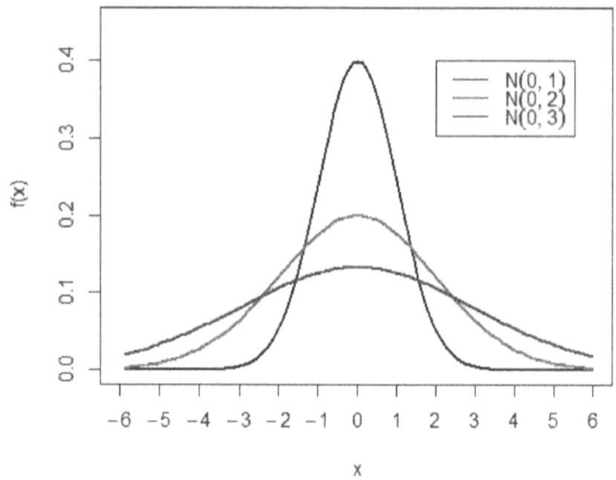

Figure 2.6 Curve of normal distribution probability density under different σ

0 and variance 1,

$$Z \sim N(0,1)$$

This special normal distribution $N(0,1)$ is called standard normal distribution, the Equation (2-5) is called standardized transformation, and Z is called standard normal deviation or Z score. The probability density function and distribution function of the standard normal distribution are denoted as $\phi(z)$ and $\Phi(z)$, let $\mu = 0, \sigma = 1$ in formulas (2-1) and (2-2).

$$\varphi(z) = \frac{1}{\sqrt{2\pi}} \mathrm{e}^{-\frac{z^2}{2}} \tag{2-6}$$

$$\Phi(z) = \int_{-\infty}^{z} \varphi(t)\mathrm{d}t \tag{2-7}$$

The probability density curve of the standard normal distribution is shown in Figure 2.7, and the area of the left tail in the figure, representing the probability of the standard normal variable taking values in $(-\infty, z)$, is the value of the distribution function $\Phi(z)$.

According to the Equation (2-7), statisticians have compiled a table for the areas of left tails under the probability density curve of standard normal distribution (Table C1 in Appendix C), that is, the corresponding values of distribution function $\Phi(z)$. Since any normal

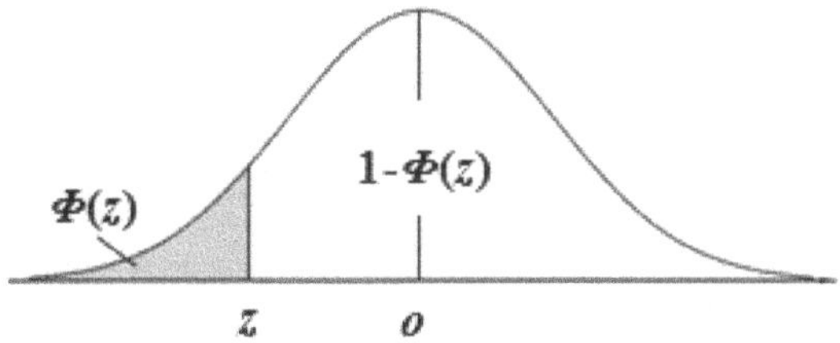

Figure 2.7 Diagram of probability density curve and distribution function of standard normal distribution

distribution can be converted into a standard normal distribution by means of standardized transformation, the values of distribution function of general normal distribution can be calculated by means of the formula (2-5) and Table C1. One thing to be aware of is that Table C1 only gives the values of $\Phi(z)$ when $z \leq 0$. Since the probability density curve of the standard normal distribution is symmetric with respect to the vertical axis at $z = 0$, the distribution function values for $z > 0$ can be obtained according to $\Phi(z) = 1 - \Phi(-z)$.

Let $Z \sim N(0, 1)$, according to the formulas (2-2) to (2-4), we can get the following equations.

$$P(-\infty < Z < b) = \Phi(b), \quad P(a \leq Z < b) = \Phi(b) - \Phi(a),$$
$$P(Z \geq b) = 1 - P(-\infty < Z < b) = 1 - \Phi(b)$$

Hence, the probability of the standard normal variable Z falling in the interval $(-1.96, 1.96)$ can be calculated.

$$\begin{aligned} P(-1.96 < Z < 1.96) &= \Phi(1.96) - \Phi(-1.96) \\ &= [1 - \Phi(-1.96)] - \Phi(-1.96) \\ &= (1 - 0.025) - 0.025 = 0.95 \end{aligned}$$

The probability that Z falls outside the interval $(-1.96, 1.96)$ is

$$P(|Z| > 1.96) = 1 - P(-1.96 < Z < 1.96) = 1 - 0.95 = 0.05$$

The probability of Z falls in the interval $(1.96, +\infty)$ is

$$\begin{aligned} P(Z > 1.96) &= 1 - P(Z < 1.96) = 1 - \Phi(1.96) \\ &= 1 - (1 - \Phi(-1.96)) = \Phi(-1.96) = 0.025 \end{aligned}$$

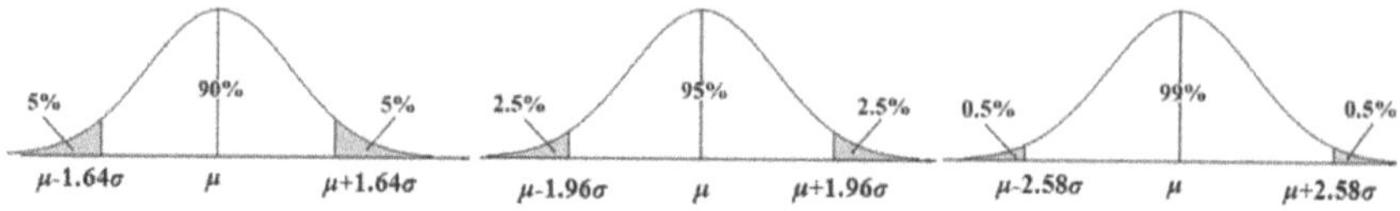

Figure 2.8 The areas under the probability density curve of normal distribution

This indicates that the area of the bilateral tails under the probability density curve with Z falling in $(-\infty, -1.96)$ or $(1.96, +\infty)$ is 0.05, and the area of right side tail at $(1.96, +\infty)$ is $\frac{0.05}{2}$=0.025. Note the significance of the value 1.96, which is one of the critical value commonly used for hypothesis testing later, another common critical value is 2.58, which represents the area of the bilateral tails under the probability density curve to the horizontal axis with Z falling in the intervals $(-\infty, -2.58)$or $(2.58, +\infty)$ is 0.01, while the area of the right side tail $(2.58, +\infty)$ is 0.005. See Figure 2.8 (take $\mu = 0$ and $\sigma = 1$).

Example 2.1. Let $X \sim N(\mu, \sigma^2)$, please try to calculate

(1) The probability of X falling in the interval $(\mu - 1.64\sigma, \mu + 1.64\sigma)$,
(2) The probability of X falling in the interval $(\mu - 1.96\sigma, \mu + 1.96\sigma)$,
(3) The probability of X falling in the interval $(\mu - 2.58\sigma, \mu + 2.58\sigma)$.

Solution: According to formula (2-5), the variables are converted into z scores following standard normal distribution, and then the probabilities can be obtained by consulting the table for standard normal distribution (Table C1).

(1) $Z_1 = \frac{(\mu - 1.64\sigma) - \mu}{\sigma} = -1.64$, $Z_2 = \frac{(\mu + 1.64\sigma) - \mu}{\sigma} = 1.64$
The probability

$$\begin{aligned} P(\mu - 1.64\sigma < X < \mu + 1.64\sigma) &= \Phi(1.64) - \Phi(-1.64) \\ &= [1 - \Phi(-1.64)] - \Phi(-1.64) \\ &= (1 - 0.05) - 0.05 = 0.90 \end{aligned}$$

(2) $Z_1 = \frac{(\mu-1.96\sigma)-\mu}{\sigma} = -1.96,\ Z_2 = \frac{(\mu+1.96\sigma)-\mu}{\sigma} = 1.96$

The probability

$$\begin{aligned} P(\mu - 1.96\sigma < X < \mu + 1.96\sigma) &= \Phi(1.96) - \Phi(-1.96) \\ &= [1 - \Phi(-1.96)] - \Phi(-1.96) \\ &= (1 - 0.025) - 0.025 = 0.95 \end{aligned}$$

(3) $Z_1 = \frac{(\mu-2.58\sigma)-\mu}{\sigma} = -2.58,\ Z_2 = \frac{(\mu+2.58\sigma)-\mu}{\sigma} = 2.58$

The probability

$$\begin{aligned} P(\mu - 2.58\sigma < X < \mu + 2.58\sigma) &= \Phi(2.58) - \Phi(-2.58) \\ &= [1 - \Phi(-2.58)] - \Phi(-2.58) \\ &= (1 - 0.005) - 0.005 = 0.99 \end{aligned}$$

Example 2.1 shows that the area under the probability density curve of normal distribution has the following properties (as shown in Figure 2.8).

- The area between the probability density curve and the horizontal axis is 1.
- The area under the probability density curve within $(\mu-1.64\sigma,\ \mu+1.64\sigma)$ is 0.90, indicating that the probability of the value falling in the range $\mu \pm 1.64\sigma$ is 0.90, and the probability of the value outside the range (the sum of the shadow areas on both sides) is 0.10, with 0.05 on each side.
- The area probability density curve within $(\mu - 1.96\sigma, \mu + 1.96\sigma)$ is 0.95, indicating that the probability of the value falling in the range $\mu \pm 1.96\sigma$ is 0.95, and the probability of the value outside the range (the sum of the shadow areas on both sides) is 0.05, with 0.025 on each side.
- The area probability density curve within $(\mu - 2.58\sigma, \mu + 2.58\sigma)$ is 0.99, indicating that the probability of the value in the range $\mu \pm 2.58\sigma$ is 0.99, and the probability of the value outside the range (the sum of the shadow areas on both sides) is 0.01, with 0.005 on each side.

In addition, similar to Example 2.1, for any normal distribution $N(\mu, \sigma^2)$, the area under the probability density curve in the interval

$\mu \pm \sigma$ is 68.27%. The area under the probability density curve in the interval $\mu \pm 2\sigma$ is 95.45%. The area under the probability density curve in the interval $\mu \pm 3\sigma$ is 99.73%.

Example 2.2. The total serum protein of normal adult females in a certain region follows a normal distribution, and 110 normal adult females in this region were observed. The sample mean of total serum protein is 72.8 g/L, and the standard deviation is 3.8 g/L. Please estimate the probability of total serum protein of normal adult females between 66.0 and 75.0 g/L in this region.

Solution: The sample mean and sample standard deviation can be used as the approximation of population mean μ and population standard deviation σ. In other words, the total serum protein (denoted by X) of the normal adult females in this region approximately follows the normal distribution of $N(72.8,\ 3.8^2)$. Make the following standardized transformation,

$$Z_1 = \frac{66.0 - 72.8}{3.8} = -1.79, Z_2 = \frac{75.0 - 72.8}{3.8} = 0.58$$

Referring to the standard normal distribution table (Table C1), it can be achieved that

$$\Phi(z_1) = 0.0367, \quad \Phi(z_2) = 1 - \Phi(-0.58) = 1 - 0.281 = 0.719$$

Therefore, the probability of serum total protein between 66.0 and 75.0 g/L is

$$P(66.0 < X < 75.0) = \Phi(z_2) - \Phi(z_1) = 0.719 - 0.0367 = 68.23\%$$

2.1.4. *The application of normal distribution*

Normal distribution is an important continuous probability distribution. Many biomedical phenomena follow normal distributions, such as the height of children of the same sex or age, the number of red blood cells, hemoglobin content and pulse rate of healthy adults of the same sex. Additionally, the size of products under normal conditions, such as the diameter, length, weight and so on, follow normal distribution approximately. Many statistical analysis methods are based on normal distribution. In addition, there are many probability distributions of random variables that take normal distribution as their limit distribution under certain conditions. Therefore, in statistics, normal distribution plays an important role in both theoretical research and practical application.

2.1.4.1. *Establishment medical reference ranges*

The medical reference range refers to the range of the observed value of an index which includes the majority of normal people. Regarding the target population, if not otherwise specified, a standard reference range generally denotes the one in healthy individuals, or without any known condition that directly affects the ranges being established under the premise of homogeneity. The "vast majority" customarily includes 90%, 95%, 99% of normal people. Reference ranges, once was called "normal ranges." However, using the term normal may not be appropriate as not everyone outside the interval is abnormal, and people who have a particular condition may still fall within this interval.

The general steps for determining a reference range for the observational indicators are as follows.

(1) According to the characteristics, background and known influencing factors of the observation indicators, the inclusion criteria and exclusion criteria of the sampling were determined. For example, in the study of reference range of the hemoglobin for normal adult women, adult women with anemia were excluded. In the study of reference range of lung ventilation, individuals with respiratory diseases should be excluded from the sample, and a certain amount of samples (generally more than 100) should be taken.
(2) Determine one or two-sided reference ranges according to the characteristics of indicators. If an index is abnormal when it is too high or too low, then the corresponding reference range should have both upper and lower limits, that is, take two-sided reference ranges. If the index is abnormal only when it is too high (such as blood lead, mercury), the one-sided reference range

should be adopted to establish the upper boundary value (upper limit). On the other hand, if an index is abnormal only when it is too low, the lower boundary value (lower limit) should be set. The reference range values should be unilateral or bilateral, usually was judged based on professional knowledge.

(3) Determine the scope: in general, the 95% reference value range is the most commonly used. The 90% or 99% reference range can also be determined according to the actual needs.

(4) According to the characteristics of data, different methods were selected to calculate the upper and lower limits of the medical reference range. The normal distribution method and percentile method were commonly used (see Table 2.1).

Before adopting the normal distribution method, the normality test of the data should be done (see Chapter 5). The sample mean $\bar{X}$ and sample standard deviation S can be used as the estimated values of population mean μ and population standard deviation σ.

The percentile method can be used to calculate the medical reference range of the variables with asymmetric or unknown type distribution. It should be noted that the sample information used by the percentile method is not sufficient. If the known indicators follow the normal distribution (or approximately follow the normal distribution after appropriate transformation), the reference range obtained

Table 2.1 The establishment of commonly used medical reference range

	Normal distribution method			Percentile method		
		One-sided			One-sided	
Reference range (%)	Two-sided	Lower limit	Upper limit	Two-sided	Lower limit	Upper limit
90	$\bar{X} \pm 1.64S$	$\bar{x} - 1.28s$	$\bar{X} + 1.28S$	$P_5 \sim P_{95}$	P_{10}	P_{90}
95	$\bar{X} \pm 1.96S$	$\bar{X} - 1.64S$	$\bar{X} + 1.64S$	$P_{2.5} \sim P_{97.5}$	P_5	P_{95}
99	$\bar{X} \pm 2.58S$	$\bar{X} - 2.33S$	$\bar{X} + 2.33S$	$P_{0.5} \sim P_{99.5}$	P_1	P_{99}

by the normal distribution method is more reliable than that by the percentile method.

Example 2.3. Estimate the 95% reference range of the total serum protein of the normal adult women in some region ($\bar{X} = 72.8$g/L, $S = 3.8$g/L).

Solution: The total serum protein of normal adult women in some region approximately follows the normal distribution, therefore, the 95% reference range should be calculate by the normal distribution method . Since too much or too little total serum protein is all abnormal, the two-sided reference range is adopted, that is to say, the upper and lower limits of the 95% reference range have to be calculated.

$$\text{lower limit} : \bar{X} - 1.96 \quad S = 72.8 - 1.96 \times 3.8 = 65.35(g/L)$$
$$\text{upper limit} : \bar{X} + 1.96 \quad S = 72.8 + 1.96 \times 3.8 = 80.25(g/L)$$

Thus, the standard reference range for this example is estimated to be 65.35–80.25 (g/L).

2.1.4.2. *Quality control*

If the experimental error is only caused by random error, and there is no error caused by some factors that have greater impact on the error, the fluctuation of the observed value should follow a normal distribution. According to this principle, the quality control of observation process can be realized.

Drawing quality control diagram is a visual and effective method of quality control (Figure 2.9). The horizontal axis of the control chart represents time, the horizontal line where $\bar{X}$ is located is the center line on the vertical axis, $\bar{X} \pm 2S$ is the upper and lower warning limit, and $\bar{X} \pm 3S$ is the upper and lower control limit. Record the observed data in chronological order, and draw points and lines on the control chart. Each data point and line shows the change of the observed data in time. If the data points are randomly distributed on both sides of the central line, the observation process is in a controlled state. If several data points cross the upper and lower control lines,

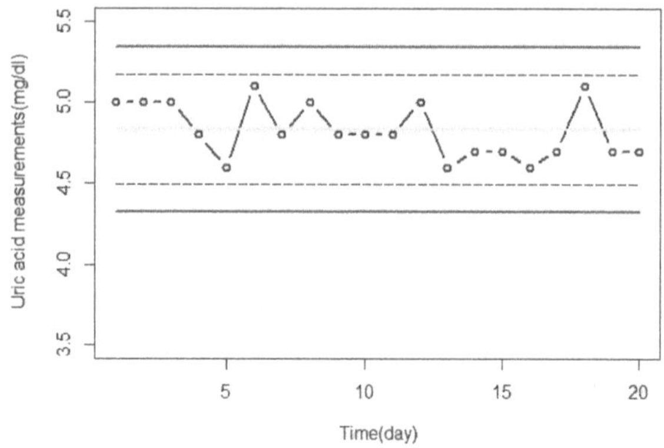

Figure 2.9 Control chart of serum uric acid measurement value

it means that there is an abnormal situation and the quality is out of control.

According to the area rule under the normal distribution curve, the probability of falling in the region $(\bar{X} - 2S, \bar{X} + 2S)$ is about 95%, while the probability of falling in the region $(\bar{X} - 3S, \bar{X} + 3S)$ is about 99%. In a measurement, the probability of falling outside the region $(\bar{X} - 3S, \bar{X} + 3S)$ is almost zero, which can be considered as an impossible event. If a certain measurement value falls outside the control limit, it is reasonable to believe that the fluctuation of data is not only caused by random error, but also there may be some non-random systematic error. It is necessary to take measures to eliminate abnormal factors in the observation process.

For example, some laboratory-made quantitative determination of uric acid in the same control serum for 20 consecutive days, and the data were obtained as follows (mg/dL).

5.0	5.0	5.0	4.8	4.6	5.1	4.8	5.0	4.8	4.8
4.8	5.0	4.6	4.7	4.7	4.6	4.7	5.1	4.7	4.7

where $\bar{X} = 4.83$ mg/dL, $S = 0.17$ mg/dL. The lower alert limit $\bar{X} - 2S = 4.49$ mg/dL, the upper alert limit $\bar{X} + 2S = 5.17$, the lower control limit $\bar{X} - 3S = 4.32$ mg/dL, the upper control limit $\bar{X} + 3S = 5.34$ mg/dL, the quality control diagram is shown in Figure 2.9.

As can be seen from Figure 2.9, each measured value is within the warning limit and randomly distributed on both sides of the central line, so it can be concluded that the measurement process is under control.

2.1.4.3. *The theoretical basis of statistical methods*

Many of the statistical methods discussed in the following chapters, such as T-test, variance analysis, regression analysis, etc., require that variables be normally distributed. For non-normal distributed data, an important way to implement statistical processing is to carry out variable transformation, so that the transformed data approximately follows the normal distribution, and then conduct statistical processing according to the normal distribution method.

In addition, the distribution of statistics, such as t distribution, χ^2 distribution, and F distribution, are derived from the normal distribution. The following binomial distribution and Poisson distribution are close to the normal distribution when the sample size is large enough. It can be seen that normal distribution plays an important role in statistics.

2.2. Binomial distribution

2.2.1. *Concept*

In biomedical studies, we need to conduct a type of "experiments" (or observations) in many cases:

(1) There are only two mutually exclusive outcomes for each experiment, such as outcomes of treatment (effective or invalid), biochemical tests (positive or negative), toxicity tests (survival or death), product inspections (qualified or unqualified), etc. Or we just focus on the status for an event A in an experiment, that is, the event occurs or not occurs (denoted by $\bar{A}$ for the opposite event).
(2) To find the regularity of the experimental outcomes, one needs to make a widely used assumption, that is, the experiments are repeated n times independently under the same conditions. For

example, same treatment strategies are conducted for n patients; biochemical tests are performed on n patients under the same conditions, toxicity tests of the same dose are conducted for n animals, and so on.

"Independence" means that the outcome for each experiment is not affected by another one. "Repeat" requires each experiment to be conducted under the same conditions, which leads to the same probability for the occurrence of event A.

(3) In n experiments, the primary focus is the number of positive outcomes. For instance, we focus on the number of cured cases among n patients receiving treatments, of the patients with positive outcomes among n patients receiving biochemical tests, of survival animals among n animals conducted toxicity tests, of qualified products among n inspected products, etc.

Independent n trials, each one of which can have only two outcomes (A or $\bar{A}$) such that the probabilities π of the outcomes do not change from one trial to another. A trial of this type is known as Bernoulli trial.

It is clear that an event A may occur $0, 1, 2, \ldots, n$ in n Bernoulli trials. A simple example is used to illustrate the probability of event A occurring $k(0 \leq k \leq n)$ times.

Example 2.4. Assume that 10% of people injected immunization vaccine will develop an uncomfortable reaction. What are the prob abilities of possible results after 3 people inject immunization vaccination?

Solution: Denote the event "suffered with uncomfortable reaction" by A. There are 3 people vaccinated, and each person will have an uncomfortable reaction after vaccination (A occurs) or not (A does not occur or $\bar{A}$ occurs). The results are independent, and the probability of occurrence of event A is 0.1 for everyone. The probability of occurrence for $\bar{A}$ is 0.9.

Denote the three people by a, b, and c, respectively. Let X denote the number of occurrence for A, where $X = 0, 1, 2, 3$. The possible results and their probabilities are given in Table 2.2.

Table 2.2 Consequences and probabilities for 3 Bernoulli trials

X	Results for a, b and c	Probabilities of results	$P(X=k)=C_3^k\pi^k(1-\pi)^{3-k}$
0	$\bar{\text{A}}$ $\bar{\text{A}}$ $\bar{\text{A}}$	$0.9\times0.9\times0.9$	$C_3^0 0.1^0(1-0.1)^{3-0}=0.729$
1	A $\bar{\text{A}}$ $\bar{\text{A}}$	$0.1\times0.9\times0.9$	$C_3^1 0.1^1(1-0.1)^{3-1}=0.243$
	$\bar{\text{A}}$ A $\bar{\text{A}}$	$0.9\times0.1\times0.9$	
	$\bar{\text{A}}$ $\bar{\text{A}}$ A	$0.9\times0.9\times0.1$	
2	A A $\bar{\text{A}}$	$0.1\times0.1\times0.9$	$C_3^2 0.1^2(1-0.1)^{3-2}=0.027$
	A $\bar{\text{A}}$ A	$0.1\times0.9\times0.1$	
	$\bar{\text{A}}$ A A	$0.9\times0.1\times0.1$	
3	A A A	$0.1\times0.1\times0.1$	$C_3^3 0.1^3(1-0.1)^{3-3}=0.001$

For example, the result of $X = 1$ implies that one of the three people, a, b or c, has an uncomfortable reaction. Then the corresponding result is A $\bar{\text{A}}$ $\bar{\text{A}}$, $\bar{\text{A}}$ A $\bar{\text{A}}$ or $\bar{\text{A}}$ $\bar{\text{A}}$ A. By the independence of Bernoulli trials and the probability multiplication formula, we have that

$$\begin{aligned}P(\text{A }\bar{\text{A}}\ \bar{\text{A}}) &= P(\text{A})P(\bar{\text{A}})P(\bar{\text{A}}) = 0.1\times0.9\times0.9 = 0.1\times0.9^2\\ &= 0.1\times(1-0.1)^2.\end{aligned}$$

Similarly,

$$P(\bar{\text{A}}\text{ A }\bar{\text{A}}) = P(\bar{\text{A}}\ \bar{\text{A}}\text{ A}) = 0.1\times0.9^2 = 0.1\times(1-0.1)^2.$$

Since $X = 1$ indicates A $\bar{\text{A}}$ $\bar{\text{A}}$, $\bar{\text{A}}$ A $\bar{\text{A}}$ or $\bar{\text{A}}$ $\bar{\text{A}}$ A (only one result occurs), on can obtain that

$$\begin{aligned}P(X=1) &= P(\text{A }\bar{\text{A}}\ \bar{\text{A}} + \bar{\text{A}}\text{ A }\bar{\text{A}} + \bar{\text{A}}\ \bar{\text{A}}\text{ A})\\ &= P(\text{A }\bar{\text{A}}\ \bar{\text{A}}) + P(\bar{\text{A}}\text{ A }\bar{\text{A}}) + P(\bar{\text{A}}\ \bar{\text{A}}\text{ A})\\ &= C_3^1 0.1^1\times(1-0.1)^2 = 0.243.\end{aligned}$$

Likewise, when the event A takes place k times, the corresponding probability is

$$P(X=k) = C_3^k 0.1^k 0.9^{3-k}, \quad k = 0, 1, 2, 3.$$

The above formulation also represents the component of Binomial expansion

$$(0.1+0.9)^3 = C_3^0 0.1^0 0.9^3 + C_3^1 0.1^1 0.9^2 + C_3^2 0.1^2 0.9^1 + C_3^3 0.1^3 0.9^0 \tag{2-8}$$

therefore, we call such a probability distribution as a binomial distribution. Considering that X where $X = 0, 1, 2, 3$, it is natural that the last column in Table 2.2 adds up to 1 (the left side of Equation (2-8) is equal to 1).

In general, for Bernoulli trials, let X denote the number of event A in n trials, and the probability distribution of X is given in the form

$$P(X = k) = C_n^k \pi^k (1-\pi)^{n-k}, \quad k = 0, 1, 2, \ldots, n \tag{2-9}$$

Where $C_n^k = \frac{n!}{k!(n-k)!}$. Then the random variable of X follows the binomial distribution, denoted by $X \sim B(n, \pi)$.

Note that the binomial distribution is a discrete distribution. The positive integer n is called as discrete parameter, and π denotes the probability of occurrence of event A.

2.2.2. *Characteristics*

1. Probability of binomial distribution

Assume that $X \sim B(n, \pi)$, then the probability distribution of X is given in Table 2.3.

Note that

(1) The sum of the probabilities for the binomial distribution is equal to 1, namely, $\sum_{k=0}^{n} C_n^k \pi^k (1-\pi)^{n-k} = (\pi + (1-\pi))^n = 1$

(2) One-sided cumulative probability

Table 2.3 Binomial probability distribution

X	0	1	...	k	...	n
$P(X)$	$C_n^0 \pi^0 (1-\pi)^{n-0}$	$C_n^1 \pi^1 (1-\pi)^{n-1}$	...	$C_n^k \pi^k (1-\pi)^{n-k}$	...	$C_n^n \pi^n (1-\pi)^{n-n}$

The probability of at most m positive cases (lower cumulative probability)

$$P(X \leq m) = \sum_{k=0}^{m} C_n^k \pi^k (1\text{-}\pi)^{n-k}$$

The probability of at least m positive cases (upper cumulative probability)

$$P(X \geq m) = 1 - P(X \leq m - 1)$$

2. Graphs of binomial distribution
Figure 2.10 are graphs of the probability distribution of binomial distribution.

3. Mean and standard deviation
Denote the number of positive outcomes by X and $X \sim B(n, \pi)$. For X, we have the population mean $\mu = n\pi$, the population

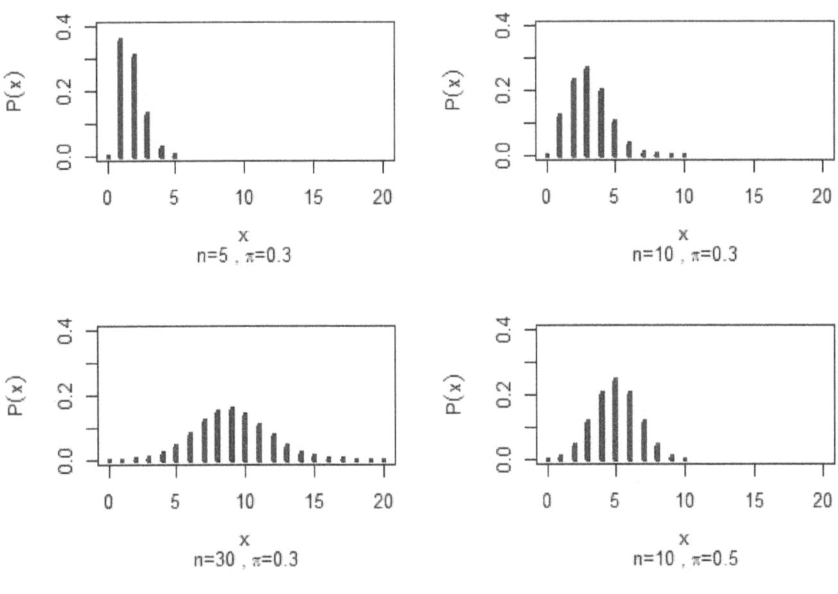

Figure 2.10 Probability distribution diagrams of binomial distributions

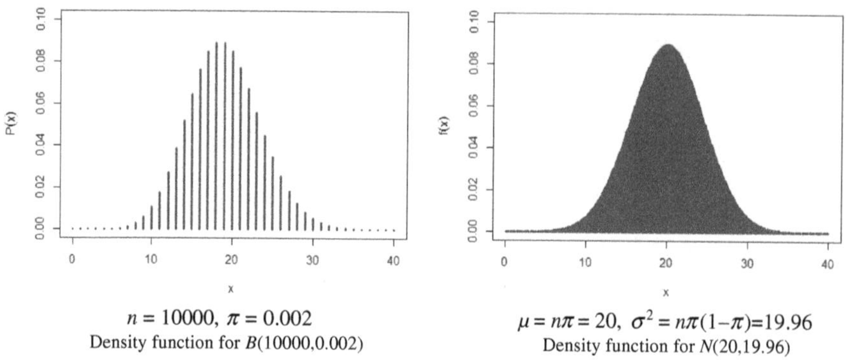

Figure 2.11 The approximation from the binomial distribution to the normal distribution

variance $\sigma^2 = n\pi(1-\pi)$ and the population standard deviation $\sigma = \sqrt{n\pi(1-\pi)}$.

4. Normal approximation
According to the central limit theorem, with a large n, $n\pi \geq 5$, or $n(1-\pi) \geq 5$, the binomial distribution converges to the normal distribution. Namely, as $n \to \infty$, the binomial distribution converges to the normal distribution $N(\mu, \sigma^2)$ where $\mu = n\pi$ and $\sigma^2 = n\pi(1-\pi)$, see the Figure 2.11.

2.2.3. *Application*

When applying the binomial distribution, we must pay attention to the three application conditions of the binomial distribution:

(1) There are a fixed number of trials n, each of which results in one of two mutually exclusive outcomes.
(2) The probability for an outcome such as death is π, then the probability for the opposite outcome should be $1-\pi$. For the unknown π, we can utilize the sample frequency p from the observations to estimate π.
(3) The outcomes of the n trials are independent, that is, the outcome of each observation is not affected by the others.

Example 2.5. It is reported that 10% of people may have an intestinal reaction to a certain drug. In order to investigate the quality of this drug, randomly selected 5 people take the drug.

(1) What is the probability that k people have an intestinal reaction?
(2) What is the probability that no more than 2 people have an intestinal reaction?
(3) What is the probability that at least 1 people has an intestinal reaction?

Solution: We know that 5 people are randomly selected to take the drug, and each person's response to the drug is independent. The probability that each person has an intestinal reaction is 0.10. Therefore, the number of people to have an intestinal reaction follows the binomial distribution $B(n, \pi)$ with $n = 5$ and $\pi = 0.10$. As a result, one can obtain that

(1) The probability that k people have an intestinal reaction is listed below

$X = k$	0	1	2	3	4	5
$P(X = k)$	0.59049	0.32805	0.07290	0.00810	0.00045	0.00001

(2) The probability that no more than 2 people have an intestinal reaction is

$$P(X \leq 2) = \sum_{k=0}^{2} P(X = k) = 0.59049 + 0.32805 + 0.07290$$
$$= 0.99144 = 99.14\%$$

That is, it is almost certain that no more than two people who take the drug will have intestinal reaction, and it is almost impossible that more than two people will respond. Therefore, if more than two people have intestinal reaction, the report of "10% response" could be questionable.

(3) The probability that at least 1 people has intestinal reaction

$$P(X \geq 1) = 1 - P(X = 0) = 1 - 0.59049 = 0.40951$$

2.3. Poisson distribution

2.3.1. *Concept*

If the possible values of random variable X are 0, 1, 2, ..., and its probability function is

$$P(X = k) = \frac{\lambda^k}{k!}e^{-\lambda}, \quad k = 0, 1, 2, \ldots \tag{2-10}$$

λ in this equation is a constant and $\lambda > 0$, $e = 2.7182\ldots$ is the base of natural logarithm, then the distribution of X is called Poisson distribution with parameter λ (Poisson's distribution), and written as $X \sim P(\lambda)$.

Now using the blood count on slide as an example to illustrate the generation mechanism of Poisson distribution. Set the average number of blood cells in the prescribed area to be λ. Take a large natural number n, to divide this area into n small lattices (Figure 2.12), then the average number of blood cells in each lattices is λ/n. (1) Because n is so big that it is impossible to have two and more blood cells on each lattice, that is to say, there is only one blood cell or no blood cells on each lattice. (2) The probability of having a blood cell on each of these lattices is the same, which is λ/n (small probability).

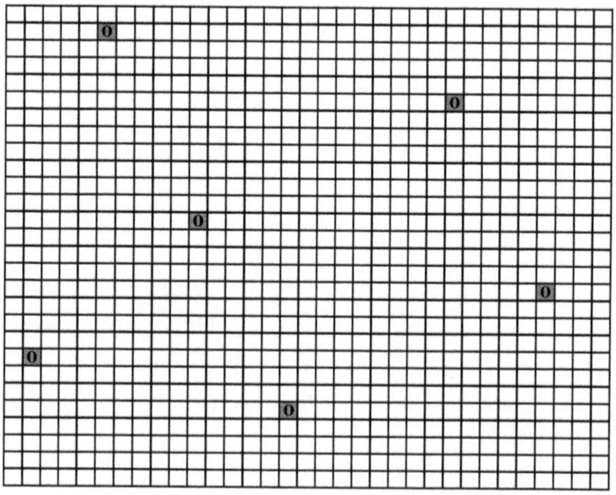

Figure 2.12 Blood count on slide

(3) The presence of blood cells in different lattices is independent of each other. So the number X of blood cells in these n lattices should satisfy the binomial distribution $B(n, \lambda/n)$, the probability function of X is

$$P(X = k) = C_n^k \left(\frac{\lambda}{n}\right)^k \left(1 - \frac{\lambda}{n}\right)^{n-k}$$

It can be proved that, when $n \to \infty$,

$$\lim_{n\to\infty} P(X = k) = \lim_{n\to\infty} C_n^k \left(\frac{\lambda}{n}\right)^k \left(1 - \frac{\lambda}{n}\right)^{n-k} = \frac{\lambda^k}{k!} e^{-\lambda}$$

It can be seen from the above deduction that Poisson distribution can be obtained as the limit of binomial distribution. In other words, if $X \sim B(n, \pi)$, when n is large and π is small, it can be assumed that X approximately follows Poisson distribution $P(\lambda)$, and $\lambda = n\pi$.

2.3.2. *Characteristics*

1. Graphs of Poisson distribution
λ is the unique parameter of Poisson distribution, it represents the average number of random events in unit time (or unit area, or unit space), namely the total mean. Given the population mean λ, according to the probability calculation formula (2-10) of Poisson distribution, the probability $P(X = k)$, $k = 0, 1, 2, \ldots$ can be obtained, thus the corresponding Poisson distribution graph is obtained (as shown in Figure 2.13). It can be seen from Figure 2.13 that the smaller the value λ, the more asymmetric the distribution is, as λ increases, the Poisson distribution tends to be symmetric.

2. The population mean is equal to the population variance
Namely $\lambda = \sigma^2$. This is an important characteristic of Poisson distribution. This characteristic can be used to preliminarily judge whether a discrete random variable follows Poisson distribution.

3. Normal approximation of Poisson distribution
When $\lambda = 20$, Poisson distribution approaches the normal distribution, when $\lambda = 50$, it can be considered that the Poisson distribution

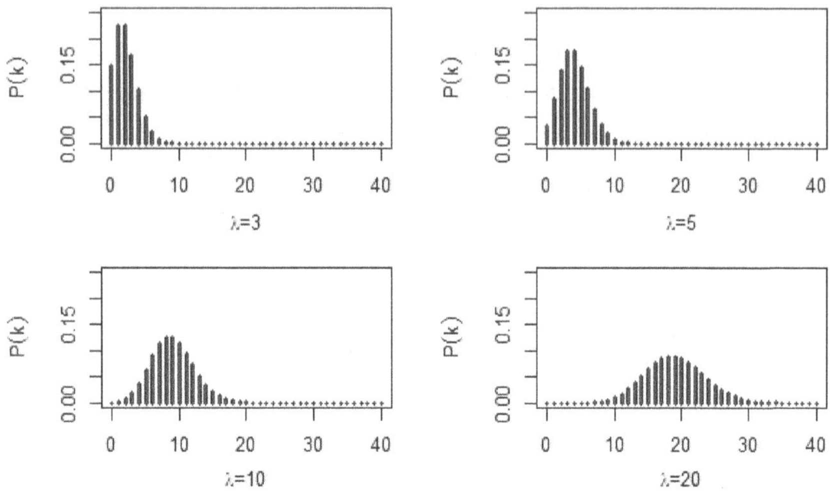

Figure 2.13 Probability distribution graphs of Poisson distribution

is normal distribution. When $\lambda \geq 20$, questions of Poisson distribution in practice can be dealt as normal distribution approximately.

4. Poisson distribution has additivity
If there are m independent random variables $X_1, X_2, \ldots, X_m$ follow the Poisson distribution with parameters $\lambda_1, \lambda_2, \ldots, \lambda_m$, respectively, then the sum of these random variables $X_1 + X_2 + \cdots + X_m$ follow Poisson distribution, and the mean of Poisson distribution is $\lambda_1 + \lambda_2 + \cdots + \lambda_m$. The additive property of independent Poisson distribution is often used in practice, combine several small independent observation units into one large observation unit, when the mean $\lambda \geq 20$, the data that follows Poisson distribution can be treated as normal distribution approximately.

For example, the number of particles per minute emitted by a known radioactive substance approximately follows Poisson distribution. Let the average number of particles per minute emitted by a radioactive substance be 5, then there is $X \sim P(5)$, now observe for 10 minutes consecutively, and consider the distribution of the number of particles emitted. Because particles emitted in the ith minute are $X_i \sim P(5)$ $(i = 1, 2, \ldots, 10)$, and each X_i is independent of each other, according to the additivity of Poisson distribution, $\sum_{i=1}^{10} X_i \sim P(50)$ can be obtained, that is, the number of particles emitted in 10 minutes still follows Poisson distribution, and the mean is 50.

2.3.3. *Application*

1. Application conditions of Poisson distribution
Since Poisson distribution can be regarded as the limit distribution of binomial distribution, application conditions of binomial distribution are also the application conditions of Poisson distribution. In addition, Poisson distribution requires a large number of trials n, and probability π of the event concerned is small.

The Poisson distribution is an important discrete probability distribution used to describe the frequency of rare events in unit space or time. In biomedical research, random variables following Poisson distribution are common. For example, the number of cases or deaths of a non-communicable disease with a low prevalence in the population, the *Escherichia coli* per liter of water, the number of blood cells in the small square of the counter, the dust per unit space, the number of patients treated in hospital outpatient per unit time, etc. In addition, the number of particles emitted by a radioactive substance per unit time, Earthquakes, volcanic eruptions, major floods, and other natural disasters, the number of calls at the switchboard and so on, also follow the Poisson distribution. It should be noted that the cases number of some rare infectious diseases can be counted as the source of infection after the first case occurs, which will affect the occurrence of subsequent cases. Therefore, it does not meet the application conditions of Poisson distribution and cannot be regarded as Poisson distribution.

For some reasons, the distribution of observed objects that are uneven in unit time, unit area, or unit volume (e.g., bacteria colonization exists in milk) does not follow Poisson distribution.

2. Probability calculation

According to Equation (2-10), the probabilities of Poisson distribution can be obtained as long as the parameters are determined. However, in most cases that follow the Poisson distribution, the distribution parameters are often unknown. In general, the corresponding sample mean calculated from the observed random sample is used as the estimated value of λ, and substitute it for λ in Equation (2-10), then calculate the probabilities when $k = 0, 1, 2, \ldots$.

Example 2.6. In order to monitor the pollution of potable water, the number of bacteria per milliliter of potable water in a community is tested, 400 in total, and the records are as follows (Table 2.4):

Table 2.4 The number of bacteria per milliliter of potable water in a community

Bacteria count in 1 mL water	0	1	2	3	Total
Frequency f	243	120	31	6	400

To analyze whether the distribution of bacteria number in potable water follows Poisson distribution. If the Poisson distribution is followed, calculate the probability and theoretical number of bacteria per milliliter of water by the Poisson distribution and intuitively compare the frequency distribution with the Poisson distribution.

Solution: The average bacterial count per milliliter of water calculated is $\bar{X} = 0.500$, the variance $S^2 = 0.496$. Two of them are very close, so the bacteria number per milliliter of water is considered to be Poisson distribution. Replace λ in Equation (2-10) with $\bar{X} = 0.500$. We have

$$P(X = k) = \frac{0.5^k}{k!} e^{-0.5}, \quad k = 0, 1, 2, \ldots$$

The calculation results are shown in Table 2.5.

It can be seen that the frequency distribution of bacteria number is quite consistent with Poisson distribution with parameter $\lambda = 0.5$,

Table 2.5 The Poisson distribution of bacteria number

Bacteria number	Actual frequency	Frequency	Probability	Theoretical frequency
0	243	0.6075	0.6065	242.60
1	120	0.3000	0.3033	121.32
2	31	0.0775	0.0758	30.32
3	6	0.0150	0.0144	5.76
Total	400	1.0000	1.0000	400.00

which further indicates that it is appropriate to describe the distribution of bacteria number in unit volume (or area) using the Poisson distribution.

2.4. Report writing

1. Medical reference range estimation
Generally, the estimation of medical reference range mainly reports the following basic contents:

(1) Target population, character, and sample size of the study.
(2) Distribution of observation indicators (normal or non-normal) and basic statistical description.
(3) Reference range, unilateral or bilateral, estimation method, and calculation results.

The following is the result report of estimating the reference range of serum total protein of normal adult women in an area of Exp. 2.3.

The serum total protein of 110 normal adult women in a district were measured. The sample mean and standard deviation were 72.8 and 3.8 g/L, respectively. Based on normal distribution, two-sided 95% reference range of serum total protein of normal adult women in this district was estimated as 65.35–80.25 g/L.

2. Applying various distributions to calculate probability
Three distributions was used to calculate the probability of events concerned, the following contents are usually required to report.

(1) Distribution of observation values (including the type of distribution and distribution parameters).
(2) The event occurrence probability of interest to the researcher, and conclusions drawn there from it. The following is the result report of Poisson distribution application of Example 2.6.

According to the data in Table 2.4, the mean and variance for number of bacteria in per milliliter of water were 0.5 and 0.496, respectively. The corresponding frequency distribution based on Poisson distribution $P(0.5)$ was showed in Table 2.5. It indicated that Poisson distribution fitted the data well.

2.5. Case discrimination

Case 2.1 In order to estimate the reference range of urinary mercury values of residents in an area, the urinary mercury values of 200 normal adults were measured as shown in Table 2.6.

The sample data was used to estimate the 95% reference range of urine mercury values of the local residents.

The following gives a variety of solutions, please judge right or wrong, and explain the reasons. If correct, please point out, if not correct, please add.

Solution 1: The sample mean and variance calculated from data were $\bar{X}$ =13.78 (μg/L) and S =11.71 (μg/L), respectively, according to the normal distribution method, in this area the two-sided 95% reference range of residents' urine mercury value is $(\bar{X} - 1.96S, \bar{X} + 1.96S) = (-9.17, 36.73)$ (μg/L).

Table 2.6 Urine mercury value of 200 normal adults in an area (μg/L)

Value of urine mercury	0∼	4∼	8∼	12∼	16∼	20∼	24∼	28∼	32∼	36∼	40∼	44∼	48∼
Number of cases	45	30	41	20	15	12	13	5	4	6	3	4	2

Solution 2: The sample mean and variance calculated from data were $\bar{X} = 13.78$ (μg/L) and S =11.71 (μg/L), respectively, because excessive mercury in urine is abnormal, only one-sided upper limit needs to be calculated. According to the normal distribution method, in this area the one-sided 95% reference range of residents' urine mercury value is $(\bar{X},\ \bar{X} + 1.64S) = (13.78, 32.98)$ (μg/L).

Solution 3: The sample mean and variance calculated from data were $\bar{X} = 13.78$ (μg/L) and $S = 11.71$ (μg/L), respectively, because excessive mercury in urine is abnormal, and values cannot be negative, the lower limit should be 0, only one-sided upper limit need to be calculated. According to the normal distribution method, in this area the one-sided 95% reference range of residents' urine mercury value is $(0, \bar{X} + 1.64S) = (0, 32.98)$ (μg/L).

Case 2.2 Twenty cases of viral mumps occurred in a population of 100,000 people in an area, and it is hoped that this will lead to an estimate of the probability that there will be at least 20 cases in a population of 100,000 people in the area. So there are solutions of some students, please judge right or wrong, and explain the reasons.

Solution 1: Randomly select one person in the area, the incidence of virulent mumps is $20/10^5$, it is considered that the number of diseases$X$among 100,000 people in this area follows Binomial distribution $B(10^5, 0.0002)$, according to the binomial distribution probability formula, the probability of having no less than 20 patients is as follows:

$$\begin{aligned} P(X \geq 20) = 1 - P(X < 20) = 1 - (&C_{100,000}^{0} 0.0002^{0} 0.9998^{100,000} \\ &+ C_{100,000}^{1} 0.0002^{1} 0.9998^{99,999} \\ &+ \cdots + C_{100,000}^{19} 0.0002^{19} 0.9998^{99,981}) = 0.52975 \end{aligned}$$

Solution 2: Prevalence of viral mumps is $20/10^5$, which is quite low, it is considered that number of cases X follows Poisson distribution that $\lambda = n\pi = 20$. Because Poisson distribution approximates normal distribution when $\lambda = 20$, so the probability of having no less than 20 cases ($X \geq 20$) is approximately

$$\begin{aligned} P(X \geq 20) &= 1 - P(X < 20) \\ &= 1 - \left(\frac{20^0}{0!} e^0 + \frac{20^1}{1!} e^1 + \frac{20^2}{2!} e^2 + \cdots + \frac{20^{19}}{19!} e^{19} \right) \\ &\approx 1 - \Phi\left(\frac{20 - 20}{\sqrt{20}} \right) = 1 - \Phi(0) = 1 - 0.5 = 0.5 \end{aligned}$$

Solution 3: Same as Solution 2, it is considered that number of cases X follows Poisson distribution that $\lambda = n\pi = 20$. According to the probability formula of Poisson distribution, the probability of having no fewer than 20 cases ($X \geq 20$) is

$$P(X \geq 20) = \frac{20^{20}}{20!} \mathrm{e}^{20} + \frac{20^{21}}{21!} \mathrm{e}^{21} + \cdots + \frac{20^{100,000}}{100,000!} \mathrm{e}^{100,000} = 0.52974$$

2.6. Computer experiments (See electronic resources exp2-1 to exp2-5)

Experiment 2.1 SPSS was used to calculate the ratio between 66.0 and 75.0 g/L of total serum protein in Case 2.2

Learn how to use SPSS function to obtain the proportion of an interval of normal distribution.

Experiment 2.2 SPSS was used to calculate the probability of Example 2.5

Learn how to use SPSS function to calculate probability.

Experiment 2.3 Demonstrating normal distribution with Excel

Understand the meaning of mean (μ) and standard deviation (σ) of normal distribution.

Experiment 2.4 Demonstrating binomial distribution with Excel

Understand the meaning of binomial distribution parameters.

Experiment 2.5 Demonstrating Poisson distribution with Excel

Understand the meaning of Poisson distribution parameters.

2.7. Frequently asked questions and summary

2.7.1. *Frequently asked questions*

1. How to determine whether a set of data is normally distributed?

There are usually several methods to determine whether a group of data follows the normal distribution: (1) According to the literature. For example, the literature reports that the body weight and vital capacity of middle school students follow normal distribution, so we can follow the literature practice. (2) Judging by experience or expertise. For example, according to professional knowledge, the number of erythrocyte, hemoglobin content, and pulse number of healthy adults of the same sex are approximately normal distribution, while the blood lead content of normal adults is approximately lognormal distribution, after logarithmic transformation, it should be approximately normal distribution. (3) Data can be tested for normality by means of statistical software (see Chapter 5).

2. Why is it inappropriate to call "medical reference range" as "normal value range"?

The medical reference range refers to the range of most individuals in physiological and biochemical data of a specific "normal" population (homogeneous population excluding diseases and related factors affecting the indicators studied). For example, 95% medical reference range only indicates that 95% of the individuals in a particular population are within this range, but it does not mean that all within this range are "normal," nor does it mean that all outside this range are "abnormal." Therefore, it is inappropriate to call "medical reference value range" as "normal value range."

2.7.2. *Summary*

1. Normal distribution is an important continuous distribution. Many medical phenomena approximately follows normal distribution, which is the theoretical basis of many statistical methods. Normal distribution $N(\mu, \sigma^2)$ is determined by μ and σ^2, where μ is the mean or expectation and σ is the standard deviation

of the distribution. When μ increases, the curve moves to the right along the X-axis, when μ decreases and the curve moves to the left along the X-axis. The larger σ is, the more dispersed the data is and the "shorter and fatter" the density curve is, in other words, the smaller σ is, the "thinner and taller" the density curve is. The Probability of a random variables falling within an interval equals to the area under its probability density curve. The probability of normal random variable X value falling within the interval $\mu \pm 1.64\sigma, \mu \pm 1.96\sigma$, and $\mu \pm 2.58\sigma$ is 90%, 95%, and 99%, respectively, or in theory, the number of observations within $\mu \pm 1.64\sigma, \mu \pm 1.96\sigma$, and $\mu \pm 2.58\sigma$ account for 90%, 95%, and 99%, respectively of total number of observations. The normal distribution law can be used to estimate medical reference range and to carry out quality control. The standard normal distribution, written as N (0, 1), is a normal distribution with a mean of zero and standard deviation of 1. Normal distribution can be transformed to standard normal distributions by the formula $Z = \frac{X-\mu}{\sigma}$, where the random variable $X \sim N(\mu, \sigma^2)$, so the probability calculation of general normal distribution can be solved by standard normal distribution table.

2. Binomial distribution with parameters n and π is the discrete probability distribution of the number of successes in a sequence of n independent experiments. The population mean of binomial distribution $B(n, \pi)$ is $n\pi$ and standard deviation is $\sqrt{n\pi(1-\pi)}$. when n is large, π is not close to 0 nor close to 1, and $n\pi$, $n(1-\pi)$ are both greater than 5, the binomial distribution $B(n, \pi)$ approximates normal distribution $N(n\pi, n\pi(1-\pi))$.
3. The Poisson distribution is also an important discrete distribution, that can be used to describe the probability distribution of the number of rare events per unit time or space. The population mean (expectation) and variance of a Poisson-distributed random variable $P(\lambda)$ are both equal to its parameter λ. When the mean of a Poisson distribution is large ($\lambda \geq 20$), it becomes similar to a normal distribution. And the normal approximation to the Poisson distribution is very useful for probability calculation.

Think and Practice

I. Best Choice

1. The observed values of a certain data are normally distributed, and theoretically there are ( ) observed values fall within the range.
   A. 68.27% B. 90% C. 95% D. 99% E. 45%
2. Under normal curve, the area from mean μ to $\mu + 1.64\sigma$ is ( ).
   A. 45% B. 90% C. 95% D. 47.5% E. 99%
3. If blood lead levels of normal people approximately **follow** logarithmic normal distribution (Written $Y = \lg X$, and S_Y is the standard deviation of Y), then the best way to calculate 95% reference range of X is ( ).
   A. $\bar{X} \pm 1.96S$ B. $P_{2.5} \sim P_{97.5}$ C. less than $\lg^{-1}(Y + 1.64S_Y)$ D. less than $\lg^{-1}(Y + 1.96S_Y)$ E. $P_5 \sim P_{95}$
4. Under the condition that the sample cases is fixed, if ( ), the more symmetric the binomial distribution is.
   A. the greater the population rate π B. the greater the sample rate p C. the smaller the population rate π D. the closer to 0.5 the population rate π E. the smaller the sample rate p
5. The number of lead workers' peripheral blood picture stippling erythrocyte on the blood slides approximately follow ( ).
   A. binomial distribution B. normal distribution C. symmetric distribution D. Poisson distribution E. None of the above is correct
6. The relationship between mean λ of Poisson distribution and standard deviation σ is ( ).
   A. $\lambda = \sigma$ B. $\lambda < \sigma$ C. $\lambda > \sigma$ D. $\lambda = \sqrt{\sigma}$ E. $\lambda = \sigma^2$

II. Essay Questions

1. What are the conditions of following binomial distribution and Poisson distribution?
2. What are the conditions of binomial distribution and Poisson distribution approximate normal distribution respectively?

III. Calculation Questions

1. It is known that the effective rate of conventional therapy for a certain non-communicable disease is 80%. Now 10 patients with this disease are treated with conventional therapy. What is the probability of cure for at least nine people?
2. According to previous statistics, the rate of chromosome abnormality of newborns in a place is 1%. What is the probability of chromosome abnormality of not less than 2 newborns in 100 newborns?
3. The height (cm) data of 110 20-year-old male youth in a city in 2010 is as follows:

173.1	166.8	172.9	175.9	172.8	170.5	174.1	174.2	175.7	173.5	173.8
168.2	173.7	184.4	174.8	172.5	174.9	174.9	174.2	173.8	176.2	180.7
170.9	165.0	176.3	174.2	179.8	174.5	180.5	171.5	178.9	171.5	176.3
166.7	170.8	168.8	177.5	174.5	183.5	182.0	170.9	173.5	177.5	177.5
181.2	177.1	172.3	176.5	174.0	174.3	174.6	172.6	171.3	173.1	178.3
176.9	170.5	174.2	177.5	176.6	182.3	172.1	169.9	179.5	175.8	176.0
178.6	180.6	175.6	173.3	168.7	174.5	178.5	171.3	172.0	173.2	174.8
168.8	176.0	182.6	169.5	177.5	180.6	181.5	175.1	165.2	168.0	180.8
175.4	169.2	170.0	171.9	176.6	178.8	177.2	173.4	168.5	177.6	176.5
175.8	164.8	175.6	180.0	176.6	176.5	177.7	174.1	180.8	170.6	179.2

(1) Try to estimate the proportion of this city's 20-year-old male youth within the height of 175.0 $\sim$ 178.0 cm.

(2) Estimate the range from 95% to 99% of city's all 20-year-old male youth in 2010.

(3) If a 20-year-old male was randomly selected in the city that year, try to estimate the probability of his height exceeding 180 cm.

Aiqin Qi, Zhongwen Zhang, Yong Gao, Fang Liu

CHAPTER 3

PARAMETER ESTIMATION

The study population of interest is usually very large, even hypothesized population (e.g., the population is all patients who will be treated). Studying the entire population is time consuming, laborious, and even impossible. Therefore, usually collect sample data that can represent the population to estimate the population parameter. Chapter 1 has learned to use the sample statistic such as sample means and sample frequency to estimate the population parameters such as population mean and population probability. These are ***point estimates*** on parameters. The point estimate does not make full use of the sample information and does not reflect the size of the sampling error. The ***interval estimate*** just overcomes these shortcomings. This chapter, first introduces the concept of sampling distribution and sampling error, second introduces several commonly used sampling distributions, and then introduces interval estimates of population mean, population probability, and population standard deviation.

3.1. Sampling distribution and standard error

From the same population, the same amount of samples are randomly selected, and one sample statistic (such as sample mean) can be calculated from each sample repeatedly extracted. For example, randomly extract n samples from a population, to calculate a sample mean according to the formula

$$\bar{X} = \sum_{i=1}^{n} \frac{X_i}{n}$$

Repeatedly extract n samples from the same population m times (usually assuming m is infinite). M sample means are obtained from m samples, and the distribution of m sample means is called ***sampling distribution***. The probability that the sample mean is exactly same as the population mean is very small. In order to measure the proximity between the sample mean and its population mean, sampling distribution plays an important role. Sampling distribution is the basis of statistical inference. The sample mean, sample frequency, and sample standard deviation will be introduced separately as follows.

3.1.1. *Sample mean*

The following is an example of casting a dice to illustrate the meaning of sampling distribution. A dice is a cube with six sides, and the points are 1, 2, 3, 4, 5, and 6. Let the random variable X denote the number of points after each throw of the dice ($X = 1, 2, 3, 4, 5, 6$) assuming that the dice is even, so the probability of each of these points occurring is $1/6$. The variable X follows uniform distribution (see Figure 3.1).

After throwing the dice indefinitely, through statistical principle determines that the population mean is

$$\mu = \sum XP(X) = 1\left(\frac{1}{6}\right) + 2\left(\frac{1}{6}\right) + 3\left(\frac{1}{6}\right) + 4\left(\frac{1}{6}\right) + 5\left(\frac{1}{6}\right) + 6\left(\frac{1}{6}\right) = 3.5$$

The population variance is

$$\sigma^2 = \sum (X-\mu)^2 P(X) = (1-3.5)^2\left(\frac{1}{6}\right) + (2-3.5)^2\left(\frac{1}{6}\right) + (3-3.5)^2\left(\frac{1}{6}\right) + (4-3.5)^2\left(\frac{1}{6}\right) + (5-3.5)^2\left(\frac{1}{6}\right) + (6-3.5)^2\left(\frac{1}{6}\right) = 2.92$$

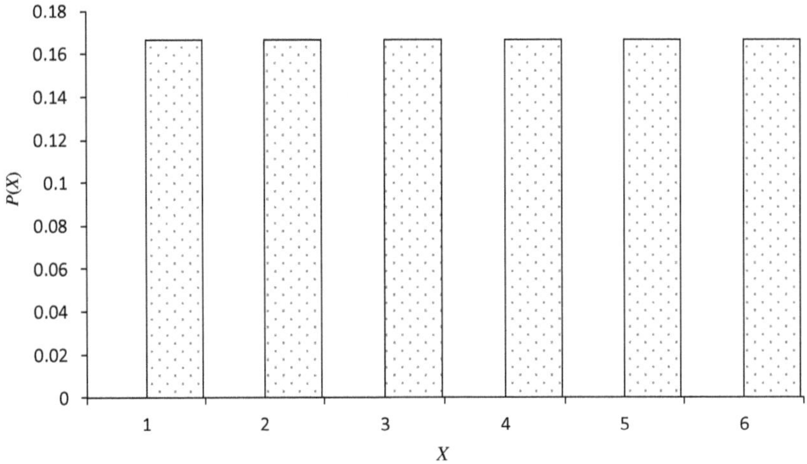

Figure 3.1 Probability distribution of random variables

Table 3.1 All possible sample means with a sample size of 2

	Dice 2					
Dice 1	1	2	3	4	5	6
1	1.0	1.5	2.0	2.5	3.0	3.5
2	1.5	2.0	2.5	3.0	3.5	4.0
3	2.0	2.5	3.0	3.5	4.0	4.5
4	2.5	3.0	3.5	4.0	4.5	5.0
5	3.0	3.5	4.0	4.5	5.0	5.5
6	3.5	4.0	4.5	5.0	5.5	6.0

The population standard deviation

$$\sigma = \sqrt{\sigma^2} = \sqrt{2.92} = 1.71$$

Throw 2 times independently. The sample size is 2, and the sample mean is calculated. Repeatedly, all possible sample mean values are shown in Table 3.1, and the probability distribution corresponding to the mean is shown in Table 3.2 (from Table 3.1), and the corresponding figure is shown in Figure 3.1.

As can be seen from Table 3.1, there are 36 possible combinations with a sample size of 2, the probability of each possibility is 1/36.

Table 3.2 Probability distribution of all samples means in Table 3.1

$\bar{X}$	1.0	1.5	2.0	2.5	3.0	3.5	4.0	4.5	5.0	5.5	6.0
$P(\bar{X})$	1/36	2/36	3/36	4/36	5/36	6/36	5/36	4/36	3/36	2/36	1/36

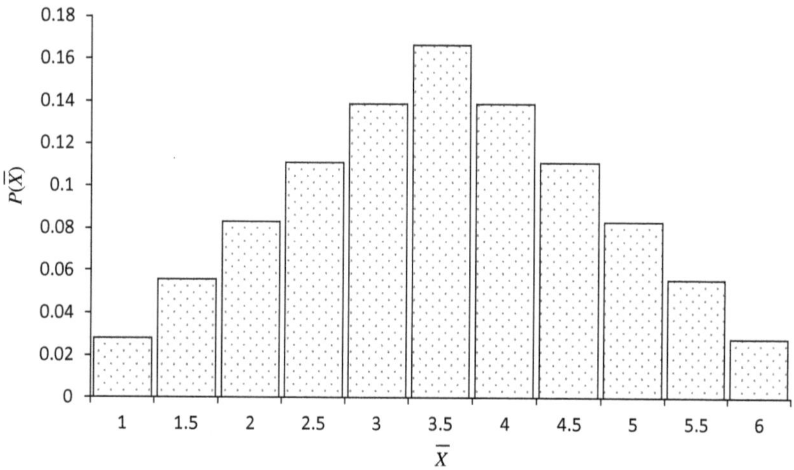

Figure 3.2 Probability distribution of sample mean

But $\bar{X}$ has only 11 possible values. That is, $1.0, 1.5, \ldots, 6.0$, of which 3.5 is the most frequent (6). Followed by 3.0 and 4.0 (5), 1.0 and 6.0 is the least frequent (1) (see Table 3.2).

As can be seen by comparing Figure 3.2 with Figure 3.1, the sampling distribution pattern of $\bar{X}$ is completely different from the probability distribution pattern of X.

The mean of $\bar{X}$ sample distribution with sample size of 2 is

$$\mu_{\bar{X}} = \sum \bar{X}P(\bar{X}) = 1.0\left(\frac{1}{36}\right) + 1.5\left(\frac{2}{36}\right) + \cdots + 6.0\left(\frac{1}{36}\right) = 3.5$$

The variance of $\bar{X}$ sample distribution with sample size of 2 is

$$\begin{aligned}\sigma_{\bar{X}}^2 &= \sum (\bar{X} - \mu_{\bar{X}})^2 P(\bar{X}) \\ &= (1.0 - 3.5)^2\left(\frac{1}{36}\right) + (1.5 - 3.5)^2\left(\frac{2}{36}\right) \\ &\quad + \cdots + (6.0 - 3.5)^2\left(\frac{1}{36}\right) = 1.46\end{aligned}$$

The standard deviation of sample mean sampling distribution is

$$\sigma_{\bar{X}} = \sqrt{\sigma^2_{\bar{X}}} = \sqrt{1.46} = 1.21$$

It can be seen that the mean of $\bar{X}$ sampling distribution is equal to the mean of X probability distribution, but the variance of sampling distribution ($\sigma^2_{\bar{X}} = 1.46$) is not equal to the variance of probability distribution ($\sigma^2 = 2.92$), and there is $\sigma^2_{\bar{X}} = \frac{\sigma^2}{2}$.

If sample size $n = 2$ is modified to $n = 5, n = 10$, or $n = 30$, then the mean of sampling distribution $\mu_{\bar{X}} = \mu = 3.5$ can be obtained. The variance is $2.92/5 = 0.584$, $2.92/10 = 0.292$, or $2.92/30 = 0.0973$, respectively. The standard deviation of sample mean is $\sqrt{2.92/5} \approx 0.7642$, $\sqrt{2.92/10} \approx 0.5404$, or $\sqrt{2.92/30} \approx 0.3120$, respectively. As can be seen, the variance of sampling distribution obtained is less than the population variance, and there is $\sigma^2_{\bar{X}} = \frac{\sigma^2}{n} < \sigma^2$, the larger the sample size is, the smaller the standard error $\sigma^2_{\bar{X}}$ is. Moreover, when there is sufficient sample size (e.g., $n \geq 30$), the sample mean obtained from random samples taken from any population will approximately follow the normal distribution. The larger the sample size is, the closer the sampling distribution is to the normal distribution. This phenomenon is statistically called central limit theorem.

In fact, if the population is originally a normal distribution, then for all n, the sampling distribution is normally distributed. If the population is non-normally distributed, $\bar{X}$ approximates a normal distribution only if n is large enough. Generally, the $\bar{X}$ sampling distribution at $n \geq 30$ is approximately normal distribution; however, if the population distribution is extremely non-normal distribution (e.g., bimodal distribution, extreme peak distribution), only if n is very large, $\bar{X}$ will be an approximate normal distribution.

In order to distinguish from the standard deviation of random variables, the standard deviation corresponding to sample statistic (such as $\bar{X}$, p) is customarily called standard error, such as the standard deviation of sample mean is referred to as standard error of mean (standard error of mean [SEM]). The standard error reflects the size of sampling error, which reflects the difference between sample statistics and population parameters, the sample statistics and the sample statistics caused by differences individuals.

If the sample comes from an infinite population (usually assumed to be the case), the standard error for sample mean is calculated as

$$\sigma_{\bar{X}} = \frac{\sigma}{\sqrt{n}} \tag{3-1}$$

If the population standard deviation is unknown (in most cases), the sample standard deviation S can be used to estimate it, where the standard error $\sigma_{\bar{X}}$ is estimated.

$$S_{\bar{X}} = \frac{S}{\sqrt{n}} \tag{3-2}$$

If the population from which the sample is derived is a finite population, computing formula for the standard error of the mean needs to be corrected, see Section 4.7.1.

3.1.2. *Difference between two sample means*

Samples were randomly and independently extracted from the two normal populations $N(\mu_1, \sigma_1^2)$ and $N(\mu_2, \sigma_2^2)$, respectively, and the sample mean was recorded as $\bar{X}_1$ and $\bar{X}_2$, respectively. Since $\bar{X}_1$, $\bar{X}_2$ follow the normal distributions $N(\mu_1, \sigma_1^2/n_1)$ and $N(\mu_2, \sigma_2^2/n_2)$, respectively, the difference $\bar{X}_1 - \bar{X}_2$ between the two sample means also follows the normal distribution, and the mean of $\bar{X}_1 - \bar{X}_2$ sample distribution is

$$\mu_{\bar{X}_1 - \bar{X}_2} = \mu_1 - \mu_2 \tag{3-3}$$

Standard error is

$$\sigma_{\bar{X}_1 - \bar{X}_2} = \sqrt{\frac{\sigma_1^2}{n_1} + \frac{\sigma_2^2}{n_2}} \tag{3-4}$$

If the original population is non-normal distribution, then when the sample size is large enough (such as $n \geq 30$ per group), according to the central limit theorem, two sample means $\bar{X}_1$ and $\bar{X}_2$ follow approximately normal distribution $N(\mu_1, \sigma_1^2/n_1)$ and $N(\mu_2, \sigma_2^2/n_2)$, respectively. The difference $\bar{X}_1 - \bar{X}_2$ follows also approximately normal distribution, and Equations (3-3) and (3-4) are still work.

1. $\sigma_1^2 \neq \sigma_2^2$
If the population variance is unknown, assuming the two population variances are unequal, the standard error of the difference $\bar{X}_1 - \bar{X}_2$ approximately equal to

$$S_{\bar{X}_1-\bar{X}_2} = \sqrt{\frac{S_1^2}{n_1} + \frac{S_2^2}{n_2}} \tag{3-5}$$

2. $\sigma_1^2 = \sigma_2^2 = \sigma_c^2$
If the population variance is unknown, assuming the two population variances are equal, the standard error of the difference $\bar{X}_1 - \bar{X}_2$ approximately equal to

$$S_{\bar{X}_1-\bar{X}_2} = \sqrt{\frac{S_c^2}{n_1} + \frac{S_c^2}{n_2}} = S_c\sqrt{\frac{1}{n_1} + \frac{1}{n_2}} \tag{3-6}$$

where S_c is pooled standard deviations, the size of the value is between S_1 and S_2, calculated by the square root of the weighted average of sample variance S_1^2 and S_2^2, that is.

$$S_c = \sqrt{\frac{(n_1-1)S_1^2 + (n_2-1)S_2^2}{(n_1-1)+(n_2-1)}} \tag{3-7}$$

3.1.3. *Sample frequency*

If the data processed is a binomial variable, then the parameter of interest is the probability of "success." The population probability of "success" denotes π, the sample frequency of "success" p is the estimated value of π. In the independent n trials, the times of "success" is denoted as X, the X follows binomial distribution, denoted as $X \sim B(n, p)$, the sample frequency

$$p = \frac{X}{n}$$

The population mean of the sample frequency p is

$$\mu_p = \pi \tag{3-8}$$

The population variance of the sample frequency p is

$$\sigma_p^2 = \frac{\pi(1-\pi)}{n} \tag{3-9}$$

The population standard deviation (the standard error of the sample frequency) is

$$\sigma_p = \sqrt{\frac{\pi(1-\pi)}{n}} \tag{3-10}$$

The standard deviation of the sample frequency p, is also called the standard error of the sample frequency, which can be used to describe the size of sampling error.

The population probability is usually unknown. At this time, if the sample data are used to calculate the sample frequency $p = X/n$ as an estimate of π, then the estimated value of σ_p is

$$S_p = \sqrt{\frac{p(1-p)}{n}} \tag{3-11}$$

In practice, when n large enough, sample frequency p not close to 0 and 1(satisfied np with $n(1-p)$ both are greater than 5), the sampling distribution of p is close to a normal distribution.

3.1.4. *Difference between two sample frequencies*

Two "successful" events X_1 and X_2, respectively follow the binomial distribution $B(n_1, \pi_1)$ and $B(n_2, \pi_2)$, the population mean of difference between two sample frequencies $p_1 - p_2$ is

$$\mu_{p_1-p_2} = \pi_1 - \pi_2 \tag{3-12}$$

1. $\pi_1 \neq \pi_2$

The population variance of $p_1 - p_2$ is

$$\sigma_{p_1-p_2}^2 = \frac{\pi_1(1-\pi_1)}{n_1} + \frac{\pi_2(1-\pi_2)}{n_2} \tag{3-13}$$

The standard deviation of $p_1 - p_2$ estimated using sample data is

$$S_{p_1-p_2} = \sqrt{\frac{p_1(1-p_1)}{n_1} + \frac{p_2(1-p_2)}{n_2}} \tag{3-14}$$

2. $\pi_1 = \pi_2 = \pi_c$
The population variance of $p_1 - p_2$ is

$$\sigma^2_{p_1-p_2} = \pi_c(1-\pi_c)\left(\frac{1}{n_1}+\frac{1}{n_2}\right) \tag{3-15}$$

The estimated value of π_c is

$$p_c = \frac{X_1 + X_2}{n_1 + n_2} \tag{3-16}$$

The estimated value of $\sigma_{p_1-p_2}$ is

$$S_{p_1-p_2} = \sqrt{p_c(1-p_c)\left(\frac{1}{n_1}+\frac{1}{n_2}\right)} \tag{3-17}$$

Whether π_1 and π_2 is equal or not, when n_1 and n_2 are large enough, p_1 and p_2 are not close to 0 and 1 (satisfied n_1p_1, $n_1(1-p_1)$ and $n_2(1-p_2)$, n_2p_2 are greater than 5). The sampling distribution of the difference between two sample frequencies $p_1 - p_2$ is close to a normal distribution.

3.2. *Z* Distribution and *t* distribution

In Chapter 2, common probability distributions such as normal distribution, binomial distribution, and Poisson distribution have been studied. Common sampling distributions are Z distribution (standard normal distribution), t distribution, F distribution, χ^2 distribution, etc., this chapter only introduces the Z distribution and the t distribution, the F distribution, and χ^2 distribution will be described in the later chapter.

3.2.1. *Z Distribution*

According to the central limit theorem, even if the population from which the sample statistic come does not follows normal distribution, when the sample size n is large enough, the sample mean is approximately following normal distribution. In Chapter 2 introduces a normal distribution, by the formula

$$Z = \frac{(X - \mu)}{\sigma}$$

The general normal distribution $N(\mu, \sigma^2)$ can be transformed to a standard normal distribution $N(0, 1)$.

Similarly, if the distribution of the simple mean $\bar{X}$ follows the general normal distribution $N(\mu, \sigma_{\bar{X}}^2)$ or $N(\mu, \sigma^2/n)$, then

$$\frac{\bar{X} - \mu}{\sigma/\sqrt{n}} \sim Z \text{ distribution} \tag{3-18}$$

3.2.2. *t Distribution*

The population standard deviation σ is usually unknown in actual research. If the population standard deviation is replaced by the sample standard deviation S, then

$$\frac{\bar{X} - \mu}{S/\sqrt{n}}$$

no longer follows Z distribution, but t distribution, denoted as

$$\frac{\bar{X} - \mu}{S/\sqrt{n}} \sim t(\nu)$$

The degree of freedom ν determines the shape of t distribution.

The British statistician Gosset published a paper under the pseudonym "Student" in 1908, proposing the theory of t distribution, so the t distribution is also called Student's t-distribution. The probability density function of the t distribution is

$$f(t) = \frac{\Gamma[(\nu+1)/2]}{\sqrt{\pi\nu}\Gamma(\nu/2)}\left(1 + \frac{t^2}{\nu}\right)^{-\frac{(\nu+1)}{2}} \quad -\infty < t < \infty$$

Where $\Gamma(\bullet)$ is a gamma function that we can calculate, $\pi \approx 3.1416$ is circular constant, ν is the degree of freedom. Taking t as abscissa, $f(t)$ as ordinate, the density curve of the t distribution can be drawn as Figure 3.3.

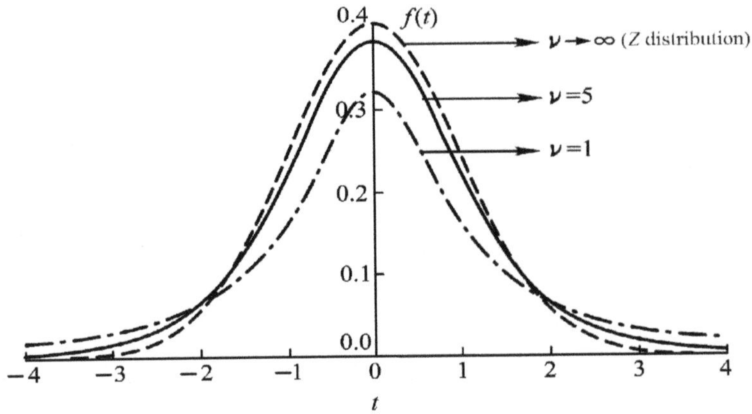

Figure 3.3 Probability density curve of t distribution with different degrees of freedom

As can be seen from Figure 3.3, for different degrees of freedom, the t distribution has different probability density curves, and its characteristics are as follows:

(1) The density curve of the t distribution is a single peak, the curve is highest at $t = 0$ and when $t = 0$ it is symmetrical about the center. The t value can be either a positive number or a negative number.
(2) Compared with the standard normal distribution, the highest point of the curve is shorter and the two tails are higher.
(3) The probability density curve of the t distribution is a cluster of curves whose morphological change is related to the degree of freedom. Once the degree of freedom is confirmed, the shape of the probability density curve is also fixed. The smaller the degree of freedom, the more dispersed the t value, the shorter and flatter the curve kurtosis and the higher the curve tail; as the degree of freedom increases, the t-distribution curve gradually approaches the standard normal distribution curve, and the limit distribution of the t-distribution is the Z-distribution (i.e., standard normal distribution).
(4) The area under the probability density curve of the t distribution has a certain regularity. For example, degrees of freedom $\nu = 9$,

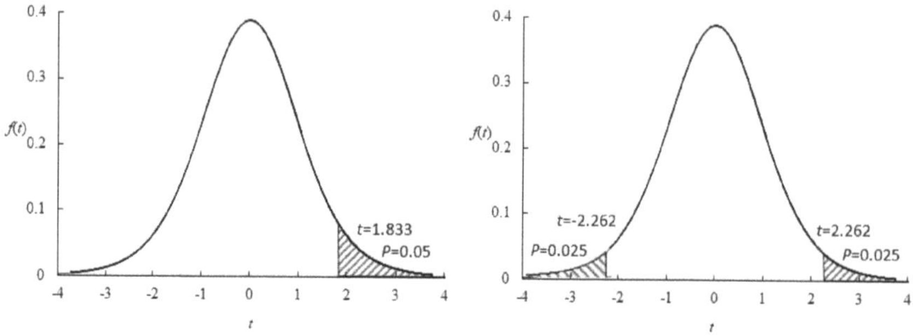

(a) (b)

Figure 3.4 When $\nu = 9$, area of the tail under the t distribution curve of one side (a) and two sides (b)

$t \leq -1.833$ or $t \geq 1.833$. The area under the curve (one side) is 0.05, see Figure 3.4(a); $t \leq -2.262$ and $t \geq 2.262$, the sum of the areas under the curve (both sides) is also 0.05 (0.025 for each of the left and right tail areas), see Figure 3.4(b).

Let α be a small probability determined in advance, by looking up t distribution critical table (Appendix C2), we can get the corresponding t critical values of one or two sides for different degrees of freedom, denoted as $t_{\alpha,\nu}$ or $t_{\alpha/2,\nu}$, respectively. α is the area under the curve where the sample statistic t is greater than or equal to $t_{\alpha,\nu}$, that is,

$$\alpha = P(t \geq t_{\alpha,\nu})$$

It is also equal to the area under the curve where absolute value of t is greater than or equal to $t_{\alpha,\nu}$, that is,

$$\alpha = P(|t| \geq t_{\alpha/2,\nu})$$

In Chapter 4, t distribution critical table (Appendix C2) is used to obtain an approximate P value corresponding to the test statistic t with the degree of freedom. The α and the P are both probability, which are the size of the tail area under the sampling distribution curve. But they are different, the α is a small probability determined in advance (usually, $\alpha = 0.05$), and the P value is the probability (random variable) corresponding to the sample statistic under the condition that the null hypothesis is established. The α is the maximum P value (constant) that is considered statistically significant, that is, the P value is less than or equal to α can be considered statistically significant.

3.3. Estimation of population parameters

According to the sampling distribution introduced above, statistical inference can be made for the corresponding population parameters (μ, π) of sample statistical $(\bar{X}, p)$. The statistical inference mainly includes two aspects: parameter estimation and hypothesis testing (significance testing). This chapter only describes the confidence interval (CI) estimates for the population parameters, and hypothesis testing will be described in the next chapter and later.

3.3.1. *Concept of confidence interval*

The parameter estimates have point estimate and interval estimate. The estimated value directly using the sample statistic as the population parameter is the point estimate, such as we use the sample mean $\bar{X}$ of the random sample directly as a point estimation value of the population mean μ. The point estimation method is simple, but it does not take into account the condition of sampling error, and the precision of the estimation is difficult to evaluate.

Interval estimations are interval ranges that contain unknown population parameters in terms of given $(1-\alpha)$, the range is called the CI of the parameter. $(1-\alpha)$ is called confidence level, it can also be expressed as $100(1-\alpha)\%$, usually 95% (also 90%, 99%). The CI is usually represented by two values, that is, the two confidence limits (CL). The smaller one is called the lower confidence limit (LCL), and the larger is called the upper confidence limit (UCL).

The practical meaning of the 95% CI for the population mean is that if 100 independent samples of the same sample size are repeatedly extracted from the same population, one CI is calculated for each sample, and in the 100 CIs, there will be approximately 95 CIs cover the population mean, and there are approximately 5 CIs that do not cover the population mean (see Figure 3.5). For a certain CI,

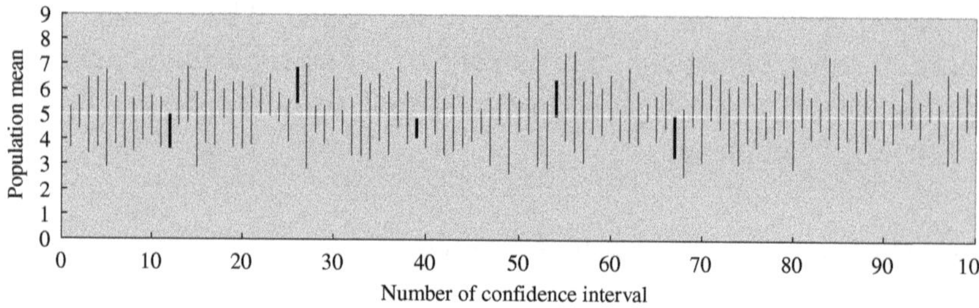

Figure 3.5 100 CIs obtained by random sampling from a normal population $N(5, 1)$

we always claim that this interval covers the population mean, but it does not completely cover the population mean. So, we add that the confidence level is 95%.

3.3.2. *Confidence interval for the population mean*

If the population standard deviation σ is known, or σ is unknown but the sample size is large enough, the CI for the population mean can be estimated by the standard normal distribution; If the population standard deviation σ is unknown, the sample standard deviation S replaces the population standard deviation σ, the CI for the population mean μ can be estimated by the t distribution.

3.3.2.1. *σ is known*

σ is known, under the general normal distribution curve, the range of CIs $(1-\alpha)$can be expressed as the middle portion of Figure 3.6.

The computing formula for two-sided $(1-\alpha)$ CI of the population mean is

$$\left(\bar{X} - Z_{\alpha/2}\sigma_{\bar{X}}, \bar{X} + Z_{\alpha/2}\sigma_{\bar{X}}\right) \tag{3-19}$$

Or abbreviated as

$$\bar{X} \pm Z_{\alpha/2}\sigma_{\bar{X}}$$

where $\bar{X}$ as the sample mean, $Z_{\alpha/2}$ is a critical value under the standard normal distribution curve for two sides, $\sigma_{\bar{X}} = \sigma/\sqrt{n}$, n is the sample size.

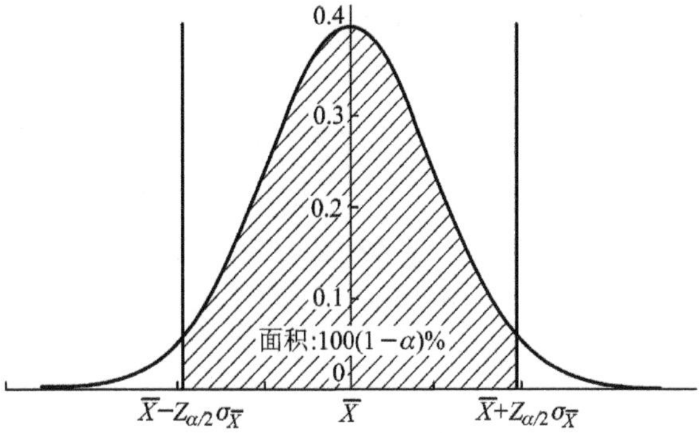

Figure 3.6 Two-sided $(1-\alpha)$ CI of the population mean

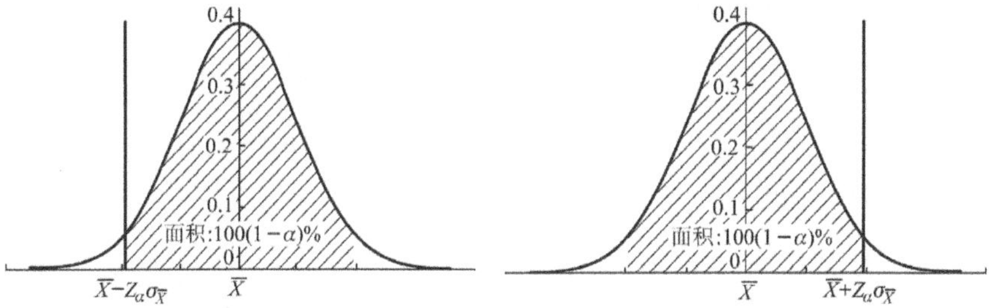

Figure 3.7 One-sided $(1-\alpha)$ CI of the population mean

Let $\alpha = 0.05$, $Z_{0.05/2} = 1.96$, the two-sided 95% CI for the population mean is

$$\left(\bar{X} - 1.96\sigma_{\bar{X}}, \bar{X} + 1.96\sigma_{\bar{X}}\right)$$

where $\sigma_{\bar{X}} = \sigma/\sqrt{n}$

σ is known, the one-sided $(1-\alpha)$ CIs of population mean can be represented as the left and right of Figure 3.7, respectively.

The computing formula for one-sided $(1-\alpha)$ CI of the population mean is

$$(\bar{X} - Z_\alpha\sigma_{\bar{X}}, +\infty) \text{ or } (-\infty, \bar{X} + Z_\alpha\sigma_{\bar{X}}) \tag{3-20}$$

where $\bar{X}$ as the sample mean, Z_α is a critical value under the standard normal distribution curve for right sided.

Let $\alpha = 0.05$, $Z_{0.05} = 1.645$, the one-sided 95% CI for the population mean is

$$(\bar{X} - 1.645\sigma_{\bar{X}}, +\infty) \text{ or } (-\infty, \bar{X} + 1.645\sigma_{\bar{X}})$$

where $\sigma_{\bar{X}} = \sigma/\sqrt{n}$. When σ is unknown but n is large enough (e.g., $n > 30$), using $S_{\bar{X}}$ replaces $\sigma_{\bar{X}}$ in formulas (3-19) and (3-20) obtain a CI for the population mean.

3.3.2.2. *σ is unknown*

When σ is unknown, the sample standard deviation S replaces σ, since $(\bar{X}-\mu)/(S/\sqrt{n})$ no longer follows the Z distribution, but follows the t distribution, the computing formula for the two-sided CI of the population mean should be modified to

$$(\bar{X} - t_{\alpha/2,\nu}S_{\bar{X}}, \bar{X} + t_{\alpha/2,\nu}S_{\bar{X}}) \qquad (3\text{-}21)$$

Or abbreviated as

$$\bar{X} \pm t_{\alpha/2,\nu}S_{\bar{X}}$$

Where $\bar{X}$ follow t distribution with $\nu = n - 1$, sample standard error $S_{\bar{X}} = S/\sqrt{n}$, $t_{\alpha/2,\nu}$ is a critical value at $\alpha/2$ area under the t-distribution curve for right sided. $t_{\alpha/2,\nu}S_{\bar{X}}$ can be called the precise of the CI, which is equal to half the width of the CI, which means how far the sample mean $\bar{X}$ is from two ends of the CI. The larger the sample size n is, the smaller the range of CI $t_{\alpha/2,\nu}S_{\bar{X}}$ is, the higher the precise (reliability) of the estimation.

σ is usually unknown, so the formula (3-12) is more commonly used than the formula (3-19).

When the population standard deviation σ is unknown, no matter whether the sample size n is large enough, the CI estimation of the population mean may be formulated (3-21), that is, the t-critical value of the t-distribution should be adopted instead of the critical value of the standard normal distribution (i.e., the Z distribution). In fact, if the population standard deviation σ is unknown, then the sampling distribution is t-distribution. Even if the sample size n is large enough, it is more exactly use the t-critical value to calculate the CI.

Example 3.1. The mean of red blood cells in 200 adult males randomly extracted was 5.00×10^{12}/L, and the standard deviation was 0.60×10^{12}/L. Please calculate the standard error of the sample mean and 95% CI for the population mean.

Solution: According to Equation (3.2), the standard error of the sample mean is

$$S_{\bar{X}} = \frac{S}{\sqrt{n}} = \frac{0.60}{\sqrt{200}} = 0.042_{(10^{12}/\mathrm{L})}$$

Because the population standard deviation is unknown, using Equation (3-21) calculate the 95% CI as follow:

$$5.00 \pm t_{0.05/2,199} S_{\bar{X}}$$

where $\nu = n - 1 = 200 - 1 = 199$, α take two-sided of 0.05, check the t critical table (Appendix Table C2),$t_{0.05/2,199} = 1.972$, $S_{\bar{X}} = 0.042$, the 95% CI for the adult male red blood cells is (3.916, 5.084) $(10^{12}/L)$.

Since the sample size is large enough, $n = 200$, so it is also possible to approximately calculate the CI using the formula (3-19). $Z_{0.05/2} = 1.96$ replace $t_{0.05/2,199} = 1.972$, and the 95% CI is (4.917, 5.083). The two intervals are very close, and the latter range is narrower, but the latter results are only approximate results.

σ is unknown. The one-sided $(1 - \alpha)$ CI of the population mean of μ is calculated as

$$(\bar{X} - t_{\alpha,\nu} S_{\bar{X}}, +\infty) \text{ or } (-\infty, \bar{X} + t_{\alpha,\nu} S_{\bar{X}}) \tag{3-22}$$

where $t_{\alpha,\nu}$ is the critical value corresponding to the right area under the t-distribution curve with a degree of freedom of ν.

3.3.3. *CIs for the difference between two population means*

Two-sided $(1-\alpha)$ CI of the difference between two population means $(\mu_1 - \mu_2)$ is

$$(\bar{X}_1 - \bar{X}_2) \pm t_{\alpha/2,\,\nu} S_{\bar{X}_1 - \bar{X}_2} \tag{3-23}$$

We can find $t_{\alpha/2,\nu}$ in Appendix C2.

When the two population variances are equal, $S_{\bar{X}_1-\bar{X}_2}$ can be calculated by the formulas (3-6) and (3-7). The degree of freedom is equal to the sum of the two sample degrees of freedom, that is,

$$\nu = (n_1 - 1) + (n_2 - 1) = n_1 + n_2 - 2 \tag{3-24}$$

When the two population variances are not equal, $S_{\bar{X}_1-\bar{X}_2}$ should be calculated using Equation (3-5). It must be noted that the t critical value $t_{\alpha/2,\nu}$ see Appendix Table C2. The formula for calculating the degree of freedom should be changed to

$$\nu = \frac{\left(S_1^2/n_1 + S_2^2/n^2\right)^2}{\frac{(S_1^2/n_1)^2}{n_1-1} + \frac{(S_2^2/n_2)^2}{n_2-1}} \tag{3-25}$$

Similarly, one-side $(1-\alpha)$ CI of the difference between the two populations is

$$\left((\bar{X}_1 - \bar{X}_2) - t_{\alpha,\nu}S_{\bar{X}_1-\bar{X}_2}, +\infty\right) \text{ or } \left(-\infty, (\bar{X}_1 - \bar{X}_2) + t_{\alpha,\nu}S_{\bar{X}_1-\bar{X}_2}\right) \tag{3-26}$$

When the sample sizes of two samples are large (such as n_1 and n_2 are larger than 30), the CI can be calculated using the above formulas (3-23) and (3-26), $t_{\alpha/2,\nu}$ and $t_{\alpha,\nu}$ replaced by $Z_{\alpha/2}$ and Z_α.

Example 3.2. To understand the effect of methotrexate on peripheral blood IL-2 levels, a doctor randomly divided 61 asthma patients into two groups, 30 cases in the control (placebo) group (n_1), 31 patients in the experimental (small doses of methotrexate) group (n_2). The mean of IL-2 in the control group was 20.00 IU/mL ($\bar{X}_1$), the standard deviation is 8.00 IU/mL (S_1); The mean of IL-2 in the treatment group was 16.00 IU/mL ($\bar{X}_2$), the standard deviation is 7.50 IU/mL (S_2). Is there a statistically significant difference between the two population means?

Solution: Let the variances of two groups equal, calculate the combined variance according to formula (3-7).

$$S_c^2 = \frac{(30-1)\times 8.00^2 + (31-1)\times 7.50^2}{30+31-2} = 60.0593$$

According to formula (3-6), then

$$S_{\bar{X}_1-\bar{X}_2} = \sqrt{60.0593\left(\frac{1}{30}+\frac{1}{31}\right)} = 1.9848$$

Let $\alpha = 0.05$, $\nu = n_1 + n_2 - 2 = 30 + 31 - 2 = 59$, according to $\nu = 60$ in the t critical table (because there is not $\nu = 59$ in Appendix Table C2, $\nu = 60$ only used instead), $t_{0.05/2,60} = 2.000$. Then calculate the two-sided 95% CI of the difference $\mu_1 - \mu_2$ between the two population means according to formula (3-23), there is $(20.00 - 16.00) \pm 2.000 \times 1.9848$ (0.0304, 7.9696) (IU/mL). The lower limit of the interval is larger than 0, that is, the interval is not included $\mu_1 - \mu_2 = 0$. The difference of peripheral blood IL-2 between the treatment group and the control group was statistically significant at $\alpha = 0.05$. It can be considered that methotrexate had an effect on peripheral blood IL-2 level.

3.3.4. *Confidence interval for population probability*

Based on the sample frequency, point estimates and interval estimates of population probability also can be made. We can use the sample frequency p to estimate the population probability π. Similar to the point estimate of the population mean, the point estimate of the population probability does not take into account the size of the sampling error, and the interval estimate of the population probability overcomes the shortcomings of the point estimate.

Using the sample data to estimate $1-\alpha$ CI of the population probability, which follow the binomial distribution. Let $\alpha = 0.05$ or 0.01, for $n \leq 50$ and p is close to 0 or 1, you can directly find the $(1-\alpha)$ CI of the population probability in Appendix Table C3 (according to the binomial distribution probability introduced in Chapter 2, the CI of the population probability can be obtained).

Example 3.3. From April to June 2003, a hospital ICU admitted 38 patients with severe SARS, including 12 deaths, Please calculate a CI for the population probability of SARS death.

Solution: Check Appendix Table C3, $n = 38$, $k = 12$, $n - k = 26$, at the cross point of k and n, obtaining the 95% CI for SARS mortality is 18% to 49% $(1 - \alpha = 0.95)$, 99% CI is $14\% \sim 54\%(1 - \alpha = 0.99)$.

When n is larger enough, sample frequency p and $1 - p$ not too small (such as np and $n(1 - P)$ more than 5), the $1 - \alpha$ CI of population probability of sample frequency p can be calculated assumed p follow approximately normal distribution.

$$(p - Z_{\alpha/2}S_p, p + Z_{\alpha/2}S_p) \tag{3-27}$$

When $\alpha = 0.05$, $Z_{0.05/2} = 1.96$, the calculation of S_p see formula (3-11).

Example 3.4. A CDC conducted anemia test on 200 primary school students in a township in 2006. There were 80 anemia patients and a detection rate of 40%, Please calculate 95% CI of the population detection rate of anemia.

Solution: In this case, $n = 200$ is relatively large, $p = 0.40$, $np = 80$ and $n(1-p) = 120$, both are larger than 5, so the CI of the population probability can be estimated using Equation (3-27).

$$p \pm Z_{\alpha/2}S_p = p \pm Z_{0.05/2}\sqrt{\frac{p(1-p)}{n}}$$

$$= 0.400 \pm 1.96\sqrt{\frac{0.400(1 - 0.400)}{200}} = (0.332, 0.468)$$

That is, the 95% CI for the detection rate of anemia in primary school students in a township is (33.2%, 46.8%).

3.3.5. *Confidence interval for the difference between the two population probabilities*

Let the two sample frequencies be p_1 and p_2, when n_1 versus n_2 are larger enough, p_1, $1 - p_1$ and p_2, $1 - p_2$ are not too small, for example, both n_1p_1, $n_1(1 - p_1)$ and n_2p_2, $n_2(1 - p_2)$ are greater than 5, the two sample frequencies can be approximated to the normal distribution, and the two sample frequency differences also follow the normal distribution. The normal approximation method is used

Table 3.3 The effective rate of a drug in the treatment of dentine hypersensitivity

Groups	Total teeth	n of effective	Effective rate (%)
Experimental	80	60	75.0
Control	70	40	57.1

to calculate the $(1-\alpha)$ CI of the differences of the two population probability,

$$\left[(p_1 - p_2) - Z_{\alpha/2}S_{p_1-p_2}, (p_1 - p_2) + Z_{\alpha/2}S_{p_1-p_2}\right] \tag{3-28}$$

where the calculation of $S_{p_1-p_2}$ see formula (3-14) or formula (3-17).

Example 3.5. A hospital dentist treats dentin hypersensitivity with a drug, using a double-fluorine coating as a control. After 1 year follow-up observation, the results shown in Table 3.3. Try to estimate the 95% CI of the differences of the two population effective rate $(\pi_2 - \pi_1)$.

Solution: $n_1 = 80, X_1 = 60, p_1 = 75.0\%; n_2 = 70, X_2 = 40, p_2 = 57.1\%$

(1) Because the effective rate difference between the two groups is large, the standard error of the difference between the two effective rates is calculated by formula (3-14),

$$S_{p_1-p_2} = \sqrt{\frac{p_1(1-p_1)}{n_1} + \frac{p_2(1-p_2)}{n_2}}$$

$$= \sqrt{\frac{60/80(1-60/80)}{80} + \frac{40/70(1-40/70)}{70}} = 0.076$$

(2) Calculate the 95% CI of the differences of two population effective rate using Equation (3-28)

$$(p_1 - p_2) \pm Z_{\alpha/2}S_{p_1-p_2} = (0.750 - 0.571) \pm 1.96 \times 0.076$$
$$= (0.029, 0.328) = (2.9\%, 32.8\%)$$

(3) Inference the lower limit of the interval is greater than 0, that is, the interval not includes $\pi_1 - \pi_2 = 0$, so the two population effective rate are different, that is, $\pi_1 \neq \pi_2$, combined with the sample frequency, the drug can be considered effective.

3.4. Report writing

This chapter is the basis of the following chapters. In addition to the CI for the population mean and the population probability, it is necessary to give a report of the CI of the regression coefficients, correlation coefficients, etc. The result reporting method of the CI is described by Example 3.2.

The results show that the mean ± SD of IL-2 for the experimental group ($n = 31$) was 16.00 IU/mL ± 7.50 IU/mL and for the control group ($n = 30$) was 20.00 IU/mL ± 8.00 IU/mL; the difference between the two groups was 4.00 IU/mL, and the 95% CI of the two population means was (0.0304, 7.9696) (IU/mL)

The results report has several points worth noting:

1. 95% CI is 95% CI, 95% is confidence level, other confidence levels (e.g., 90%, 99%) can be selected;
2. The mean difference (4.00 IU/mL) between the two groups is the point estimate of the population parameter;
3. If the range of CI is wider, it means the precision of the parameter estimation is lower, and vice versa;
4. When 95% CI does not include the population parameters, then $\alpha = 0.05$, the result is statistically significant. Specifically, in Example 3.2, if 95% CI corresponding to the difference between the two groups does not include 0 (the two population parameters are equal, the difference is 0), the difference between the two groups is statistically significant. The 95% CI of the odds ratio, the relative risk does not include 1 (when the two population parameters are equal, the odds ratio, the relative risk is 1), indicating that the results are statistically significant (see the following relevant chapters for details).

3.5. Case discrimination

Case 3.1 A researcher measured the urine lead content (mg/L) of 120 normal adults in an area as follows:

Urinary lead content	0~	4~	8~	12~	16~	20~	24~	28~	32~	36~	Total
Number of cases	14	22	29	18	15	10	6	3	2	1	120

Please using the data estimate the CI and the reference range for normal adult urine lead levels.

We can see the data from the table. $n = 120, S = 8.0031, S_{\bar{X}} = 0.7306$, an author takes the data into the formula (3.20), that is, using $\bar{X} + Z_\alpha S_{\bar{X}}$ to calculate $(1-\alpha)$ CI of the urine lead content of normal adults are $(-\infty, 14.0684)$; using $\bar{X}+Z_\alpha S$ to calculate $(1-\alpha)$ reference range of urine lead content of normal adults are $(-\infty, 26.0306)$. Is this appropriate? Why? What should we do?

Case 3.2 In the study of the efficacy of BiPAP ventilator in the treatment of chronic obstructive pulmonary disease, in order to describe whether some factors are balanced before the test, the authors list the results of blood gas analysis of patients in Table 3.4. Because the author feels that the standard deviation of his data is large, almost as large as the mean, it is unsightly to put the standard deviation in the text, so he uses "mean ± standard error" $(\bar{X} \pm S_{\bar{X}})$ instead of "mean ± standard deviation" $(\bar{X} \pm S)$ to describe the data. Is the report correctly in Table 3.4? Why?

Table 3.4 Blood gas analysis results in the experimental group and the control group before treatment $(\bar{X} \pm S_{\bar{X}})$

Group	Number of cases	Age (year)	pH	$PaCO_2$ (kPa)	PaO_2 (kPa)	SaO_2 (%)
Experimental	12	63.00 ± 4.33	7.36 ± 0.05	63.00 ± 4.33	9.25 ± 0.55	85.12 ± 1.73
Control	10	62.50 ± 3.95	7.38 ± 0.06	63.00 ± 4.33	9.16 ± 0.62	86.45 ± 2.25

Case 3.3 The average height of 12-year-old boy in a city is 140.00 cm in the past. Now, select randomly 120 cases as subjects from the 12-year-old boy in the city, the average height is 143.05 cm, and the standard deviation is 6.25 cm. Please estimate the 95% CI of the population mean for corresponding sample and determine whether the mean is different from previous years.

The answer of a student is as follows: "The point estimate value of average height of the 12-year-old boy is 143.05 cm. The 95% CI for the point estimated value is 141.92 $\sim$ 144.18 cm according to formula (3-21). Because the average height of the 12 years old boy is 140.00 cm, which does not fall within the range of 95% CI, so it can be considered that the average height of the boys of today is different from the past."

Please indicate the inadequacies in the student's response and give a correct statement.

3.6. Computer experiments

Experiment 3.1 Calculate confidence interval of Example 3.1 with SPSS

Data file: None (In order to avoid the computer prompt "Open Data File ...", we should enter a number in the SPSS data editing window).

Experiment 3.2 Calculate confidence interval of Example 4.2 in Chapter 4 with SPSS

Using **Data file:** data3-1.sav, we can obtain that the 95% CI of population mean is (20.27, 21.70).

Experiment 3.3 Using SPSS to calculate the confidence interval for the difference between the mean of the two samples

Data file: None. using Analyze ——> Compare Means ——> Independent-Samples T Test ..., Conduct independent sample t-test or using Analyze ——> Compare Means ——> Paired-Samples T Test ..., Conduct paired sample t-test. We can obtain the confidence interval of the difference between the means. See the "Comparative Mean of Two Groups" of computer experiment in Chapter 5.

Experiment 3.4 Demonstrating t distribution and Z distribution with Excel

Using **Data file:** program3-4.xls, understand the meaning of the t distribution, and grasp the relationship between the t distribution and the Z distribution.

Experiment 3.5 Demonstrate the concept of confidence interval with Excel

Using **Data file:** program3-5.xls, understand the meaning of the 95% CI.

3.7. Frequently asked questions and summary

3.7.1. *Frequently asked questions*

1. What is the accuracy and precision of the CI?

CIs have two elements of accuracy and precision. The accuracy is determined by the confidence level $(1 - \alpha)$, that is, the confidence degree of "this interval contains the population parameters" is $(1-\alpha)$. From the perspective of accuracy, the closer the confidence level is to 1, the better the accuracy is, for example, the 99% confidence level is better than 95%; the precision is half the width of the CI (i.e., $t_{\alpha/2,\nu}S_{\bar{X}}$, $Z_{\alpha/2,\nu}S_p$), meaning the distance of sample statistic (e.g., $\bar{X}$, p) and the two ends of the CI. From the perspective of precision, the narrower the CI is, the better the precision is. When the sampling error is determined, the two are contradictory. If the confidence level increases, that is, α is reduced, then the critical value of test statistic (e.g., $t_{\alpha/2,\nu}$, $Z_{\alpha/2}$) may increase, the CI will wide, resulting in a decrease in precision; conversely, lowering the confidence level, that is, reducing the accuracy, can appropriately increase the precision of the CI. In order to balance the accuracy and precision of the CI, the sample size can be appropriately increased. When the confidence level is determined, increasing the sample size can reduce the sampling error, thereby narrowing the range of CI and improving the precision of parameter estimation.

2. What is the difference between the CI and the reference range?

The CI of the population mean and the reference range of the individual values are different in meaning, purpose, and computing formula. In actual application, the two cannot be confused. See Table 3.5 for details.

Table 3.5 Differences between confidence interval and reference range

	Confidence interval	Reference range
1. Meaning	The estimate may contain a range of unknown population parameters. The degree of confidence in the range including the population parameters is $(1-\alpha)$	The fluctuation range of individual value. That is to say, the fluctuation range of anatomical, physiological and biochemical indicators of "normal people" determined according to the range $(1-\alpha)$ given in advance
2. Category	Statistical inference	Statistical description
3. Purpose	Estimate the range of unknown population parameters	It can be used as a reference for judging whether an individual's index is "normal"
4. Computing formula[a]	Normal distribution, σ is unknown: $\bar{X} \pm t_{\alpha/2,\nu} S_{\bar{X}}$ Non-normal distribution, but $n \geq 30$, there is $\bar{X} \pm Z_{\alpha/2}\sigma_{\bar{X}}$ or $\bar{X} \pm Z_{\alpha/2} S_{\bar{X}}$	Normal distribution: $\bar{X} \pm Z_{\alpha/2} S$ Non-normal distribution: $(\mathrm{p}_{100\alpha/2}, \mathrm{p}_{100(1-\alpha/2)})$

[a]This is just a two-sided computing formula. The computing formula for one-sided see next chapters detailed.

3. What is the difference and connection between standard deviation and standard error?

The standard deviation reflects the degree of dispersion of individual values around the mean, that is, reflects the difference between individual values. The standard errors described in this chapter reflect the extent to which sample statistics (such as sample mean) are spread around population parameters such as population mean.

According to formula (3.1), the standard error is less than the standard deviation; the larger the sample size, the smaller the standard error; but the standard deviation does not change significantly with the change of sample size. As the sample size increases, the standard deviation may increase or decrease. If reflect the degree of variation of the individual, the standard deviation should be used; if reflect the precision of the estimation of the population parameters by the sample statistic, a standard error or a 95% CI should be used. The difference and connection can be summarized in Table 3.6.

4. If the sample comes from a finite population, how do you make statistical inferences?

As mentioned above, statistical inference is based on an infinite population. If the population from which the sample is derived is a finite population (e.g., the sample size n is greater than 5% of the population size N), then the former standard error calculating formula should be modified appropriately, such as the calculating formula (3.1) of the standard error of mean should be changed to

$$\sigma_{\bar{X}} = \frac{\sigma}{\sqrt{n}}\sqrt{\frac{N-n}{N-1}} \tag{3-29}$$

The calculating formula (3-10) of the standard error of sample frequency should be changed to

$$\sigma_p = \sqrt{\frac{\pi(1-\pi)}{n}}\sqrt{\frac{N-n}{N-1}} \tag{3-30}$$

Table 3.6 The difference and connection between standard deviation and standard error

		Standard deviation	Standard error of sample mean
1. Difference	(1) Meaning	Describe the degree of variation in individual values. The smaller the standard deviation (large), the smaller the variation (or dispersion) of individual values (large)	Reflects the precision of the population parameter estimated and measures the magnitude of the sampling error. The smaller (larger) the standard error is, the higher (lower) the precision of the population mean estimated by the sample mean
	(2) Category	Statistical description indicator	Statistical inference indicator
	(3) Purpose (assuming following normal distribution)	Combining with the mean, describe the distribution range of individual values, often used in the estimation of medical reference ranges	Combining with the mean, at a certain confidence level, estimate a range values of covering or including the population mean, i.e., the confidence interval
	(4) Relationship with n	The larger n is, the more robust standard deviation becomes	The larger n is, the smaller the standard error is
2. Connection	(1) Standard error is proportional to the standard deviation (2) When n is certain, the larger the standard deviation, the larger the standard error		

Where N is the population size, $(N - n)/(N - 1)$ is called a finite population correction factor. When the sample size n is close to the finite population size N, $(N - n)/(N - 1)$ is close to 0, the corresponding standard error is also close to 0. In most cases, the target population is a finite population, if the population size N related to the sample size n is very large, the finite population correction factor is very close to 1, so this can usually be ignored. Only when the sample size n is less than 5% times the population size N, the above calculating formula (3.29) or (3.30) is used.

3.7.2. *Summary*

1. From the same population, the same sample sizes are sampled randomly, one sample statistic can be calculated from each sample repeatedly extracted, and the distribution of sample statistic is the sampling distribution. This chapter focuses on the Z distribution and t distribution.
2. The standard deviation corresponding to sample statistics is usually called standard error. Standard error reflects the size of sampling error, that is, the precision of estimation of the population parameter.
3. The standard error is inversely proportional to the square root of the sample size. The larger the sample size is, the smaller the sampling error is.
4. Statistical inference is based on the sampling distribution law, using sample statistics to make inferences about uncertainty of the corresponding population parameters, mainly including parameter estimation and hypothesis test. There are two kinds of parameter estimation: point estimation and interval estimation. Interval estimation is based on the confidence level $(1-\alpha)$ given in advance, to estimate a range of unknown population parameter, which is called the $(1 - \alpha)$ CI of the population parameter.
5. This chapter focuses on the CI estimation of the population mean, the difference between the two population means, the population probability, and the difference between the two population probabilities.

Think and Practice

I. Best Choice

1. Regarding the 0-centered t distribution, the wrong choice is ( ).
A. The graph of the probability density function of t distribution is a cluster of curves B. The graph of the probability density function of t distribution is a unimodal distribution C. When $\nu \to \infty$, t distribution $\to$ Z distribution D. The graph of the probability density function of t distribution is symmetric from left to right with 0 as its center E. When the ν is the same, the larger $|t|$ is, the larger the p value is
2. The mean of an indicator is $\bar{X}$, the standard deviation is S, the interval obtained by the formula $(\bar{X} - 1.96S, \bar{X} + 1.96S)$ is often called ( ).
A. 99% reference range B. 95% reference range C. 99% CI D. 95% CI E. 90% CI
3. A sample frequency p and population probability π are both known, the formula for calculating the sampling error of the sample frequency p is ( ).
A. $\sqrt{\frac{p(1-p)}{n}}$ B. $\sqrt{\frac{p(1-p)}{n-1}}$ C. $\sqrt{\frac{\pi(1-\pi)}{n}}$ D. $\sqrt{\frac{\pi(1-\pi)}{n-1}}$
E. $\sqrt{\frac{\pi(1-\pi)}{n-2}}$
4. Random sampling in the normal population with the known mean is μ, the standard deviation is σ, the probability of $|\bar{X} - \mu| >$ ( ) is 5%.
A. 1.96σ B. $1.96\sigma_{\bar{X}}$ C. $t_{0.05/2,\nu}S$ D. $t_{0.05/2,\nu}S_{\bar{X}}$
E. $t_{0.05/2,\nu}\sigma_{\bar{X}}$
5. The smaller (**C**) is, the more precision the sample estimation of population mean is.
A. CV B. S C. $\sigma_{\bar{X}}$ D. R E. Interquartile range
6. The meaning of the 95% CI is: ( )
A. The probability that this interval contains the population parameter is 95% B. The likelihood that this interval contains the population parameter is 95% C. "This interval contains the

population parameter" is 95% confidence level D. The probability that this interval contains sample statistic is 95% E. The likelihood that this interval contains sample statistic is 95%

II. Questions

1. Briefly describe the difference between standard error and standard deviation.
2. What is the central limit theorem of sampling distribution?
3. Briefly describe the difference between the CI and the range of medical reference values.
4. What is the accuracy and precision of the CI? How to coordinate the relationship between them.

III. Questions on Calculation

1. 100 first-year college students were randomly selected. The mean of fasting blood glucose was 4.5 mmol/L, and the standard deviation was 0.61 mmol/L. Try to estimate the 95% CI for the population mean of fasting blood glucose in first-year college students.
2. To investigate the enterobiasis infection in an area, among 260 cases randomly sampled, the number of infected cases is 100. Try to estimate the 95% CI for the enterobiasis infection rate.

Chuanhua Yu, Yiran Cui

CHAPTER 4

HYPOTHESIS TESTING

The confidence interval estimation introduced in Chapter 3 is to estimate the range of population parameters (such as μ or π) based on the sampling distribution of sample statistics (such as $\bar{X}$ or P). However, hypothesis testing and interval estimation are on different perspectives in statistical inference. This chapter will discuss the statistical inference of hypothesis testing through Example 4.1.

Example 4.1. In general, the mean and standard deviation of heart rate among middle school boys are 75 and 5.0 times/min (obtained from a large-scale survey), respectively. In our sample survey, we selected 100 boys who exercised regularly from a middle school. The mean of heart rate was 65 times/min. Is the heart rate of middle school boys who exercised regularly different from general middle school boys?

Solution: This example is to compare the mean of heart rate among middle school boys who exercise regularly (μ) with that of general middle school boys (μ_0); we consider a test with the null hypothesis $\mu = \mu_0$. In this case, the 100 middle school boys who exercise regularly were a sample. The reasons why the sample mean $\bar{X} = 65$ times/min differs from the given mean $\mu_0 = 75$ times/min may be (1) the heart rate among middle school boys who exercise regularly is equal to that of general middle school boys but there exists a sampling error, or (2) the heart rate of middle school boys who exercise regularly is really different from that of general middle school boys. So, we need to test whether μ is equal to μ_0 or not?

We can solve such problems by hypothesis testing. First, set up the null hypothesis: $\mu = \mu_0$, that is, the sample mean is equal to the given population mean. Then, check whether the sample data support such a null hypothesis or not and then decide either to accept or reject the null hypothesis based on the sampling distribution of sample statistics.

4.1. Steps of hypothesis testing

The basic steps of hypothesis testing are demonstrated as below with the example whether the population mean μ corresponding to the sample mean $\bar{X}$ is equal to a given population mean μ_0 or not. Generally, there are three steps:

1. Set up the statistical hypothesis and a significance level

We set up null hypothesis $H_0 : \mu = \mu_0$, that is, the two population means are equivalent and alternative hypothesis $H_1 : \mu \neq \mu_0$ (two-tailed that includes $\mu < \mu_0$ and $\mu > \mu_0$), where the difference between $\bar{X}$ and μ_0 is not only from the sampling error, but also from the actual difference between two population means.

Let the significance level $\alpha = 0.05$.

According to the professional knowledge and data characteristics, the alternative hypothesis H_1 can also be expressed as:

$$H_1\colon \mu < \mu_0, \text{ one-tailed test}$$

$$H_1\colon \mu > \mu_0, \text{ one-tailed test}$$

The choice of a one-tailed test or two-tailed test depends on the professional knowledge and data characteristics. When testing the difference in the effects of two methods (A and B), no matter which one is better, the two-tailed test is appropriate. When it is known that the effect of method A is better than or equal to that of method B, then one-tailed test should be selected. When no specific professional knowledge is listed, we choose the two-tailed test.

2. Select test methods and calculate test statistics
Based on the data type and purpose of analysis, determine the appropriate test statistics. For example, to compare the difference between the means of two samples, Z statistic is used when the population variance is known, and t statistic is used when it is unknown.

3. Statistical inference based on the values of test statistics
There are two methods to calculate P values:

(1) When statistical software (such as SPSS, SAS) is used for hypothesis testing, the exact P value can be calculated.

If $P \leq \alpha$, the conclusion is: reject H_0 and accept H_1 with the significance level α. The difference between the two means has statistical significance.

If $P > \alpha$, the conclusion is: do not reject H_0 with the significance level α. The difference between the two means has no statistical significance, that is, there is no enough evidence to reject H_0.

(2) Traditional method to calculate the P value: With a preset significance level α and given degree of freedom, find out the corresponding critical value (such as $Z_{\alpha/2}, t_{\alpha/2,v}$, etc.) of the sampling distribution (such as standard normal distribution, t distribution) which is listed in textbook and compare the critical value with the test statistic.

If the absolute value of the statistic is greater than or equal to the critical value, then we conclude $P \leq \alpha$ and reject H_0, accept H_1. There is a statistically significant difference.

If the absolute value of the statistic is less than the critical value, then we conclude $P > \alpha$ and not reject H_0. There is no statistically significant difference, that is, there is no enough evidence to reject H_0.

In the past, with few computers, the second method was often used for statistical inference. Now in a computer era, the first method is widely used for statistical inference. We can choose one of the two methods in practice.

Finally, make a professional conclusion based on the results of statistical inference and professional knowledge.

4.2. The hypothesis testing for one sample

When the standard deviation of population σ is known, use Z-test. When the standard deviation of population σ is unknown, use t-test; σ is replaced by the sample standard deviation S when H_0 is true and the statistic follows a t distribution.

4.2.1. *The Z-test for one sample mean*

When the standard deviation of population is known, choose one-sample Z-test to determine whether the population mean μ differs from a given population mean μ_0.

The Z-test is performed in the previous Example 4.1 as follows.

Solution: A two-tailed test is applied in this example according to the idea of hypothesis testing. The population mean of heart rate among middle school boys who exercise regularly is denoted by μ.

(1) Set up the statistical hypotheses and determine the significance level

H_0: The population mean of heart rate among middle school boys who exercise regularly is equal to that of general middle school boys. $\mu = \mu_0$.

H_1: The population mean of heart rate among middle school boys who exercise regularly is different from that of general middle school boys. $\mu \neq \mu_0$.

Let $\alpha = 0.05$

(2) Calculate the test statistic

When H_0 is true, the statistic Z follows the standard normal distribution.

$$Z = \frac{\bar{X} - \mu_0}{\sigma/\sqrt{n}} \tag{4-1}$$

In this example, $\bar{X} = 65$ times/min, $\mu_0 = 75$ times/min, the standard deviation $\sigma = 5.0$ times/min and the sample size $n = 100$.

(3) Determine the P value and make a conclusion
By checking the critical value table for Z-test (the row where v is ∞ in the t critical value table in Schedule 2), we know that $P < 0.001$. Compared with the significance level $\alpha = 0.05$, we reject H_0 and accept H_1. Hence, we consider that the difference between $\bar{X}$ and μ_0 is statistically significant. The 95% confidence interval of the population mean is $\bar{X} \pm 1.96\sigma_{\bar{X}} = 65 \pm 1.96 \times 5/\sqrt{100} = 64.02 \sim 65.98$ times/min. Because the upper limit of the 95% CI is less than 75 times/min (μ_0), we can conclude that the population mean of heart rate among middle school boys who exercise regularly is less than that of general middle school boys. The professional conclusion is that exercises help middle school boys improve their cardiac function.

4.2.2. *The t-test for one sample mean*

Generally, the standard deviation of population σ is unknown. If it is replaced by the sample standard deviation (S) in (4.1), the statistic in (4.1) will not follow a standard normal distribution but a t distribution. In order to test whether the population mean μ is different from a given population mean μ_0, a one-sample t-test should be used.

Example 4.2. When 100 mg drug is dissolved in 1 L of solvent, the standard concentration is 20.00 mg/L. A specific measurement method is used for the dissolution experiment, which is repeated 11 times. 100 mg of drug was dissolved in 1 L of solvent in each experiment, and the results were as follows: 20.99, 20.41, 20.10, 20.00, 20.91, 22.41, 20.00, 23.00, 22.00, 19.89, and 21.11. Is the sample mean of concentration of the drug measured by this method equal to the standard concentration?

Solution: The standard concentration $\mu_0 = 20.00$ mg/L and the sample size $n = 11$ are known. Then we can get the sample mean of concentration $\bar{X} = 20.98$ mg/L and standard deviation $S = 1.068$ mg/L.

(1) Set up the statistical hypotheses and determine the significance level

H_0: The population mean of concentration of the drug measured by this method is equal to the standard concentration. $\mu = \mu_0$.
H_1: The population mean of concentration of the drug measured by this method is different from the standard concentration. $\mu \neq \mu_0$.

Let $\alpha = 0.05$.

(2) Select test methods and calculate test statistics

Because the standard deviation of population σ is unknown, one-sample t-test is used. The statistic is

$$t = \frac{\bar{X} - \mu_0}{S/\sqrt{n}} \tag{4-2}$$

When H_0 is true, the statistic follows the t distribution with the degree of freedom $\upsilon = n - 1$.

In this example,

$$t = \frac{20.98 - 20.00}{1.068/\sqrt{11}} = 3.056, \quad \nu = 11 - 1 = 10$$

(3) Determine the P value and conclusion

By checking up the critical value table for t-test (in Schedule C2), we know that $0.01 < P < 0.02$. Compared with the significance level $\alpha = 0.05$, we reject H_0 and accept H_1, indicating that there is a statistically significant difference. The difference between the sample mean and the population mean is 0.98 mg/L. The 95% *CI* of the population mean is $\bar{X} \pm t_{0.05/2,\upsilon}\, S_{\bar{X}} = 20.98 \pm 2.2228 \times 1.068/\sqrt{11} = 20.26 \sim 21.70$ mg/L. Because the lower limit of 95% *CI* is higher than the standard concentration (20.00 mg/L), we conclude that the population mean of concentration of the drug measured by this method is higher than the standard concentration. The professional conclusion is that the measuring method is not accurate because the mean of concentration of the drug is higher than the standard concentration.

When the sample size is large enough, that is, the degree of freedom is large enough, $t_{\alpha/2,v} \approx Z_{\alpha/2}$; for example, $t_{0.05/2,100} = 1.98 \approx Z_{0.05/2} = 1.96$, and then the critical value of the standard normal distribution can be used approximately.

The above is a two-tailed test. If the population mean of concentration measured by the method is no less than the standard concentration such as in Example 4.2, then a one-tailed test should be used. The alternative hypothesis is H_1: $\mu > \mu_0$; whereas the alternative hypothesis is H_1: $\mu < \mu_0$.

Note: The significance of P value and test statistic t for one-tailed t test

When H_0 is true, the statistic following the t distribution with the degree of freedom $\nu = 10$ and the significance of P value for one-tailed test are shown in Figure 4.1.

By checking up the critical value table for t-test (in Schedule C2), we can get the one-tailed critical values of t distribution are $t_{0.01,10} = 2.764$ and $t_{0.005,10} = 3.169$. The absolute value of sample statistic t is 3.056 and $t_{0.01,10} < t < t_{0.005,10}$. Thus, we get $0.005 < P < 0.01$ and reject H_0, accept H_1, indicating that the difference is statistically significant. The professional conclusion is that the population mean

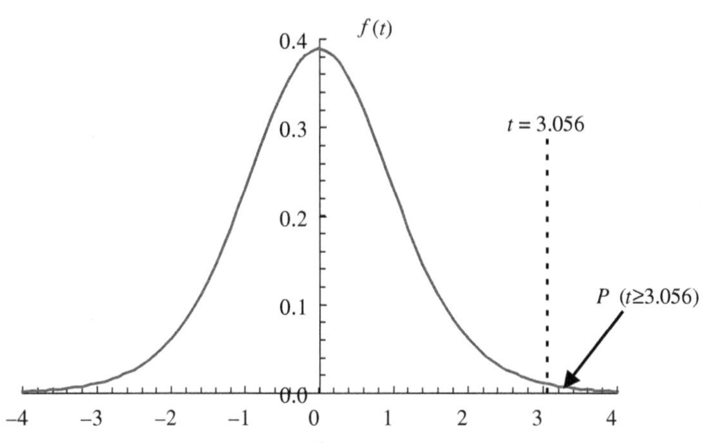

Figure 4.1 The significance of the test statistic t and P value for one-tailed test

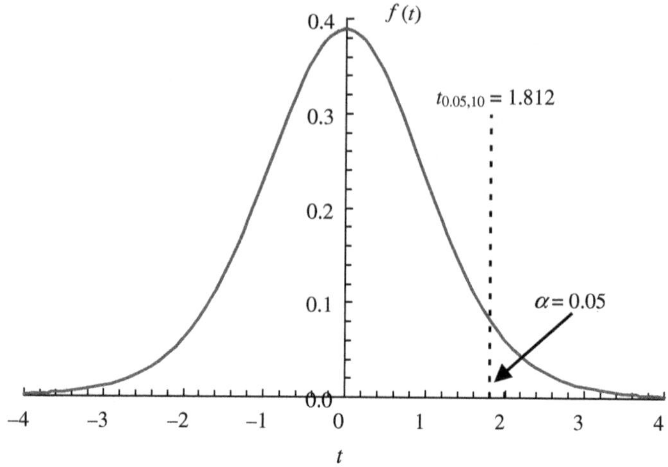

Figure 4.2 The significance of one-sided critical value t and α

of concentration measured by this method is higher than the standard concentration.

When H_0 is true, the one-tailed critical value of t statistic following the t distribution with the degree of freedom $\nu = 10$ and the significance of α are shown in Figure 4.2. The significance level in this example is 0.05. It is a one-tailed test and $H_1 : \mu > \mu_0$, hence the area under the t distribution curve and with statistic t greater than or equal to (i.e., on the right side of) the critical value is 0.05.

4.2.3. *Hypothesis testing for probability of one sample*

If a random variable X follows the binomial distribution $X \sim B(n, \pi)$, the cumulative probability function can be calculated as follows:

$$P(X \leq k) = \sum_{X=0}^{k} P(X) = \sum_{X=0}^{k} \frac{n!}{X!(n-X)!}\pi^X(1-\pi)^{n-X} \tag{4-3}$$

or

$$P(X \geq k) = \sum_{X=k}^{n} P(X) = \sum_{X=k}^{n} \frac{n!}{X!(n-X)!}\pi^X(1-\pi)^{n-X} \tag{4-4}$$

The value of probability P is calculated directly for hypothesis testing (see Chapter 3).

If n, π and $(1-\pi)$ are large enough, for example, both $n\pi$ and $n(1-\pi)$ are greater than 5, the sample probability p is approximately normal distributed and a Z-test for probability of one sample can be used.

Example 4.3. 150 staff were randomly selected from the department of infectious diseases in a certain area for HBV serological tests, of which 35 were positive. It is known that the positive rate in the local general population is 17.00%. Is the positive rate of local staff of the department of infectious diseases higher than the positive rate of the general population?

Solution: It is known from the professional knowledge that the positive rate of local staff is not lower than the positive rate in the general population, so a one-tailed test is applied. The population probability π_0 is 0.17 and the sample size n is 150. The sample probability is

$$p = \frac{X}{n} = \frac{35}{150} = 0.2333$$

Because both $n\pi_0$ and $n(1-\pi_0)$ are greater than 5 in this example, the Z-test approximation is used.

(1) Set up the statistical hypotheses and determine the significance level

H_0: $\pi = \pi_0 = 0.17$. The positive rate of HBV among the staff of the department of infectious diseases is equal to that of the general population.
H_1: $\pi > \pi_0 = 0.17$. The positive rate of HBV among the staff of the department of infectious diseases is higher than that of the general population.
$\alpha = 0.05$ (one-tailed test)

(2) Calculate the test statistic:

$$Z = \frac{p - \pi_0}{\sigma_p} = \frac{p - \pi_0}{\sqrt{\pi_0(1-\pi_0)/n}} \quad (4\text{-}5)$$

When H_0 is true, the statistic follows the standard normal distribution approximately.

In this example, we calculate the test statistic

$$Z = \frac{p - \pi_0}{\sqrt{\pi_0(1 - \pi_0)/n}} = \frac{0.2333 - 0.1700}{\sqrt{0.17(1 - 0.17)/150}} = 2.065$$

(3) Determine the P value and conclusion
By checking the critical value table for Z-test (the row where v is ∞ in the t critical value table in Schedule 2), we know that $0.01 < P < 0.001$. Compared with the significance level $\alpha = 0.05$, we reject H_0 and conclude that the difference between P and π_0 is statistically significant and that the overall positive rate of HBV among staff is higher than that of the general population. The professional conclusion is that the positive rate of HBV among the staff of the department of infectious diseases is higher than that of the general population.

4.3. Two types of errors in hypothesis testing

Although the hypothesis testing can answer the question of whether μ and μ_0 are equal or not, it is possible to make mistakes whether rejecting (accepting the opposite hypotheses) or not rejecting the null hypotheses.

4.3.1. *Type I error*

If the null hypothesis H_0 is actually true but we reject it because of the test statistic calculated from the sample data, then an error occurred. The error that rejects the correct null hypothesis is called the type I error. The probability of type I error is controlled to be lower than α.

In order to control the possibility of such an error, a small probability α is usually preset in advance as a test level for statistical inference. If the probability of observed and even more extreme situation (P value) is less than or equal to α, then the event of the null hypothesis is considered to be rare in a specific sampling study. Therefore, we reject H_0 and infer that the difference is statistically significant. The probability of type I error is less than or equal to α. If the probability of a more extreme situation (P value) is greater than α, then we do not reject H_0, and conclude that the difference is not statistically significant.

4.3.2. *Type II error*

Another type of error in hypothesis testing is called type II error. That is, the null hypothesis H_0 is not true (H_1 is true) but we do not reject it because of the test statistic calculated from the sample data, then a type II error occurs. The probability of type II error is controlled to be lower than β.

4.3.3. *Power*

The probability of rejecting an incorrect H_0 is called power of test in statistics. It is the probability of correctly recognizing the difference (rejecting the null hypothesis $H_0 : \mu = \mu_0$ when $H_1 : \mu \neq \mu_0$ is true) between two population parameters. The power of test is limited by $1 - \beta$, that is, the power of test must not be lower than $1 - \beta$. In general, the power of test should not be lower than 0.8.

In hypothesis testing, we should take into account both the type I error (α) and type II error (β). If the type I error is set small, it will increase the type II error and reduce the power of test. On the contrary, if the type II error is set small, improving the power of test will increase type I error. In order to reduce α and β simultaneously, the only way is to increase the sample size and reduce the sampling error.

The above contents about the two types of errors can be summarized in Table 4.1 and Figure 4.3.

4.3.4. *The factors influencing the power*

In practice, sometimes a new medicine is not only effective, but also more efficient than known routine medicine (such as 15%). However, due to the small sample size, it is possible to obtain a large P value (i.e., the difference is not statistically significant), which cannot support the conclusion that the new medicine is superior to the routine

Table 4.1 Two types of errors

The truth	The conclusion of hypothesis testing	
	Reject H_0	Not reject H_0
H_0 is true	Type I error The probability of type I error is less than α	Correct
H_0 is false	Correct The correct probability (power of test) is greater than $1-\beta$	Type II error The probability of type II error is less than β

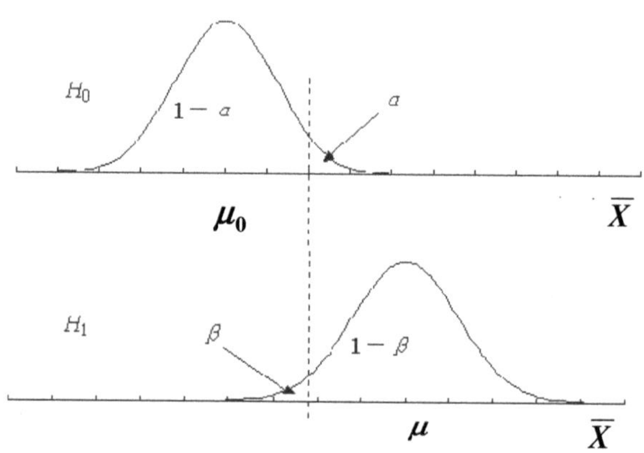

Figure 4.3 The two types of errors (one-tailed Z-test)

medicine. Why does this happen? It is related to the elements influencing the power of test. The following is an example formula of a one-sample Z-test to analyze the four elements influencing the power of test.

$$Z = \frac{\bar{X} - \mu_0}{\sigma/\sqrt{n}}$$

(1) The greater the difference between the population parameters is, the larger the power of test is.

In the one-sample Z-test for one sample mean, $\delta = \mu - \mu_0$. The larger $|\delta|$ is, the larger the absolute difference $|\bar{X} - \mu_0|$ between the sample mean and a given population mean is. Under the same conditions,

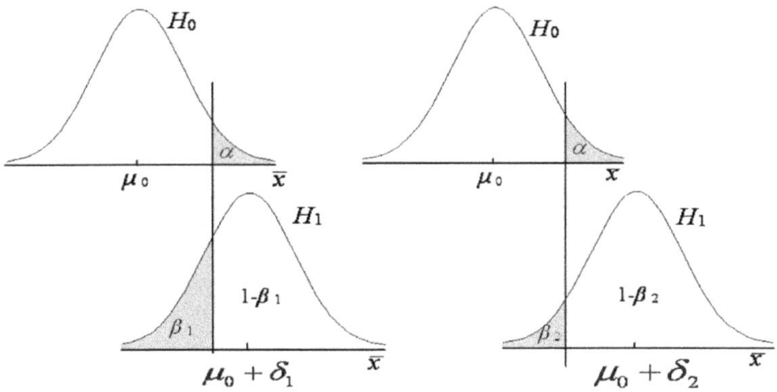

Figure 4.4 The relationship of power and difference between population means

the larger $|\delta|$ is, the larger $|\bar{X} - \mu_0|$ is, as well as the sample statistic Z. Hence, it is more likely to reject H_0 and conclude that the difference between the sample mean and the given population mean is statistically significant. In addition, as shown in Figure 4.4, when the other elements keep the same, if $\delta_2 > \delta_1$, then $(1 - \beta_2) > (1 - \beta_1)$.

(2) The smaller the variation among individuals (standard deviation) is, the greater the power of test is.

When the variation among individuals becomes smaller (i.e., the standard deviation $\sigma = \sigma_0$ becomes smaller), the denominator in the Z-test formula becomes smaller and the statistic Z becomes bigger. Therefore, it is more likely to reject H_0 and conclude that the difference between the sample mean and the given population mean is statistically significant. As shown in Figure 4.5, when other elements are kept the same, the smaller the difference among individuals (standard deviation) is, the smaller $\sigma_{\bar{x}}$ is and the greater the power of test is.

(3) The larger the sample size is, the greater the power of test is

In the Z-test for one sample mean, the sample size n is inversely proportional to σ. When other conditions are the same, the larger n is, the smaller $\sigma_{\bar{X}}$ is, the larger the sample statistic Z is, and the more likely it is to reject H_0 and conclude that the difference between the two populations is statistically significant (shown in Figure 4.5).

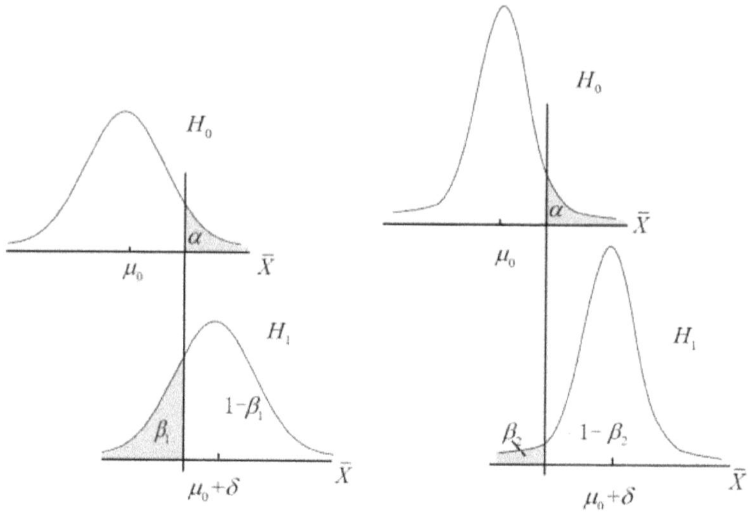

Figure 4.5 The relationship of power and standard error

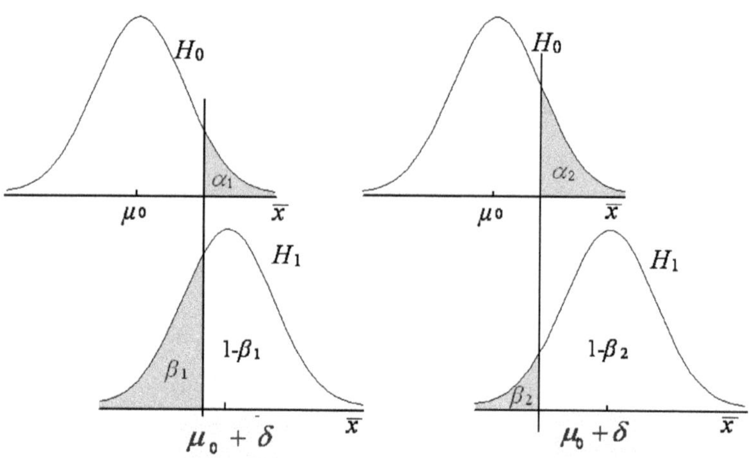

Figure 4.6 The relationship of power and test level α

(4) The greater the test level α (the probability of type I error) is, the greater the power of test is.

The power of test when $\alpha = 0.05$ is larger than the power when $\alpha = 0.01$. Because the larger α is, the smaller the critical value of

Z-test is, and it is easier to reject H_0. Figure 4.6 shows that when the other elements are kept the same, the greater the test level α is, the greater the power of test is. When $\alpha_2 > \alpha_1, (1-\beta_2) > (1-\beta_1)$. Among the four elements influencing the power above, the difference between population parameters δ, the standard deviation of population σ, and the test level α are usually relatively fixed. The element that can be adjusted is the sample size. So, if the power of test is not large enough, increasing the sample size is a good choice.

4.4. Report writing

The report of hypothesis testing for one sample includes the following contents:

(1) Basic statistical description of the sample.
(2) The purpose of the hypothesis testing and the design method.
(3) The method of hypothesis testing, one-tailed or two-tailed test, the significance level, the test statistic, and its P value.
(4) The 95% confidence interval of the population parameter.

The following reports are the results of the t-test for one sample mean in Example 4.2 and the Z-test for one sample probability in Example 4.3.

Example 4.2. The standard concentration of the solution of the drug was 20 mg/L. Based on the data of 11 solutions measured by a method, the mean and the standard deviation were 20.98 and 1.068 mg/L, respectively. A two-tailed t-test showed that the population mean of the measurements was statistically higher than the standard concentration and that a systematic error existed ($t = 3.056$; $\nu = 10$; $0.01 < P < 0.02$; 95% CI $= 20.26$–21.7 mg/L.

Example 4.3. To determine whether the positive rate of HBV serological test for staffs from the departments of infectious diseases was higher than that of general population (17%), 150 staffs were randomly selected to have the serological tests which resulted in 35 positives. The sample positive rate was 23.33%. A one-tailed Z-test showed that the positive rate for staffs of the departments of infectious diseases was statistically higher than that of the general population ($Z = 2.056$; $0.01 < P < 0.025$; 95% CI = 18.23%–28.38%).

4.5. Case discrimination

Case 4.1 In order to compare the efficacy of a new medicine (measured by mean μ) with that of a routine medicine μ_0, 25 patients were randomly selected, and the sample mean $\bar{X}$ was calculated and a t-test was applied. The null hypothesis was $\mu = \mu_0$, the alternative hypothesis was $\mu \neq \mu_0$, and the significance level was 0.01. The value of statistic t was large through to reject the null hypothesis. What does "rejecting the null hypothesis" mean? Do you think the following statements are right?

(1) You absolutely reject the null hypothesis that the population means are equal.
(2) The probability that the null hypothesis is true is 1%.
(3) You absolutely prove the alternative hypothesis that the population means are different.
(4) The probability that the alternative hypothesis is true is 99%.
(5) If you decide to reject the null hypothesis, the probability of error is 1%.
(6) You get a reliable finding: assuming that the experiment is repeated many times, the chance that you get statistically significant results is 99%.

Tips: For similar questions, Haller and Kruss (2002) asked 30 teachers of statistics, 44 students of statistics, and 39 psychologists in 6 psychological departments in Germany. All the students of statistics, 35 psychologists, and 24 teachers of statistics believed that at least one of them was correct; 10 teachers of statistics, 13 psychologists, and 26 students of statistics believed that the fourth statement was correct. (See *Statistical Science*, 20 (3): 223–230, 2005.)

Case 4.2 The qualified rate of a medical device manufactured by a factory has been 80% for many years. Recently, 20 medical devices were selected to be tested, 13 of which were qualified, and the qualified rate was 65%. A week later, 15 medical devices were selected and tested, 10 of which were qualified, and the qualified rate was 66.7%. The Z-test was carried out to compare the two results with the given population qualified rate (80%) separately. The results showed that the null hypothesis was not rejected, and the conclusion was that the qualified rate did not decrease. Then, the two samples were combined and the mean of combined sample was compared with the given population qualified rate (80%) by Z-test. The result showed that the null hypothesis was rejected and the conclusion was that the qualified rate decreased. Please comment on the two different conclusions.

4.6. Computer experiments

Experiment 4.1 Hypothesis testing for the mean of one sample

Analyze the data from Example 4.2 by SPSS.

Experiment 4.2 Hypothesis testing for the probability of one sample

Analyze the data from the Example 4.3 by SPSS.

Experiment 4.3 Comprehensive experiment of hypothesis testing

The statistical inference includes the interval estimation and hypothesis testing. Hypothesis testing is the foundation and core of statistics. Through this experiment, students can understand the basic ideas, steps of hypothesis testing, the concepts of two types of error and power of test in hypothesis testing. (The data file: program4-3.xls.)

4.7. Frequently asked questions and summary

4.7.1. *Frequently asked questions*

1. What is the difference between α and P in hypothesis testing?

α is a small probability (e.g., 0.05) preset as the critical value to control the type I error. If the probability of an even more extreme situation (P value) is less than α, it is considered that the situation of null hypothesis is not possible to appear. Therefore, reject H_0 and conclude that there is a statistically significant difference.

The P value is the probability of observed or even more extreme situation when H_0 is true. The P value is also a random variable, that is, different samples can obtain different P values.

2. The results of hypothesis testing showed that $P > \alpha$. Can we say the probability of making a mistake when we accept H_0 is very small?

No, because only the probability of type I error is controlled to be lower than α in hypothesis testing. When $P > \alpha$, H_0 cannot be rejected. However, the probability of type II error is unknown.

3. If the P value is very small in hypothesis testing, can we say that there is a great difference between the population means?

P value is the probability of observed or even more extreme situation when H_0 is true. It is not only related to the difference between the actual values of means, but also the sampling error. So, we cannot judge the difference between the population means only by P value.

4.7.2. *Summary*

1. Hypothesis testing is a logical process of statistical inference of the population based on the limited information provided by the sample. It is a choice of two opposing hypotheses for the study population.
2. The steps of hypothesis testing: Set up the hypotheses → Calculate the test statistic → Determine the P value and make a conclusion.
3. The basic ideas of hypothesis testing: Given that "a small probability event is unlikely to occur in a single sample." Once it occurs, it takes a certain risk to reject the null hypothesis, but the probability of error is controlled to be less than α.
4. There are type I error and type II error in hypothesis testing.
5. According to the results of hypothesis testing, the conclusion cannot be absolutely correct, and attention should be paid to the combination with professional knowledge.

Think and Practice

I. Best Choice

1. When the sample means are compared by t-test, the following significance levels are taken. The case with the smallest type II error is ( ).
A. $\alpha = 0.01$ B. $\alpha = 0.05$ C. $\alpha = 0.10$ D. $\alpha = 0.20$
E. $\alpha = 0.30$
2. In a hypothesis testing comparing one sample mean with a given population mean, the results are $t = 3.24$, $t_{0.05(v)} = 2.086$, $t_{0.01(v)} = 2.845$. The correct conclusion is ( ).
A. The sample mean is different from the given population mean.
B. The sample mean differs greatly from the given population mean. C. The population mean corresponding to the sample mean differs greatly from the given population mean. D. The population mean corresponding to the sample mean is equal to the given population mean. E. The population mean corresponding to the sample mean is different from the given population mean.
3. The steps of hypothesis testing are ( ).
A. Set up the hypotheses, select and calculate the test statistic, determine the P value and make a conclusion. B. Set up the null hypothesis and alternative hypothesis, determine the significance level C. Determine the one-tailed or two-tailed test, select t-test or Z-test, estimate the type I error and type II error D. Calculate the value of statistic, determine P value, and make a conclusion.
E. None of the above is correct.
4. When t-test is used to compare one sample mean with a given population mean, the correct statement is ( ).
A. The larger the statistic t is, the larger the difference between the two population means is. B. The larger the statistic t is, the smaller the difference between the two population means is.
C. The larger the statistic t is, the more reasonable to believe that the two population means are not equal. D. The P value is equal to α. E. The P value is not equal to α and always lower than α.

II. Questions for Reflection

1. Discuss the relationship and difference between α and P in hypothesis testing.
2. Discuss the relationship and difference between hypothesis testing and confidence interval.
3. How to correctly choose one-tailed or two-tailed test?
4. Discuss the significance and relationship of the two types of errors.
5. Describe the concept of power of a test and factors that influence power.
6. Briefly describe the basic ideas of hypothesis testing.

III. Questions on Calculation

1. The mean of hemoglobin in general adult males is 140 g/L. A researcher randomly selected a sample of 25 adult males from the plateau area for examination. The mean of hemoglobin of the sample was 155 g/L with a standard deviation of 25 g/L. *Question*: Is the population mean of hemoglobin among adult males living in the plateau area higher than that of general adult males?
2. Generally, the cure rate of a disease treated with routine treatment is 45%. Now a new treatment method has been used and 180 patients with the disease were randomly selected and treated with the new treatment, 117 of which were cured. *Question*: Is there a difference between the effect of the new treatment and routine treatment?

Aihua Lin, Guiming Gao

CHAPTER 5

COMPARISON OF MEANS BETWEEN TWO GROUPS

This chapter covers hypothesis testing, the second of two general areas of statistical inference. The other is parameter estimation discussed in the preceding chapter. Hypothesis testing involving the difference between two population means is frequently employed in medical research. For example, if we aim to examine whether the average weight of primary school students from Beijing city differs from that in Guangdong city, the convenient approach is to conduct a random sample from each region and then make hypothesis testing based on sample means. From the type of design, two samples include two independent samples and paired samples. From the statistical method, there is parametric test and non-parametric test. This chapter will introduce how to make statistical inference for quantitative variables between two groups.

5.1. Hypothesis testing: The difference of means between two groups

5.1.1. *Two independent samples t test*

[Example 5.1] Researchers were interested in the effect of a new drug to anemia patients. 20 patients with anemia were randomly allocated into two groups after approval by the ethics committee and informed consent of the participants. One group was treated with the new drug and the other with the conventional drug. The hemoglobin increase (g/L) in two groups were shown in Table 5.1

Table 5.1 Hemoglobin increase (g/L) among patients with anemia in two groups

Group	Hemoglobin increase (g/L)									
New drug	30.5	21.4	25.0	34.5	33.0	32.5	29.5	25.5	24.4	23.6
Conventional drug	19.5	19.0	13.0	24.7	21.5	22.0	19.0	15.5	24.5	23.4

(See data5-1.sav). Can we conclude that the average increase of hemoglobin among anemia patients with the new drug is different from the conventional drug?

[**Analysis**] The above study aims to compare whether the difference of two population means is significant. That is, whether $\mu_1 = \mu_2$ stands or not. Based on the knowledge of sampling error, two sample means are likely to be unequal under the condition that two population means are equal. Hypothesis testing, which plays a fundamental role in statistics literature, will serve to solve this question.

Hypothesis testing involving the difference of means between two groups will be discussed in three different contexts. ① Choose t test when either of two independent random samples have been drawn from a normally distributed population and the two groups have equal variances. ② Choose correction t test, also called t' test, when either groups two independent random samples have been drawn from a normally distributed population and the two groups have unequal variances. ③ Choose Wilcoxon rank-sum test when at least one sample is not normally distributed.

Normality test and homogeneity of variance test are the implicit assumptions of t test. It is necessary that such tests are carried out prior to comparison of two population means. So we will perform normality test and homogeneity of variance test firstly.

5.1.1.1. *Normality test*

If the sample size in each group is greater than or equal to 50, we can assume the sample is approximately normally distributed. Otherwise, normality tests need be conducted to explore whether the sample has been drawn from a normally distributed population such as Example 5.1. Moment test and W test (Shapiro-Wilk W test) are two commonly used methods of testing normality. The moment test is more conservative while the W test is more sensitive. In addition, Kolmogorov-Smirnov test (K-S test) and D test can also be served to explore the normality. The calculation process of the above methods is complicated and laborious that is why it is mostly implemented with computer packages. Let us state the three-step procedure of normality test.

(1) State the hypothesis and significance level

There are two statistical hypotheses involved in hypothesis testing, which should be stated explicitly. The null hypothesis is the hypothesis to be tested, designated by the symbol $\mathrm{H_0}$. In general, the null hypothesis is set up for the express purpose of being discredited. In the testing process the null hypothesis may be rejected or not. The null hypothesis is not rejected means the data on which the test is based does not provide sufficient evidence of rejection. The testing procedure leads to rejection means the data at hand is not compatible with the null hypothesis. The alternative hypothesis is a statement that is believed to be true if the sample data rejects the null hypothesis, designated by $\mathrm{H_1}$. Usually the alternative hypothesis and the research hypothesis are the same and in fact the null hypothesis and alternative hypothesis are used interchangeably.

The term level of significance reflects the fact that hypothesis tests are sometimes called significance tests, and a computed value of the test statistic that falls in the rejection region is said to be significant. The level of significance, designated by α, specifies the area under the curve of the distribution of the test statistics that are above the values on the horizontal axis constituting the rejection region. The decision as to which values go into the rejection region and which ones go into the non-rejection region is made on the basis of the desired level of significance.

H_0: The sample is from a normally distributed population.
H_1: The sample is from a non-normally distributed population.
$\alpha = 0.10$

The more frequently encountered values of α are 0.01, 0.05 and 0.10. While we prefer to make a conclusion that "Reject the null hypothesis" in the normality test and homogeneity test of variance, so the test level α can be relatively larger, usually set as 0.10. In this book, the significance level is uniformly set at 0.05, exception to 0.10 level while performing the normality test and the test for homogeneity of variance.

(2) Calculate the test statistic

The test statistic is computed from the sample data. As we will see that the test statistic serves as a decision maker, since the decision to reject or not to reject the null hypothesis depends on the magnitude of the test statistic.

Here we refer to the output of SPSS (Statistical Package for Social Science) directly.

New drug group $W = 0.928$, $p = 0.431$
Conventional drug group $W = 0.933$, $p = 0.479$

(3) Determine the p value and make a decision

The p value is the probability that the computed value of a test statistic is at least as extreme as a specified value of the test statistic when the null hypothesis is true. A small p value indicates that the sample results are not likely to have occurred. If $p > \alpha$, we should say the null hypothesis is "Not reject" Otherwise, if $p < \alpha$, we should say the null hypothesis is "Reject" then the reverse alternative hypothesis is usually true.

In this example, we cannot reject H_0 and we may conclude that the two samples both come from normally distributed population at 0.10 significance level.

5.1.1.2. *Test for homogeneity of variance*

The test statistic of homogeneity of variance is F, and the formula is

$$F = \frac{S_1^2}{S_2^2}, v_1 = n_1 - 1, v_2 = n_2 - 1 \tag{5-1}$$

The terms of the formula are defined as follows: S_1^2 represents the larger sample variance and S_2^2 represents the smaller sample variance. ν_1 and ν_2 represents degrees of freedom, which is equal to n − 1 corresponding to the larger variance and smaller variance respectively.

The three-step procedure for homogeneity of variance test are as follows.

Solution:

(1) State the hypothesis and significance level

$$H_0 : \sigma_1^2 = \sigma_2^2, H_1 : \sigma_1^2 \neq \sigma_2^2$$
$$\alpha = 0.10$$

(2) Calculate the test statistic

$$F = \frac{S_1^2}{S_2^2} = \frac{4.56^2}{3.82^2} = 1.426 \quad \upsilon_1 = 10 - 1 = 9, \quad \upsilon_2 = 10 - 1 = 9$$

(3) Determine the p value and make a decision

$P = 0.261$, we cannot reject H_0 and conclude that the two population variances are equal at 0.10 significance level.

In addition to the F test, the Levene test and the Bartlett test are also commonly used in the test for homogeneity of variance. When the sample follows normal distribution, the F test and the Bartlett test can be used. Comparing the latter, the Levene test is more robust because of the independence of the type of distribution. To add on, the F test can only be used for test for homogeneity of variance between two populations while the Levene test and the Bartlett test can be served for more than two populations. The default method for performing the test for homogeneity of variance by SPSS is Levene test.

5.1.1.3. *t test for two independent samples*

As we have learned from the above procedure, the data in Example 5.1 meets the assumption of normality and homogeneity of variance.

Thus it is reasonable to conduct t test. The test statistic for testing $\mathrm{H}_0 : \mu_1 = \mu_2$ is given by

$$t = \frac{\overline{X}_1 - \overline{X}_2}{\sqrt{S_c^2(\frac{1}{n_1} + \frac{1}{n_2})}} \tag{5-2}$$

When H_0 is true, the test statistic is distributed as Student's t with degrees of freedom $\mathrm{n}_1 + \mathrm{n}_2 - 2$. The terms of the equation (5-2) are defined as follows: $\overline{X}_1$ and $\overline{X}_2$ represents two sample means respectively. The denominator in the equation is the standard error of the difference of means $(\overline{X}_1 - \overline{X}_2)$, which pool the sample variances by means of the following formula:

$$S_c^2 = \frac{S_1^2(n_1 - 1) + S_2^2(n_2 - 1)}{n_1 + n_2 - 2}$$

The basic steps of t test in Example 5.1 are as follows.

Solution:

(1) State the hypothesis and significance level

$$H_0 : \mu_1 = \mu_2, H_1 : \mu_1 \neq \mu_2$$

$$\alpha = 0.05$$

(2) Calculate the test statistic

$$t = \frac{\overline{X}_1 - \overline{X}_2}{\sqrt{S_c^2(\frac{1}{n_1} + \frac{1}{n_2})}} = \frac{27.99 - 20.21}{\sqrt{\frac{4.56^2(10-1)+3.82^2(10-1)}{10+10-2} \times (\frac{1}{10} + \frac{1}{10})}}$$
$$= 4.137$$

(3) Determine the p value and make a decision

Generally, there are two ways to get p value. One is to look up the critical value at the specified significance level and then compare it with the test statistic. If the critical value is greater than the test statistic, $p < \alpha$. If the critical value is less than the test statistic, $p > \alpha$. Another is to obtain the exact p value based on the result by the computer software. The former is advantageous in the past and it allows a decision to be made without the calculation of a probability, but it was deficient for reporting results. With the development of computer packages and promulgation of guidelines of strengthening the reporting of medical studies, reporting the exact p value is a fundamental requirement of journals while submitting a manuscript.

For t test of the above example, $p < 0.05$ using t critical value table, since the computed value $4.137 > t$ critical value 2.101 with degrees of freedom 18 (See Appendix table 2), or $p = 0.001$ using the computer. Based on the data, we can conclude that the average hemoglobin increase in anemia patients treated with new drug is significantly higher than that in the conventional drug. We can also draw the same conclusion from the 95% confidence interval (CI) for the difference (3.829–11.731).

5.1.2. *t′ test for two independent samples*

When two independent simple random samples have been drawn from normally distributed populations with unequal population variances, the test statistic for testing $H_0 : \mu_1 = \mu_2$ is given by

$$t' = \frac{\overline{X}_1 - \overline{X}_2}{\sqrt{\frac{S_1^2}{n_1} + \frac{S_2^2}{n_2}}} \tag{5-3}$$

Degrees of freedom can be computed by the following equation

$$\nu = \frac{\left(\frac{S_1^2}{n_1} + \frac{S_2^2}{n_2}\right)^2}{\frac{\left(\frac{S_1^2}{n_1}\right)^2}{n_1-1} + \frac{\left(\frac{S_2^2}{n_2}\right)^2}{n_2-1}} \tag{5-4}$$

[Example 5.2] The study aimed to a study was to identify the effects of vanadyl sulfate on blood glucose concentration in diabetic cataract rats. One focus was to determine if there were different levels of blood glucose in diabetic cataract rats with and without vanadyl sulfate. 100 diabetic cataract rats were divided into two groups. The following summarized the researchers' main findings (See data5-2.sav). Is there sufficient evidence to claim that vanadyl sulfate has a role in blood glucose concentration in diabetic cataract rats? Let $\alpha = 0.05$.

With Vanadyl sulfate $n_1 = 50$, mean glucose $= 6.5$ mmol/L, standard deviation $= 1.35$ mmol/L

Without Vanadyl sulfate $n_1 = 50$, mean glucose $= 13.2$ mmol/L, standard deviation $= 4.20$ mmol/L

[**Analysis**] This example involves the comparison of the mean of two independent samples. We can assume that the two samples approximately follow the normal distribution because the sample size in each group is 50. However, the test for homogeneity of variance results shows that the two population variances are not equal ($F = 9.679$, $p < 0.001$) at 0.10 significance level. Therefore, the t' test should be performed.

Solution:

(1) State the hypothesis and determine the test level

$$H_0 : \mu_1 = \mu_2, H_1 : \mu_1 \neq \mu_2$$
$$\alpha = 0.05$$

(2) Calculate the test statistic

$$t' = \frac{\overline{X_1} - \overline{X_2}}{\sqrt{\frac{S_1^2}{n_1}} + \sqrt{\frac{S_2^2}{n_2}}} = \frac{13.2 - 6.5}{\sqrt{\frac{4.20^2}{50} + \frac{1.35^2}{50}}} = 10.745$$

$$\nu = \frac{\left(\frac{S_1^2}{n_1} + \frac{S_2^2}{n_2}\right)^2}{\frac{\left(\frac{S_1^2}{n_1}\right)^2}{n_1 - 1} + \frac{\left(\frac{S_2^2}{n_2}\right)^2}{n_2 - 1}} = 59.02 \approx 59$$

(3) Determine the p value and make a decision

$P < 0.001$ from the SPSS output. Based on the data, we may conclude that the diabetic cataract rats with and without vanadyl sulfate may have differing blood glucose concentration, which is lower in the diabetic cataract rats with vanadyl sulfate. We can also make the same conclusion from the 95% CI for the difference (5.452, 7.948).

5.1.3. *Rank-sum test of two independent samples*

5.1.3.1. *Introduction of nonparametric test*

The statistical inference procedures are classified as parametric statistics and nonparametric statistics. An example of a parametric statistical test is the widely used t test and analysis of variance that we will discuss in the proceeding chapter. The most common uses of parametric test include testing a hypothesis about a single population mean and the difference among two or more than two population means. In each case, our interest was focused on estimating or testing a hypothesis about one or more population parameters. One of the assumptions underlying the valid use of this test is that the sampled population or populations are at least approximately normally distributed. When the underlying assumptions are violated or one wishes to perform a test without making assumptions about the sampled population, nonparametric test may be applied.

Three advantages of nonparametric statistics may be summarized from the above discussion: ① They could allow for the test without making assumptions about the sampled population or the form of the sampled population is unknown. ② Nonparametric procedures may be applied when the data being analyzed consists merely of rankings or classifications. ③ Nonparametric procedures tend to be computationally easier and consequently more quickly applied than parametric procedures.

Although nonparametric statistics enjoy the above advantages, their disadvantages must also be pointed out: ① The use of nonparametric procedures results in a waste of data information when the data can be handled with a parametric procedure. ② The application of some of the nonparametric tests may be laborious for large samples.

Wilcoxon rank sum test is one kind of nonparametric tests frequently used, which can be applied in the comparison of two independent samples, including the quantitative variable and ordinal variable. For example, we could use a rank transformation on the data by replacing the original data prior to analysis. The rank or the order of the data and the test statistic can be computed easily, which does not dependent on the distribution of population.

5.1.3.2. *Wilcoxon rank-sum test*

[Example 5.3] Physicians wish to know whether pneumonia patients and normal people differ with respect to their serum ferritin concentration. 10 pneumonia patients and 16 normal people were randomly selected and their serum ferritin concentration (μg/L) was measured (See data5-3.sav). Can we conclude that the pneumonia patients and normal people differ with respect to their serum ferritin concentration from this data? Let $\alpha = 0.05$.

Pneumonia patients: 3168237174457492199515599238

Normal people:

17717234471325447524729468432774443 95

[Analysis] As was pointed out in the previous section of this chapter,

this case covers the comparison of two independent samples. So t test is the first method we will consider. Prior to t test, we should explore the normality and homogeneity of variance. The results of normality test indicates that the sample with pneumonia patients follows the normal distribution: $W = 0.919$, $P = 0.345$, while the sample with normal people violates the assumption, $W = 0.748$, $P = 0.001$ at 0.10 significance level. Therefore, the Wilcoxon rank sum test should be applied to determine whether two independent samples were selected from populations having the same distribution.

In statistics, Wilcoxon rank-sum test also called the Mann-Whitney U test, or Mann–Whitney-Wilcoxon (MWW),developed by Mann and Whitney. Unlike the t-test it does not require the assumption of normal distributions.

Solution:

(1) State the hypothesis and determine the test level

H_0: The distributions of both populations are equal, or $M_1 = M_2$
H_1: The distributions of both populations are not equal, or $M_1 \neq M_2$
$\alpha = 0.05$

Where M_1 and M_2 is the median of a population of serum ferritin concentration in pneumonia patients and normal people, respectively.

(2) Calculate the test statistic

To compute the test statistic, we put the observations from both groups to one set and assign numeric ranks to all the observations, beginning with 1 for the smallest value and ending with $n_1 + n_2$ for the largest value. Tied observations are assigned a rank equal to the mean of the rank positions for which they are tied if they belong to different groups. For example, 68 appears not only in the group with pneumonia patients, but also in the group with normal people. So we should pool the rank of 11 and 12, which is $(11 + 12)/2 = 11.5$. Another tied observation in this example is 47, which appears three times in the group with normal people. We can pool the rank of 6, 7 and 8, which is equal to 7, or use the rank positions 6, 7 and 8. Add up the ranks for the observations which come from sample 1 and sample 2 respectively and get $T_1 = 183.5$, $T_2 = 167.5$. The results of this step are shown in Table 5.2.

The rank reflects the level of the original data, so the analysis to the original observation can be transformed into the analysis to the rank. When H_0 is true, the two samples come from the same population. So the expected rank value for each data is $(n_1 + n_2 + 1)/2$. It can be proved that the rank sum T_1 of sample 1 is symmetrically distributed at its expected value $n_1(n_1 + n_2 + 1)/2$ when H_0 is true. Generally when H_0 is false, T_1 will be far from its expected value $n_1(n_1 + n_2 + 1)/2$. Similarly, we can prove that the rank sum T_2 of sample 2 have the same nature and the expected value is $n_2(n_1 + n_2 + 1)/2$. In Example 5.3, the computed value T_1 is 183.5, summing up the rank of each observations in the sample 1 together. The computed value T_2 is 167.5, summing up the rank of each observations in sample 2.

Theoretically, the rank sum in either of the group can be the test statistic. For convenience, we usually choose the rank sum with smaller sample size as the test statistic consulting significance tables, here we chose 183.5 as the test statistic value.

Table 5.2 Original data and ranks, Example 5.3

Pneumonia patients		Normal people	
Serum ferritin concentration	Rank	Serum ferritin concentration	Rank
31	1	177	17
68	11.5	172	15
237	19	34	2
174	16	47	7
457	23	132	14
492	24	54	10
199	18	47	7
515	25	52	9
599	26	47	7
238	20	294	22
		68	11.5
		43	3.5
		277	21
		44	5
		43	3.5
		95	13
Rank sum $T_1 = 183.5$		Rank sum $T_2 = 167.5$	

(3) Determine the p value and make a decision

There are two approaches of obtaining p value. One is to look up T critical values from the distribution of the test statistic given in Appendix table 8 for various levels of α. The other is to look up Z critical values based on normal distribution given in Appendix table 1.

(1) Look up T critical value table: In the case of small samples, for example n_1 or $n_2 - n_1$ is less than 10, the distribution is tabulated. When Appendix 8 T critical value table with $n_1 = 10$, $n_2 - n_1 = 6$ and $\alpha = 0.05$, we find the critical value of T to be 97–173. Compared the test statistic value 183.5 with this range, we can make conclusion $p > \alpha$ if the computed test statistic is within the critical value range. Or else if the computed test

statistic is beyond the critical value range, we can make conclusion $p < \alpha$. About Example 5.3, 183.5 falls beyond the range of 97–173, so $p < \alpha$. From the sample data we may conclude that the population distribution of serum ferritin in pneumonia patients and normal people are significantly different.

(2) Large-sample approximation: It will be applied when either n_1 or $n_2 - n_1$ is greater than 10, thereby we cannot use Appendix table 10 to obtain the critical values. In this case, we may compute the Z value and compare the result with critical value of the standard normal distribution.

$$Z = \frac{|T - n_1(n_1 + n_2 + 1)/2| - 0.5}{\sqrt{n_1 n_2 (n_1 + n_2 + 1)/12}} \qquad (5\text{-}5)$$

In the formula (5-5), 0.5 is a continuous correction number, which will be applied when $n_1 < 100$ or $n_2 < 100$.

Formula (5-5) is not corrected for ties and is applicable when there are no ties in the data. If there are ties in ranks, especially when the proportion of ties in ranks is larger than 25%, the formula (5-5) will yield the biased results hence the Z value should be corrected.

$$Z_c = Z/\sqrt{c} \qquad (5\text{-}6)$$

Where, $c = 1 - \sum (t_j^3 - t_j)/(N^3 - N)$

In formula (5-6), $N = n_1 + n_2$, t_j is the number of subjects sharing rank j. As shown in Table 5.2, 43 and 68 appears twice, 47 appears three times, so $t_1 = 2$, $t_2 = 2$, $t_3 = 3$.

As seen from the SPSS output for example 5-3, $Z = 2.559$ and p value $= 0.011$, it can be concluded that the serum ferritin concentration in pneumonia patients and normal people are significantly different. The mean rank is 18.35 in pneumonia patients and 10.47 in normal population, and we can make conclusion that the pneumonia patients have higher serum ferritin concentration. It is also worth to mention that ties can be ignored if the number of ties is small, especially if there are no large tie bands. The computer statistical packages will use the correctly adjusted formula as a matter of routine by default.

5.2. Hypothesis test for paired samples

In our previous discussion involving the difference of means between two groups, it is assumed that the samples are independent. Another method frequently employed for assessing the effectiveness of a treatment or experimental procedure is to make dependent samples or paired samples. A hypothesis test based on this type of data is known as the paired comparisons test.

The objective of paired comparisons tests is to eliminate a maximum number of sources of extraneous variation by making the pairs similar with respect to as many variables as possible. Paired observations may be obtained in a number of ways: ① Pairs may be formed by matching individuals of some characteristics, for example the same age or state of illness, which is closely related to the measurement of interest, and then the pairs are assigned randomly to receive either treatment or placebo. ② Pairs of twins or siblings may be assigned randomly to two treatments in such a way that members of a single pair receive different treatments. ③ The same subjects may be measured before and after receiving some treatment, such as the blood pressure with hypertensive patients before and after taking medicine. ④ The specimen to be analyzed may be divided equally so that one-half is analyzed by one method and the other half is analyzed by the other while comparing two methods of analysis.

Instead of performing the analysis with individual observations, we use the difference between pairs of observations as the interest variable.

When the difference between pairs of observations comes from a normally distributed population, the test statistic for testing hypothesis about the population mean difference μ_d is

$$t = \frac{\overline{d}}{S_d/\sqrt{n}}, \quad \nu = n - 1 \tag{5-7}$$

Where $\overline{d}$ is the sample mean difference, S_d is standard deviation of sample differences and n is number of pairs. When H_0 is true, the test statistic is distributed as Student's t with n − 1 degrees of freedom.

The following example illustrates the procedures involved in the paired comparisons test.

5.2.1. *Paired t test*

[Example 5.4] To explore the inhibitory effect of a new anticancer drug on transplanted sarcoma S180 in mice, 20 mice were assigned randomly to treatment group or control group after matching sex, body weight and litter. The tumor weights of mice were measured after the experiment and the results are shown in Table 5.3 (See data5-4.sav).We wish to know if this data provides sufficient evidence to conclude that the new anticancer drug inhibits the growth of transplanted sarcoma S180 in mice. Let $\alpha = 0.05$.

Here, we may obtain the differences in one of the two ways: by subtracting the tumor weight in the treatment group from the control group or by subtracting the tumor weight in the control group from the treatment group. Let us obtain the differences by subtracting the tumor weight in the treatment group from the control group. The differences are listed in Table 5.3.

[Analyze] The present example covers the comparison of paired samples. Hypothesis testing involving it will be introduced in two different contexts. ① Choose paired t test when the difference between pairs of observations comes from a normally distributed population. ② Choose Wilcoxon signed-rank test when the differences between pairs of observations do not come from a normally distributed population.

Based on the result of normality tests from the SPSS output, $W = 0.893$, $p = 0.185$, we may conclude that the differences of the

Table 5.3 Tumor weight in two groups (g)

Group	1	2	3	4	5	6	7	8	9	10
Control	0.80	0.74	0.31	0.48	0.76	0.65	0.72	0.68	0.39	0.53
Treatment	0.47	0.42	0.38	0.44	0.38	0.43	0.39	0.71	0.32	0.41
Difference	0.33	0.32	−0.07	0.04	0.28	0.22	0.33	−0.03	0.07	0.12

pairs follow a normal distribution at 0.10 significance level, so paired t test is applicable here.

Solution:

(1) State the hypothesis and determine the test level

$$H_0 : \mu_d = 0, H_1 : \mu_d \neq 0$$

$$\alpha = 0.05$$

(2) Calculate the test statistic

$$t = \frac{\bar{d}}{S_d/\sqrt{n}} = \frac{0.171}{0.1658/\sqrt{10}} = 3.262, \quad v = 10 - 1 = 9$$

(3) Determine the p value and make a decision

$P = 0.010$ from the SPSS output, this data provides sufficient evidence to conclude that the new anticancer drug inhibits the growth of transplanted sarcoma S180 in mice at 0.05 significance level. We can also make the same conclusion from 95% *CI* for μ_d(0.052,0.290).

5.2.2. *Wilcoxon signed-rank test*

Wilcoxon signed-rank test differs from the Wilcoxon rank-sum test, although both are nonparametric and involve summation of ranks. The Wilcoxon signed-rank test is applied to matched or dependent samples while the Wilcoxon rank-sum test is applied to independent samples. The following example illustrates the procedures of Wilcoxon signed-rank test.

[**Example 5.5**] The urine samples from 12 workers in the medical instrument factory were divided equally so that one-half is analyzed by ion exchange method and one-half is analyzed by distillation method. The mercury concentration in urine was measured as follows (See data5-5.sav). Can we perceive any difference in average urinary mercury between the two methods? Let $\alpha = 0.05$.

[**Analyze**] The present example involves the comparison of paired samples. So paired t test is the first method we consider. Prior to paired t test, we should run the normality tests for the difference of

Table 5.4 The mercury concentration in urine measured by two methods(mg/L)

Number	Ion exchange	Distillation
1	0.200	0.320
2	0.020	0.015
3	0.010	0.030
4	0.382	0.424
5	0.723	0.789
6	0.876	0.721
7	0.035	0.014
8	0.023	0.020
9	0.940	0.051
10	1.201	1.115
11	0.408	0.612
12	1.256	1.078

pairs, which indicates the assumptions underlying the paired t test are violated at 0.10 significance level, $W = 0.703$, $p = 0.001$, so Wilcoxon signed-rank test may be performed to test the null hypothesis that the median difference is 0.

In Wilcoxon signed-rank test, the median difference should follow symmetrical distribution centered on 0, if there is no difference between the two methods. We may obtain the differences of pairs, the positive difference and the negative difference is marked as "+" and "–" respectively. In a random sample of matched pairs, we would expect the rank sum "+" and "–" to be about equal, which can be proved to be near to n(n+1)/4. If there are more "+" or more "–" than the expected, we will entertain some doubts about the truth of the null hypothesis.

Solution:

(1) State the hypothesis and determine the test level

$$H_0 : M_d = 0, H_1 : M_d \neq 0$$

$$\alpha = 0.05$$

Where M_d is the median of the differences of pairs.

Table 5.5 Signs of difference in urinary mercury concentration and ranks

Pair(1)	Ion exchange (2)	Distillation (3)	Difference (4) = (2) − (3)	Rank of $\|d\|$ (5)	Signed rank (6)
1	0.200	0.320	−0.120	8	−8
2	0.020	0.015	0.005	2	2
3	0.010	0.030	−0.020	3	−3
4	0.382	0.424	−0.042	5	−5
5	0.723	0.789	−0.066	6	−6
6	0.876	0.721	0.155	9	9
7	0.035	0.014	0.021	4	4
8	0.023	0.020	0.003	1	1
9	0.940	0.051	0.889	12	12
10	1.201	1.115	0.086	7	7
11	0.408	0.612	−0.204	11	−11
12	1.256	1.078	0.178	10	10
				$T_+ = 45$; $T_- = 33$	

(2) Calculate the test statistic

As a first step in determining the value of the test statistic, we should compute the difference and determine which differences of pairs are above zero and which ones are less than zero. If we assign a plus sign to the positive difference and a minus to the negative difference, we have the results shown in Table 5.5.

(1) Calculate the difference of each pairs. See column (4) in Table 5.5.
(2) Rank the differences from the smallest with 1 to the largest with n based on the absolute value of the difference. Note that tied differences with absolute value are assigned an equal rank, and don't rank at all when the difference is 0.
(3) Calculate the rank sum. We could obtain the T_+ (adding up all the plus ranks) and T_- (adding up all the minus ranks).

The test statistic for the sign test is either the observed number of plus signs or the observed number of minus signs. For simplicity, we choose the smaller rank sum as the test statistic.

(3) Determine the p value and make a decision

There are two ways to obtain p value. One is to look up critical values from the distribution of the test statistic given in Appendix table 7. The other is to look up Z critical values based on normal distribution given in Appendix table 1.

(1) Look up T critical value of Wilcoxon signed rank test. When n is less than 50, the distribution is tabulated. When we enter Appendix 7 T critical value table with $n = 12$, $\alpha = 0.05$ (two-sided), we find the critical value of T to be 13–65. Compared the test statistic value 33 with this range, we observe 33 falls within this range, then $p > \alpha$. We can also refer to the SPSS output $p = 0.638$ to draw the conclusion. From the sample data we may conclude that there is no difference in the average level of urine mercury concentration between the two methods.

(2) Large-sample approximation: It will be applied when n is greater than 50, thereby we cannot obtain the critical values by Appendix table 7. In this case, we may compute the Z value and compare the result with critical values of the standard normal distribution.

$$Z = \frac{|T - \mu_T|}{\sigma_T} = \frac{|T - n(n+1)/4|}{\sqrt{n(n+1)(2n+1)/24}} \tag{5-8}$$

When $n < 50$, the test statistic need to be corrected as follows:

$$Z = \frac{|T - \mu_T| - 0.5}{\sigma_T} = \frac{|T - n(n+1)/4| - 0.5}{\sqrt{n(n+1)(2n+1)/24}} \tag{5-9}$$

Formula (5-8) and (5-9) are applicable when there are no ties in the data. If there are ties in ranks, the Z value should be corrected.

$$Z_c = \frac{|T - n(n+1)/4| - 0.5}{\sqrt{\frac{n(n+1)(2n+1)}{24} - \frac{\sum(t_j^3 - t_j)}{48}}} \tag{5-10}$$

Where, t_j is the number of subjects sharing rank j. N is the number of pairs. Strictly speaking, n the number of pairs minus the number of difference zero because we don't rank 0 at all.

5.3. Hypothesis test for Poisson distribution data

Poisson distribution is a discrete probability distribution that expresses the probability of a given number of events occurring in a fixed interval of time or space in terms of probability theory and statistics. We have studied its properties in the proceeding chapter. The following statements introduce the comparison of Poisson distribution data.

5.3.1. *Hypothesis test of two samples with poisson distribution when the observation units are equal*

[Example 5.6] In the study of colony experiment, two kinds of formulations were made into solid culture medium in 3 plates mixed with 1 ml gastric juice containing *Helicobacter pylori*.72 hours later, the number of *Helicobacter pylori* colonies in each sample was counted. Assuming that the number of *Helicobacter pylori* colonies follows a Poisson distribution, can we conclude that the mean number of *Helicobacter pylori* colonies cultured by two growth medium are different? Let $\alpha = 0.05$.

$$A14,\ 21,\ 16B12,\ 10,\ 8$$

[Analysis] Based on the knowledge of Poisson distribution, it is approximate to a normal distribution when $\lambda \geq 20$. And one interesting feature of Poisson distribution is that the mean and variance are equal, represented by the symbol λ. So we can designate it as N (λ, λ). Assume that X_1 and X_2 represents the observation of two samples with Poisson distribution, X_1 and X_2 are both approximate to the normal distribution, noted as N $(\lambda_1,\ \lambda_1)$ and N $(\lambda_2,\ \lambda_2)$ when X_1 and X_2 are larger enough. It can be inferred that $\lambda_1 - \lambda_2$ are also approximate to the normal distribution N $(\lambda_1 - \lambda_2,\ \lambda_1 + \lambda_2)$.

When the null hypothesis H_0: $\lambda_1 = \lambda_2$ is true, $X_1 - X_2$ follows a normal distribution, designated as $N(0,\ \lambda_1 + \lambda_2)$. Furthermore, it can be inferred that $(\lambda_1 - \lambda_2)/\sqrt{\lambda_1 + \lambda_2}$ follows a standard normal distribution N(0,1) approximately. In view of λ_1 and λ_2 unknown in most of the cases, so we may replace them with the sample observation X_1 and X_2. Then the test statistic is as follows when the observation units are equal:

$$z = \frac{X_1 - X_2}{\sqrt{X_1 + X_2}} \tag{5-11}$$

Solution:

(1) State the hypothesis and determine the test level

$$H_0 : \lambda_1 = \lambda_2, H_1 : \lambda_1 \neq \lambda_2$$
$$\alpha = 0.05$$

(2) Calculate the test statistic

Totally, 51 *Helicobacter pylori* colonies were observed in A growth medium and 30 *Helicobacter pylori* colonies were observed in B growth medium. X_1 and X_2 are both larger than 20 so we can refer to equation (5-11) to compute the test statistic value.

$$z = \frac{X_1 - X_2}{\sqrt{X_1 + X_2}} = \frac{51 - 30}{\sqrt{51 + 30}} = 2.333$$

(3) Determine the p value and make a decision

We enter Appendix 1 Z critical value table and get $Z_{(0.05/2)} = 1.96$. Abiding by the decision rule, we can reject the null hypothesis since $2.333 > 1.96$. There is significant difference in the number of *Helicobacter pylori* colonies between the two kinds of growth media, and the number of *Helicobacter pylori* colonies cultured in A growth medium was more than that in B growth medium.

5.3.2. *Hypothesis test of two samples with Poisson distribution when the observation units are not equal*

[Example 5.7] The radioactivity of the two specimens was measured by isotope method. The first specimen was measured for

10 minutes and the particle number was 1 500. The second specimen was measured for 20 minutes and the particle number was 2 400. The researcher wants to know whether the radioactivity of the two specimens are same under the condition that they are measured for the same time.

[Analysis] Equation (5-11) is reasonable when the observation units of two samples are the same. That is to say, Equation (5-11) cannot be used for this case.

From the previous introduction about Poisson distribution, we can infer:

$$\frac{X_1}{n_1} \sim N\left(\frac{\lambda_1}{n_1}, \frac{\lambda_1}{n_1^2}\right), \frac{X_2}{n_2} \sim N\left(\frac{\lambda_2}{n_2}, \frac{\lambda_2}{n_2^2}\right)$$

$$\frac{X_1}{n_1} - \frac{X_2}{n_2} \sim N\left(\frac{\lambda_1}{n_1} - \frac{\lambda_2}{n_2}, \frac{\lambda_1}{n_1^2} + \frac{\lambda_2}{n_2^2}\right) \quad (5\text{-}12)$$

When the null hypothesis H_0:$\frac{\lambda_1}{n_1} = \frac{\lambda_2}{n_2}$ is true, $\frac{X_1}{n_1} - \frac{X_2}{n_2}$ follows a normal distribution

$$\frac{X_1}{n_1} - \frac{X_2}{n_2} \sim N\left(0, \frac{\lambda_1}{n_1^2} + \frac{\lambda_2}{n_2^2}\right)$$

In the similar way, we can infer the equation of test statistic when the observation units are not equal:

$$Z = \frac{\overline{X}_1 - \overline{X}_2}{\sqrt{\frac{\overline{X}_1}{n_1} + \frac{\overline{X}_2}{n_2}}} \sim N(0, 1) \quad (5\text{-}13)$$

Solution:

(1) Establish the hypothesis and determine the test level

$$H_0 : \frac{\lambda_1}{n_1} = \frac{\lambda_2}{n_2} \; H_1 : \frac{\lambda_1}{n_1} \neq \frac{\lambda_2}{n_2}$$

$$\alpha = 0.05$$

(2) Calculate the test statistic

$$\overline{X}_1 = 150, n_1 = 10; \overline{X}_2 = 120, n_2 = 20$$

$$Z = \frac{\overline{X}_1 - \overline{X}_2}{\sqrt{\frac{\overline{X}_1}{n_1} + \frac{\overline{X}_2}{n_2}}} = \frac{150 - 120}{\sqrt{\frac{150}{10} + \frac{120}{20}}} = 6.547$$

(3) Determine the p value and make a decision

We enter Appendix 1 Z critical value table and get $Z_{(0.05/2)} = 1.96$. Abiding by the decision rule, we can reject the null hypothesis since $6.547 > 1.96$, which shows that the radioactivity of the two specimens differ under the condition that they are measured at the same time. With the information $\overline{X}_1 > \overline{X}_2$, We can conclude that the particle numbers of the first specimen were larger than that of the second.

5.4. Report writing

Generally speaking, the results report of comparison of two population means should cover statistical description and statistical inference. Report $\overline{X} \pm S$ when the sample comes from a normal distribution and $M(P_{25}–P_{75})$ when the sample comes from a skewed distribution. The contents of statistical inference include α, test statistic, p value and 95% CI. For Example 5.1, we should report as follows.

Two samples meet the assumptions of normal distribution(*Shapiro-Wilk* test: $p_1 = 0.431$, $p_2 = 0.479$) and equal population variances ($F = 1.345$, $p = 0.261$). Thereby, two independent samples t test is performed and the results indicate a statistical difference between two population means at significant level 0.05, $t = 4.137$,

Table 5.6 Average hemoglobin increase in two groups ($\overline{X} \pm S$)

Groups	N	The hemoglobin increase(g/L)
New drug group	10	27.99 ± 4.56
Conventional drug group	10	20.21 ± 3.82

$p = 0.001$. The average hemoglobin increase is higher in new drug group, which could be observed from the $\mu_1 - \mu_2$ and 95% *CI* 7.780 (3.829–11.731).

5.5. Case discrimination

[Case 5.1] The researcher wants to evaluate effect of two drugs on obese patients, and 20 obese patients with BMI$\geq$ 28 kg/m^2 were divided into two groups randomly. The weights before and after 2 months of medication were given in the following table in each groups (See Table 5.7).

(1) The researcher adopted paired *t*test to analyze the changes of pre-post medication of two groups separately. The results showed the difference was significant either in group A ($t = 30.76$, $p = 0.013$) or in group B ($t = 3.701$, $p = 0.005$). It is concluded that two drugs are effective to obese patients.
(2) The researcher performed two independent t test further to compare the mean weight after treatment between two groups ($t = 0.490$, $p = 0.630$). Based on the result, it is concluded the curative effect in the two drugs is not significantly different.

Do you consider the analysis and the conclusion reasonable? Please give your reason.

[Case 5.2] An experiment study designed to explore the influence of hypoxia on HIF-1a,BNIP3 mRNA and protein expression of trophoblast. The mean level and standard deviation for the two samples

Table 5.7 Body weight of obese patients before and after taking medicine (kg)

Medicine		1	2	3	4	5	6	7	8	9	10
A	Before	75.6	61.2	67.8	77.2	73.2	65.4	80.0	74.4	82.6	68.6
	After	71.0	60.2	63.6	72.0	74.6	60.8	69.4	77.4	75.1	59.3
B	Before	69.4	89.9	66.8	63.4	70.0	86.6	90.4	74.8	67.4	84.4
	After	60.8	90.2	56.7	60.3	69.4	78.4	77.5	76.6	58.2	75.4

Table 5.8 The expression nutrient cells HIF-1a, BNIP3 mRNA and protein under hypoxia

Groups	n	HIF-1a mRNA	BNIP3 mRNA	HIF-1a protein	BNIP3 protein
Normoxic	3	1.014 ± 0.204	1.015 ± 0.216	0.576 ± 0.035	0.890 ± 0.055
Anoxic	3	1.118 ± 0.067	1.885 ± 0.455	0.814 ± 0.042	1.321 ± 0.076
t		2.921	1.700	0.518	0.765
P		0.449	0.040	0.002	0.001

were as follows and t test was used to compare the difference. How do you evaluate the analysis procedure?

5.6. Computer experiments

[Experiment 5.1] Using SPSS software to implement two independent sample t test (See electronic resources exp5.1)

[Experiment 5.2] Using SPSS software to implement correction t test (See electronic resources exp5.2)

[Experiment 5.3] Using SPSS software to implement Wilcoxon rank sum test (See electronic resources exp5.3)

[Experiment 5.4] Using SPSS software to implement paired-samples t test (See electronic resources exp5.4)

[Experiment 5.5] Using SPSS software to implement Wilcoxon signed-rank test (See electronic resources exp5.5)

5.7. Frequently asked questions and summary

5.7.1. *Frequently asked questions*

1. Can we conclude that, the smaller the p value is, the larger the mean difference of two samples is while comparing two population means by t test?

A p value is defined as the probability that the computed value of a test statistic is at least as extreme as a specified value of the test statistic when the null hypothesis is true. The smaller the p value is, the more likely we are to refuse the null hypothesis and accept the alternative hypothesis. From the equation of t test, it is easier to discover p value is not only determined by the mean difference of two samples but also the sample size. As long as the sample size is large enough, we can get a smaller p value even with smaller mean difference. So we emphasize that a smaller p value does not imply that the mean difference is large.

2. In view of the fact that it is more likely to perceive the difference by one-sided test than two-sided test, we had better to choose one-sided test. Do you agree with this opinion? Why or why not?

Take 0.05 test level as an example, the critical value with one-sided probability of 0.05 is sure larger than two-sided probability of 0.05 at the same degrees of freedom, so we can perceive the significant difference and then draw the conclusion of rejection. An author may prefer to see this conclusion, but this is not a reason for us to choose one-sided test. Whether one-sided test or two-sided test adopted is based on the research aim and professional background. Using a medical treatment as an example. Suppose there are two groups, one is drug and the other is placebo. The researcher may have sufficient evidence to support a drug performs better than a placebo, then one-sided test, strictly speaking, superiority test can be applied. Suppose two groups represent different drugs, the researcher may have no evidence to prove which drug performs better, then two-sided test will be applied. Two-sided test is applied in most practical situations, exception to pre-market clinical trial.

3. The researcher carried out t test to compare the difference among more than two population means. How do you evaluate the analysis?

This method is inappropriate. There are two fundamental reasons. Firstly, it goes against the study design and cannot compare the overall difference. Secondly, the combination probability of committing type I error will increase to $1-(1-0.05)^n$ (N represents the times of multiple comparisons) if we adopt multiple comparisons using t test. Since the probability of type I error is 0.05 while doing t test each time, let $\alpha = 0.05$.

5.7.2. *Summary*

While comparing the mean of two independent samples, the choice of test statistic dependents on the model assumptions, including normality and homogeneity of variances. Just as we have discussed in the previous section. ① Choose t test when each of two independent random samples have been drawn from a normally distributed population and the two populations have equal variances. ② Choose correction t test when each of two independent random samples has been drawn from a normally distributed population and the two populations have unequal variances. ③ Choose Wilcoxon rank-sum test when at least one sample is not normally distributed.

About the paired samples, the choice of test statistic dependents on the normality of paired-difference. ① Choose paired t test when the difference between pairs of observations comes from a normally distributed population. ② Choose Wilcoxon signed-rank test when the difference between pairs of observations does not come from a normally distributed population.

The statistical significance should not be confused with professional significance and they have notable differences. When $\alpha = 0.05$, we may make statistical conclusion that the difference is significant with $p < 0.05$ and the difference is not significant with $p > 0.05$. Professional significance seek to provide professional explanation for the differences observed in basic medicine/clinical medicine/biology. This margin is actually mean difference, usually pre-specified, which may distinguish patients with different groups or different stages of disease progression. Brief summary, statistical significance is a necessary condition for professional significance.

Think and Practice

1. Best Choice

1. Which one can reflect the margin of the difference while comparing the difference between the two population means? ( )
   A. t value B. p value C. F value D. 95% CI of the mean difference E. none of the above

2. If the data comes from normal distribution and the population variance are not equal in the comparison of two independent sample means, we should apply ( )
A. Wilcoxon rank-sum test. B. correction t test. C. t test. D. paired-samples t test. E. Wilcoxon signed-rank test.
3. The null hypothesis of Wilcoxon rank-sum test can be stated as ( )
A. two sample rank sums are equal. B. two population distributions are the same. C. two sample distributions are the same. D. two population Wilcoxon rank-sum test. E. two population means are equal.
4. The choice for non-parametric test ( )
A. depends on study aim and distribution of the observations. B. can be determined after calculating the test statistic and drawing preliminary conclusions. C. depends on which statistical conclusion satisfy with professional theory. D. depends on which p value is smaller. E. can be used directly in any case since it does not have strict requirements for data.
5. The test statistic T in Wilcoxon rank-sum test is ( )
A. the smaller rank sum. B. the larger rank sum. C. the rank sum corresponding to smaller sample size. D. the rank sum corresponding to larger sample size. E. either one is okay
6. The significant difference in comparing two population means indicate ( )
A. the difference between two population means has practical significance. B. the difference between two sample means has practical significance. C. the difference of two sample/population means has practical significance. D. two population means are significantly different. E. two sample means are significantly different.
7. The null hypothesis of paired t test is ( )
A. two sample means are equal. B. two population means are equal. C. the population mean difference of pairs is 0. D. the median of the difference of pairs is 0. E. the distributions of two populations are the same.

8. Compared with two independent t test, the advantage of Wilcoxon rank-sum test include ( )
   A. wide application. B. higher test power. C. the test result is more accurate. D. making full use of data information. E. the probability of making false negative result is lower.
9. In Wilcoxon rank-sum test, the smallest observation is 0.5, which appears twice in group A and one time in group B. How to assign a rank to the observation 0.5? ( )
   A. assign rank 0.5 to all B. assign rank 2 to all C. assign rank 1 to all D. assign rank 1, 2, and 3 respectively E. assign rank 3 to all
10. Null hypothesis of Wilcoxon signed-rank test is ( )
    A. the distributions of two populations are same. B. two population means are equal. C. the median of the difference of pairs is 0. D. the mean difference of pairs is 0. E. the distributions of two samples are the same.

2. Questions for Reflection

1. How do you compare the difference of two independent samples? Please list the possible methods and their applications.
2. Why should we assign the average rank when the tired observations appear in different groups, however not assign the average rank when the tired observations appear in the same group?
3. What is the relationship and difference between the hypothesis test of two independent sample means and the confidence interval of the difference of the mean?

3. Questions on Calculation

1. The purpose of a study is to examine whether the average weight of the left kidney is the same with the right. The research collected the following data from autopsy specimens. Does this data provide sufficient evidence to allow you to conclude that, in general, the average weight of the left kidney is same with the right? Let $\alpha = 0.05$.

Table 5.9 Weight of kidneys in 16 autopsy specimens(g)

Number	Left kidneys	Right kidneys	Number	Left kidneys	Right kidneys
1	170	150	**9**	105	125
2	155	145	**10**	145	135
3	130	120	**11**	155	150
4	115	100	**12**	110	125
5	235	222	**13**	140	150
6	125	115	**14**	145	140
7	130	120	**15**	95	115
8	105	100	**16**	136	126

An experiment was designed to observe the effect of local hyperthermia on transplanted tumor in mice. The survival time was collected. Does this data provide sufficient evidence to allow you to conclude that the two populations differ with respect to survival time?

Experimental group	10	12	14	15	15	17	18	20	26	80	
Control group	2	3	6	7	8	9	10	12	12	13	30

References

[1] Kang, L, Jia, H. *Medical Statistics* [M]. Beijing: People's Medical Publishing House; 2018.

[2] Xiaosong, L, Feng, C, Yuantao, H, Meina, L. *Health Statistics* [M]. Beijing: People's Medical Publishing House; 2017.

[3] Song, W, Faming, P. *SPSS Statistical Analysis* [M]. Beijing: Tsinghua University Publishing House; 2014.

[4] Wentong, Z. *A Foundation for Statistical Analysis by SPSS.* (3rd ed.) [M]. Beijing: Higher Education Publishing House; 2017.

Yongli Yang and Xuezhong Shi

CHAPTER 6

COMPARISON OF MEANS AMONG MULTIPLE GROUPS

In work, we often encounter the comparison of quantitative data among more than two groups, for which test, Wilcoxon rank-sum test shown in Chapter 5 cannot be used. Instead, we should use one-way analysis of variance (ANOVA) and Kruskal–Wallis test introduced in this chapter. One-way ANOVA is a parametric test, and Kruskal–Wallis test is a non-parametric test, which can be regarded as an extension of Wilcoxon rank-sum test.

6.1. One-way ANOVA

6.1.1. *Case study*

Example 6.1. To study the effect of beverage with tea polyphenols on anti-acute hypoxia, 60 Wistar mice were randomly divided into a control group and the other 3 groups with low, medium, and high doses, 15 mice for each, and treated once a day respectively. The control group was treated by 0.25 mL of distilled water, and the groups with low, medium, and high doses were treated by the beverage at the content of 2.0 g/kg, 4.0 g/kg, 8.0 g/kg dissolved in 0.2–0.3 mL of distilled water, respectively. The hypoxia tolerance survival time was measured for each, and the results were shown in Table 6.1. The purpose of this is to test the differences in effects of different doses of tea polyphenols on prolonging the survival times of mice under hypoxia.

Table 6.1 Hypoxia tolerance survival time of mice in different groups/min

Groups	Hypoxia tolerance survival time (X_{ij})								n_i	$\bar{X}_i$	S_i
Control group ($i = 1$)	21.31	23.14	27.28	19.54	18.03	24.03	22.82	18.72			
	23.46	20.34	26.98	19.56	17.39	24.37	16.01		15	21.545	3.427
Low dose group ($i = 2$)	20.16	24.49	21.32	19.46	25.63	28.81	18.74	18.42			
	26.13	25.24	20.23	22.47	29.38	20.16	22.51		15	22.877	3.556
Medium dose group ($i = 3$)	35.07	28.11	24.74	29.79	22.68	23.01	28.32	29.04			
	24.33	33.97	21.86	28.65	25.13	34.44	31.69		15	28.055	4.381
High dose group ($i = 4$)	30.23	36.84	38.61	27.13	28.79	33.24	31.68	28.29			
	38.47	35.10	28.01	23.37	28.44	34.22	35.08		15	31.833	4.537
Total									60	26.078	5.698

Example 6.2. Some researchers studied the blood lipid levels of government officers in Beijing. After 3 age intervals for Young, Middle, and Old were well defined, 10 male officers were randomly selected in each age interval respectively, and their total cholesterol (TC) levels (mmol/L) were measured. The results were as follows:

Young age group	5.00	4.85	4.93	5.18	4.95	4.78	5.18	4.89	5.07	5.21
Middle age group	5.12	5.13	4.89	5.20	4.99	5.14	5.16	4.98	5.16	5.25
Old age group	5.24	5.26	5.23	5.10	5.31	5.23	5.21	4.98	5.15	5.19

Question: Is there any difference in average content of TC among the 3 age groups?

Analysis: In the study design, Example 6.1 was a completely randomized experimental study, in which the subjects were randomly assigned to different treatment groups. The 4 groups of data could be regarded as 4 samples representing different populations, to infer whether the 4 population means were equal; Example 6.2 was an observational study, and the subjects were randomly selected from 3 groups to measure a certain index for comparison, and to infer whether their population means were equal.

Can we draw a conclusion by using t-test or Wilcoxon rank-sum test in Chapter 5 when comparing quantitative data among multiple groups similar to that we have done in Examples 6.1 and 6.2? No! Because the tests in Chapter 5 can only be used to compare two means at a time, and the probability of making the first type of error is controlled at a prescribed level (i.e., a predetermined value), and the probability of not making the first type of error is $(1 - 0.05) = 0.95$. If one would use t-test to compare 4 groups, then 6 times of t tests were needed; when these tests were carried out independently, the probability of not making first type of error was $0.95^6 = 0.7351$, and the probability of making the first type of error was $1 - 0.7351 = 0.2649$, much higher than prescribed figure 0.05. In theory, with the increase of the times of comparison, the total probability of making the first type of error will increase and tend to 1. Therefore, it is not suitable to use t-test for multiple times. The same problem exists for Wilcoxon rank-sum test.

In research design, the design with only one treatment factor is called single factor design, whose subjects are randomly selected is a completely randomized design. If the univariate data obtained from an experiment with completely randomized design meet the requirements of homogeneity of variance and following normal distributions, then the method called ANOVA can be used, including one-way ANOVA, two-way ANOVA, and multivariate ANOVA. The one-way ANOVA introduced in this section is used to test whether the population means corresponding to different levels of a single factor under a completely randomized design are equal each other.

6.1.2. *The basic idea of ANOVA*

The same basic idea is shared by all types of ANOVA. It will be introduced below through the one-way completely random design.

Supposing the subjects are randomly divided into g groups; the subjects in i-th group receive the i-th treatment ($i = 1, 2, \ldots, g$), the sample size of the i-th group is n_i, and the total sample size is $N(N = \sum n_i)$. X_{ij} is used to indicate the j-th ($j = 1, 2, \ldots, n_i$) observation of the i-th treatment group. $\bar{X}_i$ shows the mean of the

Table 6.2 Expression for the results of an experiment with completely randomized design

Treatment	X_{ij}			
1st treatment group	X_{11}	X_{12}	$\cdots$	X_{1n1}
2nd treatment group	X_{21}	X_{22}	$\cdots$	X_{2n2}
$\vdots$	$\vdots$	$\vdots$	$\vdots$	$\vdots$
g treatment group	X_{g1}	X_{g2}	$\cdots$	X_{gng}

i-th treatment group, $\bar{X}$ stands for the grand mean of the observations. The experimental results are usually summarized by a table like Table 6.2.

1. Decomposition of variation

The basic idea of ANOVA is to make the variation of all observations decomposed into several components according to the design and needs, then analyze respectively. Now we will analyze the data X_{ij} shown in Tables 6.1 and 6.2.

(1) Total variation

The hypoxia tolerance survival times after gavage of 60 Wistar mice were different. This kind variation is called total variation. The variation included both random errors (individual differences and measurement errors in mice) and effects of different treatments (4 different doses of tea polyphenols) on the hypoxia tolerance survival time. It reflected the total variation within the observed values of all individuals. The size was expressed by SS_T, the sum of squares of the total deviation

$$\mathrm{SS}_T = \sum_{i=1}^{g}\sum_{j=1}^{n_i}(X_{ij} - \overline{X})^2 \tag{6-1}$$

From Equation (6-1), we can see that the size of SS_T is related to dispersion of the data, the more dispersion, the greater SS_T; at the same time, SS_T is also related to the number of samples, specifically, to the total degrees of freedom of the sample, $\nu_T = N - 1$.

The bigger ν_T the greater SS_T.

(2) Between-groups variation

Owing to the different levels of treatment, the survival time of the 4 groups may differ (with different sample averages $\bar{X}_i$) and this variation is called between-groups variation. It reflects the differences among the 4 groups of treatment (if the treatments do work) and also includes random errors (including individual differences and measurement errors). The size can be expressed by SS_B, which is the sum of the squared deviation of the sample mean $\bar{X}_i$ from the total mean $\bar{X}$. The formula is

$$\mathrm{SS}_B = \sum_{i=1}^{g} n_i(\overline{X_i} - \overline{X})^2 \tag{6-2}$$

Degree of freedom between groups $\nu_B = g - 1$

It can be seen from Equation (6-2) that when the corresponding population means of the 4 groups are equal, when the 4 groups of data come from the same population, when the mean of each group and the total mean $\bar{X}$ are the point estimates of the same population mean, the differences among them are small and only subject to sampling error, so the variation among groups is small; when the population means corresponding to the 4 different groups are different, when the sample mean of each group is the estimated value of its own population mean, the total mean $\bar{X}$ is the weighted average of the 4 population means. So the difference between the sample mean and the total mean $\bar{X}$ not only contains sampling error, but also contains the estimated value of treatment effect. Therefore, when the 4 population means are different, the variation among groups SS_B will increase.

(3) Within-groups variation

The survival time of hypoxia-tolerant mice within each group was different. This variation was called within-groups variation. The within-groups variation only reflects random error, so it is also called variation of error. The within-groups variation can be expressed by the sum of squares of the differences between the measured values

X_{ij} in the group and the group mean $\bar{X}_i$. The formula is:

$$\mathrm{SS}_W = \sum_{i=1}^{g}\sum_{j=1}^{n_i}(X_{ij} - \overline{X_i})^2 = \sum_{i=1}^{g}(n_i - 1)S_i^2 \tag{6-3}$$

Degree of freedom within groups $\nu_W = N - g$

(4) Decomposition of total variation

$$\begin{aligned}
\mathbf{SS}_T &= \sum_{i=1}^{g}\sum_{j=1}^{n_i}(X_{ij} - \overline{X})^2 = \sum_{i=1}^{g}\sum_{j=1}^{n_i}(X_{ij} - \bar{X}_i + \bar{X}_i - \overline{X})^2 \\
&= \sum_{i=1}^{g}\sum_{j=1}^{n_i}[(X_{ij} - \bar{X}_i)^2 + (\bar{X}_i - \overline{X})^2 + 2(X_{ij} - \bar{X}_i)(\bar{X}_i - \overline{X})] \\
&= \sum_{i=1}^{g}\sum_{j=1}^{n_i}[(X_{ij} - \bar{X}_i)^2 + \sum_{i=1}^{g}\sum_{j=1}^{n_i}(\bar{X}_i - \overline{X})^2 \\
&\quad + \sum_{i=1}^{g}\sum_{j=1}^{n_i}2(X_{ij} - \bar{X}_i)(\bar{X}_i - \overline{X})
\end{aligned}$$

The third item can be proved to be 0:

$$\sum_{i=1}^{g}\sum_{j=1}^{n_i}2(X_{ij} - \bar{X}_i)(\bar{X}_i - \overline{X}) = 2\sum_{i=1}^{g}[(\bar{X}_i - \overline{X})\sum_{j=1}^{n_i}(X_{ij} - \bar{X}_i)]$$

However, $\sum_{j=1}^{n_i}(X_{ij} - \bar{X}_i) = (\sum_{j=1}^{n_i}X_{ij}) - n_j\bar{X}_i = n_j\bar{X}_i - n_j\bar{X}_i = 0$

$$\begin{aligned}
\mathbf{SS}_T &= \sum_{i=1}^{g}\sum_{j=1}^{n_i}(X_{ij} - \overline{X})^2 = \sum_{i=1}^{g}\sum_{j=1}^{n_i}(X_{ij} - \bar{X}_i)^2 + \sum_{i=1}^{g}\sum_{j=1}^{n_i}(\bar{X}_i - \overline{X})^2 \\
&= \sum_{i=1}^{g}\sum_{j=1}^{n_i}(X_{ij} - \bar{X}_i)^2 + \sum_{i=1}^{g}n_i(\bar{X}_i - \overline{X})^2
\end{aligned}$$

It can be seen that the total variation can be partitioned into two parts.

$$\mathbf{SS}_T = \mathbf{SS}_B + \mathbf{SS}_W \tag{6-4}$$

Correspondingly, the total degree of freedom is decomposed into two parts: the degrees of freedom between groups and the degrees of freedom within groups.

$$\nu_T = \nu_B + \nu_W \tag{6-5}$$

2. Comparison of variation

Between-groups variation and within-groups variation are related to degree of freedom, so that they cannot be compared directly. In order to reduce the influence of the degrees of freedom, dividing the sum of squared deviations (SS) by its degrees of freedom, the corresponding mean square (MS) is obtained. The formulas of between-groups mean square and within-groups mean square are:

$$\mathrm{MS}_B = \frac{\mathrm{SS}_B}{\nu_B} \tag{6-6}$$

$$\mathrm{MS}_W = \frac{\mathrm{SS}_W}{\nu_W} \tag{6-7}$$

From Equations (6-3) and (6-7), when there are only two groups, the within-groups mean square is just the combined variance in the t-test for two independent samples, so the within-groups mean square can be understood as the joint estimate of the variance of error, so the within-groups mean square has nothing to do with whether H_0 is true or not.

Statistic F is defined as the ratio of the between-groups mean square divided by within-groups mean square

$$F = \frac{\mathrm{MS}_B}{\mathrm{MS}_W} \tag{6-8}$$

When $H_0 : \mu_1 = \mu_2 = ... = \mu_g$ holds, the samples of each treatment group are from the same population, without the effect of treatment factors, the between-groups variation and within-groups variation are similar, and they only reflect the random error. Since MS_B and MS_W are close, in most cases, F is randomly fluctuating around 1. It can be proved that when H_0 holds, F follows an F distribution with the numerator degree of freedom $\nu_1 = g - 1$ and the denominator degree of freedom $\nu_2 = N - g$. On the contrary, when H_0 does not hold, the means of g groups are not the same, in most cases MS_B will be relatively bigger, while MS_W is unrelated to whether H_0 is true or not, so the corresponding F value will be relatively bigger as well. It is necessary to check the table for F distribution (Table C5) for ANOVA to get the corresponding P values, and then make inference according to the test level α.

In the Table for F distribution, the vertical label is the numerator degree of freedom ν_1, and the horizontal label is the denominator degree of freedom ν_2; given $\alpha = 0.01$ or $\alpha = 0.05$ one can get the critical value $F_{\alpha(\nu_1,\nu_2)}$. If the calculated F value is greater than or equal to $F_{\alpha(\nu_1,\nu_2)}$, then $P \leq \alpha$. In such a case, if H_0 holds, it is almost impossible to have current data, henceforth, we will reject H_0, taking H_1 and concluding that $\mu_1, \mu_2, \ldots, \mu_g$ are not all equal; otherwise, if $P > \alpha$, then we will not reject H_0.

6.1.3. *Steps of ANOVA*

Now we will use Example 6.1 to introduce the steps of one-way ANOVA.

(1) Establish hypotheses and determine test level

H_0: The 4 population means are equal.
H_1: The 4 population means are not all equal (At least one mean is different from the others).
$\alpha = 0.05$

(2) Calculate the test statistics

According to the formula (6.1)∼(6.8), that is, the formula in Table 6.3 and the data on the right side of Table 6.1, the ANOVA table in Table 6.4 can be obtained directly by statistical software SPSS.

$$\begin{aligned}\text{SS}_T &= (21.31 - 26.078)^2 + (23.14 - 26.078)^2 + \cdots \\ &\quad + (35.08 - 26.078)^2 = 1915.800,\end{aligned}$$

$$\nu_T = 60 - 1 = 59$$

Table 6.3 Calculation formula for ANOVA under completely randomized design

Source of variation	Sum of squares of mean deviation SS	Degree of freedom ν	Mean square MS	F value
Between-groups variation	$\sum_{i=1}^{g} n_i(\overline{X_i} - \overline{X})^2$	$g - 1$	$\frac{SS_B}{\nu_B}$	$\frac{MS_B}{MS_W}$
Within-groups variation	$\sum_{i=1}^{g}\sum_{j=1}^{n_i}(X_{ij} - \overline{X_i})^2$	$N - g$	$\frac{SS_W}{\nu_W}$	
Total variation	$\sum_{i=1}^{g}\sum_{j=1}^{n_i}(X_{ij} - \overline{X})^2$	$N - 1$		

Table 6.4 The results of ANOVA

Source of variation	SS	ν	MS	F	P
Between-groups	1017.41	3	339.14	21.14	< 0.01
Within-groups	898.39	56	16.04		
Total	1915.80	59			

$$SS_B = 15 \times (21.545 - 26.078)^2 + \cdots + 15 \times (31.833 - 26.078)^2 = 1017.410,$$

$$\nu_B = 4 - 1 = 3$$

$$SS_W = 1915.800 - 1017.410 = 898.390, \quad \nu_W = 60 - 4 = 56$$

The results of ANOVA are shown in Table 6.4.

(3) Determine the P value and make decision

When $\nu_1 = 3$, $\nu_2 = 56$, Looking up the table for F distribution (Table C5.1), because there is no corresponding value of $F_{0.01(3,56)}$ in the table, using a smaller degree of freedom and closest to 56 instead, we get $F_{0.01(3,50)} = 4.20$, and $P < 0.01$. According to $\alpha = 0.05$, reject H_0, accept H_1; it can be concluded that different doses of tea polyphenol health beverage had different effects on prolonging the average survival time of mice under hypoxia.

with corresponding degrees of freedom.

$$F = \frac{(N-g)\sum_{i=1}^{g} n_i(\overline{Z}_i - \overline{Z})^2}{(g-1)\sum_{i=1}^{g}\sum_{j=1}^{n_i}(Z_{ij} - \overline{Z}_i)^2} \quad \nu_1 = g-1 \quad \nu_2 = N-g \tag{6-9}$$

among which $N = \sum n_i$, g stands for the number of groups, and deviations Z_{ij} is usually calculated by Equation (6-10)

$$Z_{ij} = \left|X_{ij} - \overline{X}_i\right| \tag{6-10}$$

in which $\overline{X}_i$ is the arithmetical average of the i group.

Example 6.3. Please use Levene method to test the homogeneity of variance of materials shown in Example 6.1.

(1) Establishing hypotheses and determining significance levels

H_0: $\sigma_1^2 = \sigma_2^2 = \sigma_3^2 = \sigma_4^2$, The 4 population variances are all equal.
H_1: The 4 population variances are different.
$\alpha = 0.10$

(2) Calculating test statistics

Firstly, the original observation formula X_{ij} (6-10) of Example 6.1 was converted into the corresponding deviation Z_{ij}, and then one-way ANOVA was performed. The detailed calculation steps are omitted here, and only the final calculation results are listed. $F = 0.76$, $P = 0.5253$.

(3) Making a conclusion

$F = 0.76, P = 0.5253$, according to $\alpha = 0.10$, we fail to reject H_0, it can be considered that the 4 population variances are homogeneous.

6.1.6. *Residual graph method for examining preconditions*

Two basic assumptions of variance analysis, especially the simplest, intuitive, and effective method to judge the homogeneity of variance, are residual plots. Variance analysis of data from different design has different formulas for calculating residuals, such as variance analysis of complete randomized design. From Equation (6-3) $SS_W = \sum_i \sum_j (X_{ij} - \bar{X}_i)^2$, the calculation formula of residual is:

$$e_{ij} = X_{ij} - \bar{X}_i \tag{6-11}$$

Figure 6.1 is an example of 6.1 data residual diagram made by computer SPSS software. The longitudinal axis represents the residual, the horizontal axis of Figure 6.1(a) represents the group, and the horizontal axis of Figure 6.1(b) represents the predicted value.

The criterion of judging whether the data conform to the condition of ANOVA from the residual graph is: if the scattered points randomly go up and down the horizontal line of 0, and there is no special structure, there is no abnormal point, it can be considered to meet the requirements. From Figure 6.1, we can roughly estimate that the data of 6.1 satisfy the precondition of variance analysis.

6.1.7. *Data transformation*

For some data which obviously deviate from the conditions of normality and homogeneity of variance, the data can be transformed to meet the requirements of variance analysis, t-test, or other statistical methods. Data transformations, that is, making some function transformation on the original data, change the form of data distribution, but do not change the relationship between groups of data. The disadvantage is that the interpretation of the analysis results is not intuitive. Commonly used data transformation methods are:

1. Logarithmic transformation
   Logarithmic transformation is to take the natural logarithm or commonly used logarithm to the original data. The transformation formula is:

$$X' = \ln(X + a) \tag{6-12}$$

   a equals to 0 or positive. The transformation is applicable to:

   (1) Lognormal distribution data, such as antibody titer data, disease incubation period, pesticide residues in food, vegetables, fruits, etc.

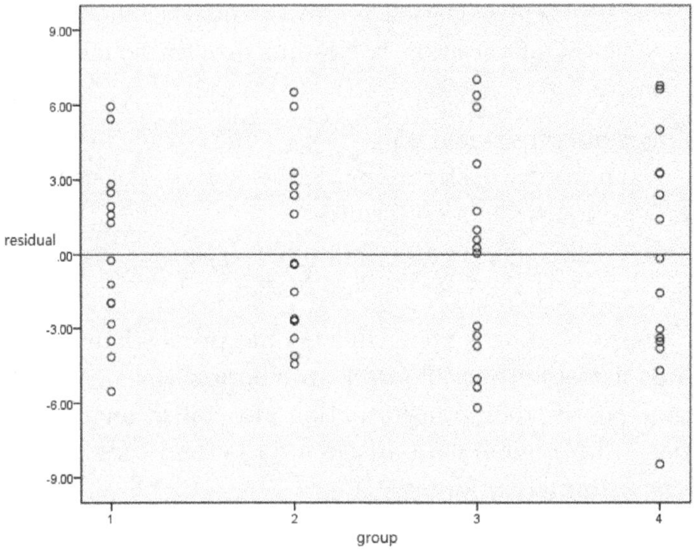

(a)

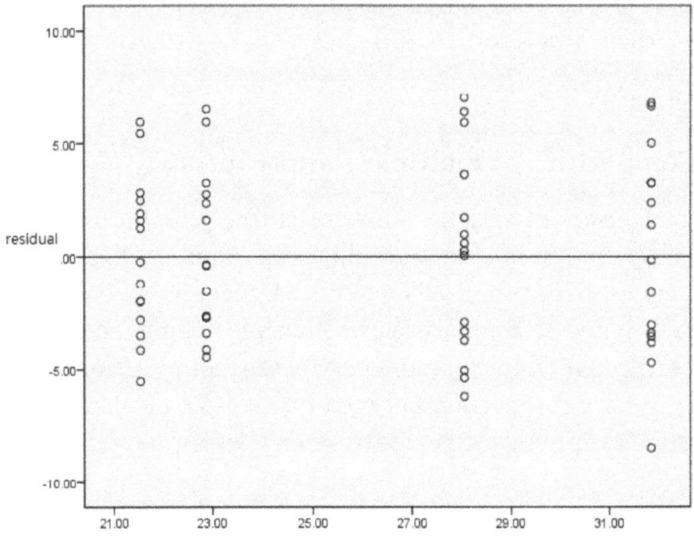

(b)

Figure 6.1 Residual graph of Example 6.1 data

(2) The standard deviation is proportional to the mean, or the coefficient of variation is close to or even equal to a certain constant.

2. Square root transformation
   The square root transformation is the square root of the original data. The transformation formula is

$$X' = \sqrt{X} \quad \text{or} \quad X' = \sqrt{X + 0.5} \tag{6-13}$$

   The transformation is applicable to data proportional to variance, such as data that obey Poisson distribution.
3. Arcsine square root transformation also called angular transformation. The original data are square root and then the anti-sine. The transformation formula is

$$X' = \arcsin \sqrt{X} \tag{6-14}$$

   The transformation is applicable to percentage data such as, $X = 0.46$, then according to (6.14) it can be transformed to $X' = \arcsin \sqrt{0.46} = 0.75$.

6.2. Comparison of multiple sample means

If the conclusion of variance analysis is to reject H_0 but accept H_1, it can only be considered that the total number of populations is not all equal. If you want to know which mean is different, you need to make a pairwise comparison, or multiple comparisons of multiple samples. The pairwise comparison between sample means cannot use the t test of the comparison between two sample means. Here are two commonly used multiple comparison methods.

6.2.1. *LSD-t test*

The least significant difference t-test, is used to test the difference between the mean value of a pair or several pairs of professional items of special significance, whether the total mean of $\bar{d}_{ij} = \bar{X}_i - \bar{X}_j (i \neq j)$ is "0". Even if the results of variance analysis are not enough for us to think that the difference between groups is statistically significant, they can be used for LSD-t test. The LSD-t test is

$$\text{LSD}-t = \frac{|\bar{X}_A - \bar{X}_B|}{S_{X_A - X_B}} = \frac{|\bar{X}_A - \bar{X}_B|}{\sqrt{\text{MS}_W\left(\frac{1}{n_A} + \frac{1}{n_B}\right)}}, \quad v = \nu_{\text{error}} \qquad (6\text{-}15)$$

if LSD-$t \geq t_{\alpha/2,\nu}$, that is when $|\bar{X}_A - \bar{X}_B| \geq t_{\alpha/2,\nu}\sqrt{\text{MS}_W(\frac{1}{n_A} + \frac{1}{n_B})}$, it is thought that according to α standard, the population mean of μ_A and μ_B is different after comparison $t_{\alpha/2,\nu}\sqrt{\text{MS}_W(\frac{1}{n_A} + \frac{1}{n_B})}$ is called minimum meaningful difference, written as LSD. obviously, when the sample size of each group is the same, LSD $= t_{\alpha/2,\nu}\sqrt{\frac{2\text{MS}_W}{n}}$.

In the above formulas, $\bar{X}_A$, $\bar{X}_B$ is the sample mean of two comparison groups. MS_{error} is the mean square of error in the ANOVA, and n_A, n_B is the sample content of the two comparison groups, ν is the degree of error freedom in the ANOVA, and the critical value obtained from the boundary table when the degree of error freedom is the level. When the difference between the two mean is greater than or equal to the time, the difference is statistically significant.

Example 6.4. Making a pairwise comparison of the means of the data shown in Example 6.1 using LSD

H_0: $\mu_A = \mu_B$, the population mean of the two comparison groups is equal.
H_1: $\mu_A \neq \mu_B$, the population mean of the two comparison groups is not equal.
$\alpha = 0.05$

The sample size is equal in each case, so

$$\text{LSD}_{0.05} = t_{0.05/2,56}\sqrt{\frac{2\text{MS}_W}{n}} = 2.000 \times \sqrt{\frac{2 \times 16.043}{15}} = 2.925$$

$$\text{LSD}_{0.01} = t_{0.01/2,56}\sqrt{\frac{2\text{MS}_{\text{error}}}{n}} = 2.660 \times \sqrt{\frac{2 \times 16.043}{15}} = 3.890$$

The absolute value of the mean difference between the comparison groups is compared with LSD. The results are as follows:

$$\left|\bar{X}_{\text{control-group}} - \bar{X}_{\text{low-dose-group}}\right| = |21.545 - 22.877|$$
$$= 1.331 < \text{LSD}_{0.05}, P > 0.05$$
$$\left|\bar{X}_{\text{control-group}} - \bar{X}_{\text{middle-dose-group}}\right| = |21.545 - 28.055|$$
$$= 6.510 > \text{LSD}_{0.01}, P < 0.01$$
$$\left|\bar{X}_{\text{control-group}} - \bar{X}_{\text{high-dose-group}}\right| = |21.545 - 31.833|$$
$$= 10.288 > \text{LSD}_{0.01}, P < 0.01$$
$$\left|\bar{X}_{\text{low-dose-group}} - \bar{X}_{\text{middle-dose-group}}\right| = |22.877 - 28.055|$$
$$= 5.179 > \text{LSD}_{0.01}, P < 0.01$$
$$\left|\bar{X}_{\text{low-dose-group}} - \bar{X}_{\text{high-dose-group}}\right| = |22.877 - 31.833|$$
$$= 8.957 > \text{LSD}_{0.01}, P < 0.01$$
$$\left|\bar{X}_{\text{middle-dose-group}} - \bar{X}_{\text{high-dose-group}}\right| = |28.055 - 31.833|$$
$$= 3.778 > \text{LSD}_{0.05}, P < 0.05$$

According to the $\alpha = 0.05$ standard, except the low dose group and the control group, there were significant differences in prolonging the survival time of hypoxia tolerance between the other groups.

The difference between LSD-t test and two independent sample tests is that in LSD-test, the combined mean square is the error mean square in the ANOVA, and the degree of freedom is the error freedom in the ANOVA. The minimum significant difference method is simple to calculate, but it has some shortcomings, that is, the more the number of comparisons is, the greater the probability of type I error is.

6.2.2. *Bonferroni correction*

If each test level is α', and we conducted m times, when H_0 is true, the cumulative probability of the first type of error is $\alpha'' \leq m\alpha'$.

Set $m\alpha' = \alpha$, then

$$\alpha' = \frac{\alpha}{m} \tag{6-16}$$

It can make the cumulative probability of the first kind of error after multiple comparisons are not exceeding. This is the Bonferroni correction for multiple comparisons. Bonferroni correction is the most conservative of the two-to-two comparisons and is suitable for all two-to-two comparisons, including multiple mean comparisons and multiple frequency comparisons. When the number of comparisons is small, this method is more effective; when the number of comparisons is large, for example, the conclusion is conservative because of the lower selection of test level.

Example 6.5. Please make a pairwise comparison of the 4 population mean of the materials shown in Example 6.1 cases that were considered statistically significant after variance analysis.

(1) Establishing test hypothesis and determining test level

H_0: $\mu_A = \mu_B$, The population mean of any two comparison groups is equal.
H_1: $\mu_A \neq \mu_B$, The population mean of any two comparison groups is not equal.

For the 4 population mean make a pairwise comparison, compare it for $m = C_4^2 = 4(4\text{-}1)/2 = 6$ times and the test level for each comparison is $\alpha' = \alpha/m = 0.05/6 = 0.0083$

(2) Calculating test statistics

According to the result of Equation (6.17) and Example 6.1 list Table 6.5

$$t = \frac{\bar{X}_A - \bar{X}_B}{S_{\bar{X}_A - \bar{X}_B}} = \frac{\bar{X}_A - \bar{X}_B}{\sqrt{\mathrm{MS}_W(\frac{1}{n_A} + \frac{1}{n_B})}} \quad \nu = \nu_{\mathrm{error}} \tag{6-17}$$

among which, $\mathrm{MS}_W = 16.04$ and $\nu_W = 56$ are chosen from the variance analysis table (Table 6.4).

Table 6.5 Pairwise comparison of Example 6.1

Comparison groups A vs. B (1)	Mean difference $\bar{X}_A - \bar{X}_B$ (2)	Standard error $S_{\bar{X}_A - \bar{X}_B}$ (3)	t (4)	P (5)
1 ⇆ 4	−10.2880	1.4625	7.03	<0.001
1 ⇆ 3	−6.5100	1.4625	4.45	<0.001
1 ⇆ 2	−1.3314	1.4625	0.91	0.20∼0.40
2 ⇆ 4	−8.9566	1.4625	6.12	<0.001
2 ⇆ 3	−5.1786	1.4625	3.54	<0.001
3 ⇆ 4	−3.7780	1.4625	2.58	0.01∼0.02

(3) Determine P value, determine the result

The above t values and degrees of freedom 56 are checked in the distribution boundary table (Table C2) to obtain the P values of each comparison group, which are listed in the last column of Table 6.5 (approximated by the corresponding values of degrees of freedom 60 in the distribution boundary table).

According to the $\alpha' = 0.0083$ standard, test 1 and 4, 1 and 3, 2 and 4, 2 and 3, all these tests reject H_0, indicating that there were significant differences between the high-dose group and the control group, the middle-dose group and the control group, the high-dose group and the low-dose group, the middle-dose group and the low-dose group; but there was no significant difference between the low-dose group and the control group, the high-dose group and the middle-dose group.

Example 6.6. Performing ANOVA and Pairwise comparisons to the data shown in Example 6.2

Firstly, the Levene test is used to test the homogeneity of variance, $F = 1.94, P = 0.16$, which means the homogeneity of variance. And the scattered points of the residual graph have no special structure, which accords with the precondition of the ANOVA, so the ANOVA is feasible. The analysis is shown in Table 6.6.

There was a statistically significant difference in the mean TC content among the three age groups ($F = 5.90, P = 0.008$), and further pairwise comparisons showed a statistically significant difference

Table 6.6 6.2 Data on total cholesterol content of male workers in different age groups in Beijing (mmol/L)

Groups	Cases	$\bar{X} \pm S$	F value	P value
Young age group	10	5.00 ± 0.15		
Middle age group	10	5.10 ± 0.11	5.90	0.008
Old age group	10	5.19 ± 0.09		

between the youth group and the elderly group (Bonferroni correction $P < 0.01$, LSD-t test $P = 0.002$) while there was no significant difference between the young age group and the middle age group, the middle age group and the old age group.

6.3. Kruskal–Wallis test

6.3.1. *Comparison of multiple samples*

In the ANOVA, the data need to meet the two basic conditions described in Section 6.1.4. However, the actual scientific research data often cannot meet these conditions, for example, many data for partial peak are distributed, the variance of a group in many groups is too large or too small, observation indicators are ordered classification variables, etc. At this time we cannot use variance analysis, but non-parametric Kruskal–Wallis test can be used. Similar to the Wilcoxon rank-sum test, this method can be regarded as an extension of the Wilcoxon rank-sum test, which can be used to test whether multiple samples come from the same population. The idea of Kruskal–Wallis test to solve the problem of multiple samples is to mix the size $n_1, n_2, \ldots, n_k$ of the sample into a data set, rank the data in the order from small to large, each observation has its own rank in the mixed data set, if there is the same value, then take the average value of the rank. The rank of the observation X_{ij} is R_{ij}, rank sum of all observations in the same group, then we will get $R_i = \sum_j^{n_i} R_{ij}, i = 1, \ldots, g$. If the zero hypothesis (H_0 : g population have the same distribution) holds, the rank of g samples should be evenly distributed, and the deviation between the actual average rank of each sample $\bar{R}_i$ and the average rank of all data $(N+1)/2$ should be small. If a big difference lies in these $\bar{R}_i$, we can reject the null hypothesis. Based on the above principle, the test statistic constructed by K–W test is

$$H = \frac{12}{N(N+1)}\sum_{i=1}^{g} n_i(\bar{R}_i - \bar{R})^2 = \frac{12}{N(N+1)}\sum_{i=1}^{g}\frac{R_i^2}{n_i} - 3(N+1) \tag{6-18}$$

Among which,

$$N = \sum_{i=1}^{g} n_i, \bar{R} = \frac{1}{N}\sum_{i=1}^{k} R_i = \frac{N+1}{2}$$

where R_i is the sum of the ranks of the ith sample, g is represents the number of samples, N is the sum of the sample sizes, and n_i is the size of the ith sample.

It can be verified that the Wilcoxon rank-sum test of the two groups is a special case of the Kruskal–Wallis statistic H in these two groups.

When there is more rank persistence, the test statistic H can be corrected into H_c.

$$H_c = \frac{H}{1 - \sum(t_j^3 - t_j)/(N^3 - N)} \tag{6-19}$$

In the formula, t_j stands for the number j individual.

When the sample size is large, if H_0 is true, H approximately obeys the χ^2 distribution when the degree of freedom equals $g-1$; when the sample size is small, the rank-sum test H boundary table (Schedule C6) can be consulted; if the H value exceeds the boundary value, H_0 can be rejected.

Example 6.7. Four dehydration methods were used for the same sample. Each method was repeated five times. The results are shown in Table 6.7. Is there any difference in the dehydration rate among the 4 methods?

Because this case is percentage data and does not conform to normal distribution, it is not suitable to use variance analysis and Kruskal–Wallis test can be used.

Table 6.7 The dehydration rate among 4 methods

Method 1		Method 2		Method 3		Method 4	
Dehydration rate/%	Rank	Dehydration rate/%	Rank	Dehydration rate/%	Rank	Dehydration rate/%	Rank
1.6	9.5	1.5	6	1.4	5	1.0	1
1.7	14	1.6	9.5	1.6	9.5	1.1	2
1.9	17	1.6	9.5	1.6	9.5	1.2	3
1.9	17	1.7	14	1.7	14	1.3	4
2.0	19.5	2.0	19.5	1.9	17	1.6	9.5
R_i	77		58.5		55		19.5
n_i	5		5		5		5
$\bar{R}_i$	15.4		11.7		11		3.9

(1) Establishing test hypothesis

H_0: The population dewatering rate of the 4 dehydration methods is the same.

H_1: The population dewatering rate of the 4 dehydration methods is different. $\alpha = 0.05$.

(2) Rank: The data of each group will be mixed and ranked from small to large, the same values are assigned an average rank. The rank and rank sum of the 4 groups of unified sorting are shown in Table 6.7

(3) Computation and results are obtained by Equation (6-18):

$$H = \frac{12}{20(20+1)}\left[\frac{77^2}{5} + \frac{58.5^2}{5} + \frac{55^2}{5} + \frac{19.5^2}{5}\right] - 3(20+1) = 9.89$$

Due to the existence of many same ranks, the statistics H in formula (6.19) is modified to statistics H_c.

$$H_c = \frac{H}{1 - \sum(t_j^3 - t_j)/(N^3 - N)}$$

$$= \frac{9.89}{1 - \frac{(6^3-6)+(3^3-3)+(3^3-3)+(2^3-2)}{20^3-20}} = 10.23$$

$$\nu = 4 - 1 = 3$$

(4) Determine the P value, and draw conclusion
According to the χ^2 distribution boundary table (Table C4), $P < 0.05$, the dehydration rates of the 4 dehydration methods are different or different in general distribution according to the $\alpha = 0.05$ standard, reject H_0 but accept H_1.

6.3.2. *Pairwise comparisons among multiple groups*

After Kruskal–Wallis rank-sum test, when the inference is to reject H_0, multiple comparisons between groups are needed to make different inferences about each two population distributions.

Example 6.8. Pairwise comparisons of 4 dehydration rate methods shown in Example 6.7.

(1) Establishing test hypothesis

H_0: The overall distribution of dehydration rate is the same between the i group and the j group.
H_1: The population distribution of dehydration rate is different between the i group and the j group.
$\alpha = 0.05$

(2) Calculating the test statistics and determining the P value when R_i and R_j are set to stand for the rank sum of the i group and the j group, the mean rank difference is $\bar{R}_i$ and $\bar{R}_j$. $\left|\bar{R}_i - \bar{R}_j\right|$ is used to represent the absolute value of the mean rank difference, and the standard deviation of the mean rank difference is

$$\sigma_{\bar{R}_i - \bar{R}_j} = \sqrt{\frac{N(N+1)}{12}\left(\frac{1}{n_i} + \frac{1}{n_j}\right)} \tag{6-20}$$

When the normal approximation method is used, the test statistic is

$$Z_{ij} = \frac{\left|\bar{R}_i - \bar{R}_j\right|}{\sigma_{\bar{R}_i - \bar{R}_j}} \tag{6-21}$$

Table 6.8 Pairwise comparison between 4 groups

Comparison groups (1)	$\lvert\bar{R}_i - \bar{R}_j\rvert$ (2)	$\sigma_{\bar{R}_i-\bar{R}_{j_i}}$ (3)	z_{ij} (4)	P value (5)
Method 1 & 2	3.7	3.74	1.00	0.1587
Method 1 & 3	4.4	3.74	1.18	0.1190
Method 1 & 4	11.5	3.74	3.07	0.0011
Method 2 & 3	0.7	3.74	0.19	0.4247
Method 2 & 4	7.8	3.74	2.09	0.0183
Method 3 & 4	7.1	3.74	1.90	0.0287

The data of Table 6.7 are fitting into Equation (6-21), and the Z_{ij} values of three comparison pairs are obtained respectively.

$$Z_{1,2} = \frac{\lvert\bar{R}_1 - \bar{R}_2\rvert}{\sqrt{\frac{N(N+1)}{12}\left(\frac{1}{n_i} + \frac{1}{n_j}\right)}} = \frac{\lvert 15.4 - 11.7\rvert}{\sqrt{\frac{20(20+1)}{12}\left(\frac{1}{5} + \frac{1}{5}\right)}} = 0.99$$

$Z_{1,3} = 1.18$, $Z_{1,4} = 3.07$, $Z_{2,3} = 0.19$, $Z_{2,4} = 2.09$, $Z_{3,4} = 1.90$

(3) The adjustment of significance level

Pairwise comparisons of 4 samples require Bonferroni correction. Comparison times $m = 4(4-1)/2 = 6$; setting test standard $\alpha = 0.05$, test standard after correction $\alpha' = 0.05/6 = 0.0083$.

The boundary value $Z_{0.0083} = 2.40$ of the multiple tests is obtained from Table C1. When the results were $Z_{ij} \geq 2.40$, deciding whether the difference between the i group and the j group was statistically significant.

The results of pairwise comparison of the data in Tables 6.7 are shown in Tables 6.8. There is no significant difference between the other methods except for the difference between the first method and the fourth method.

6.4. Report writing

When the results of multiple sets of quantitative data are shown, the following contents are usually reported:

(1) Statistical description results of each group.
(2) The type of design and the purpose of hypothesis testing.
(3) Test level and unilateral or bilateral tests.
(4) The hypothesis test method, test statistic and its P value of multiple sets of quantitative data.
(5) Multiple comparison methods and results.

Take Example 7.1 as an example to introduce the writing of the result report.

In order to study the effect of tea polyphenol beverage on acute lack of oxygen, 60 Wistar mouse were randomly assigned to one of 4 treatment groups: control, low-dose, medium-dose. and high-dose, 15 for each. After 40 days, the tolerable length of time for lack of oxygen was measured (Table 7.1). The (mean $\pm$ standard deviation)s of the 4 groups were (21.54 ± 3.43)min, (22.88 ± 3.56)min, (28.06 ± 4.38)min and (31.83 ± 4.54)min respectively. 95% CI for means were (19.47, 23.62), (20.81, 24.95), (25.98, 30.13), (29.76, 33.91) min, respectively.

One-way ANOVA resulted in $F = 21.14$, $P < 0.01$; further analysis with LSD-t test revealed that except length of time of low-dose group was not significantly greater than that of control group, the differences on prolonging the tolerable length of time for lack of oxygen between any other two groups were statistically significant ($P < 0.05$).

6.5. Case discrimination

Case 6.1 The serum luteinizing hormone (IU/L) levels in patients with ovarian dysfunction were determined by gynecology in a hospital. The results are as follows:

Ovarian dysplasia 42.50 38.31 35.76 33.60 31.38

Thalamic amenorrhea 6.71 3.32 4.59 1.67 10.51 2.96 11.82 3.86 8.26 2.63 2.20

Pituitary amenorrhea 4.50 2.75 11.14 5.98 1.90 5.43 11.05 22.03

The researchers conducted pairwise comparisons by means of t-test for 3 times. The conclusion is that the content of luteinizing

Table 6.9 Days of survival after inoculation of 3 different bacteria in mice

Type of bacteria	Cases	$\bar{x} \pm s$	F value	P value
A Bacteria	5	5.40 ± 2.70		
B Bacteria	5	7.20 ± 3.11	4.53	0.034
C Bacteria	5	13.40 ± 6.43		

hormone in serum of ovarian dysplasia is higher than that of thalamic amenorrhea and pituitary amenorrhea. Is this operation proper? Why? What is the right operation?

Case 6.2 A researcher randomly divided 15 mice into three groups to compare the survival days of mice inoculated with three different bacteria. The experimental data are as follows

A Bacteria	2	4	5	7	9
B Bacteria	4	5	7	8	12
C Bacteria	8	9	10	17	23

The researchers analyzed the data by ANOVA (Table 6.9), and then LSD test showed that there were significant differences between C and A bacteria, C and B bacteria, but no significant differences between B and C bacteria.

Is this statistical processing correct? Why? What is the right thing to do?

Case 6.3 Three drugs were used to kill *Oncomelania hupensis* in a certain area, and 200 live *O. hupensis* were used each time. The mortality rate of each batch of *O. hupensis* was counted as follows (%):

I	46.5	39.5	40.5	32.5	49.5	30.0
II	36.0	29.0	20.5	22.5	16.5	26.0
III	24.0	8.5	9.2	6.5		

The researchers analyzed the data directly by variance analysis, $F = 17.06, P < 0.001$; and then corrected by Bonferroni, the effects of the three drugs differed from one another ($P < 0.05$).

Is this statistical processing correct? Why? What is the right thing to do?

6.6. Computer experiments (See exp6-1 to exp6-3 in digitized resource)

Experiment 6.1 Variance analysis for the data of Example 6.1 by SPSS

To master variance analysis of multiple sets of quantitative data and pairwise comparison of mean by SPSS.

Experiment 6.2 Kruskal–Wallis analysis for the data of Example 6.3 by SPSS

To master implementation of Kruskal–Wallis rank-sum test for multiple sets of quantitative data by SPSS.

6.7. Frequently asked questions and summary

6.7.1. *Frequently asked questions*

1. Why is it not suitable for direct analysis of multiple quantitative data?

The data of variance analysis should satisfy two premises: (1) each sample is independent random sample and obeys normal distribution; (2) the total variance of each sample is equal, that is, homogeneity of variance. Therefore, in the ANOVA for multiple groups of quantitative data, the homogeneity of variance and the normality of each sample should be tested first, then the ANOVA should be carried out and further pairwise comparisons should be made if necessary. Otherwise, if the condition of variance analysis is not satisfied, data transformation is needed to satisfy the condition of variance analysis, or Kruskal–Wallis rank-sum test should be selected.

2. If the comparison of the mean of three samples by ANOVA has statistical significance, in multiple comparisons appeared the "$\mu_1 = \mu_2$ no rejection, $\mu_1 = \mu_3$ no rejection, but reject $\mu_2 = \mu_3$" results, how to explain the results? Why?

According to the basic principle of hypothesis testing, the result can be interpreted in this way: there is reason to believe $\mu_2 \neq \mu_3$, but there is no reason to believe $\mu_1 \neq \mu_2$ and $\mu_1 \neq \mu_3$. Because statistical conclusions are established in a certain probability sense, they cannot be recursively determined in a deterministic mathematical way. The result can neither be interpreted as: μ_1 is between μ_2 and μ_3; nor will the result be interpreted like the following: if $\mu_2 = \mu_1$, and $\mu_1 = \mu_3$, then $\mu_2 = \mu_3$.

3. Whether is it necessary to find statistical significance after ANOVA, and then make pairwise comparisons of the mean?

Generally speaking, when statistical significance is found using ANOVA, then pairwise comparison between the means should be made, but not absolute. When statistical significance is found using ANOVA, making pairwise comparisons between the mean values later are unplanned comparisons. There are many methods of mean pairwise comparisons, perhaps more than ten kinds, but these methods are not mature. Some statistics experts suggest that some multiple comparisons should not depend on the results of ANOVA. In addition, there are conditions that the data are statistically significant with ANOVA, but not statistically significant with pairwise comparisons, or the data is not statistically significant with ANOVA and some means are statistically significant with pairwise comparisons, these two phenomena often occur in the condition that P value is close to the prescribed α level, it should be particularly careful to make the conclusion.

4. There are many multiple comparison methods. Is it possible to use all kinds of methods? Is it reasonable that we report the results of the method with a good P value?

There are many methods of multiple comparisons, and even some statistical results are inconsistent when using multiple comparisons, which actually involves the choice of pairwise comparisons of multiple means. Various methods are used, and selective reporting P value is inappropriate. Pairwise comparisons should be selected according to the purpose of the study. In confirmatory studies, it is advisable to plan pairwise comparisons between certain means at the design stage based on research purposes. For example, LSD or Dunnett tests are optional. LSD method is more sensitive, but the first kind of error may increase, suitable for research whose groups are smaller and only interested in some specific groups; Dunnett test is suitable for multiple comparisons of mean differences between $k - 1$ experimental groups and one control group. Bonferroni correction method or SNK-q test is often used in exploratory research when multiple mean pairwise comparisons are decided only after several hints of unequal mean are obtained by hypothesis testing without prior consideration or expectation at the research and design stage. SNK-q test is often used to compare the two mean values of multiple samples; Bonferroni method is simple and widely used in different occasions, but the conclusion is conservative.

6.7.2. *Summary*

1. The comparison between three or more means can be made by using ANOVA to test whether multiple samples come from the same population; it can also be used in the bilateral test between two means, where the result is completely equivalent to the t−test; this chapter introduces the simplest one-way ANOVA in ANOVA, which can be used in the complete random design, the experimental study and the observational study of multiple general random sampling.
2. The basic idea of variance analysis is to compare the mean variance of the treatment groups with the mean variance of the standard error. For completely random design data, the sum of squared deviations and their degrees of freedom of all observations are decomposed into two parts: inter-group variation and intra-group variation, which are explained respectively by processing factors and random errors. By comparing the mean squares of different sources of variation, statistical inferences are made with the help of F distribution to infer whether treatment factors have an impact on the experimental results.
3. The thought for comparing multiple sets of quantitative data: first, homogeneity of variance and normality test of various samples.

If it fits the homogeneity of variance, and all samples were subject to normal distribution, we choose one-way ANOVA. There are usually two ways to deal with the data which obviously deviate from normality and homogeneity of variance: one is to improve its hypothesis by some form of data transformation; the other is to use Kruskal–Wallis rank-sum test instead of parametric statistical method. If the ANOVA or rank-sum test results are statistically significant, it is necessary to select the appropriate method (such as Bonferroni, LSD method, etc.) for pairwise comparison.

Think and Practice

I. Questions for Reflection

1. What are the basic ideas and application conditions of variance analysis?
2. What is the basic process of statistical processing when comparing multiple sets of quantitative data?

II. Questions on Calculation

1. According to Table 6.10, does typhoid or pertussis vaccination after infection with poliovirus in rats affect survival days? If the answer is positive, make a multiple comparison (compared to the control group).
2. 18 patients with epidemic encephalitis B were randomly divided into three groups, using monoclonal antibodies, thymic peptides, and Ribavirin treatment, the observation index is fever clearance time after treatment, the results are shown in Table 6.11.

Table 6.10 Survival days of each group of rats after vaccination (days)

Groups	Days to live (d)									
Control	8	9	10	10	10	11	12	12	14	16
Typhoid	5	7	8	9	9	10	10	11	11	12
Pertussis	6	6	7	8	8	9	9	10	10	11

Table 6.11 Fever clearance time of three treatment groups of epidemic encephalitis B patients

Treatment group	Fever time/day					
Monoclonal antibody group	0	2	0	0	5	9
Thymic peptide group	32	13	6	7	10	2
Ribavirin group	0	11	15	11	3	1

Question: Are there any differences between the three groups of treatment outcomes?

Jiu Wang, Hongwei Sun

CHAPTER 7

COMPARISON OF DISTRIBUTIONS OF CATEGORICAL VARIABLES

Qualitative variables refer to unordered categorical variables and ordered categorical variables. For example, blood type (A, B, O, AB), and gender (male, female) are unordered categorical variables, and efficacy (cure, improvement, inefficacy, death) and drug dose (high dose, medium dose, low dose) are ordered categorical variables. This chapter introduces the comparison methods commonly used for data of qualitative variables.

7.1. Basic concepts of the chi-square test

7.1.1. *Examples*

Example 7.1. To compare the effectiveness of venlafaxine and fluoxetine in the treatment of senile depression, 60 patients with similar conditions were randomly divided into two groups and treated with two drugs, respectively. The results are shown in Table 7.1.

A qualitative variable, namely treatment effect, is involved in Table 7.1, and it takes "value" either effect or not effect. The question we are going to address now is whether the overall effective rates of the two medications are the same or not. This type of problem is usually solved by the chi-square test.

Example 7.2. Peripheral blood and venous blood samples were collected for hepatitis b antigen test. To compare the overall positive rate of the 2 samples, please refer to Table 7.2.

Table 7.1 Comparison of efficacy of venlafaxine and fluoxetine in the treatment of depression

Groups	Effect n (%)	Not effect n (%)	Total
Venlafaxine	19 (63.33)	11 (36.67)	30
Fluoxetine	15 (50.00)	15 (50.00)	30
Total	34 (56.67)	26 (43.33)	60

Table 7.2 Results of hepatitis b antigen tests for peripheral blood and venous blood (case number)

	Peripheral blood		
Venous blood	Positive	Negative	Total
Positive	47	3	50
Negative	7	243	250
Total	54	246	300

Example 7.2 is subject to the paired design. The paired results of hepatitis b antigen tests for peripheral blood and venous blood of each patient can be summarized into Table 7.2. In order to compare the overall positive rates between the 2 samples, peripheral blood and venous blood, the paired chi-square test is usually used.

Example 7.3. The three preparations of fosfomycin were used to treat the patients with skin and soft tissue infection. To study whether the three preparations had the same overall cure rate or not, the observed data are shown in Table 7.3.

The outcome measure in Table 7.3 is a qualitative variable, which may take one of two possible "values": cure or not cure. And there are 3 groups, ointment-A group, ointment-B group and powder group. In general, to compare the data of a qualitative variable among more than 2 groups, chi-square tests are usually used; and in case there exists significant difference, appropriate pairwise comparisons may be performed accordingly.

Table 7.3 Effects of different preparations of fosfomycin on skin and soft tissue infection

Preparation	No. of cured	No. of not cured	Total	Cure rate (%)
Ointment-A	47	19	66	71.21
Ointment-B	24	1	25	96.00
Powder	159	44	203	78.33

Table 7.4 Occupational distributions of the three ethnic samples (number of cases)

	Occupation				
Nationality	Cadre	Worker	Farmer	Others	Total
Han	20	56	62	7	145
Hui	14	40	32	11	97
Man	18	28	45	8	99
Total	52	124	139	26	341

Example 7.4. To study the occupational distributions of Han, Hui, and Man residents, three ethnic samples of 145, 97, and 99 people were surveyed. The results are shown in Table 7.4.

In Table 7.4, the qualitative variable "occupation" has four possible "values": cadre, worker, farmer, and others; and there are 3 frequency distributions within 3 groups of Han, Hui, and Man, respectively. The aim was to compare the occupational distributions of different ethnic groups. For unordered multi-category data like those in Table 7.4, the chi-square test is usually used to compare different groups.

7.1.2. *Distribution of chi-square*

Chi-square distribution is a probability distribution of a continuous random variable (Figures 7.1 and 7.2). If random variables $X_1, X_2, \cdots, X_n$ independently follow standard normal distribution respectively, then random variable $Y = \sum_{i=1}^{n} X_i^2$ follows the chi-square distribution with degree of freedom n, denoted as $Y \sim \chi^2(n)$.

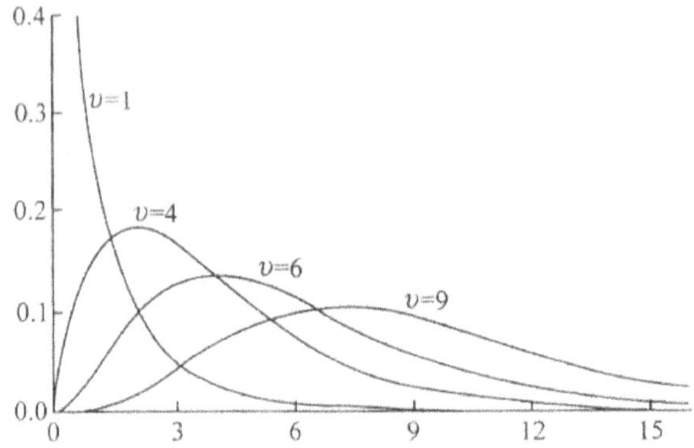

Figure 7.1 The probability density curves of the chi-square distribution ($v = 1, 4, 6, 9$)

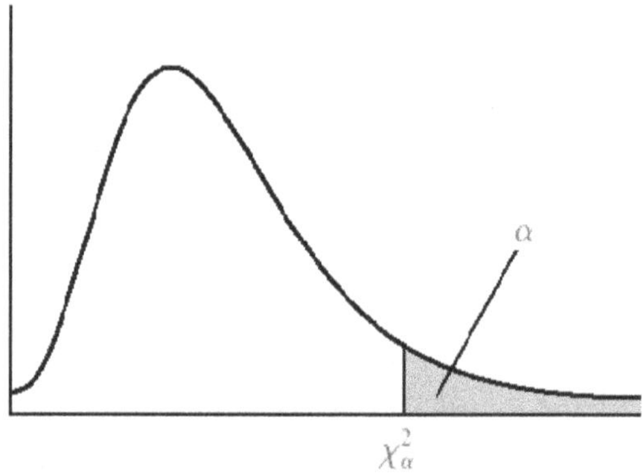

Figure 7.2 Critical value of the chi-square distribution

The shape of the chi-square distribution depends on the degree of freedom. The critical value of chi-square distribution with degree of freedom v is denoted as $\chi^2_\alpha(v)$ or $\chi^2_{\alpha,v}$ (Appendix Table C1.4).

7.1.3. *Basic concept of chi-square tests*

The chi-square (denoted as χ^2) test examines differences in rates or proportions. The main components are as follows:

Null hypothesis (H_0): There are no differences between the two population rates (or proportions).

Alternative hypothesis (H_1): There are some differences between the two population rates (or proportions).

To determine whether there is a difference between the two population rates (or proportions), we can calculate the chi-square (χ^2) statistic, using the following formula:

$$\chi^2 = \sum \frac{(\text{Observed} - \text{Expected})^2}{\text{Expected}} \qquad v = (R-1)(C-1) \qquad \text{(7-1)}$$

A chi-square statistic which reflects the deviation between the observed and theoretical frequencies can be calculated using Formula (7-1). And the v can also be calculated: where R is the number of rows and C is the number of columns.

Note: This formula measures the difference between the observed and expected frequencies under the condition that null hypothesis is true. The larger the difference between the two values is, the larger the chi-square statistic will be and the more likely the observed patterns will be to have a statistically significant difference from the expected patterns. In the minimum limit, if all observed values equal the expected values, then the chi-squared statistic simply equals 0. It has been demonstrated that when null hypothesis is true, the chi-square statistic approximately follows the chi-square distribution.

7.2. Two samples chi-square tests

7.2.1. *Two-independent samples chi-square tests*

The data for chi-square tests are summarized using cross tabulations as shown in Table 7.1. These tables are sometimes called frequency or contingency tables. Table 7.5 is called a 2×2 table with four cells (or fourfold table) because each variable has two levels.

In a fourfold table, one variable (usually the treatment) forms the rows and the other variable (usually the attribute) forms the columns. For example, the treatment (venlafaxine, fluoxetine) would form the rows and the effect (yes, no) would form the columns in Table 7.1. The four internal cells of the table show the counts for each of the attribute/treatment groups; for example, cell "a" shows the number who satisfy treatment A and effective (attribute positive).

Table 7.5 General form of a fourfold table

Treatment	Attribute Positive	Negative	Total
A	a	b	$n_1 = a + b$
B	c	d	$n_2 = c + d$
Total	$m_1 = a + c$	$m_2 = b + d$	$n = a + b + c + d$

As mentioned previously, chi-square tests are used to test whether the frequency of an attribute in 2 independent groups is significantly different in case of large sample size.

Table 7.5 is the data of two sample frequencies. First, assume that

Null hypothesis: The proportions of effect in the venlafaxine group and the fluoxetine group are the same. $\pi_1 = \pi_2$

Alternative hypothesis: The proportions of effect in the two groups are different. $\pi_1 \neq \pi_2$

Under the assumption of null hypothesis, the overall proportion of the 2 groups should be approximately equal to the combined estimated frequency $\pi \approx m_1/n$. Thus, the positive expected count of group i is calculated as $T_{i1} = n_i\pi = n_i m_1/n$, and the negative expected count of group i is calculated as $T_{i2} = n_i(1-\pi) = n_i m_2/n$.

The expected count of each cell in the fourfold table, also known as the theoretical frequency, T_{ij}, is calculated by the following formula:

$$T_{ij} = \frac{n_i m_j}{n} \quad (i = 1, 2;\ j = 1, 2) \tag{7-2}$$

where n is the sample size, n_i is the sum of the cases in row i, and m_j is the sum of the cases in column j.

If the sample size, n, is greater than or equal to 40 and the smallest theoretical frequency, T_{ij}, is greater than or equal to 5, then the special formula for Pearson's chi-square statistic is as follows

$$\chi^2 = \frac{(ad - bc)^2 \cdot n}{(a+b)(c+d)(a+c)(b+d)} \tag{7-3}$$

A correction would be made to the calculation of Pearson's chi-square (Yates continuity correction) in case of sample size, n, is greater than or equal to 40, and the smallest theoretical frequency is $1 \leq T_{ij} < 5$. Continuity correction formula for the chi-square statistic of a fourfold table data:

$$\chi^2 = \frac{(|ad - bc| - 0.5n)^2 n}{(a+b)(c+d)(a+c)(b+d)} \tag{7-4}$$

When $n < 40$ and theoretical frequency $T_{ij} < 1$, then an alternative procedure called Fisher's exact probabilities should be used for 2×2 tables. Although this method does not belong to the chi-square test category, it can be supplementary to the chi-square test.

The fourfold table of the four elements of a, b, c, and d is stochastic, since the total values of the rows and columns are fixed. The null hypothesis states that the observed frequencies or more extreme frequencies can occur by chance.

When H_0 holds with a fixed number of total values (row and column), the probability is:

$$P_i = \frac{(a+b)!(c+d)!(a+c)!(b+d)!}{a!b!c!d!n!} \tag{7-5}$$

where P_i is the probability of the i-th fourfold table, and a, b, c, and d are the four observed frequencies of the i-th fourfold table.

The P value of a statistical hypothesis test is "the probability of getting a value of the present or more extreme than that observed by chance alone, if the null hypothesis is true."

Resolution

In Example 7.1, theoretical frequencies T_{ij} can be calculated: $T_{11} = 17$, $T_{12} = 13$, $T_{21} = 17$, $T_{22} = 13$ using Formula (7.2). The sample size n is greater than 40 and all theoretical frequencies T_{ij} are greater than 5. Therefore, the chi-square statistic can be calculated according to Formula (7-3).

The following steps show the chi-square test for Example 7.1:

(1) Set the hypotheses and the test level.

Null hypothesis: $\pi_1 = \pi_2$, the overall effective rates of the two medications are the same.

Alternative hypothesis: $\pi_1 \neq \pi_2$, the overall effective rates of the two medications are different.

$\alpha = 0.05$

(2) Calculate the chi-square statistic.

The chi-square statistic is $\chi^2 = 1.086$, and the degree of freedom v is equal to 1.

(3) Calculate the P value and make a conclusion.

Check the critical value corresponding to $\nu = 1$ (Appendix Table C1.4), $\chi^2_{0.05,1} = 3.84$. Since the larger the value is, the smaller the probability P value is, in this case $\chi^2 = 1.086 < \chi^2_{0.05,1}$, so $P > 0.05$.

At the test level of $\alpha = 0.05$, null hypothesis could not be rejected, and the difference is not statistically significant. Therefore, the efficacy of venlafaxine and fluoxetine in the treatment of senile depression could not be considered to be different.

7.2.2. *Paired design chi-square tests*

Example 7.2 was subject to the paired design. The objective was to compare the overall positive rates between the 2 samples, peripheral blood and venous blood. Such data form is called a paired fourfold table, and its general form is shown in Table 7.6.

To compare the population proportions of the paired samples, rather than independent samples, McNemar's test formula should be used.

McNemar's test is generally used when the data consist of paired observations. As shown in Table 7.6, the frequencies "a" and "d" are the numbers of consistent test, while the frequencies "b" and "c" are the numbers of inconsistent test. Therefore, it is only necessary to examine whether the data "b" and "c" are the same or not to test the difference of population proportions between two paired samples.

Table 7.6 General form of paired design 2 × 2 contingency table

	Variable 2		
Variable 1	+	−	Total
+	a	b	$n_1 = a + b$
−	c	d	$n_2 = c + d$
Total	$m_1 = a + c$	$m_2 = b + d$	$n = a + b + c + d$

When $b + c \geq 40$, Formula (7-6) can also be used to calculate the McNemar's chi-square statistic:

$$\chi^2 = \frac{(b - c)^2}{b + c} \qquad v = 1 \tag{7-6}$$

When $b + c < 40$, use Formula (7-7) to calculate the McNemar's chi-square statistic:

$$\chi^2 = \frac{(|b - c| - 1)^2}{b + c} \qquad v = 1 \tag{7-7}$$

Resolution

(1) Establish the test hypotheses and set the test level.

Null hypothesis: $\pi_1 = \pi_2$, the positive rates tested by two kinds of methods are the same.

Alternative hypothesis: $\pi_1 \neq \pi_2$, the positive rates tested by two kinds of methods are different.

$\alpha = 0.05$

(2) Calculate the test statistics

In Table 7.2, $b + c = 3 + 7 = 10 < 40$, Formula (7-7) should be used to calculate statistic:

$$\chi^2 = \frac{(|b - c| - 1)^2}{b + c} = \frac{(|3 - 7| - 1)^2}{3 + 7} = 0.90, \quad v = 1$$

(3) Calculate the P value and make a conclusion.

Check the critical value corresponding to degree of freedom 1 (Appendix Table C1.4), $\chi^2_{0.05,1} = 3.84$. In this case $\chi^2 = 0.90 < \chi^2_{0.05,1}$, therefore $P > 0.05$.

At the test level of $\alpha = 0.05$, H_0 cannot be rejected, and the difference is not statistically significant. There is no significant difference in the positive rate of HBsAg between peripheral blood and venous blood.

7.3. Chi-square tests for $R \times 2$ tables

The objective of Example 7.3 is to test whether the overall cure rates of the 3 groups are the same or not. Table 7.3 can be collated into a $R \times 2$ contingency table, where R is the number of rows. The general form is shown in Table 7.7.

In general, chi-square tests are used to compare such data of a qualitative variable among more than 2 groups. And in case there exists significant difference, appropriate pairwise comparison may be performed accordingly.

In a chi-square test for $R \times 2$ contingency table, the theoretical frequency cannot be smaller than 1. Moreover, any theoretical frequencies below 5 cannot exceed 1/5 of cells. Otherwise, the contiguous rows or columns must be combined with smaller frequencies to

Table 7.7 Completely random design of $R \times 2$ contingency table (frequency)

	Attributes		
Groups	1	2	Total
1	A_{11}	A_{12}	n_1
2	A_{21}	A_{22}	n_2
...	...	...	...
R	A_{R1}	A_{R2}	n_R
Total	m_1	m_2	n

avoid throwing off the rows or columns with the smaller frequencies. Another alternative is to use Fisher's exact test. However, the best method is to increase the sample size.

Resolution

(1) Set the hypotheses and the test level.

Null hypothesis: $\pi_1 = \pi_2 = \pi_3$, that is, the overall cure rates of the three preparations are the same.

Alternative hypothesis: Not all of π_1, π_2, and π_3 are equal, that is, not all of the overall cure rates of the three preparations are the same.

$$\alpha = 0.05$$

(2) Calculate the chi-square statistic.

The overall cure rates of each group are the same, which should be approximately equal to the mean cure rate when the null hypothesis is true. Formula (7-1) can still be used for the $R \times 2$ contingency table, and Formula (7-2) is used for the calculation of theoretical frequency.

A formula for $R \times 2$ contingency tables can be derived as the following from Formula (7-1):

$$\chi^2 = n\left(\sum_{i=1}^{R}\sum_{j=1}^{2}\frac{A_{ij}^2}{n_i m_j} - 1\right) \tag{7-8}$$

where n is the sample size, A_{ij} is the actual frequency of each cell, n_i is the total count of the row i, m_j is the total count of the column j, and R is the number of rows.

The degrees of freedom can be calculated as

$$v = (R - 1)(C - 1) \tag{7-9}$$

Example 7.3 meets the application conditions of Formula (7-8), and the statistic calculated is $\chi^2 = 6.454$, and degree of freedom $v = (3 - 1)(2 - 1) = 2$.

(3) Calculate the P value and make a conclusion.

Check the critical value corresponding to $df = 2$ (Appendix Table C1.4), $\chi^2_{0.05,2} = 5.99$. χ^2=6.545 > $\chi^2_{0.05,2}$, therefore, $P < 0.05$.

At the test level of $\alpha = 0.05$, reject null hypothesis and accept alternative hypothesis, the difference is statistically significant, and it can be concluded that the overall cure rates of the three preparations are different.

For the chi-square test for multiple independent samples, the rejection of null hypothesis indicates that not all of the overall recovery rates of each group are the same. To test which two groups differ, appropriate pairwise comparison should be performed accordingly.

To avoid the increase of type I error, Bonffroni method is used to calibrate the level of test in pairwise comparison of multiple group proportions. If the original test level is α, and k times (the maximum value of k is $R(R-1)/2$, that is, comparisons are made between each two groups) pairwise comparisons needs to be made between R groups, then the test level of pairwise comparison should be $\frac{\alpha}{k}$.

In Example 7.3, three times pairwise comparisons are required for 3 groups. The original test level is $\alpha = 0.05$, the test level of the pairwise comparisons should be $\alpha = 0.05/3 = 0.0167$, and the test results are shown in Table 7.8.

Table 7.8 Pairwise comparison of the overall cure rates of the three preparations

Control group	Fourfold	Table	χ^2	P	Test result
Ointment-A and ointment-B	47 24	19 1	6.497	0.011	*
Ointment-A and powder	47 159	19 44	1.409	0.236	—
Ointment-B and powder	24 159	1 44	(correction)	0.067	—

the "*" indicates that the difference is statistically significant; and the "—" indicates that the difference is not statistically significant.

Thus, the overall cure rates of the ointment-A group and the ointment-B group are different.

7.4. Chi-square tests for $R \times C$ tables

7.4.1. *Chi-square tests for unordered $R \times C$ tables*

Example 7.4 is subject to unordered multi-category data. Generally, if a qualitative variable has C possible "values," with frequency distribution of R independent groups, then it can be collated into an $R \times C$ contingency table (Table 7.9).

According to the type of grouping variables and the objective of the study, $R \times C$ contingency tables can be divided into: unordered contingency tables, one-way ordered contingency tables, and two-way ordered contingency tables. Different analytical methods are used for different types of data or different analytical purposes.

Example 7.4 surveys the occupational distributions of Han, Hui, and Man residents. The aim is to compare the occupational distributions of different ethnic groups. The qualitative variables "nationality" and "occupation" are unordered multi-category data. The chi-square test of unordered multi-categorical data should be used.

For the unordered contingency table data, the chi-square test for the frequency distribution among multiple samples can be performed according to Formula (7-1), and its v follows Formula (7-9).

Table 7.9 General form of an $R \times C$ contingency table

	Attributes (or levels)				
Groups	1	2	⋯	C	Total
1-st group	A_{11}	A_{12}	⋯	A_{1C}	n_1
2-nd group	A_{21}	A_{22}	⋯	A_{2C}	n_2
⋯	⋯	⋯	⋯	⋯	⋯
R-th group	A_{R1}	A_{R2}	⋯	A_{RC}	n_R
Total	m_1	m_2	⋯	m_C	n

Formula (7-1) is also called the fundamental formula for the contingency tables, which can be modified to Formula (7-10), also called the general equation, for unordered contingency table data:

$$\chi^2 = n\left(\sum_{i=1}^{R}\sum_{j=1}^{C}\frac{A_{ij}^2}{n_i m_j} - 1\right) \tag{7-10}$$

where n is the sample size, n_i is the total of the i-th row, m_j is the total count of the j-th column, and A_{ij} is the actual frequency of the i-th row and the j-th column.

Resolution

The chi-square test for Example 7.4 can be performed using the fundamental formula.

(1) Set the hypotheses and the test level.

Null hypothesis: The overall occupational proportions among the three ethnic groups are the same.

Alternative hypothesis: The overall occupational proportions among the three ethnic groups are different or not all the same.

$\alpha = 0.05$.

(2) Calculate the test statistic.

$\chi^2 = 8.80$ and degree of freedom $v = (3-1)(4-1) = 6$ according to Formula (7-1).

(3) Calculate the P value and make a conclusion.

Check the critical value corresponding to $df = 6$ (Appendix Table C1.4), $\chi^2_{0.05,6} = 12.59$. In this case $\chi^2 = 8.80 < \chi^2_{0.05,6}$, therefore, $P > 0.05$.

At the test level of $\alpha = 0.05$, null hypothesis cannot be rejected and the difference is not statistically significant. It can be concluded that the overall occupational proportions among the three ethnic groups are the same.

In a chi-square test for $R \times C$ contingency tables, the theoretical frequency cannot be smaller than 1. Moreover, any theoretical frequencies below 5 cannot exceed 1/5 of cells. Otherwise, the contiguous rows or columns must be combined with smaller frequencies to avoid throwing off the rows or columns with the smaller frequencies. Another alternative is to use Fisher's exact test. However, the best method is to increase the sample size.

The theoretical frequencies of Example 7.4 are 22.1, 52.7, 59.1, 11.1, 14.8, 35.3, 39.5, 7.4, 15.1, 36.0, 40.4, and 7.5, respectively. All theoretical frequencies are greater than 5.

7.4.2. *Chi-square tests for ordered $R \times C$ tables*

Example 7.5. To compare the efficacy of three therapies, 400 patients were randomly assigned to three treatment groups, and the efficacy data were collected and shown in columns (1)–(5) of Table 7.10.

An ordered variable, namely treatment effect, is involved in Table 7.10, and it takes "value" not effect, improved, excellent, or cure. The grouping variable is unordered. Table 7.10 is a one-way ordered contingency table. The question we are going to address now is whether the overall efficacy of the three treatments is the same or not. This type of problem is usually solved by the rank-sum test.

During the rank-sum test for ordered multi-category data, firstly uniformly rank the data and compute the rank sum, and then the H value statistic can to be calculated according to Formula (7-11):

$$H = \frac{12}{N(N+1)} \sum \frac{R_i^2}{n_i} - 3(N+1) \tag{7-11}$$

where $N = \sum n_i$ is the sample size; n_i is the number of observations for group i; R_i is the rank sum of group i.

Formula (7-11) is appropriate for the cases of few ties or no ties; otherwise, the corrected H_c value should be calculated by Formula (7-12).

$$H_c = \frac{H}{c} \tag{7-12}$$

where $c = 1 - \sum (t_j^3 - t_j)/(N^3 - N)$, t_j is the number of the same ranks at the j-th time.

Table 7.10 Comparison of efficacy of three treatment groups

Efficacy	Number of cases				Rank scope	Average rank	Sum of ranks		
(1)	Group A (2)	Group B (3)	Group C (4)	Total (5)	(6)	(7)	Group A (8)	Group B (9)	Group C (10)
Not effect	18	22	20	60	1∼60	30.5	549	671	610
Improve	22	28	24	74	61∼134	97.5	2145	2730	2340
Excellent	52	30	24	106	135∼240	187.5	9750	5625	4500
Cure	96	36	28	160	241∼400	320.5	30,768	11,538	8974
Total	188	116	96	400	80,200	—	43,212	20,564	16,424

If the number of treatment groups $k = 3$, and $n_i \leq 5$ for each group, the H-threshold table can be used to obtain the H-threshold with probability $P = 0.05$ and $P = 0.01$; if $k \geq 4$, and $n_i \geq 5$ for each group, then H approximates the chi-square distribution of $v = k - 1$, the critical value can be obtained by checking Appendix Table C1.4.

Resolution

The rank-sum test procedure for Example 7.5 is as following:

(1) Set the hypotheses and the test level.

Null hypothesis: The overall efficacy of the three treatment groups are the same.

Alternative hypothesis: Not all of the overall efficacy of the three treatment groups are the same.

$\alpha = 0.05$

(2) Calculate the test statistic

The calculation of the three groups of rank sums is shown in columns (6)–(10) of Table 7.10. The test statistic is calculated by Formula (7-11): $H = 23.01$. Since the total count of each level is the number of average ranks, and there are many ties, the corrected H_c value should be calculated by using Formula (7-12): $c = 0.91$, $H_c = 25.29$.

(3) Calculate the P value and make a conclusion.

In this example, the number of treatment groups k is equal to 3, and the number of cases per group $n_i \geq 5$, so when H_0 holds, it approximates the chi-square distribution of $v = k - 1 = 3 - 1 = 2$. Check Appendix Table C1.4, $\chi^2 = 25.29 > \chi^2_{0.05,2}$, therefore, $P < 0.05$.

Reject H_0 and accept H_1 at the level of $\alpha = 0.05$, the difference is statistically significant. It can be concluded that not all of the overall efficacy of the three treatment groups are the same. To know which groups are different, appropriate pairwise comparisons are required.

7.5. Chi-square tests for high-dimension $R \times C$ tables

For high-dimension contingency table data, it is necessary to check whether there is a statistical correlation between the row variable and the column variable in the two-way $R \times C$ table after controlling for confounding factors (stratification variables). To solve such questions, the Cochran–Mantel–Haenszel chi-square (χ^2_{CMH}) test is usually performed.

Example 7.6. To study the association between cardiovascular diseases and smoking, a case-control study was conducted to investigate the smoking status of 665 cardiovascular patients and 480 controls. Considering that age may be a confounding factor, the results stratified by age are shown in Table 7.11. The question was to test whether cardiovascular diseases is related to smoking after stratification by age.

Table 7.11 Case-control study of age-stratified cardiovascular diseases and smoking

		Smoking		
Age	Cardiovascular	Yes	No	Total
$<$50 years old	Case	144	81	225
	Contrast	56	43	99
	Sub-total	200	124	324
$\geq$50 years old	Case	176	264	440
	Contrast	120	261	381
	Sub-total	296	525	821
Total		496	649	1145

Analysis. Example 7.6 involves two binary variables, namely age and smoking. The purpose is to analyze the effects of whether the cardiovascular disease is related to smoking after stratification by age. This type of question is usually solved by the CMH chi-square test.

The CMH chi-square test is commonly used for high-dimensional contingency tables, the purpose is to test

Null hypothesis: Row variables X of any layer are not related to column variables Y.

Alternative hypothesis: At least one layer X has a statistical correlation with Y.

When the null hypothesis holds, the CMH chi-square statistic is approximately equal to the distribution of chi-square. However, when the row variables X are inconsistent with the column variables Y of each layer, the χ^2_{CMH} statistic is less effective.

According to the type of X and Y, χ^2_{CMH} statistics can be divided into the following categories:

(1) General association statistic: appropriate for row variables X and column variables Y are unordered categorical variables. The purpose is to test whether there is a correlation between X and Y. For a one-dimension $R \times C$ contingency table, χ^2_{CMH} is equal to $\frac{n-1}{n}\chi^2_p$, and χ^2_P is a Pearson χ^2 statistic; for a high-dimension $R \times C$ contingency table, χ^2_{CMH} is equal to Pearson χ^2 statistic corrected with the stratification variable. The v is $(R-1)\times(C-1)$.

(2) Analysis of variance statistic: also known as row means score statistic, which is appropriate for column variables Y is ordered categorical variables. In this case, the average score of the column variables Y in each row can be obtained, with the null hypothesis is that the average scores of the rows for all layers are equal. For a one-dimensional $R\times C$ contingency table, the test is equivalent to the analysis of the variance of the average score of each row of variables Y. If the score is calculated by rank, it is equivalent to the Kruskal–Wallis test. The v is $(R - 1)$.

(3) Correlation statistic: appropriate for both X and Y are ordered categorical variables. For a one-dimension $R \times C$ contingency table, the CMH statistic is χ^2_{MH}; for high-dimensional $R \times C$ contingency tables, χ^2_{CMH} is the statistic that corrects the effect of the stratification variable. Both χ^2_{MH} and χ^2_{CMH} have v of 1.

Because the calculation of χ^2_{CMH} statistics is very complicated, it is usually performed by statistical software.

For a 2×2 layer table data, let $h = 1, 2, \ldots, q$ be the stratification variables and their values. The general form for the h-th layer fourfold table is shown in Table 7.12.

Table 7.12 General form of the h-th layer of fourfold table in the stratified data

	Attributes		
Treatments	Positive	Negative	Total
Group A	a_h	b_h	n_{h1}
Group B	c_h	d_h	n_{h0}
Total	m_{h1}	m_{h0}	n_h

where a_h, b_h, c_h, d_h are the actual frequencies of the four cells of the h-th layer.

Then the χ^2_{CMH} statistic can be calculated as follows:

$$\chi^2_{\mathrm{CMH}} = \frac{\left[\sum_{h=1}^{q} (a_h - E(a_h))\right]^2}{\sum_{h=1}^{q} \mathrm{Var}(a_h)}, v = 1 \tag{7-13}$$

where $E(a_h)$ and $\mathrm{Var}(a_h)$ are the theoretical frequency and its variance respectively corresponding to the first column of the first row of the layer h based on the H_0, which can be calculated as following:

$$E(a_h) = \frac{n_{h1} \cdot m_{h1}}{n_h} \tag{7-14}$$

$$\mathrm{Var}(a_h) = \frac{n_{h1} \cdot n_{h0} \cdot m_{h1} \cdot m_{h0}}{n_h^2(n_h - 1)} \tag{7-15}$$

Resolution

The CMH chi-square test process of Example 7.6:

(1) Set the hypotheses and the test level.

Null hypothesis: Cardiovascular disease in all age groups are not correlated to smoking.

Alternative hypothesis: At least in one age group the cardiovascular diseases is correlated to smoking.

$\alpha = 0.05$

(2) Calculate the test statistic.

Calculate $E(a_h)$ and $\mathrm{Var}(a_h)$ of layer $h(h = 1, 2)$ according to Formulas (7-14) and (7-15):

$$E(a_1) = \frac{225 \times 200}{324} = 138.89,$$

$$\mathrm{Var}(a_1) = \frac{225 \times 99 \times 200 \times 124}{324^2 \times (324 - 1)} = 16.29$$

$$E(a_2) = \frac{440 \times 296}{821} = 158.64,$$

$$\mathrm{Var}(a_2) = \frac{440 \times 381 \times 296 \times 525}{821^2 \times (821 - 1)} = 47.13$$

Calculate the CMH statistic according to Formula (7-13):

$$\chi^2_{\mathrm{CMH}} = \frac{\left[\sum_{h=1}^{q} (a_h(E - a_h))\right]^2}{\sum_{h=1}^{q} \mathrm{Var}(a_h)}$$

$$= \frac{[144 \times (138.89 - 144) + 176 \times (158.64 - 176)]^2}{16.29 + 47.13} = 59.78$$

(3) Calculate the P value and make a conclusion.

Check the boundary value table for chi-square with $v = 1$, $P < 0.001$. At the test level of $\alpha = 0.05$, reject H_0 and accept H_1, it can be concluded that cardiovascular disease is correlated to smoking after controlling for age.

In addition, for stratified case-control study or cohort study data, the Breslow–Day test is usually used to test the effect value (OR or RR) of each layer. If the homogeneity hypothesis is not rejected, it can be inferred that whether the exposure factor is related to the disease from the results of CMH chi-square test. If relevant, the Mantel–Haenszel method can be used to estimate the OR or RR value and its confidence interval. Otherwise, if the homogeneity hypothesis is rejected by the Breslow–Day test, there exists an interaction between the stratification variable and the exposure factor. In this case, the CMH chi-square test cannot solve the question, and multivariate logistic regression analysis should be performed.

In Example 7.6, the result of the Breslow–Day test was $P = 0.833$, and the overall OR value of smoking in cardiovascular and cerebrovascular diseases in the two age groups was considered to be homogeneous; the Mantel–Haenszel method was used to estimate OR and the confidence interval was 1.43 (1.12–1.83).

7.6. Report writing

The appropriate reporting format of comparison of qualitative data should include sufficient information to address the following:

1. Aim of the analysis and the type of study design.
2. Basic statistical description of qualitative data.
3. Method of hypothesis test, test level (one-side or two-side), test statistic, and its P value.

For example, the result of Example 7.1 can be reported as below:

To compare the effects of venlafaxine and fluoxetine in the treatment of senile depressions, 60 patients with senile depressions were randomly assigned into two groups, respectively treated with two medications. The result of the treatment are shown in Table 7.1. For data analysis, the chi-square test was applied.

The chi-square test showed that at the two-side test level of $\alpha = 0.05$, the difference of the overall effective rates between venlafaxine and fluoxetine groups was not statistically significant ($\chi^2 = 1.086$, $v = 1$, $P = 0.297$).

7.7. Case discrimination

Case 7.1 A researcher surveyed the positive rates of hepatitis b surface antibody (HbsAg) in four groups of participants, and wanted to compare the positive rates of the three types of patients with healthy participants. The data are shown in Table 7.13.

Please discuss the following questions in this case:

1. The chi-square test for a 4×2 contingency table data was performed, is it correct?

Table 7.13 The positive rates of hepatitis b surface antibody (HbsAg) in four categories of people

Groups	Positive cases	Negative cases	Total	Positive rate (%)
Liver cancer patients	17	159	176	9.66
Hepatitis patients	18	160	178	10.11
Esophageal cancer patients	5	142	147	3.40
Healthy participants	3	151	154	1.95
Total	43	612	655	6.56

Table 7.14 Effects of the two treatments on neonatal hypoxic-ischemic encephalopathy (number of cases)

	Effects			
Groups	Excellent	Efficacy	Inefficacy	Total
Observation group	58	44	18	120
Control group	56	43	35	134
Total	114	87	53	254

2. Collate the HbsAg test results of each type of patients respectively with healthy people into the fourfold table, and three times of fourfold table chi-square tests were performed, is it correct?

Case 7.2 In the paper titled "Therapeutic effect of fructose diphosphate sodium in the treatment of neonatal hypoxic-ischemic encephalopathy," in order to study the efficacy of fructose diphosphate sodium in the treatment of neonatal hypoxic-ischemic encephalopathy, patients were randomly assigned into observation group and control group, respectively treated with sodium fructose diphosphate and citicoline. The effects were divided into three categories: ineffective, effective, and excellent (Table 7.14).

The original author used the special chi-square test formula for the contingency table. The results were: $\chi^2 = 4.74, P < 0.05$. The difference between the two groups was considered statistically significant.

Please discuss the following questions in this case:

1. What is the purpose of the original author's analysis? What is the problem with the chi-square test?
2. Which statistical method should be used to solve this question? And why?

7.8. Computer experiments

Experiment 7.1 Comparison of binary data between two independent groups: Example 7.1

There are two methods according to the input format of data.

Experiment 7.2 Comparison of paired binary data between the two groups: Example 7.2

The data file data7-2.sav is used to compare the data of paired fourfold table.

Experiment 7.3 Comparison of multi-category unordered data between independent multi-groups: Example 7.4

The data file data7-3.sav is used to complete the comparison of multi-groups and multi-category data.

Experiment 7.4 Comparison of multi-category ordinal data between independent multi-groups: Example 7.5

The data file data7-4.sav is used to complete the comparison of multi-groups ordered multi-category data.

Experiment 7.5 Stratified comparison of binary data between two independent groups: Example 7.6

The data file data7-5.sav is used to complete the stratified comparison of the independent binary data.

7.9. Frequently asked questions and summary

7.9.1. *Frequently asked questions*

1. Can the ordinary fourfold chi-square formula be used to test the difference for paired design data?

Table 7.15 Hepatitis b antigen test results of peripheral blood and venous blood (number of cases)

Testing sample	Testing result		Total
	Positive	Negative	
Venous blood	50	250	300
Peripheral blood	54	246	300
Total	104	496	600

The completely random design data requires that the two sets of data must be two independent samples. Because the paired design data are dependent, it can only be sorted into the format of Table 7.15.

Accordingly, the fundamental chi-square formula for fourfold table cannot be used to test the difference of paired design data. When performing a difference test on a paired fourfold table, the chi-square test Formulas (7-6) and (7-7) should be used.

2. For multiple-groups binary data and unordered multi-category data, can it be tested separately by converting into multiple fourfold table data?

No, it is wrong. Because it will destroy the original design, and more importantly, increase the probability of type I error. For example, for the 3×3 contingency table, the test level of $\alpha = 0.05$ is taken. If the data are converted into multiple fourfold tables, the tests should be performed 9 times, so the probability of type I error will increase to $1 - (1 - 0.05)^9 = 0.37$.

Therefore, to avoid the increase of type I error, Bonffroni method should be used to calibrate the level of test in pairwise comparison of multiple group proportions. If the original test level is α, and k times pairwise comparisons needs to be made between R groups, then the test level of pairwise comparison should be α/k.

7.9.2. *Summary*

1. Qualitative data are usually organized into the format of contingency tables.

2. The simplest contingency table is a 2×2 table, also known as a fourfold table. According to the type of design, the data are organized into the corresponding fourfold table, and the corresponding statistical method should be selected for analysis.
3. When choosing the chi-square test, the requirements for the sample size and the theoretical frequencies should be taken into account.
4. For the chi-square test for multiple independent samples, the rejection of null hypothesis indicates that not all of the overall rates of each group are the same. To test which two groups differ, appropriate pairwise comparison should be performed accordingly.
5. The CMH chi-square test is commonly used for high-dimensional contingency tables data. Note that the homogeneity hypothesis need be met; otherwise, if the homogeneity hypothesis is rejected, there exists an interaction between the stratification variable and the exposure factor. In this case, the CMH chi-square test cannot solve the question, and multivariate logistic regression analysis should be performed.
6. The chi-square test is not a panacea for all contingency tables. For example, the rank-sum test is the most appropriate method for ordered categorical data. For two-way ordered contingency table data, you can choose the chi-square test, linear trend test and other methods. For high-dimensional contingency table data, there are logarithmic linear model and logistic regression model.

Think and Practice

I. Best Choice

1. Which method commonly used in statistical inference of qualitative data? ( )
   A. t test B. Normality test C. F test D. χ^2 test E. t' test
2. To compared the incidence of binary data between the two groups, and the total number of samples was 100, then the degree of freedom of χ^2 test is ( ).
   A. 1 B. 4 C. 95 D. 99 E. 100

3. Which method should be used in the comparison of ordinal data? ( )
   A. t test B. χ^2 test C. F test D. Normality test E. Rank-sum test

II. Questions for Reflection

1. Briefly describe the data types applicable to the χ^2 test.
2. How many types of design for the two groups of binary data. What is the corresponding test method?
3. What data is suitable for testing with rank-sum test? Briefly describe the rank-sum test procedure.

III. Questions on Calculation

1. A hospital observed the serum anti-platelet antibodies of 28 patients with liver cirrhosis and 14 patients with aplastic anemia, and the results were: 2 of patients with liver cirrhosis were positive, and 5 of patients with aplastic anemia were positive. Is there any difference in the positive rates of anti-platelet antibodies between the two groups of patients?
2. A total of 100 patients with leptospirosis were diagnosed serologically by indirect immune antibody test and microscopic agglutination test at the same time. The results are shown in Table 7.16. Is there any difference in the positive rates between the two methods?
3. To study the effects of two different treatment and training programs on weight loss in obese patients, and the results are shown

Table 7.16 Comparison of test results of the two methods (number of cases)

	Micro-agglutination		
Indirect immunofluorescence	+	−	Total
+	66	11	77
−	6	17	23
Total	72	28	100

Table 7.17 Effects of weight loss from two therapeutic programs (number of cases)

Therapeutic programs	Powerful effect	General effect	Bad effect	Total
A	16	22	8	46
B	28	17	5	50
Total	44	39	13	96

Table 7.18 Therapeutic effects of three Chinese herbal prescriptions on osteoporosis (number of cases)

Groups	Valid	Invalid	Total
Prescription A	18	6	24
Prescription B	12	14	26
Prescription C	11	15	26
Total	41	35	76

in Table 7.17. Are the two treatment training programs the same for weight loss in obese patients?

4. To compare the therapeutic effects of three traditional Chinese medicine prescriptions on osteoporosis, and the results are shown in Table 7.18. Is there any difference in the therapeutic effects of the three prescriptions?

Xiangtong Liu, Yanxia Luo, Xiaonan Wang

CHAPTER 8

ANALYSIS OF ASSOCIATION

In medical research, it is common to analyze the relationship between two random variables; for example, whether linear relationships exist between height and weight, body temperature and pulse, blood pressure and age, and the strength of these relationships. In this chapter, we discuss the linear relationships between two quantitative variables and two qualitative variables. Generally, a linear relationship between two continuous random variables is called a linear correlation or simple correlation, and a relationship between two categorical variables is called an association.

8.1. Overview

8.1.1. *A correlation study between the height and weight of children*

Example 8.1. The heights and weights of 10 school-aged children are shown in Table 8.1. Please try to analyze the correlation between height (cm) and weight (kg).

This study analyzes the correlation between height (X) and weight (Y).

The linear correlation between two variables can be analyzed using two distinct approaches. The first is to study whether an "association" or a linear association between the two variables exists and, if so, the degree of this association. If two continuous random variables X and Y change according to the same relationship, the direction and

Table 8.1 The height and weight of 10 school-aged children

No.	1	2	3	4	5	6	7	8	9	10
Height/ cm (X)	149.35	167.64	146.30	170.69	161.54	164.59	155.45	158.50	149.35	152.40
Weight/ kg (Y)	30.84	42.64	33.11	44.00	36.29	40.82	32.66	35.38	33.11	31.75

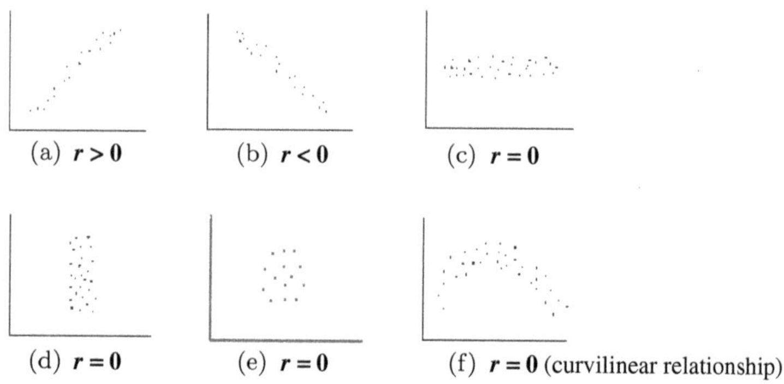

Figure 8.1 Typical patterns of a scatter plot

the degree of the potential linear relationship between them can be described using a linear correlation analysis. The second is to study the "dependence" between the two variables; that is, how much the dependent variable changes when the independent variable changes by one unit. This can be described using linear regression, as outlined in Chapter 9.

8.1.1.1. *The type of correlation*

1. Positive correlation: Y increases linearly as a function of X (Figure 8.1(a)).
2. Negative correlation: Y decreases linearly as a function of X (Figure 8.1(b)).
3. Zero correlation: Y does not vary linearly as a function of X (Figure 8.1(c–e)).

4. Nonlinear correlation: Y changes curvilinearly as a function of X (Figure 8.1(f)). In such cases, it is not suitable to analyze the linear correlation between the two variables.

8.1.1.2. *Correlation coefficient*

One can broadly determine whether a linear or a curvilinear correlation between two variables exists by considering a scatter plot. However, this subjective approach does not allow one to accurately determine the strength of this correlation. Rather, the strength of the correlation between two continuous random variables is described by the correlation coefficient. The correlation coefficient of a population is referred to as the population correlation coefficient, and is denoted by ρ. Analogously, the correlation coefficient of a sample is referred to as the sample correlation coefficient and is denoted by r. The correlation coefficient ranges between -1 and 1. The closer the coefficient to 1 or -1, the stronger the correlation. When the coefficient is equal to 0, there is no correlation. When the coefficient is positive, it indicates a positive correlation; when the coefficient is negative, it indicates a negative correlation; and when the coefficient is 0, it indicates 0 correlation.

8.2. The correlation analysis of two continuous random variables

8.2.1. *Analysis*

For Example 8.1, our analysis is broadly organized as follows.

1. Statistical description. Is there a correlation between the height and the weight of school-age students? If so, is this a linear or a nonlinear correlation? If it is linear, what is the strength of the correlation, and is it a positive or a negative correlation?
2. Statistical inference. If a linear correlation exists, is it statistically significant? Similarly, is the degree of this correlation statistically significant?

3. Statistical application. If a linear correlation exists, how can one interpret its direction and strength on the basis of professional knowledge?

8.2.2. *Pearson's correlation*

Let X and Y represent two variables. Pearson's product-moment correlation coefficient, or more simply the correlation coefficient, can be used to describe the relationship between these two variables if they are random, independent, linearly related, and obey a bivariate normal distribution.

8.2.2.1. *Calculation of Pearson's product-moment correlation coefficient*

For a sample, Pearson's product-moment correlation coefficient is computed as

$$r = \frac{\sum(X - \overline{X})(Y - \overline{Y})}{\sqrt{\sum(X - \overline{X})^2 \sum(Y - \overline{Y})^2}}. \tag{8-1}$$

If two variables are closely related, the sum of the products of the average deviations of the observed values of the two variables is not close to 0. Conversely, if two variables are not closely related, the sum of the products of the average deviation of the observed values of the two variables is very close to 0. These products are also influenced by the units of X and Y. The covariance is thus calculated after standardization of X and Y.

8.2.2.2. *Hypothesis test for Pearson's product-moment correlation coefficient*

The sample Pearson's product-moment correlation coefficient (r) between two variables is theoretically an estimate of the population correlation coefficient (ρ). The population correlation coefficient has the following features:

1. ρ is unitless, and $-1 \leq \rho \leq 1$;
2. $\rho > 0$ corresponds to a positive correlation, and $\rho < 0$ corresponds to a negative correlation;

3. the closer the value of $|\rho|$ to 1, the stronger the correlation, and the closer the value of $|\rho|$ to 0, the weaker the correlation.

Different samples from the same population will generate different sample correlation coefficients. Thus, the correlation coefficients of samples (r) are heterogeneous random variables. We are interested in testing the hypothesis that the population correlation coefficient (ρ) is equal to 0. More precisely, we consider a hypothesis test with the following null and alternative hypotheses:

$$H_0 : \rho = 0, \quad H_1 : \rho \neq 0$$

This test is performed as follows.

1. Compute the test statistic
$$t = \frac{r - 0}{S_r} = \frac{r}{\sqrt{(1 - r^2)/(n - 2)}}, \qquad \nu = n - 2, \qquad \text{(8-2)}$$
where, as above, r denotes the sample correlation coefficient. When H_0 holds, this statistic follows the t distribution with $\nu = n - 2$ degrees of freedom.
2. Compute the P value using a t table (Appendix Table C12) with the required degrees of freedom, or using statistical software. The bigger the value of $|t|$, the smaller the P value. Similarly, the smaller the value of $|t|$, the larger the P value. If $P \leq 0.05$, reject H_0 and accept H_1. This indicates that a statistically significant linear correlation between the two variables exists. Conversely, if $P > 0.05$, do not reject H_0. This indicates that a statistically significant linear correlation between the two variables does not exist (on the basis of the current data).

8.2.2.3. *Confidence interval for Pearson's product-moment correlation coefficient*

A confidence interval for the population correlation coefficient (ρ) can be constructed as follows.

The sample correlation coefficient (r) is limited to the interval $[-1, 1]$, and does not follow a normal distribution. Thus an inverse hyperbolic tangent transformation is first applied to r. It is possible to show that z is approximately distributed according to the normal distribution $N\left(\tanh^{-1}\rho, \frac{1}{\sqrt{n-3}}\right)$. The $(1-\alpha)$ confidence interval for $\tanh^{-1}\rho$ is thus given by:

$$\tanh^{-1}\rho : \left(\tanh^{-1} r - Z_{\alpha/2}\frac{1}{\sqrt{n-3}}, \tanh^{-1} r + Z_{\alpha/2}\frac{1}{\sqrt{n-3}}\right). \tag{8-4}$$

That is,

$$\tanh^{-1}\rho : \quad (z_1, z_2),$$

where

$$z_1 = \tanh^{-1} r - Z_{\alpha/2}\frac{1}{\sqrt{n-3}}, \quad z_2 = \tanh^{-1} r + Z_{\alpha/2}\frac{1}{\sqrt{n-3}} \tag{8-5}$$

Let

$$\tanh^{-1}\rho_1 = z_1, \quad \tanh^{-1}\rho_2 = z_2.$$

Then

$$\rho_1 = \frac{e^{2z_1}-1}{e^{2z_1}+1} \quad \rho_2 = \frac{e^{2z_2}-1}{e^{2z_2}+1}. \tag{8-6}$$

Thus the $(1-\alpha)$ confidence interval for the population correlation ρ is given by

$$\rho : (\rho_1, \rho_2). \tag{8-7}$$

8.2.2.4. *Case study*

(1) Scatter plot. The weights and heights of school-age students are observed to follow a linear trend (Figure 8.2). In particular, taller students tend to have a larger weight, indicating that the relationship between the height and weight of students is in a positive direction.
(2) Pearson's product-moment correlation coefficient. The correlation coefficient is calculated as

$$r = 0.929.$$

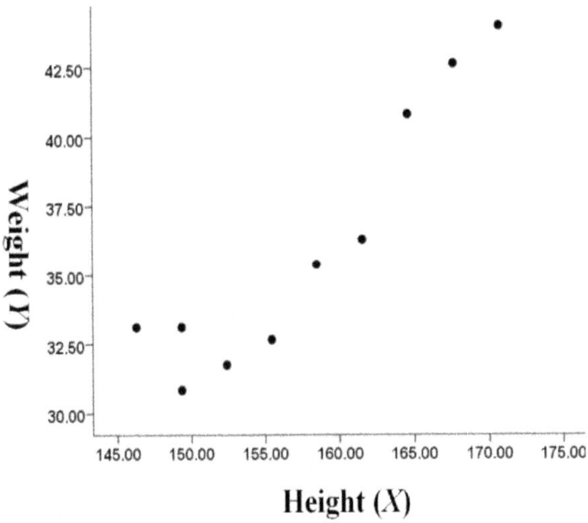

Figure 8.2 The scatter plot of Example 8.1

(3) Hypothesis test. We test the hypothesis that the correlation coefficient of the population (ρ) is 0

$$H_0 : \rho = 0, \quad H_1 : \rho \neq 0, \quad \alpha = 0.05$$

The test statistic is calculated as

$$t = 7.10.$$

From the t distribution table (Appendix Table C12), we find $t_{0.001/2,8} = 0.5041$, $t > t_{0.001/2,8}$, and $P < 0.001$. This indicates that there is a statistically significant positive correlation between the height and weight of school-age students.

(4) Confidence interval. After the inverse hyperbolic tangent transformation, the 95% confidence interval for $\tanh^{-1} \rho$ is computed according to Equation (8-4) as

$$(0.910, 2.392).$$

The 95% confidence interval for the population correlation coefficient (ρ) is then calculated according to Equation (8-6) as

$$(0.721, 0.983).$$

8.2.3. *Spearman's rank correlation*

If the variables X, Y do not obey the bivariate normal distribution, the population distribution is unknown, there are unknown values, or the data is classified, it is preferable to use the rank correlation to characterize the degree and the direction of correlation.

8.2.3.1. *Calculation of Spearman's rank correlation coefficient*

Example 8.2. The cost (RMB) of each patient per day and the time (days) of participating in a family plan are shown in Table 8.2. Is the cost correlated with the participating time?

The basic idea of rank correlation is to transform the original data into rank data. More precisely, rank the observed values of the variables X and Y, letting p_i denote the rank of X_i, and q_i denote the rank of Y_i. If there is more than one occurrence of a particular observed value, assign the average rank. Spearman's rank correlation coefficient (r_s) is then computed using Formula (8-1), replacing X_i, Y_i with p_i, q_i, respectively.

8.2.3.2. *Hypothesis test for Spearman's rank correlation coefficient*

We require a hypothesis test to determine whether the sample rank correlation coefficient is statistically significant. As for the product-moment correlation coefficient, the hypothesis test for the rank

Table 8.2 The cost (RMB) of each patient per day and the time (days) of participating in a family plan for 10 patients

No.	Time (X)	Rank (p_i)	Cost (Y)	Rank (q_i)	Difference (d_i)
1	10	1	516	10	−9
2	150	10	122	3	7
3	143	9	82	1	8
4	25	2	262	7	−5
5	132	8	135	4	4
6	65	3	300	9	−6
7	118	6	86	2	4
8	129	7	268	8	−1
9	70	4	203	6	−2
10	92	5	164	5	0

correlation coefficient is specified by

$$H_0: \rho = 0, \quad H_1: \rho \neq 0, \quad \alpha = 0.05.$$

When $n \leq 50$, this test is carried out by checking the threshold table for r_s (Appendix Table C13). In particular, one should reject H_0 if the sample rank correlation coefficient is greater than the threshold. When $n \geq 50$, one can also use the t-test (Equation (8-2)) to test the hypothesis.

8.2.3.3. *Case study*

(1) Preliminary analysis. Neither the time nor the cost obeys a normal distribution. Thus, we opt to use Spearman's rank correlation to analyze the degree of correlation. After transforming the time and the cost into their ranks, the Spearman's product-moment correlation coefficient r_s is computed as

$$r_s = -0.770.$$

(2) Hypothesis test. We test the hypothesis that the Spearman's correlation coefficient of the population is equal to 0. From the threshold table for r_s, we find $r_{0.05,10} = 0.648$, $|r_s| > r_{0.05,10}$, $P < 0.05$. Alternatively, the t-test yields $t = 3.410$, $P < 0.05$. We therefore conclude that there exists a statistically significant negative correlation between the cost per day and the participating time.

8.2.4. *Discussion of the correlation*

(1) It can be inferred that two variables are "linearly correlated" if the corresponding scatter plot demonstrates a linear trend, and the null hypothesis is rejected when the hypothesis test for the correlation coefficient being equal to 0 is conducted. However, this does not imply that there is any biological association between the two variables, or that they are casually related. Indeed, it is simply an analysis of the mathematical characteristics of the two variables, and does not consider the sequence of time, or any possible biological association between the two variables. It may be the case that the correlation is an adjoint correlation, due to the change in another variable.

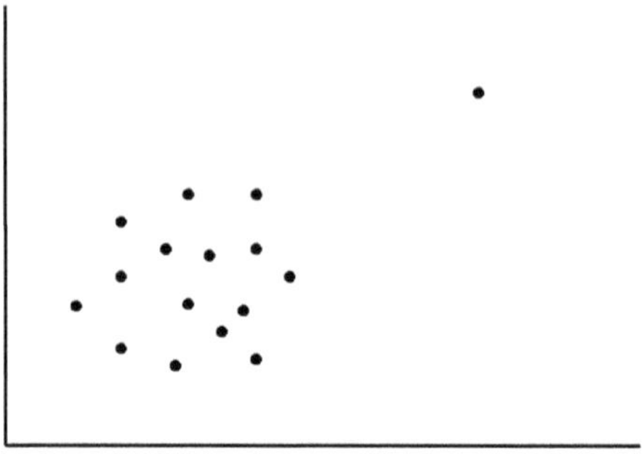

Figure 8.3 One should exercise caution when outliers are present

(2) It cannot be concluded that two variables are "irrelevant" simply on the basis that the hypothesis that the population correlation coefficient $\rho = 0$ is accepted in the hypothesis test. One should verify whether the sample size is large enough (i.e., if the power of the test is large enough). The curvilinear correlation should then be analyzed via a scatter plot, and whether a stratified analysis is suitable. Once these considerations have been made, the conclusion should be "according to the current data, one cannot consider these two variables to be linearly correlated."

(3) The outlier problem may occur in correlation analysis (Figure 8.3). In this situation, the data must be checked against the original database. If there are no errors in the data, the analysis should then be performed both with and without the outlier. Further, the analysis must describe the management of the outlier and only cautious conclusions can be drawn.

8.3. Association analysis for two categorical variables

The relationship between two categorical variables is different from the relationship between two continuous variables. In particular, the calculations and hypothesis tests differ from those used in linear correlation analysis for continuous random variables. However, their purpose and significance are consistent. Association analysis can be used to describe the association between categorical variables, and to test independence attributes of the two variables using the χ^2 test for categorical data.

8.3.1. *Association analysis for* 2 × 2 *cross-classification data*

A random sample of size n can be cross classified using two binary characteristics (attributes). These can be used to form a 2×2 cross-classification data table, also referred to as a 2×2 contingency table.

Example 8.3. To analyze the relationship between behavior type and coronary heart disease, a research group collected data for 3154 participants. The researchers classified the subjects as either type A (more ambitious, enterprising and competitive) or type B (more calm, easy, and not flustered) according to their behaviors. Thus two attributes were recorded for each subject: occurrence of coronary heart disease and behavior type. These data are shown in Table 8.3. Try to analyze the association of the two attributes.

The random sample, with a sample size of $n = 3154$, is classified according to two attributes. If the probability distribution of one attribute is independent from the probability distribution of the other attribute, these two attributes are independent. Otherwise, there is an association between these two attributes.

For the purpose of analysis, it is useful to transform the counts in Table 8.3 to probabilities (Table 8.4). In this table, A_{ij} denotes the frequency of the attributes (A_i, B_j) with π_{ij} its joint probability;

Table 8.3 The relationship between behavior type and coronary heart disease

Behavior type (Attribute A)	Coronary heart disease (Attribute B) Yes (1)	No (2)	Total
Type A (1)	178	1411	1589
Type B (2)	79	1486	1565
Total	257	2897	3154

Table 8.4 The general form and probabilities of a 2 × 2 cross-classification frequency table

	Attribute B		
Attribute A	1	2	Total
1	A_{11} (π_{11})	A_{12} (π_{12})	n_1 (π_{r1})
2	A_{21} (π_{21})	A_{22} (π_{22})	n_2 (π_{r2})
Total	m_1 (π_{c1})	m_2 (π_{c2})	n

n_i denotes the frequency of the attribute A_i with π_{ri} its marginal probability; and m_j denotes the frequency of the attribute B_j with π_{cj} its marginal probability.

In terms of probability, two attributes are independent if their joint probability is equal to the product of their two marginal probabilities. That is,

$$\pi_{ij} = \pi_{ri}\pi_{cj}, \quad ij = 1, 2.$$

We are interested in the following hypotheses:

H_0: Attributes A and B are independent of each other,
H_1: Attributes A and B are associated with each other.

This independence test is used to analyze whether the equation $\pi_{ij} = \pi_{ri}\pi_{cj}$ holds. It utilizes the χ^2 statistic

$$\chi^2 = \sum_{i.j} \frac{(A_{ij} - T_{ij})^2}{T_{ij}},$$

where A_{ij} is the observed frequency and T_{ij} is the expected frequency. When H_0 holds, this statistic follows a χ^2 distribution.

The theoretical or expected frequency is calculated as follows. Under H_0, it is assumed that $\pi_{ij} = \pi_{ri}\pi_{ej}$. Because the probabilities π_{ri} and π_{ej} are unknown, they are approximated by the sample frequencies

$$\pi_{ri} \approx \frac{n_{ri}}{n}, \quad \pi_{cj} \approx \frac{n_{ej}}{n}.$$

It follows that

$$\pi_{ij} = \pi_{ri}\pi_{ej} \approx \left(\frac{n_{ri}}{n}\right)\left(\frac{n_{ej}}{n}\right), \quad ij = 1, 2.$$

Under H_0, the expected frequency T_{ij} is thus approximated as

$$T_{ij} = n\pi_{ij} \approx \frac{n_{ri} \cdot n_{ej}}{n}, \quad ij = 1, 2.$$

This formula is identical to the formula in Chapter 7 (Formula (7.2)). When calculating the expected frequency, we replace the two independent parameters (π_{r1} and π_{c1}) with their sample estimates. Note that π_{r2} and π_{c2} are not independent, because

$$\pi_{r2} = 1 - \pi_{r1}; \quad \pi_{c2} = 1 - \pi_{c1}$$

Thus the degrees of freedom of the aforementioned χ^2 distribution is $\nu = 4 - 1 - 2 = 1$ or $\nu = (2 - 1)(2 - 1) = 1$.

The independence test for cross-classification data and the hypothesis test used to compare the frequencies of two independent samples use the same χ^2 test formula, theoretical frequency calculation formula, and degree of freedom calculation formula. In particular, the 2×2 table simplification formula (Formula 7.3) provided in Chapter 7 still applies:

$$\chi^2 = \sum \frac{(A - T)^2}{T} \tag{8-8}$$

$$\chi^2 = \frac{(ad - bc)^2 \cdot n}{(a + b)(c + d)(a + c)(b + d)} \tag{8-9}$$

where A is the observed frequency and T is the expected frequency. Under H_0, this statistic follows the χ^2 distribution as above.

We now apply these methods to the data in Example 8.3. In particular, we consider the hypothesis test:

H_0: Behavior type and coronary heart disease are independent of each other,

H_1: Behavior type and coronary heart disease are associated with each other.

$\alpha = 0.05$

Substituting the relevant values from Table 8.3 into Formula (8-9), we have

$$\chi^2 = \frac{(178 \times 1486 - 79 \times 1411)^2 \times 3154}{1589 \times 1565 \times 257 \times 2897} = 39.900,$$

$$\chi^2 > \chi^2_{0.005,1}, \quad P < 0.005.$$

It follows that there is a statistically significant association between behavior type and coronary heart disease.

We are also interested in the degree of this association. There are many metrics that can be used to determine the degree of correlation between two attributes. We consider the association coefficient (r), given by

$$r = \sqrt{\frac{\chi^2}{\chi^2 + n}}. \tag{8-10}$$

In the current example, this is calculated as

$$r = \sqrt{\frac{\chi^2}{\chi^2 + n}} = \sqrt{\frac{39.90}{39.90 + 3154}} = 0.112.$$

For a 2×2 contingency table, the association coefficient r is between 0 and $\sqrt{0.5}$. The larger the value, the higher the degree of association. The hypothesis test of whether the association coefficient is equal to 0 is equivalent to the independence test of two attributes described above.

8.3.2. *Association analysis for 2 × 2 paired data*

Example 8.4. Imaging examinations (A) and biochemical tests (B) were performed on 103 patients. The results were divided into disease (+) and normal (−). The data are shown in Table 8.5. Analyze the association between the test results for methods A and B.

Table 8.5 Comparison of two test results

	Method B		
Method A	$B+$	$B-$	Total
$A+$	50	15	65
$A-$	8	30	38
Total	58	45	103

The design and data format in this example are the same as those in the paired design χ^2 test described previously. In Chapter 7, the McNemar test was used to determine whether the positive rates of the two methods were equal. If we are interested in whether there is any association between the results of the two methods, however, we are required to do an association analysis of the two attributes. We thus compute

$$\chi^2 = \frac{(50 \times 30 - 15 \times 8)^2 \times 103}{65 \times 38 \times 58 \times 45} = 30.43.$$

We also have $\chi^2_{0.05,1} = 3.84$, $P < 0.05$. We thus conclude that there is a statistically significant association between the two methods.

We can also compute the association coefficient as

$$r = \sqrt{\frac{\chi^2}{\chi^2 + n}} = \sqrt{\frac{30.43}{30.43 + 103}} = 0.477.$$

We note that these paired data permit both a frequency comparison and an association analysis, and that the data sorting in each case is completely consistent. However, the method of calculation is different due to different analysis purposes. When comparing frequency, the McNemer test only tests for inconsistent paired data (see Chapter 7).

8.3.3. *Association analysis for multi-category data*

Example 8.5. Studies have shown that people of different nationalities have different blood types. The distribution of the blood types

Table 8.6 The blood type distribution of different nationalities

	Blood type				
Nationality	O	A	B	AB	Total
American	450	410	100	40	1000
Chinese	300	250	350	100	1000
Norwegian	190	250	40	20	500
Total	940	910	490	160	2500

of 2,500 people with different nationalities is shown in Table 8.6. Is nationality associated with blood type?

The "association" and "comparison" mentioned above represent two different types of problems and two different designs. We have previously encountered comparisons of the frequency distributions of multiple groups.

In this example, we first determine the population of the three nationalities. We then investigate the blood type distribution. Finally, we analyze whether the blood type distribution for the three nationalities is different. The 2500 cases in this example are obtained from a survey, and thus can be regarded as a random sample among the population.

We utilize cross-classification according to two attributes (nationality and blood type) and the frequency statistic to analyze whether there is an association between the two attributes. After a derivation similar to that for 2×2 cross-classification, one obtains a χ^2 formula identical to the formula for the comparison of the multiple groups in Chapter 7. That is,

$$\chi^2 = n\left(\sum\sum \frac{A_{ij}^2}{n_{ri}n_{ej}} - 1\right), \quad \nu = (R-1)(C-1), \qquad \text{(8-11)}$$

where n is the total number of cases, A_{ij} is the observed frequency of cell (i, j); n_i and m_j are the total number of cases for row i and column j, R is the number of rows and C is the number of columns.

For example 8.5, the association analysis corresponds to the following hypothesis test:

H_0: Blood type and nationality are independent of each other.
H_1: Blood type and nationality are associated with each other.
$\alpha = 0.05$

Substituting the relevant values from Table 8.5 into Formula (8-9), we obtain $\chi^2 = 332.97$. Furthermore, we have $\nu = (3-1)(4-1) = 6$, $\chi^2_{0.05,6} = 12.59$, $\chi^2 > \chi^2_{0.05,6}$, $P < 0.05$. We thus reject the null hypothesis, and conclude that there is a statistically significant association between blood type and nationality.

We can also calculate the association coefficient, which now ranges between 0 and $\sqrt{1 - \frac{1}{\min(R,C)}}$, where R is the number of rows and C is the number of columns. In this case, we obtain

$$r = \sqrt{\frac{\chi^2}{\chi^2 + n}} = \sqrt{\frac{332.97}{332.97 + 2500}} = 0.343$$

Similar to the χ^2 test for the comparison of multiple frequencies, this test is not applicable if the expected frequency is less than 5 in more than 1/5 of the grid cells, or any single expected frequency is less than 1. In this case, the closest attribute can be properly merged, but some information will be lost.

For two ordered multi-category variables, we can use the Spearman's rank correlation method for analysis.

8.4. Report writing

The "report writing" contains the content of a correlation analysis, including:

(1) Descriptive statistics of each indicator, such as sample size, mean, and standard deviation of continuous data, frequency and proportion of classified data.
(2) The process of correlation or association analysis, such as whether the scatter plot indicates a linear correlation trend, the size of the correlation coefficient and its 95% confidence interval,

the hypothesis test method, test statistic, and P value. If a data transformation is performed, the reason for and method of the transformation should be explained.

(3) The statistical conclusion (whether correlation exists and the degree of correlation).

The result report for the Pearson's product-moment correlation coefficient of the two continuous random variables in Example 8.1 is as follows.

Data from 10 school-age children were collected to investigate the correlation between height and weight. The average height of the 10 school-age children was 157.58 cm ($S = 8.39$), and the average weight was 36.06 kg ($S = 4.76$). A linear trend was observed in a scatter plot of the data (Figure 8.2). Pearson's product-moment correlation coefficient was computed as $r = 0.929$ ($t = 7.10$, $P < 0.001$, 95% CI $=[0.721, 0.983]$. These results indicate that the heights and weights of school-age children are positively correlated.

The result report for the association analysis of the two categorical variables in Example 8.3 is as follows.

Data from 3154 participants were collected to investigate the association between behavior type and coronary heart disease. There were 178 coronary heart disease patients with type A behavior and 79 patients with type B behavior (Table 8.3). Pearson's χ^2 test was conducted to analyze the association, yielding $\chi^2 = 39.900$, $P < 0.001$, $r = 0.112$. These results indicate that there is an association between behavior type and coronary heart disease.

8.5. Case discrimination

Case 8.1 A study was conducted on the relationship between blood glucose, blood lipids, the prevalence of fatty liver disease and diabetes grade (i.e., normal blood glucose, impaired glucose tolerance, or type II diabetes). The indicators were expressed as mean ± standard deviation, and the statistical analysis was conducted by comparing two groups of independent samples. The results showed that there were statistically significant differences in blood glucose, triglyceride,

Table 8.7 Blood biochemistry and the prevalence of fatty liver disease among people with three blood glucose levels

		Blood glucose (mmol/L)				
Group	Cases	On an empty stomach	After a meal	Triglyceride (mmol/L)	Total cholesterol (mmol/L)	Prevalence of fatty liver disease (%)
Normal blood glucose	87	5.0 ± 0.5	5.6 ± 1.0	0.9 ± 0.3	3.0 ± 0.9	48.3
Impaired glucose tolerance	62	6.5 ± 0.5	8.2 ± 1.3	2.1 ± 1.0	4.6 ± 0.8	69.4
Type II diabetes	68	8.3 ± 2.6	12.5 ± 3.4	2.6 ± 1.5	5.1 ± 0.8	83.8

total cholesterol, and the prevalence of fatty liver disease among the three groups (data and statistical results are shown in Table 8.7). With the development of normal blood glucose toward impaired glucose tolerance and type II diabetes, the indicators of blood glucose, triglyceride, total cholesterol, and fatty liver disease prevalence were all increased. The differences were statistically significant. It was concluded that blood glucose level, triglyceride, total cholesterol, and the prevalence of fatty liver disease were positively correlated with decreased glucose tolerance and type II diabetes.

After performing t-tests, pairwise comparison of the P values of all indicators in the normal blood glucose group, the impaired glucose tolerance group and the type II diabetes group were all <0.05.

Questions: is the purpose of the study consistent with the design method? What type of design is this study, and is there a better design? What kind of statistical analysis method is most suitable for this design? What is wrong with the statistical analysis method in this example? Can the statistical analysis result in this example lead to the conclusion in this example? If not, what conclusions can be draw? What is wrong with the statistical expression in this example?

Table 8.8 The results of the rating scales

Scale	Grader	Patient 1	Patient 2	Patient 3	Patient 4	Patient 5
1	A	86	90	73	88	78
2	B	45	47	39	42	40

Case 8.2 A researcher was interested in evaluating the consistency of the severity score of one disease using two scales. Grader A used scale 1 and Grader B used scale 2 to score the same group of patients (5 people). The results are shown in Table 8.8. The researchers used the Pearson χ^2 to calculate the correlation coefficient of the two scores in Excel, and the correlation coefficient was very high (0.8663). They therefore concluded that the two scales were consistent.

Questions: (1) Is the purpose of this study consistent with the design method? Is there anything wrong with the design in this example? (2) Can Pearson's product-moment correlation coefficient be used in this example? Is the calculation correct? Is it true?

Case 8.3 A researcher was interested in studying the relationship between the oral dose of a certain drug and the blood drug concentration. The oral doses were set as 1, 2.5, 5, 7.5, 10, 15, 20, 30 (mg). Three animals (24 in total) from each group were used for testing, and blood samples were taken 1 hour after taking the drug to test the blood drug concentration (Table 8.9). A scatter plot (Figure 8.4) was produced in SPSS, and the Pearson's product-moment correlation coefficient between the oral drug dose and the blood drug concentration was calculated as 0.979. After the hypothesis test, the P value was <0.001. It was concluded that oral drug dose was positively linearly correlated with blood drug concentration.

Questions: What are the characteristics of the two variables in this example? Can Pearson's product-moment correlation coefficient be calculated? If so, what is wrong with the calculation method and procedure? Is the calculation correct? Can the conclusion of this example be deduced?

Table 8.9 Different oral dosages and corresponding blood concentrations

Oral dose (mg)	Blood concentration (mmol/L)	Oral dose (mg)	Blood concentration (mmol/L)
1	0.3	10	2.8
1	0.4	10	3
1	0.3	10	3
2.5	0.6	15	4.5
2.5	0.6	15	4.5
2.5	0.7	15	4.3
5	1	20	8.3
5	1	20	8
5	1.1	20	7.8
7.5	1.8	30	15.2
7.5	1.9	30	14.2
7.5	2	30	13.8

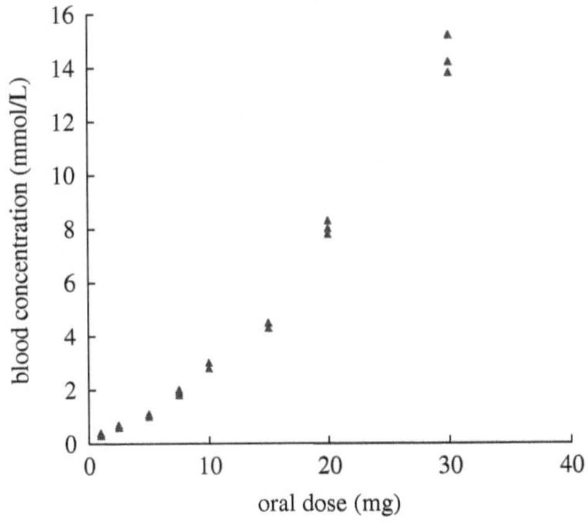

Figure 8.4 Scatter diagram of the relationship between oral dose of drugs and blood drug concentration

8.6. Computerized experiments

Experiment 8.1 Calculation of the Pearson's product-moment correlation coefficient.

Using the **data file** data8-1.sav (use the data in Example 8.1 as the raw data), plot a scatter diagram and calculate the Pearson's product-moment correlation coefficient.

Experiment 8.2 Calculation of the Spearman's rank correlation coefficient.

Using the **data file** Data8-2.sav (use the data in Example 8.2 as the raw data), calculate the Spearman's rank correlation coefficient.

Experiment 8.3 Association analysis for multi-categorical data.

Using the **data file** Data8-3.sav (use the data in Example 8.5 as the raw data), conduct the association analysis for multi-categorical data.

Experiment 8.4 Correlation analysis between economic income and happiness: stratifying and merging of scatter plots.

Using the **data file** Data8-4.sav, calculate the Pearson's product-moment correlation coefficient between rural annual income and happiness, and plot scatter diagrams. Compare the three kinds of scatter diagrams, the correlation coefficients, and their P values.

Experiment 8.5 Association analysis for two groups.

Change the design in Example 8.3 to a comparison between two groups (coronary heart disease and non-coronary heart disease). Change the number of people in the two groups in the case that the total number of people remaining unchanged, and the proportion of types A and B in the two groups is unchanged. Observe the changes in the association coefficient after changing the data in Excel.

8.7. Frequently asked questions and summary

8.7.1. *Frequently asked questions*

1. Are all data suitable for correlation analysis?

Correlation analysis requires that both variables are random variables. Thus, if the values of X are artificially decided, calculating the correlation coefficient is not appropriate. Calculating the Pearson's product-moment correlation coefficient also requires that the data follow a bivariate normal distribution. Finally, there are different types of data (e.g., continuous, categorical), which imply different methods to describe the relationship between variables (e.g., correlation analysis, association analysis).

2. The correlation coefficient and the results of the hypothesis test are automatically given in the program. Why is it still necessary to plot a scatter diagram?

While it is true that some studies report the correlation coefficient and the results of the hypothesis test without plotting a scatter diagram, this may lead to the conclusion of a linear correlation between two variables even when a linear relationship does not exist. Furthermore, without a scatter diagram, it may not be easy to determine whether the data have any outliers, or whether the data are stratified. Therefore, before conducting any correlation analysis, a scatter diagram must be plotted to confirm the existence of a linear relationship between the two variables of interest. The correlation coefficient can then be computed, and the hypothesis test performed.

3. If the mean values of a particular indicator are different between two groups, does it imply that this indicator is related to the grouping factor?

It should be noted that "correlation" is a statistical term with a very specific meaning. In this sense, it is important to distinguish between the somewhat colloquial phrase "the means of some indicator are related to grouping" and the more statistically precise phrase "the linear correlation between an indicator and grouping variables", which refer to two different concepts.

Indeed, the fact that the means of a particular indicator between two groups are different cannot, in itself, be considered as evidence of a correlation between the indicator and the grouping factor. Rather, if the difference of the two mean values is statistically significant, one can simply consider the overall level of the two groups to be different. The conclusion of linear correlation can only be obtained via a correlation analysis or an association analysis. Grouping factors are usually set artificially (non-randomly) and are thus unsuitable for correlation analysis.

4. The statistical test shows that the population correlation coefficient is not 0, and the P value is very small. Does this imply that the relationship between variables is very close?

The P value of the statistical test refers to the probability that, when the population correlation coefficient is 0, the population correlation coefficient is equal to or greater than the current sample correlation coefficient. If the P value is small, it means that, when the population correlation coefficient is 0, it is unlikely to exceed the current sample correlation coefficient. It is therefore unlikely that the population correlation coefficient is 0. However, small the P value, one can only conclude from the statistical test that the population correlation coefficient is not 0.

When the sample size is small, no statistically significant results may be obtained even if the absolute value of the sample correlation coefficient is close to 1. Conversely, when the sample size is large, the null hypothesis can be rejected even for a relatively small correlation coefficient. For example, if the sample size is greater than 50, $P < 0.05$ can be obtained by $r = 0.279$. Conversely, if the sample size is 5, $P > 0.05$ will be obtained even if $r = 0.870$.

5. Are all data suitable for Spearman's rank correlation, since this method has no requirement on the nature of data?

Spearman's rank correlation is indeed regarded as a universal correlation method in some literature. Spearman's rank correlation can be used for any type of data, but this may result in a loss of information and decreased efficacy. Correlation intensity indicators should therefore be selected according to the type of data and applicable conditions. When the two variables are continuous random variables, the Pearson's product-moment correlation coefficient is usually used.

6. Is it correct to use formula $r_s = 1-(6\sum d_i^2)/[n(n^2-1)]$ to calculate the Spearman's rank correlation coefficient?

When there are no ties in rank, the result obtained via this formula is identical to the result obtained through the formula for the Pearson's product-moment correlation coefficient based on rank. However, it is generally inappropriate to use this formula when there are more ties in rank.

7. Is there any difference in design between the $R \times 2$ table or the $R \times C$ table for multi-group comparison, and the $R \times C$ table in this chapter?

The $R \times 2$ table or the $R \times C$ table for multi-group comparison contains completely random design data. The groups or categories (e.g., three nationalities) are fixed first, and the adjustment of the number of cases in each group is not affected by the other groups. One can then investigate the frequency distribution (e.g., blood type distribution) of each group, and analyze whether the frequency distributions of the three groups are different.

The data in the $R \times C$ table in this chapter is the result of a survey, and can be regarded as a sample from a population. The sample size is fixed, and a change in the number of cases of one category of an attribute (e.g., American nationality) implies a reverse change in the number of cases of the other categories of that attribute (e.g., Chinese nationality, Norwegian nationality). The frequencies are counted according to cross-classification of two attributes (e.g., nationality and blood type). One can therefore determine whether the two attributes are independent.

8.7.2. *Summary*

1. Correlation is an indicator that measures the correlation or the association between two variables. The two variables in the correlation study must both be random variables.
2. Before performing a correlation analysis, a scatter diagram must be plotted to verify whether there is a linear relationship between the two variables, whether there are any outliers, and whether the data is stratified. When reporting the results, the inclusion of the scatter diagram and a summary of its characteristics is recommended.
3. Correlation analysis methods for two continuous variables include Pearson's product-moment correlation and Spearman's rank correlation. The former requires: (1) both variables are random variables; (2) the data follow a bivariate normal distribution;

(3) the samples are independent; (4) there is a linear trend between the two variables. The latter is used when the data do not follow a normal distribution or the data are ranked data. The calculation methodology for the two methods is consistent, but the rank correlation method uses the rank rather than the raw data in calculations. After computing the correlation coefficient, a hypothesis test should be performed, and a confidence interval for the population correlation coefficient should be calculated.

4. Categorical data for association analysis includes two kinds of data: binary data and multiple categorical data. Independence for both classes of data is tested using the χ^2 test. If the test rejects the hypothesis that the two variables are independent, the association coefficient can be calculated.
5. The correlation or association is simply a measure of the numerical correlation or association between two variables, and does not imply the existence of a biological association or causation between the two variables. The correlation may just be an adjoint correlation.
6. The association analysis for categorical data should be distinguished from the comparative study for rates. The purpose, design, and meaning of these two methods are different.

Thinking and Practice

I. Best Choice

1. When making a hypothesis test for the simple correlation coefficient, the statistical conclusion for $t > t_{(v)}$ is ( ).
   A. The two variables are not correlated B. The two variables are linearly correlated C. The two variables are not linearly correlated D. The two variables are not curvilinearly correlated, but must be linearly correlated E. None of the above
2. The calculation of product-moment correlation coefficient requires ( ).
   A. Y to be a normal variable, while X does not have to be normal
   B. X to be a normal variable, while Y does not have to be normal
   C. Both variables to be normally distributed D. Both variables

to be measurements E. Y to be quantitative, while X can be any type of data

3. To perform the association analysis for a frequency table of two categorical variables, we can use the ( ).
   A. Product-moment correlation B. Rank correlation C. Association coefficient D. Linear correlation E. All of the above
4. The t test result for a sample correlation coefficient r was $P < 0.01$, indicating that ( ).
   A. the two variables have high correlation B. r comes from a highly correlated population C. r comes from a population whose population correlation coefficient is 0 D. r comes from a population whose population correlation coefficient is not 0 E. r comes from a population whose population correlation coefficient is greater than 0

II. Calculation and Analysis

1. A school randomly selected 18 students and measured their intelligence quotients (IQ), together with their total scores in mathematics and literature. These data are shown in Table 8.10. Try to calculate the correlation coefficients between mathematics scores and IQ, literature scores and IQ, and mathematics scores and literature scores. In each case, test whether the population correlation coefficient is 0. Can we say that being good at mathematics may be *caused* by being good at literature, and vice versa?

Table 8.10 The intelligence quotients, mathematics scores, and literature scores of 18 students

No.	1	2	3	4	5	6	7	8	9
Mathematics scores (X)	78	84	61	52	93	89	98	98	65
Literature scores (Y)	83	76	70	58	82	78	89	95	61
IQs (Z)	95	100	100	75	105	97	110	120	76
No.	**10**	**11**	**12**	**13**	**14**	**15**	**16**	**17**	**18**
Mathematics scores (X)	73	48	45	67	75	95	88	99	81
Literature scores (Y)	75	53	43	70	78	97	92	92	88
IQs (Z)	92	61	60	88	96	125	113	126	102

Table 8.11 Ranks of 10 admission applications from two teachers

No. of applications	1	2	3	4	5	6	7	8	9	10
Ranks from teacher A	6	10	5	1	7	2	8	9	3	4
Ranks from teacher B	7	8	5	4	6	3	9	10	1	2

Table 8.12 Prevalence of arthritis in 100 middle-aged couples

Middle-aged wives	Middle-aged husbands		
	Ill	Not ill	Total
Ill	16	24	40
Not ill	24	36	60
Total	40	60	100

2. Ten applications for admission to graduate school were ranked by two teachers (Table 8.11). Are the ranks of the two teachers correlated?
3. The prevalence of arthritis in 100 middle-aged couples is shown in Table 8.12. Try to analyze whether the prevalence of arthritis in husbands and wives are associated.

III. Thinking

1. In 1988, a sampling survey was performed to study the prevalence of malnourishment in children between the ages of 0 and 7 (Table 8.13). Suppose a doctor is interested in whether age and the prevalence of malnourishment are related. Which statistical method do you think should be used and why?
2. Please look up domestic medical literature with the theme of correlation analysis or association analysis published within the last 3 years, and read at least three articles carefully. You are advised

Table 8.13 The prevalence of malnourishment in children between the ages of 0 and 7

Age/years	0~	1~	2~	3~	4~	5~	6~7
Prevalent number	98	278	86	29	59	82	34
Prevalence/%	15.7	11.7	12.9	7.4	8.9	7.3	5.1

to select one paper each on Pearson correlation, Spearman correlation, and association analysis. Summarize the improper points if any.

3. When discussing scatter diagrams, it was noted that caution should be exercised when stratification is present, as the results of stratification may significantly differ from the overall analysis. Please give an example or two to illustrate this phenomenon.

Jing Gu, Qinghai Liu, Li Ling

CHAPTER 9

SIMPLE LINEAR REGRESSION

The occurrence, development and changes in biomedical phenomena result from mutual restriction and the influence of many factors under certain conditions. For example, there are many influencing factors for high blood pressure, such as age, gender, family history, diet, smoking, alcoholism, and psychology. In adolescence, a person's height in general increases with age, but is also influenced by elements such as parental height and nutrition. Determining the main influencing factors and the size of their effects are the questions with which we are concerned. In this chapter, the basic idea of regression analysis is introduced through a simple linear regression model with only one influencing factor. Multiple regression analysis is introduced in Chapter 19.

9.1. Summary

9.1.1. *Study on the factors influencing the concentration of the air pollutant nitric oxide*

Example 9.1. To study whether the concentration of nitric oxide (NO) in atmospheric pollutants is affected by vehicle flow rate, climatic condition, and other factors, we choose a location in each of 24 cities with similar industrial levels, and count the number of vehicles passing per unit of time (1000). We also measure the average temperature (°C), air humidity (%), wind speed (m/s), and NO concentration (ppm) in the atmosphere at a given (low) altitude. The data are shown in Table 9.1.

Table 9.1 Monitoring data for atmospheric NO concentration at 24 urban locations

NO concentration (Y)	Vehicle flow (X_1)	Air temperature (X_2)	Air humidity (X_3)	Wind speed (X_4)	NO concentration (Y)	Vehicle flow (X_1)	Air temperature (X_2)	Air humidity (X_3)	Wind speed (X_4)
0.066	1.300	20.0	80	0.45	0.005	0.948	22.5	69	2.00
0.076	1.444	23.0	57	0.50	0.011	1.440	21.5	79	2.40
0.001	0.786	26.5	64	1.50	0.003	1.084	28.5	59	3.00
0.170	1.652	23.0	84	0.40	0.140	1.844	26.0	73	1.00
0.156	1.756	29.5	72	0.90	0.039	1.116	35.0	92	2.80
0.120	1.754	30.0	76	0.80	0.059	1.656	20.0	83	1.45
0.040	1.200	22.5	69	1.80	0.087	1.536	23.0	57	1.50
0.120	1.500	21.8	77	0.60	0.039	0.960	24.8	67	1.50
0.100	1.200	27.0	58	1.70	0.222	1.784	23.3	83	0.90
0.129	1.476	27.0	65	0.65	0.145	1.496	27.0	65	0.65
0.135	1.820	22.0	83	0.40	0.029	1.060	26.0	58	1.83
0.099	1.436	28.0	68	2.00	0.099	1.436	28.0	68	2.00

Data source: selected from Jiqian Fang, Ed., *Health Statistics*, 5th edition, People's Medical Publishing House.

The purpose of this study is to explore the factors influencing NO concentration, and to provide ideas for controlling air pollution. The difference from the previous chapter is that instead of talking about how variables are correlated, we are looking at how one variable (such as the concentration of NO in the air) is affected by other variables (such as vehicle flow). This kind of problem is analyzed statistically using a linear regression model (linear regression).

A linear regression model is adopted to investigate the influence of vehicle flow on the concentration of NO in the air, which is usually analyzed from the following three aspects:

1. Statistical description: a regression equation is used to describe the quantitative relationship between two variables.
   (1) Does the concentration of NO increase when vehicle flow increases?
   (2) Is this a linear trend or a nonlinear trend?
   (3) How can we use the regression equation to describe quantitatively the influence of vehicle flow on the NO concentration?
   (4) What is the average increase in NO concentration when the vehicle flow increases by 1000?
2. Statistical inference: a hypothesis test is used to infer whether the average NO concentration changes as the vehicle flow changes.
   (1) Is the influence of vehicle flow on NO concentration statistically significant?
   (2) What is the contribution of vehicle flow to NO concentration?
3. Statistical applications: using models for statistical prediction or control.
   (1) How can we predict the average NO concentration from vehicle flow?
   (2) How can we control the NO concentration by controlling the vehicle flow?

9.1.2. *Basic concepts*

Linear regression models play an important role in statistical analysis, with the goal to assess the relationship between the explanatory and response variables. The analysis of influencing factors in regression models uses the previously mentioned ideas of variance analysis. Many statistical methods, such as multiple regression and logistic regression, have been developed on the basis of linear regression.

9.1.2.1. *Regression analysis and simple linear regression*

Regression analysis is a statistical analysis method for studying relationships between variables. If height increases with age, then the heights of different individuals of the same age may be higher or lower, fluctuating around a certain average level. However, the general trend is to "return" to the average height and generally not deviate too far. If we link the average height of each age group in a line, then we obtain a regression line. The word "regression" is derived from the mean regression phenomenon proposed by Francis Galton, a British statistical geneticist, in the study of genetic characteristics. In regression analysis, the simplest case is a model that contains only two variables with a dependence relationship. One variable (the response variable) changes depending on the changes in another variable (the explanatory variable). When the trend in these changes is linear, it is called simple linear regression. When more than one independent variable is involved, it is called multiple linear regression.

9.1.2.2. *Explanatory variables and response variables*

In regression analysis, if Y changes with changes in $X_1, X_2, \ldots, X_m$, then Y is called the response variable or the dependent variable. The variables $X_1, X_2, \ldots, X_m$ are called explanatory variables or independent variables. We usually regard factors as independent variables. A response variable Y is a random variable that changes according to some rule. An explanatory variable X can be a random variable, or it can be controlled or selected. In the relationship between age and height, age is the independent variable and height is the dependent variable. In Example 9.1, NO concentration is the dependent variable, while vehicle flow, air temperature, air humidity and wind speed are the independent variables that may affect NO concentration.

9.2. Simple linear regression analysis steps

9.2.1. *Describing the relationship between two variables quantitatively*

9.2.1.1. *Scatter plots*

The first step in regression analysis is to draw a scatter plot, which can be used to visually investigate the relationship between two variables. Its purpose is to see whether there is a trend between the two variables, whether this trend is linear or nonlinear, and whether there are outliers that deviate from the trend. In Example 9.1, vehicle flow (X) is plotted on the horizontal axis and NO concentration (Y) is plotted on the vertical axis. The scatter plot is shown in Figure 9.1.

Figure 9.1 shows that NO concentration increases linearly with an increase in vehicle flow. However, NO concentration can vary greatly for similar vehicle flows, indicating that NO concentration may be influenced by other known or unknown factors, such as wind speed and air temperature. That is, the relationship between two variables described by regression analysis is not the familiar one-to-one functional relationship, but involves some uncertainty.

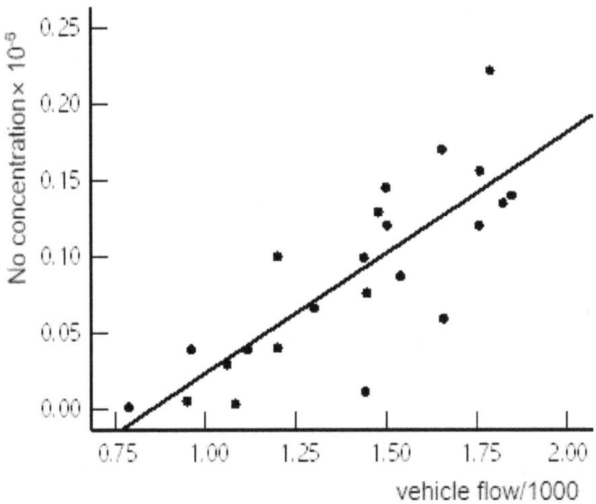

Figure 9.1 Scatter plot of NO concentration against vehicle flow

9.2.1.2. *Simple linear regression model*

In practical applications, simple linear regression is used to describe the relationship between dependent variables and independent variables quantitatively. The general expression for a linear regression model is

$$\mu_{Y|X} = \beta_0 + \beta X, \tag{9-1}$$

where $\mu_{Y|X}$ is the mean of Y corresponding to a certain value of X, and β_0 is the intercept of the regression line on the Y-axis. The statistical significance of β_0 is that it is the average value of Y when $X = 0$. The interpretation of the intercept must be consistent with reality. For example, in a regression equation linking the age of infants and the height of infants, the intercept represents the average length of the newborn (age 0). However, in a regression analysis of weight and height, the intercept cannot be interpreted as the average weight when the height is 0.

The parameter β is the regression coefficient of the population, which gives the slope of the regression line. The statistical significance of β is that for every unit of increase (or decrease) in X, the mean of Y, $\mu_{Y|X}$, changes by β units.

If $\beta > 0$, then the changes in Y and X have the same trend.

If $\beta < 0$, then Y and X have an inverse linear trend.

If $\beta = 0$, then Y and X have no linear regression relationship (this does not mean that they have no other relationship).

For a fixed value of X, the relationship between an observed value Y and the mean $\mu_{Y|X}$ is

$$Y = \mu_{Y|X} + \varepsilon, \tag{9-2}$$

where $\varepsilon \sim N(0, \sigma^2)$ is the residual.

Because β_0 and β are unknown in the linear regression model, they need to be estimated from sample values. Let the estimated values of β_0 and β be b_0 and b. The linear regression equation for a sample is

$$\hat{Y} = b_0 + bX. \tag{9-3}$$

In Equation (9-3), $\hat{Y}$ is the estimated value of the mean $\mu_{Y|X}$ of Y for a fixed value of X, b_0 is the sample intercept, b is the sample regression coefficient, and $Y - \hat{Y}$ is the residual.

9.2.1.3. *Least squares estimation of model parameters*

When there is a linear trend between two variables, a straight line can be drawn through their scatter plot visually, but the result is highly subjective. Using least squares estimation (LSE), we can calculate an "optimal" line. The idea is to find a line that minimizes the sum of squares of the longitudinal distance $(Y - \hat{Y})$ between the observed point and the line, which is called the sum of squared residuals and is written SS_{residual}. The smaller the sum of squared residuals, the better the representation of the scatter plot by the regression line. This method is based on least squares regression and therefore, is called ordinary least-squares regression (OLS regression). The estimation (b_0 and b) of β_0 and β can be achieved using calculus to find an extreme value:

$$b = \frac{\sum(X - \bar{X})(Y - \bar{Y})}{\sum(X - \bar{X})^2}, \quad b_0 = \bar{Y} - b\bar{X}. \tag{9-4}$$

In Equation (9-4), the denominator is the sum of squares of the mean deviation of X. while the numerator is the sum of the product of the mean deviations of X and Y.

Using Equation (9-4), the parameters β_0 and β for Example 9.1 are

$$b = 0.1584 \quad \text{and} \quad b_0 = -0.1353.$$

Thus, the estimated simple linear regression equation is

$$\hat{Y} = -0.1353 + 0.1584X.$$

Having obtained the simple linear regression equation, the regression line can be graphed on the scatter plot. The regression line can also be directly generated using statistical software (see Figure 9.1), and passes through $(\bar{X}, \bar{Y}) = (1.4035, 0.0871)$.

The result ($b = 0.1584$) shows that NO concentration increases as vehicle flow rate increases, more specifically, that the average NO concentration increases by 0.1584 ppm for every 1000 vehicles.

9.2.2. *Preconditions for linear regression analysis*

Linear regression analysis requires that the data are linear, independent, normally distributed, and have equal variance.

(1) Linear means that the response variable Y and explanatory variable X have a linear change trend. That is, if X increases or decreases by one unit, then the average change in Y remains the same. If the average change in Y increases or decreases as X increases, then the relationship should be modeled with a nonlinear equation. In general, scatter plots can be used to investigate whether two variables have a linear trend.

(2) Independence refers to the independence of any two observation values. That is, the value of an observation is not affected by other observations. In medical research, there are a large number of non-independent data, such as longitudinal observation data, repeated measurement data, and family research data. Whether a dataset meets the independence requirement can be judged by professional knowledge and experience, and can also be determined statistically. For data that do not meet the independence requirement, statistical analysis methods for non-independent data should be used, such as ANOVAs for repeated measurement data or multilevel models introduced in later chapters of this book.

(3) Normal distribution means that, for a given value of X, the observed values of Y follow a normal distribution. This is equivalent to the residual error following a normal distribution. Whether the residuals follow a normal distribution can be investigated using a residual diagram or a normal probability diagram.

(4) Equal variance means that the total variance in the Y values is equal for different X values. Whether the data meet the requirement of equal variance can also be determined using a residual diagram.

For the convenience of description, the conditions for using a simple linear regression model can be abbreviated as LINE (linearity, independence, normal distribution, and equal variance). Figure 9.2 is a schematic representation of these assumptions.

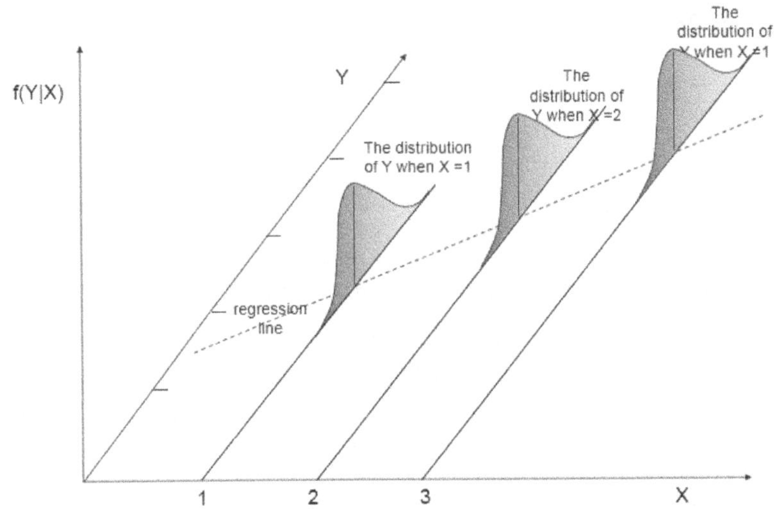

Figure 9.2 Three-dimensional diagram of the assumptions of the linear regression model

9.2.3. *Statistical significance of the regression equation*

The above regression equation and the regression line are only statistical descriptions of the relationship between the response and explanatory variables in the sample. Whether this relationship is statistically significant can be determined using hypothesis testing. The hypothesis test has two aspects: testing whether the regression model is established (model test) and testing whether the regression coefficient β is 0 (parameter test). The former uses variance analysis, while the latter uses a t-test.

9.2.3.1. *Hypothesis test of the regression equation*

As with the analysis of variance for comparing multiple means, the sum of squares of the total deviation in regression analysis can be decomposed into two parts:

$$\sum(Y-\bar{Y})^2=\sum(\hat{Y}-\bar{Y})^2+\sum(Y-\hat{Y})^2. \tag{9-5}$$

This equation can also be expressed as follows:

$$SS_{\text{total}}=SS_{\text{regression}}+SS_{\text{residual}} \tag{9-6}$$

The corresponding degrees of freedom and their relationship are

$$\nu_{\text{total}} = n - 1, \quad \nu_{\text{regression}} = 1, \quad \nu_{\text{residual}} = n - 2,$$
$$\nu_{\text{total}} = \nu_{\text{regression}} + \nu_{\text{residual}}.$$

The sum of squares of the three deviations in Equation (9-6) has the following different meanings.

SS_{total}: $\sum(Y - \bar{Y})^2$ is the sum of squared deviations of Y, and represents the total variance of the dependent variable Y.

$SS_{\text{regression}}$: $\sum(\hat{Y} - \bar{Y})^2$ is the sum of squares for regression. This reflects the component of the total variation of Y that can be explained by the linear relationship between Y and X by introducing X into the model. The larger the regression sum of squares, the stronger the regression effect.

SS_{residual}: $\sum(Y - \hat{Y})^2$ is the sum of squared residuals, and represents the influence of factors other than X on Y. That is, it is the component of the total variation of Y that cannot be explained by the linear relationship between X and Y, and represents random errors in Y after considering regression. As mentioned in the least squares method, the closer each observed point in the scatter diagram is to the regression line, the smaller the residual error, which means that the value of SS_{residual} is smaller and the regression effect is better.

The variances or mean squares corresponding to the three types of variation are:

$$MS_{\text{total}} = SS_{\text{total}}/\nu_{\text{total}}, \quad MS_{\text{regression}} = SS_{\text{regression}}/\nu_{\text{regression}},$$
$$MS_{\text{residual}} = SS_{\text{residual}}/\nu_{\text{residual}}.$$

If the value X in the population does not contribute to Y, then the value of $MS_{\text{regression}}$ and MS_{residual} shall be close. However, if X contributes to Y in the population, then $MS_{\text{regression}}$ will reflect more than random error, that is, $MS_{\text{regression}}$ must be much larger than MS_{residual}. The extent to which this is considered statistically significant can be inferred from the F-statistic:

$$F = \frac{SS_{\text{regression}}/\nu_{\text{regression}}}{SS_{\text{residual}}/\nu_{\text{residual}}} = \frac{MS_{\text{regression}}}{MS_{\text{residual}}}. \tag{9-7}$$

When the null hypothesis is established, the F-statistics follow the F-distribution for the degrees of freedom $(\nu_{\text{regression}}, \nu_{\text{residual}})$. After obtaining the F-statistic, we check the F-boundary value table to find the P value, and make a conclusion according to the test level (α).

An ANOVA was performed on the regression equation for Example 9.1 as follows.

H_0: The population regression equation is not established or the independent variable X in the population has no contribution to the dependent variable Y.

H_1: The population regression equation is established or the independent variable X in the population contributes to the dependent variable Y.

$\alpha = 0.05$

The results of variance analysis using the SPSS software are shown in Table 9.2.

As can be seen from Table 9.2, $P < 0.0001$, according to the $\alpha = 0.05$ level, the regression equation between NO concentration and vehicle flow can be considered statistically significant.

9.2.3.2. *Hypothesis test of the regression coefficient*

Even if the regression coefficient β is zero, the existence of sampling error means that the sample regression coefficient b is not necessarily zero. It is still necessary to test whether β is zero. Testing a regression coefficient usually uses the t-statistic.

Table 9.2 Analysis of variance of a simple linear regression model

Sources of variation	SS	*df*	MS	*F*	*P*
Regression	0.0530	1	0.0530	41.376	<0.0001
Residual	0.0282	22	0.0013		
Total variation	0.0812	23			

$H_0 : \beta = 0$
$H_1 : \beta \neq 0$
$\alpha = 0.05$

$$t = \frac{b - 0}{S_b}, \quad \nu = n - 2 \tag{9-8}$$

$$S_b = \frac{S_{Y.X}}{\sqrt{\sum(X - \bar{X})^2}} \tag{9-9}$$

$$S_{Y.X} = \sqrt{\frac{SS_{\text{residual}}}{n - 2}} \tag{9-10}$$

In these equations, $S_{Y.X}$ is the standard deviation of residuals of the regression, and S_b is the standard error of the sample regression coefficient. When the null hypothesis is established, the t-statistic Equation (9-8) follows a t-distribution with $n - 2$ degrees of freedom.

Because there is only one independent variable in a simple linear regression model, the ANOVA for the regression model is equivalent to a t-test of the regression coefficient, with $t = \sqrt{F}$.

Following the above example, we calculate that the following:

$$S_{Y.X} = 0.0358, \quad S_b = 0.0246,$$

$$t = 0.1584/0.0246 = \sqrt{41.376} = 6.432, \quad \nu = n - 2 = 22.$$

The condition $P < 0.0001$ was obtained from the statistical value for t, and H_0 was rejected at the $\alpha = 0.05$ level. Therefore, the regression coefficient was considered to be statistically significant.

Note: for the same group of data subject to a bi-variate normal distribution, if both correlation analysis and regression analysis are done at the same time, then the t-test of the correlation coefficient is equivalent to the t-test of the regression coefficient, and $t_r = t_b$.

9.2.3.3. *Interval estimation for the regression coefficient*

The regression coefficients obtained above are sample estimates. It is also necessary to estimate the confidence interval for the regression coefficient β. It is known that S_b is the standard error of the sample regression coefficient b (see Equation (9-9)), thus, the bilateral $1 - \alpha$

confidence interval for the regression coefficient β is

$$b \pm t_{\alpha/2,\upsilon} S_b. \tag{9-11}$$

In the above example, we calculated $b = 0.1584$, $S_b = 0.0246$, $\nu = 22$, and $t_{0.05/2,22} = 2.074$, so the bilateral 95% confidence interval for the regression coefficient is

$$0.1584 \pm 2.074 \times 0.0246 = (0.1074, 0.2095).$$

The confidence interval can be used to answer the hypothesis test question. When the $(1-\alpha)$ confidence interval does not contain 0, the total regression coefficient β is not equal to 0 at the $(1-\alpha)$ level.

9.2.4. *Finding the size of the effect of vehicle flow on NO concentration*

A common misunderstanding is that a larger regression coefficient indicates a greater influence of the independent variable(s) on the dependent variable(s). The size of the regression coefficients for X and Y are related to the units or sizes of the two variables, but do not indicate the size of the effect. The coefficient of determination was introduced to investigate the proportion of variation caused by X in the total variation of Y.

The coefficient of determination is an important statistic in regression analysis. It is defined as the ratio of the sum of squares for regression to the total sum of squares, and is denoted by R^2:

$$R^2 = \frac{SS_{\text{regression}}}{SS_{\text{total}}}. \tag{9-12}$$

Because $SS_{\text{regression}} \leq SS_{\text{total}}$, R^2 is between 0 and 1. Its numerical value reflects the contribution of the independent variables to the regression effect, that is, the percentage of the total variation in Y that the regression relationship can explain (variance account formula (VAF)), the percentage VAF that can be explained by the total variance of Y. The coefficient of determination also reflects the fitting effect of a regression model, and is often used as a goodness of fit indicator. It is left to the reader to show that, when both X and Y

are random variables, the coefficient of determination is equal to the square of the correlation coefficient (r).

For the above example, the values of SS_{total}, $SS_{\text{regression}}$, and SS_{residual} are shown in Table 9.2, from which we can calculate

$$R^2 = \frac{SS_{\text{regression}}}{SS_{\text{total}}} = \frac{0.0530}{0.0812} = 0.6527 = 65.27\%.$$

This indicated that 65.27% of the total variation in NO concentration is related to vehicle flow.

9.2.5. *Statistical applications*

9.2.5.1. *Confidence interval for the mean*

The $(1-\alpha)$ confidence interval for the mean $\mu_{Y|X}$ of Y for a given value of X is

$$\hat{Y} \pm t_{\alpha/2,(n-2)} S_{\hat{Y}}. \tag{9-13}$$

In Equation (9-13), $S_{\hat{Y}}$ is the standard error of $\hat{Y}$, which can be calculated according to the following formula:

$$S_{\hat{Y}} = S_{Y.X}\sqrt{\frac{1}{n} + \frac{(X_i - \bar{X})^2}{\sum(X - \bar{X})^2}}. \tag{9-14}$$

For example, when the vehicle flow is 1300, $\hat{Y} = 0.0707$, and the 95% confidence interval for the mean value of the NO concentration is

$$\begin{aligned} &0.0707 \pm 2.074 \times 0.0358\sqrt{\frac{1}{24} + \frac{(1.3 - 1.4035)^2}{2.1124}} \\ &= (0.05465 \sim 0.08675) \times 10^{-6} \end{aligned}$$

9.2.5.2. *Prediction intervals for individual values*

Prediction is one of the important applications of regression analysis. It is commonly used in medicine to calculate the interval containing $(1-\alpha)$ of the individual values Y for a given X value (prediction factor). The $(1-\alpha)$ prediction interval for Y is calculated using the formula

$$\hat{Y} \pm t_{\alpha/2,(n-2)} S_Y, \tag{9-15}$$

where S_Y is the standard deviation of Y:

$$S_Y = S_{Y.X}\sqrt{1 + \frac{1}{n} + \frac{(X_i - \bar{X})^2}{\sum(X - \bar{X})^2}}. \tag{9-16}$$

When n is fairly large and X_i is very close to $\bar{X}$, $S_Y \approx S_{Y.X}$.

For example, when the vehicle flow is 1300, $\hat{Y} = 0.0707$, and the 95% prediction interval for the NO concentration is

$$0.0707 \pm 2.074 \times 0.0358\sqrt{1 + \frac{1}{24} + \frac{(1.3 - 1.4035)^2}{2.1124}}$$
$$= (0.0000 \sim 0.1467) \times 10^{-6}$$

Note: the confidence interval for the mean is different from the prediction interval for individual values. The former is the interval for the mean $\mu_{Y|X}$ of Y when X takes a certain value. The latter is the possible interval for Y for a given value of X. Figure 9.3 illustrates the regression line (solid line), the confidence interval band for the mean (short dashed line), and the individual value prediction interval band (long dashed lines). It can be seen from the figure that the individual value prediction interval band is wider than the confidence interval band.

9.2.5.3. *Statistical control*

According to the air pollution index classification, when the air quality status does not exceed grade II, the NO content in the air should not exceed $(0.100 \sim 0.150) \times 10^{-6}$. To reduce the NO concentration in the air, the city plans to control vehicle flow appropriately.

According to the regression equation $\hat{Y} = -0.1353 + 0.1584X$ and the above criteria, we obtain the following results.

When $Y_1 = 0.100 \times 10^{-6}$, $X_1 = (Y_1 - b_0)/b = (0.100 + 0.1353)/0.1584 = 1.485(\times 1000)$.
When $Y_2 = 0.150 \times 10^{-6}$, $X_2 = (Y_2 - b_0)/b = (0.150 + 0.1353)/0.1584 = 1.801(\times 1000)$.

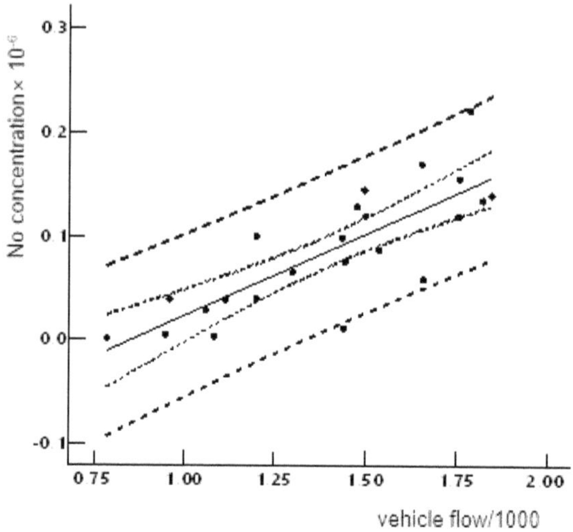

Figure 9.3 Regression line, confidence interval for the mean and prediction interval for individual values

The vehicle flow of the city should be controlled within 1500 vehicles per unit time.

Exceeding this vehicle flow may lead to slight pollution. Moderate air pollution may occur when vehicle flow is greater than 1800 vehicles per unit time. Of course, the degree of pollution may also be affected by wind speed, air temperature, and other factors. Using a multiple linear regression model should increase the accuracy of statistical control.

9.3. Report writing

Simple linear regression analysis usually requires reporting the following.

(1) Purpose of the analysis.
(2) Estimation method for fitting simple linear regression equations.
(3) Discussion of whether the data meet the conditions for using simple linear regression.
(4) Parameter estimation results.
(5) Goodness of fit for the model and hypothesis testing.
(6) Professional interpretation of the results.

Table 9.3 Parameter estimation of regression model

Model	Unstandardized coefficients B	Std. Error	Standardized coefficients	t	P
Intercept	−0.1353	0.035		−3.829	<0.001
X	0.1584	0.025	0.808	6.432	<0.001

Use the analysis of NO concentration and vehicle flow as an example to write a report for using simple linear regression.

Table 9.3 shows the result of parameter estimation of linear regression model between NO in air (Y) and motor vehicle flowrate (X), including regression coefficients, standard errors, standardized coefficient, and the results of hypothesis tests.

Table 9.3 suggest that the average density of NO may increase with the motor vehicle flow rate ($R^2 = 0.6527$, $P < 0.0001$). The regression line of NO concentration versus motor vehicle flow was plotted in Figure 9.1.

9.4. Case discrimination

Case 9.1 Age and height prediction study

The heights of boys and girls aged 4–18 were recorded in a certain place (as shown in Table 9.4). Describe the relationship between average height and age of boys and girls, and predict the height of boys and girls at 10.5, 16.5, 19, and 20 years old.

The SPSS software was used for regression analysis of height and age, with the results shown in Tables 9.5 and 9.6.

After fitting the simple linear regression model, the t-test results indicated that the models were statistical significant. The R^2 results indicated that the fitting effect was very good and therefore, we make the following conclusions.

1. The average height of boys and girls increases linearly with age. For each year of increase in age, the average height of boys and

Table 9.4 Survey data for average height against age for boys and girls in a certain place

Age (years)	Average height (cm)		Age (years)	Average height (cm)		Age (years)	Average height (cm)	
	Boys	Girls		Boys	Girls		Boys	Girls
4.0	102.1	101.2	8.0	126.8	126.3	14.0	162.5	157.1
4.5	105.3	104.5	9.0	132.2	131.8	15.0	166.1	157.7
5.0	108.6	107.6	10.0	136.6	137.9	16.0	169.0	158.7
5.5	111.6	110.8	11.0	142.3	144.1	17.0	170.6	158.9
6.0	116.2	115.1	12.0	147.2	150.0	18.0	170.7	158.9
7.0	122.5	121.1	13.0	156.3	155.1			

Data file:case data9-1.sav

Table 9.5 Results of simple linear regression analysis for height and age for boys

	Estimated value	Standard error	t	P
Constant	83.7363	1.8824	44.4839	<0.001
Age	5.2748	0.1676	31.4798	<0.001

$F = 990.98$, $R^2 = 98.5\%$

Table 9.6 Results of simple linear regression analysis for height and age for girls

	Estimated value	Standard error	t	P
Constant	88.4326	3.2800	26.9611	<0.001
Age	4.5340	0.2920	15.5290	<0.001

$F = 241.15$, $R^2 = 94.1\%$

girls increases by 5.27 and 4.53 cm, respectively, so boys grow faster than girls.

2. According to the regression equation, the average heights of boys in this area at 10.5 years old, 16.5 years old, 19 years old, and 20 years old were 139.12, 170.77, 183.96, and 189.23 cm,

respectively. The average heights of girls aged 10.5, 16.5, 19, and 20 were 136.04, 163.24, 174.58, and 179.11 cm, respectively.

For the above analysis results, consider the following questions.

(1) Does the analysis process conform to the basic steps of regression analysis?
(2) Can the regression model reflect changes in trend in the data?
(3) Is it reasonable to make the predictions given according to the regression equation?
(4) Is it true that boys grow faster than girls?

Case 9.2 Study of serum transferrin in patients with anemia

To study the effect of a new drug on anemia patients, 20 patients with anemia were randomly divided into two groups. One group was treated with the new drug, and the other group was treated with conventional drugs. The increase in hemoglobin (g/L) was measured to study whether the increases in hemoglobin were different when using the new drugs versus the conventional drugs to treat anemia patients.

Dr. Zhang used a t-test to compare the increases in hemoglobin after treatment with the different drugs. The mean increase in hemoglobin with the new drugs was $\bar{Y}_1 = 27.99$, the mean increase in hemoglobin with the conventional drugs was $\bar{Y}_2 = 20.21$, and the t-test gave a value of $t = 4.137$ for $\bar{Y}_1 - \bar{Y}_2 = 7.78$.

Dr. Wang decided to use linear regression analysis. Two variables were involved in these data. The dependent variable Y, which was a continuous variable, was the increase in hemoglobin. The treatment factor, which was a binary variable, was taken as the independent variable X, with the new drug group coded as $X = 1$ and the conventional drug group coded as $X = 0$. The data were converted into bi-variate form (see Table 9.7). After analysis, the obtained regression equation was $\hat{Y} = 20.21 + 7.78X$, with $t = 4.137$.

According to the analysis of the two doctors, please think carefully:

(1) Are the methods used by Dr. Zhang and Dr. Wang to analyze the data correct?

Table 9.7 Results for anemia patients treated with two different drugs

Number	Y	X	Number	Y	X	Number	Y	X	Number	Y	X
1	19.5	0	6	22.0	0	11	30.5	1	16	32.5	1
2	19.0	0	7	19.0	0	12	21.4	1	17	29.5	1
3	13.0	0	8	15.5	0	13	25.0	1	18	25.5	1
4	24.7	0	9	24.5	0	14	34.5	1	19	24.4	1
5	21.5	0	10	23.4	0	15	33.0	1	20	23.6	1

Data file:case data9-2.sav

(2) Can regression analysis replace the t-test for the mean of two individuals?
(3) Based on this case study, what is the relationship between regression analysis and the t-test?

9.5. Computer experiments

Experiment 9.1 The calculations in Example 9.1 should be done using SPSS.

Draw a scatter plot, and observe whether there are linear trends and outliers. Fit a simple linear regression model, write the regression equation and test your results. Explain the ANOVA analysis table and parameter estimation results.

Experiment 9.2 Use SPSS to perform the calculations for Case 9.1.

Estimate the linear trend from the scatter plot. Compare the results of linear and nonlinear fitting and goodness of fit. Choose the best type of modeling curve, giving a reasonable explanation.

9.6. Frequently asked questions and summary

9.6.1. *Frequently asked questions*

(1) Identifying and handling outliers

In practice, the identification of outliers in a dataset should be completed before statistical analysis to avoid errors and wasted effort. Some "statistical lies" are caused by analysts including outliers in the

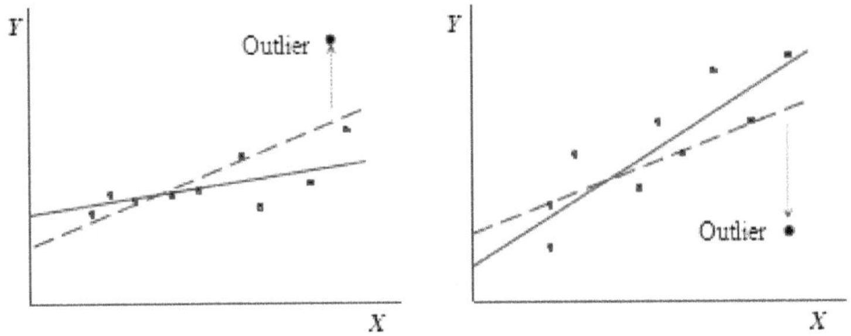

Figure 9.4 Influence of outliers on regression analysis

analysis, which may exaggerate or weaken the actual effect as shown in Figure 9.4. The dotted line represents the regression line when the outlier is included. Recognizing outliers can be achieved using scatter plots, which are simple, intuitive, and effective, or using relevant statistics (such as residuals, generalized squared distance, etc.). Scatter plots provide a visual representation of which data points are possible outliers.

Once possible outliers have been found, it is not advisable to delete them hastily. The process by which the possible outliers were found should be carefully reviewed. If they were obtained experimentally, the experiment should be repeated several times. Only when an outlier is caused by human factors, such as experimental error or incorrect records, should deletion or replacement with the correct data be considered. If careful examination reveals that outliers in the data are caused by the nature of the individuals, then these data should be studied further and may yield unexpected findings.

(2) Variables that do not have a linear relationship

In complex biomedical phenomena, the relationship between two variables may be nonlinear in many cases, such as the relationship between drug concentration in the blood and time, the growth curve, and dose–response. If simple linear regression is used to analyze nonlinear data, the results will distort the actual relationship between variables. In practice, curve fitting is used instead. Some common types of curve are:

(1) The exponential curve, also known as the exponential growth curve, can be used to model bi-variate data where the dependent variable Y increases (or decreases) more quickly as the independent variable X increases.
(2) The polynomial curve, adding the terms b_2X^2 and b_3X^3 into the simple linear model gives quadratic and cubic polynomial curves. Polynomials are good choices for fitting curves.
(3) The logistic curve, also known as the Pearl-Reed curve, has an elongated "S" shape. It is mostly used in studies on development, dynamic rates, dose–response relationships, and population. The logistic model mentioned in the following chapters fits data with a logistic curve.
(4) The hyperbola is similar to the exponential curve, but is suitable for analyzing data with a greater degree of curvature, such as interphase data for muscle tension and neurophysiological strength.

The SPSS software can perform a wide variety of curve fitting for researchers. In practice, several different curves should be applied to a scatter plot. Determining the final curve type is based on the following principles. ① A larger R^2 value indicates a better fit. However, it is not necessary to pursue goodness of fit excessively. For example, in the case of a polynomial model, using a higher degree polynomial will increase the R^2 value but also complicates interpretation. ② Consider whether the type of curve agrees with the professional interpretation. ③ If two curves have similar measures for goodness of fit, choose the curve that is easiest to explain and simplest to express.

(3) Combining batches of data to fit a linear regression model

In practice, the X and Y variables often come from two batches of data, which cannot be easily combined for regression analysis. The individuals analyzed should come from the same population to ensure homogeneity. If two batches of data come from two different subgroups, it is possible to draw unrealistic conclusions. As shown in Figure 9.5, the solid point and the hollow point represent two batches

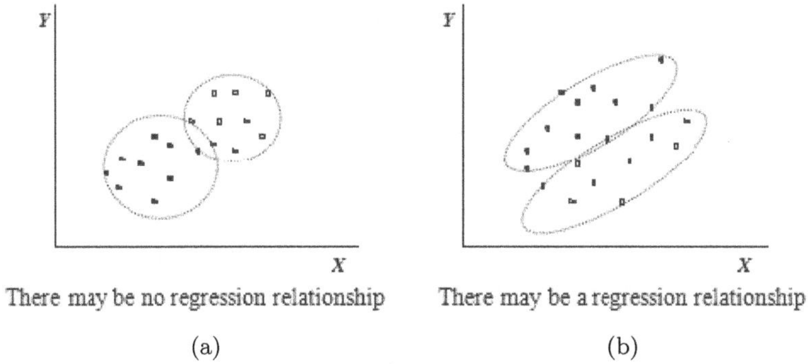

Figure 9.5 Influence of combining two batches of data on regression

of data respectively. In Figure 9.5(a), there is no actual regression relationship in either batch of data, but merging the batches of data suggests that there is a regression relationship. In Figure 9.5(b), each batch of data may have a regression relationship, which are lost by merging the data. The existence of two subgroups is a confounding factor that can affect regression relationships.

9.6.2. *Summary*

1. Simple linear regression refers to a linear regression model with a single independent variable. It is used to describe a linear relationship between the values of the dependent variable and the independent variable. In practical applications, the relationship between the two variables should have practical significance. Regression analysis should not be used for two unrelated phenomena.
2. The steps for performing simple linear regression analysis are: ① draw a scatter plot to investigate whether there is a linear trend between the two variables and to identify potential outliers; ② estimate the regression coefficient and intercept; ③ apply a hypothesis test to the regression coefficient and/or the regression equation; ④ determine the regression equation and draw the regression line; ⑤ apply the regression results.

3. A simple linear regression equation includes an intercept and a regression coefficient, and usually uses LSE. The appropriate hypothesis test for regression analysis is variance analysis of the regression equation and a t-test for the regression coefficient.
4. Decomposing the total variation of Y is helpful for understanding simple linear regression analysis. That is, the sum of squared deviations of Y (SS_{total}) can be decomposed into the sum of squares for regression ($SS_{\text{regression}}$) and the sum of squared residuals (SS_{residual}).
5. The main uses of linear regression analysis are prediction and control. In practical applications, it should be noted that the regression equation cannot be extended at will. That is, the applicability of a regression equation is in general limited to the observed values of the independent variable, unless there is sufficient reason to believe that it is valid outside this interval. Otherwise, prediction and control should be restricted to the observed interval.
6. When two variables have a nonlinear relationship, fitting with a nonlinear regression equation can be considered. Commonly used types of curve include exponential curves, polynomial curves, hyperbolae, and logistic curves.

Think and Practice

I. Questions for Reflection

1. Briefly describe the process of simple linear regression analysis.
2. Briefly describe the differences and similarities between linear regression analysis and linear correlation.

II. Questions on Calculations

1. In Example 9.1, take NO concentration as the dependent variable and wind speed ($X4$) as the independent variable. Use statistical software to complete the following analysis.
   (1) Find a simple linear regression equation to describe the relationship between NO concentration and wind speed.
   (2) Test your hypothesized regression equation and regression coefficient.

Table 9.8 Correlation variables and predicted values

X	Y	$\hat{Y}$	e	X	Y	$\hat{Y}$	e	X	Y	$\hat{Y}$	e
1.30	0.07	0.0707	−0.0047	1.20	0.10	0.0548	0.0452	1.12	0.04	0.0415	−0.0025
1.44	0.08	0.0935	−0.0175	1.48	0.13	0.0986	0.0304	1.66	0.06	0.1271	−0.0681
0.79	0.00	−0.0108	0.0118	1.82	0.14	0.1531	−0.0181	1.54	0.09	0.1081	−0.0211
1.65	0.17	0.1265	0.0435	1.44	0.10	0.0922	0.0068	0.96	0.04	0.0168	0.0222
1.76	0.16	0.1429	0.0131	0.95	0.01	0.0149	−0.0099	1.78	0.22	0.1474	0.0746
1.75	0.12	0.1426	−0.0226	1.44	0.01	0.0929	−0.0819	1.50	0.15	0.1017	0.0433
1.20	0.04	0.0548	−0.0148	1.08	0.00	0.0365	−0.0335	1.06	0.03	0.0327	−0.0037
1.50	0.12	0.1024	0.0176	1.84	0.14	0.1569	−0.0169	1.44	0.10	0.0922	0.0068

(3) According to the above results, calculate the 95% confidence interval for the regression coefficient.

(4) For a wind speed of 1.50 m/s, calculate the 95% prediction interval and the 95% confidence interval for NO concentration, and illustrate the significance of these intervals.

2. The following table presents some results of regression analysis for a case study. The four columns are the independent variable (X), the dependent variable (Y), the estimated value of $Y(\hat{Y})$, and the residual $e(Y - \hat{Y})$. Use correlation analysis to investigate the relationship between the four columns, and analyze and explain the numerical values and the statistical significance of the relationship (Table 9.8).

Yanbo Zhang, Yuantao Hao

Part II

Design and Implementation of Bio-medical Research

CHAPTER 10

SAMPLING SURVEY

With the changed of medical model and disease spectrum, it has become an important issue in the field of public health to explore the occurrence and progression of life and other health events in population. However, it is impossible to observe every individual in one study due to limited resources. Usually, we can obtain a sample that is a part of individuals sampled from the population randomly. And then the characteristics of the population can be inferred based on the sample information. Such research is called sampling survey. The basic concepts and methods in sampling survey research will be mainly introduced in this chapter.

10.1. Introduction

Same as other study, sampling survey research must have a clear objective. From the view of statistics, there usually are two main objectives for sampling survey research. One is to estimate the population parameters, such as the total cholesterol (TC) level of people in a certain area. The other is to understand the relationship between different variables, such as the relationship between living conditions, lifestyles, etc., and hypertension.

Example 10.1. It was verified that blood lipids was an independent risk factor of cardiovascular disease, and serum TC was an important indicator of clinical lipid. How to assess the serum TC level for a certain population by sampling survey, to provide the latest information for the prevention and treatment of blood lipids?

Example 10.2. Bronchial asthma is one of the most common chronic respiratory diseases. Knowing the prevalence is of great reference for interventions against asthma. How to estimate the prevalence of asthma for people aged 14 or over in a certain area through a sampling survey?

Example 10.3. It was verified that social support was related to health status of the elderly in numerous studies. Knowing the social support of the elderly plays a great role in improving the health status of the elderly. Besides objective, visible, or practical support, social support also includes subjective emotional support. How to measure the social support for the elderly in a sampling survey?

The above examples concern the estimation of population mean and proportion, and the measurement of subjective outcomes. The following topics will be introduced which related to the three examples. How to extract individuals from the population (sampling method)? How to infer population characteristics (parameter estimation) based on the sample information? How to measure subjective outcomes? How to perform quality control in the sampling survey?

10.2. Sampling method

Randomization is an important principle to ensure that the sample taken is representative of the population. Sampling methods are classified as probability sampling and non-probability sampling based on randomization or not. It is called probability sampling that every unit in the population has an equal probability of being sampled in the sampling process. Otherwise it is called non-probability sampling. The common probability sampling methods include simple random sampling, systematic sampling, stratified random sampling, and cluster sampling. Convenience sampling, judgment sampling, quota sampling, and snowball sampling are common non-probability sampling methods. Due to limited spaces, only probability sampling methods are introduced in this chapter.

10.2.1. *Simple random sampling*

As name suggests, simple random sampling is a method of selecting the sample at random completely. Generally, simple random sampling is such a technique that each individual in the population has an equal chance and likelihood of being selected in the sample. Simple random sampling is a very basic type of sampling method. It is usually divided into three steps. Firstly, a list of all the individuals from the population is prepared. Then each individual is assigned a specific number (e.g., there are N members then they will be numbered from 1 to N) based on a certain rule. Finally, individuals are selected to be a part of the sample based on random numbers, which are usually from random number tables and random number generator software.

Example 10.4. For the purpose of the research in Example 10.1, 684 patients would be randomly selected from 25,416 physical examiners with complete information. Firstly, a list of all the physical examiners having complete information was made. Then sequential numbers were assigned to each examiner $(1, 2, 3, \ldots, 25{,}416)$ according to physical examination order. Finally, 684 random numbers between 1 and 25,416 were generated in a random number generator. Examiners whose numbers match the 684 random numbers were selected in the sample.

The advantage of simple random sampling is simple and easy to implement. In addition, it is easy to estimate the sampling error as well. However, it is a costlier method of sampling as it requires a complete list of all potential respondents to be available, especially for a larger population. Otherwise, it is difficult to ensure the representative when the variation is large and the sampling ratio is small.

10.2.2. *Systematic sampling*

Systematic sampling is selecting every "rth" individual to be a part of the sample based on the sequence numbers that are assigned to individuals according to a certain rule. Systematic sampling process includes several steps. Similar to simple random sampling, a list of all individuals from the population and their specific number are prepared firstly. Then the sampling interval r is determined. $r =$ Number of individuals in population/Number of individuals in sample. The starting point k between 1 and r is selected randomly. Finally, individuals with numbers of $k, k + r, k + 2 \times r, k + 3 \times r, \ldots$, are selected as the sample.

Example 10.5. For the purpose of the research in Example 10.1, the researcher wanted to select 500 physical examiners from 20,000 medical examiners with complete information. Firstly, a list of all the physical examiners having complete information was made and sequential numbers were assigned to each examiner $(1, 2, 3, \ldots, 20{,}000)$ according to physical examination order. Then the sampling interval was calculated, $r = 20{,}000/500 = 4$. A random number k between 1 and 4 was generated. Finally, the examiners with numbers of $k, k + 4, k + 2 \times 4, k + 3 \times 4, \ldots$, and $k + 499 \times 4$ were extracted.

The advantages of systemic sampling are simple and time-saving, and the sampling error is smaller than simple random sampling. The disadvantage is less protection from sampling bias especially when there exists certain tendency between the individuals (such as periodic changes).

10.2.3. *Stratified random sampling*

Stratified random sampling is a method of sampling from a population, which can be partitioned into sub-populations (strata) according to the main characteristics (such as age, gender, illness, etc.). Then simple random sampling or systematic sampling is applied within each sub-population. The diversification within each stratum will be much lesser than the diversification that exists in the target population. There are two stratified sampling strategies, proportionate allocation and optimum allocation (or disproportionate allocation).

Proportionate allocation uses a sampling fraction in each of the sub-population that is proportional to that of the population.

It means that the sample size is larger for a sub-population with larger number of individuals, and smaller with smaller number of individuals. For optimum allocation, the sampling fraction of each stratum is proportionate to both the proportion (as above) and the standard deviation of the variable. Larger number of individuals are selected in the sub-population with greater variability or larger number of individuals.

Example 10.6. In Example 10.1, it is known that the blood lipid level are different for people with different age groups. Stratified random sampling should be performed to select the sample. The examiners with complete information were divided into four strata according to age, such as $\leq$29 years old, 30$\sim$39 years old, 40$\sim$49 years old, and $\geq$50 years old. Simple random sampling was applied in each stratum.

The advantage of stratified random sampling is that the sampling error is small than simple random sampling since the individuals of the sample are chosen from every strata. In addition, each stratum can be analyzed independently and compared with each other. The disadvantage is that investigation and analysis are troublesome when there are a large number of strata.

10.2.4. *Cluster sampling*

Cluster sampling is a sampling method based on groups. With cluster sampling, the researcher divides the population into K separate groups, called clusters. Then, a simple random sample of k clusters is selected from K separate groups. In other words, the sampling unit is a cluster, not an individual. Each cluster should be a small-scale representation of the population. The clusters should be mutually exclusive and collectively exhaustive, such as villages, workshops, classes, and company. For example, in order to investigate the health status of residents in a certain area, villages are selected randomly, and all residents in the selected villages are surveyed. If the diversification between groups is small, and k is large, then the representativeness of the samples is good.

Example 10.7. For the purpose of the study in Example 10.2, the communities or villages in the area were numbered, and about 6 communities or villages were randomly selected. All residents aged 14 or over in the selected communities and villages were investigated.

The advantages of cluster sampling is that it is easy to organize and control quality of survey. It can be cheaper than other sampling plans, for example, fewer travel expenses and administration costs. The disadvantage is that the sampling error is higher than other sampling methods.

Above four sampling methods are listed in ascending order by the sampling error as follows, stratified random sampling, systematic sampling, simple random sampling and cluster sampling.

10.2.5. *Multistage sampling*

The above four methods can be used alone or in combination. The method of dividing the entire sampling process into several stages is called multistage sampling. Multistage sampling can be considered as a complex form of cluster sampling because it involves dividing the population into groups (or clusters). Firstly, the population is divided into several groups, which are called primary sampling units. Then a sampling method is used to extract a part of the primary units. The extracted primary units are divided into several sub-samplings unit, then a part of the secondary units are extracted by a sampling method from each of the extracted primary units. This process is repeated until there is no unit need to be divided.

Example 10.8. In Example 10.2, firstly, the areas were divided as urban, suburban and remote suburb based on the administrative district. In each stratum, a simple random sampling was used to extract the district or county. Then simple random sampling was carried out to extract streets or towns in the selected district or county. And finally, simple random sampling was used to extract communities or villages in the selected streets or towns. All residents aged 14 or above in the selected community or village were as research subjects.

10.3. Population parameter estimation

Same as experimental studies, the population parameter estimation in sampling survey includes point estimation and interval estimation. Sample mean ($\bar{X}$) and proportion (p) are the point estimations for population mean and proportion, respectively. The interval estimation of the population mean can be calculated by $(\bar{X} - t_{\alpha/2,n-1}S_{\bar{X}}, \bar{X} + Z_{\alpha/2}S_{\bar{X}})$, $(\bar{X} - Z_{\alpha/2}S_{\bar{X}}, \bar{X} + Z_{\alpha/2}S_{\bar{X}})$, and $(\bar{X} - Z_{\alpha/2}\sigma_{\bar{X}}, \bar{X} + Z_{\alpha/2}\sigma_{\bar{X}})$. While the interval estimation of the population proportion can be obtained from population proportion table or calculating by $(p - Z_{\alpha/2}S_p, p + Z_{\alpha/2}S_p)$. However, the sampling errors of different methods are quite different. There is no special standard error calculation formula for systematic sampling. Researchers can estimate the standard error for systematic sampling according to simple random sampling. It is difficult to estimate the sampling error for non-probability sampling. This chapter only introduces the estimation of the standard error of mean and proportion for simple random sampling, stratified random sampling and cluster sampling (see Tables 10.1 and 10.2).

Example 10.9. In Example 10.4, 684 physical examiners were selected by simple random sampling, the mean and standard deviation of serum TC were 4.75 and 1.14 mmol/L, respectively. Please try to estimate the 95% confidence interval of the serum TC for the examiners.

According to the standard error estimation formula in Table 10.1,

$$S_{\bar{X}} = \frac{S_X}{\sqrt{n}} = \frac{1.14}{\sqrt{684}} = 0.044\,(\text{mmol/L}).$$

Since $n = 684$ (large sample), $(\bar{X} - Z_{\alpha/2}S_{\bar{X}}, \bar{X} + Z_{\alpha/2}S_{\bar{X}})$ was used to estimate the confidence interval. So the 95% confidence interval

Table 10.1 Standard error ($S_{\bar{X}}$) estimation of mean for the three sampling methods

Sampling methods	Infinite population	Limited population
Simple random sampling	$\frac{S_X}{\sqrt{n}}$	$\sqrt{1-\frac{n}{N}}\frac{S_X}{\sqrt{n}}$
Stratified random sampling	$\sqrt{\sum_{i=1}^{k}\left(\frac{n_i}{n}\right)^2\left(\frac{S_{X_i}}{\sqrt{n_i}}\right)^2}$	$\sqrt{\sum_{i=1}^{k}\left(\frac{n_i}{n}\right)^2\left(\left(1-\frac{n_i}{N_i}\right)\frac{S_{X_i}}{\sqrt{n_i}}\right)^2}$
Cluster sampling	$\sqrt{\frac{1}{k(k-1)}\sum_{i=1}^{k}\left[\frac{n_i}{\bar{n}}(\bar{X}_i-\bar{X})\right]^2}$	$\sqrt{\frac{1-k/K}{k(k-1)}\sum_{i=1}^{k}\left[\frac{n_i}{\bar{n}}(\bar{X}_i-\bar{X})\right]^2}$

Note: N is the number of individuals in the population, i is the number of strata (clusters) in the stratified (cluster) sampling, n_i is the sample size of the i-th stratum (cluster), and k is the number of strata or the number of selected clusters. $\bar{n}$ is the average sampling size for the k strata (clusters), N_i is the number of individuals for the i-th stratum, S_{X_i} is the standard deviation of the i-th stratum, K is the number of clusters in the population, and $\bar{X}_i$ is the sample mean of the i-th cluster, $\bar{X}$ is the sample mean of all the k clusters (same as the following table).

Table 10.2 Standard error (S_p) estimation of proportion for the three sampling methods

Sampling methods	Infinite population	Limited population
Simple random sampling	$\sqrt{\frac{p(1-p)}{n-1}}$	$\sqrt{\left(1-\frac{n}{N}\right)\frac{p(1-p)}{n-1}}$
Stratified random sampling	$\sqrt{\sum_{i=1}^{k}\left(\frac{n_i}{n}\right)^2\left(\frac{p_i(1-p_i)}{n_i-1}\right)}$	$\sqrt{\sum_{i=1}^{k}\left(\frac{n_i}{n}\right)^2\left(\left(1-\frac{n_i}{N_i}\right)\frac{p_i(1-p_i)}{n_i-1}\right)}$
Cluster sampling	$\sqrt{\frac{1}{k(k-1)}\sum_{i=1}^{k}\left[\frac{n_i}{\bar{n}}(p_i-\bar{p})\right]^2}$	$\sqrt{\frac{1-k/K}{k(k-1)}\sum_{i=1}^{k}\left[\frac{n_i}{\bar{n}}(p_i-\bar{p})\right]^2}$

Note: p_i is the sample proportion of the i-th stratum (cluster), $\bar{p}$ is the sample proportion of all the k clusters.

Table 10.3 The results of TC test for examiners stratified random sampled with different age

Age (year)	Number of individuals	TC (mmol/L) Mean	Standard deviation
≤29	132	4.34	0.95
30∼39	122	4.71	0.93
40∼49	210	4.72	0.92
≥50	220	5.06	0.88
Total	684	4.75	0.97

of the serum TC for the examiners was $(\bar{X} - 1.96S_{\bar{X}}, \bar{X} + 1.96S_{\bar{X}})$, that was (4.66, 4.84) mmol/L.

Example 10.10. In Example 10.6, the physical examiners were selected by stratified random sampling. The results were shown in Table 10.3. Please try to estimate the 95% confidence interval for the serum TC of the examiners.

The standard error estimation was as follows.

$$S_{\bar{X}} = \sqrt{\sum_{i=1}^{k}\left(\frac{n_i}{n}\right)^2\left(\frac{S_{X_i}}{\sqrt{n_i}}\right)^2}$$
$$= \sqrt{\left(\frac{132}{684}\right)^2\left(\frac{0.95}{\sqrt{132}}\right)^2 + \left(\frac{122}{684}\right)^2\left(\frac{0.93}{\sqrt{122}}\right)^2 + \left(\frac{210}{684}\right)^2\left(\frac{0.92}{\sqrt{210}}\right)^2 + \left(\frac{220}{684}\right)^2\left(\frac{0.88}{\sqrt{220}}\right)^2}$$
$$= 0.035\ (\text{mmol/L})$$

Same as Example 10.9, the 95% confidence interval of the serum TC was $(\bar{X} - 1.96S_{\bar{X}}, \bar{X} + 1.96S_{\bar{X}})$, that was (4.68, 4.82) mmol/L.

Example 10.11. In Example 10.7, residents aged 14 or over were selected by cluster sampling to investigate the prevalence of asthma. The investigation results were shown in Table 10.4. Please try to estimate the 95% confidence interval for asthma prevalence of residents aged 14 or over.

Table 10.4 The results of asthma prevalence for different community or village

ID of community or village	Number of individuals surveyed	Number of individuals with asthma	Prevalence of asthma (%)
1	19,204	204	1.06
2	19,264	214	1.11
3	4492	53	1.18
4	4692	55	1.17
5	4898	78	1.59
6	5097	83	1.63
Total	57,647	687	1.19

The standard error estimation was as follows.

$$S_p = \sqrt{\frac{1}{k(k-1)}\sum_{i=1}^{k}\left[\frac{n_i}{\bar{n}}(p_i - \bar{p})\right]^2}$$

$$= \sqrt{\frac{1}{6(6-1)}\left\{\left[\frac{19204}{57647/6}(0.0106 - 0.0119)\right]^2 + \cdots + \left[\frac{5097}{57647/6}(0.0163 - 0.0119)\right]^2\right\}}$$

$$= 0.00079$$

For the data approximately followed normal distribution, so the 95% confidence interval of asthma prevalence was: $(p - 1.96S_p, p + 1.96S_p)$, that was (0.0104, 0.0134).

In the above examples, for the convenience of calculation, we did not take the correction number $1 - \frac{n}{N}$ or $1 - \frac{k}{K}$ into consideration for finite population. In practical applications, if $N \gg n$, or $K \gg k$, the correction has little effect, otherwise the correction is needed for the finite population. The sampling error estimation for the cluster sampling listed in Tables 10.1 and 10.2 are applicable only to the case of simple random sampling of clusters. If the difference between clusters is large, it is not appropriate to use simple random sampling, the better way is to use other sampling methods such as probability proportional to size (PPS) and so on, and the sampling error estimation also adopts the corresponding method.

10.4. Design of survey instrument

In a sampling study, the outcome measurement (namely survey instrument) is questionnaire. Questionnaire is a series of questions related to the objectives of the study. Such a questionnaire consisting of indicators reflecting a conceptual framework, is known as the scale. The scale is used to measure a state, behavior, or attitude of a subject. In biomedical research, the scale is a commonly used, simple, and feasible measurement instrument, especially for outcomes that cannot be accurately measured such as frail, pain, etc., and subjective feelings of the subjects. Scale is a standardized measurement instrument, with more strictly development process, including more rigorous reliability and validity evaluation. So, scale can be considered as a special type of questionnaire. The construction (development) of general questionnaire (named questionnaire for short) and the scale will be introduced in the following sections.

10.4.1. *Questionnaire development*

Questionnaire is also known as interview questionnaire form. The investigator or target person fill in the form according to questions.

10.4.1.1. *Composition of questionnaire*

1. Title: The subject of the study. It should be simple and clear, such as "Health status questionnaire for middle-aged intellectuals."
2. Survey items: The survey items are the core part of questionnaire. It is made up of questions that can be understood and replied by target population. It usually includes the following three parts:

   (1) Background information: Age, gender, ethnicity, marital status, educational level, occupation, etc. of subjects.
   (2) Outcomes: Primary outcomes and secondary outcomes of the study, such as serum TC value in Example 10.1.
   (3) Verification items: Name, telephone number, and other information of subjects, as well as name of the investigator and the interview time, etc. These are mainly used for verification and further tracking.

3. Instructions of the form: It refers to a specific description of the contents of the questionnaire, which gives a clear explanation and definition for the outcomes and related variables. This will enable investigators and respondents to clearly respond to the questions or answers in the questionnaire.

10.4.1.2. *Steps of questionnaire development*

1. Making outline of questionnaire

Making main contents of questionnaire based on the objective, time, scope, subjects, and analysis method of the survey.

2. Determining survey items

According to the outline, specifying the contents of questionnaire. Then determining the interview questions, variables to be measured and information related to the study.

3. Preparing and sequencing questions

Specifying questions based on survey items and determining the sequence according to importance, logic, and filling methods of questions.

4. Pre-investigation and modifying the questionnaire

Administrating the draft questionnaire in a small sample size. Assessing the applicability of the questionnaire, and revising it until it is perfected.

10.4.1.3. *Design of questions*

1. Type of question

Based on the answering ways, questions were divided as open-ended, closed-ended, and semi-closed questions.

(1) Open-ended questions

The respondents are not given any restrictions to some specified options. They can reply freely based on their own understanding. For example, "What is the main problem with your health?" "How do you think about current medical services?" and so on.

Advantages: It is easy to motivate the respondents for the comfortable atmosphere between investigators and respondents, and obtain more information.

Disadvantages: Respondents are usually "not on the topic," and the responses may not be within the expected scope. It is difficult to arrange and analyze data for the diverse responses. Respondents are apt to reject to reply due to the costly time and energy on thinking for the question.

(2) Closed-ended questions

The responses are limited to the specified options, such as "yes" and "no," as well as "high school or above," "junior high school," "primary school or below" for "the level of education."

Advantages: The response rate is high due to easily understanding and replying. For the standardized reply, it is easy to encode, arrange, and analyze. As to sensitive issues, like income, etc., for the options are presented in a hierarchical manner, it is also easy to be accepted by respondents.

Disadvantages: Some information, which is not covered by the options may be omitted. The respondent may respond the question at a guess and will. So the information collected may not always reflect the real situation.

(3) Semi-closed questions

This type of question combines the closed-ended question with open-ended question. For "the hospital which you visit mostly (single choice)," options are "provincial hospitals," "municipal hospitals," "district hospitals," "community medical service stations," and an open option "others (please specify)."

Advantages: It can not only avoid the "not on the topic" for open questions, but also compensate the limitation of closed-ended questions.

Disadvantages: Respondents are apt to choose the specified options, and the proportion of "Other" is usually underestimated.

2. Principles for question preparation

(1) Words should be simple, straightforward and easy to be understood, avoiding "jargons" with which only the professionals are familiar.
(2) Questions or options should always be clear. Ambiguous questions are avoided, because it will lead to vague replies. The meaning of words such as "often," "occasionally," and "sometimes" should be clearly defined. For example, "often" is defined as "once a week or above" in a survey.
(3) Questions covering two issues and double negative questions should be avoided. For example, "Do you smoke or drink?" focus on two issues, smoking and drinking. As an example of double negative question, "How do you think about that preventing tumors is not impossible?" It is difficult for respondents to reply these questions.
(4) Induced questions should be avoided. For example, respondents are apt to reply "You don't smoke, don't you?" with "No, I don't." So, there is bias for these kinds of questions.
(5) Personal privacy issues should be treated with care. It is advisable to adopt methods such as object transfer and assumption method to eliminate the worries of the respondents. For example, "Some people deem that AIDS is caused by dirty sex. While others disagree it. Which point do you agree with?" As another example, "If family planning policy is not implemented in our country, how many children would you like?"

3. The principle for questions sequence

(1) Be logical. The arrangement of questions should conform to people's logical thinking habits. The basic information, such as age, gender, education level, family situation, etc., are usually arranged forward, proceeding with primary research outcomes and related indicators, such as illness, treatment, and others.
(2) From general to specific. Questions about special issues should be arranged to follow the questions about general issues.
(3) From easy to difficult. The questions easy to reply should come first before the difficult ones.

(4) From familiar to unfamiliar. Questions with which the subjects are familiar should be arranged before the questions the subjects are unfamiliar with.
(5) Properly arrange the sensitive questions. The sensitive questions should be usually placed after the other questions. But when there are a few sensitive questions, they should be dispersed among other questions to reduce the sensitivity and rejection rate.

10.4.1.4. *Cautions in questionnaire development*

1. The questionnaire should be divided into several parts, such as general information, dietary, illness, others.
2. In case to be readable and importable by the computer, all questions should be encoded, such as $A1, A2, \ldots, An$. If the questions also have sub-questions, "_" or other symbols and numbers should be added. For example, question A1 contains three sub-questions, which can be encoded as $A1\_1, A1\_2, A1\_3$, respectively.
3. The options for all closed-ended questions should be encoded. The encoding of each option for different closed-ended questions should be consistency, such as "No" is encoded as "0" and "Yes" is encoded as "1." "unknown," "not clear" and so on should be encoded as "999" and other impossible numbers.
4. Researchers should pay attention to the number of questions. Amount of investigations have shown that an interview should be finished in less than 30 minutes. If the interviewing time exceeds 30 minutes, the quality of respondents' reply might decline. So the number of questions should be limited within 50. In large-scale investigation, the questionnaire always contains several scales, so the number of questions is inevitably beyond 50. Corresponding measures must be taken to ensure the investigation quality, while the interviewing time should still be controlled within 1 hour.

10.4.1.5. *Examples of questionnaire*

Example 10.12. The attitude of medical workers to medical insurance were surveyed in a certain area. Parts of the questionnaire were shown in Table 10.5.

Table 10.5 Questionnaire on the attitude of medical workers to medical insurance in a certain area

Medical insurance is the combination of accumulated personal savings and social co-ordination of insurance. Insurance premiums payment are composed of the country, department, and individuals. One part of insurance premiums is a personal account fund, which is managed by individual. The remaining part is a social co-ordination fund, which is managed by the medical insurance institutions uniformly. So, it is given a full role to bring the personal relief and social common relief to individuals. This questionnaire anonymously asks your attitude to medical insurance. Please answer all the questions. There are several options for each question, please choose one option based on your true situation.

We look forward to your sincere cooperation, thank you!

GENERAL INFORMATION

A1, Age (years) □□

A2, Gender 1 male 2 female □

A3, Department 1 Internal Medicine 2 Surgery 3 Gynecology 4 Pediatrics 5 Administration 6 other □

A4, Education Level 1 primary school 2 junior high school 3 senior high/secondary school 4 college school or above □

PLEASE INDICATE YOUR ATTITUDE TO THE FOLLOWING HEALTH INSURANCE ISSUES.

B1, How do you think about the current health insurance policy □
1 very reasonable 2 reasonable 3 neither reasonable nor unreasonable 4 unreasonable 5 very unreasonable

B2, In your opinion, who has benefited most from health insurance? □
1 country 2 department 3 individual 4 Hospital 5 None

B3, Would you like to participate in health insurance? □
1 very willing 2 willing 3 neither willing nor unwilling 4 unwilling 5 very unwilling

......

Fill in date Check signature Verification date

10.4.2. *Scale development*

10.4.2.1. *Classification and construction of scale*

The scale can be divided as categorical scale, ordinal scale, isometric scale, and ratio scale according to the level, units, and reference points of measurement. According to the application scope, it is divided as universal scale and specific scale. Generally, the scale is composed of several domains, which refer to the conceptual framework of measurement. For example, the WHO quality of life scale WHOQOL-100 contains six domains, such as physical, psychological, level of independence, social relationships, environment, and spirituality. Each domain is composed of several facets, and each of them is actually composed of items related to the evaluation characteristics. For example, in WHOQOL-100, the physical domain includes three facets that are pain and discomfort, energy and fatigue, sleep and rest. Each facet can contain several items. Item is actually question, with which the different aspects of situation about subjects are measured. For example, each facet of WHOQOL-100 consists of four items. The hierarchy structure of scale can be represented by Figure 10.1.

10.4.2.2. *Steps of scale development*

(1) Determination of the intended population. The target population should be identified at the beginning of the scale development. The scale should be ascertained to be universal or specific according to the purpose of the study. A universal scale is developed for the general population, and a specific scale is developed for a specific group of people (the elderly, diabetics, etc.).

The research team of scale development should include relevant experts and practitioners in the field of research. For instance, in the

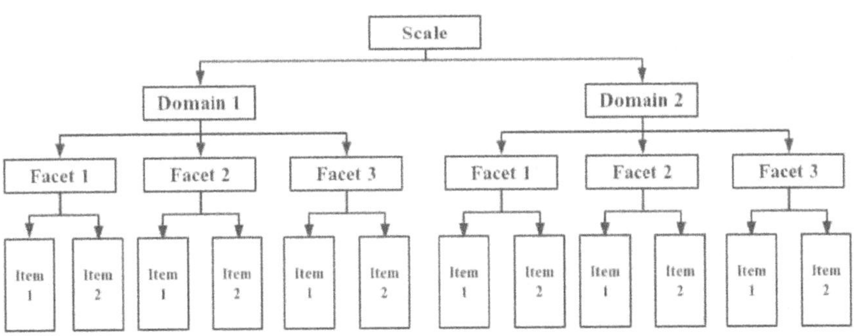

Figure 10.1 Hierarchy structure of the scale

process of development the scale of satisfaction on the service of the aged care institutions. The research team should include members of the civil affairs and health department members, medical workers, elderly caregivers, and institutional managers, etc., and should also include the target of the service, who are in different levels of disability among the elderly and their families. The research team can be divided as a Nominal Group and a Focus Group (also known as a core group). The members of Nominal Group should be more extensive, and composed of people who can represent the target group. In addition to the professionals in the fields, there must be quantitative intended subjects, and they are mainly responsible for the presentation of the items. While for the Focus Group, which needs to be more specialized and responsible for the specific scale development work.

(2) Definition and decomposition of measurement concepts

Conceptual framework of measurement, namely the operable definition of measurement concept and its decomposition, is formed to explore the domains and facets of the scale based on literature. The operable definition and its composition of the measurement concepts are given by the Focus Group. Such as "What is the concept of satisfaction?" "What domains and facets are included in satisfaction measurement" "What are the meaning and connotation of each domain and facet?" etc. This step needs to be fully discussed within the Focus Group and reviewed by the Expert Group.

(3) Generation of item pool. The Focus Group explained the definition and content of the measured concepts, domains, and facets to the Nominal Group. Then the Nominal Group independently put forward items using interview method (30–50 intend subjects) and derivation method (based on the measurement conceptual framework, writing items based on professional knowledge and experience) and literature reviews (reading literatures and related scales, extracting items). Then the items are discussed in each Focus Group (3–6 core groups, 6–8 persons each group). Finally, the proposed scale items are collated and aggregated to form item pool.

As the item pool generated, the form and response options of the items, that is, the response scale of item, should be determined. Most of the response scales adopt linear or equidistant rank scale. The former gives a line segment with a scale (e.g., 0–10), and the respondent marks at the line segment to indicate the scores. The latter consists of some equidistant words regarding levels such as very poor, poor, neither poor nor good, good, and very good. The isometric grading scale method was founded by Likert (1932). It mainly consists of 3-point, 5-point, and 7-point method, among which 5-point method is the most commonly used. In addition, there is an unequal scale of rank, with which the degree of the alternative words is not completely equidistant. For unequal scale of rank, it often requires response scale analysis to determine the corresponding score of each option.

(4) Development of the pilot form of the scale. The layout of the pilot form, including the frontispiece, instructions, informed consent, and the item sequence, should be determined firstly. Then all the items are administrated in 5–10 subjects educated moderately selected from the target population and the general population, respectively. The items are selected roughly to construct the pilot form of the scale in terms of the degree of difficulty and responsiveness and so on for items inquiry. Eventually, 40–50 subjects from the target population and the general population were chosen for field testing respectively. Items would be revised once again according to the feedback from the respondents in the field testing to form the questionnaire including the pilot form of the scale.

(5) Administration the pilot form of the scale in target population, and selecting items to form the refined pilot of the scale. A representative sample in the target population is selected. The proportion of gender, age, education level, region, etc., should be close to that of the population. After data collection, if it is found that the composition of the sample is greatly different from that of the population, correction (such as standardization) should be carried out. Regarding the sample size, Kendall had proposed that as a rough working criterion, the sample size should be 5–10 times the number of variables. For a scale with 20 items, at least 100 individuals should be tested.

The pilot form of the scale was refined after variety of statistical item selecting methods, as well as the expert opinions.

(6) Field survey with refined scale and psychometric assessment of the refined scale. Representative sample from the target population (who did not participate in the pilot survey) was selected interviewed with a questionnaire containing the refined scale. The suitability, language fluency, reliability, validity, acceptability, and responsiveness of the scale were evaluated quantitatively.

(7) Form the final draft of the scale. On the basis of the validation, the refined pilot form of the scale was modified and improved to be the final draft of the scale. If necessary, the modified scale shall be assessed and modified and improved again until the assessment of psychological properties is good.

(8) Composition of the scale's user manual. Complete scale's user manual includes the introduction (background, objective, intended application, funding), development process, scale description (scale format, instructions, scoring method), results of scale validation, advice of application (the purpose of the scale, cautions, the copyright owner, and their contact information), references and appendix.

10.4.2.3. *Statistical methods for item selection*

A good item should hold the characteristics of strong importance, good representativeness, high sensitivity and strong independence, as well as a certain operability and acceptability, in accordance with the requirements of social ethics. The statistical methods available for item selection are as follows.

(1) Correlation coefficient

The correlation coefficients between each item and the domain are calculated. This method select items from representative and independent perspective. Items, which have large correlation coefficient with own domain and small correlation coefficient with other domains, should be retained in the scale.

(2) Dispersion tendency

This method select items on the view of sensitivity. Standard deviation or coefficient of variation is often used to indicate the variation of an item. The smaller the variation is, the worse the discrimination ability is, and the less sensitive to the differences of the tested subjects is.

(3) Principal component analysis and factor analysis

The items are selected based on a representative perspective. According to the results of principal component or factor analysis (see Chapter 24), the items with greater loading on each factor should be retained in the scale.

(4) Discrimination analysis

The items are selected from a discriminating perspective. For example, the score of each item was tested by t-test with health status as the grouping variable, and the items that could distinguish patients from healthy people were selected. Logistic regression or stepwise discrimination can also be used, but the influence of correlation between items on the results should be cared.

(5) Cronbach's α coefficient

The items are selected from the perspective of internal consistency. The Cronbach's α coefficient of a certain facet is calculated and compared the changes in the coefficients after removing one of the items. If α coefficient increases after an item deletion, the item should be deleted, otherwise it should be retained.

(6) Test–retest reliability

The items are selected on the view of stability. Items with high test–retest reliability should be retained. However, it should be noted that the time between the two measurements should not be too long, and it is assumed that the relevant conditions of the respondent (such as the characteristics measured by the scale) do not change during the two tested time.

(7) Item response theory (IRT)

IRT is a mathematical model that represents the relationship between the subjects' response to an item and the item parameters. Items are selected according to item parameters, item characteristic curves, the individual-item graph, the fitting of the item to the model, the amount information of the item, and the differential item function in different groups. See Chapter 29 for details.

In practical applications, the results of different item selection method are not always the same. It can be combined to determine the retention and deletion of items.

Example 10.13. In the process to develop "Multidimensional Functional Health for old adults," 60 items in the pilot form of the scale were comprehensively selected according to 6-item screening methods. The selection results of 10 items in the domain of social relationship were shown in Table 10.6. The number of deletions per item was accumulated. The 5 items with the lowest number of deletions were retained to construct the final scale.

10.4.3. *Scale assessment*

The refined pilot form of the scale can be considered as the final draft of the scale, only when it is verified reliable, valid and responsiveness. Otherwise, it should be modified and assessed again.

1. Reliability

The term reliability refers to stability and consistency of the scale. It can be considered as the variation of the measured value, which is caused by random errors in the measuring process. The commonly used reliability indexes include test–retest reliability, split-half reliability and Cronbach's α coefficient.

(1) Test–retest reliability

Test–retest reliability is a measure of consistency of the scale. Individuals are asked to take the same scale twice at different times. The correlation coefficient (r) of the two scores is calculated. The larger the r is, the more reliable the scale is. Generally, it is required to

Table 10.6 Selection results of items in the domain of social relationship in "Multidimensional Functional Health for old adults"

Item	Cronbach's α	Correlation coefficient	Factor loading	Discrimination parameter	Average information amount	Delphi importance rating	Number of deletions
S1	0.005^b	0.305^b	0.233^b	0.79^b	0.159^b	4.5833	5
S2	−0.024	0.706^b	0.489^b	1.54^b	0.571^b	4.2500	4
S3	−0.026	0.686^b	0.820	1.67^b	0.656^b	4.2500^b	4
S4	−0.029	0.708	0.547^b	1.69^b	0.671^b	4.5000	3
S5[a]	−0.031	0.704^b	0.698^b	2.76	1.230	4.4167	2
S6	−0.033	0.631^b	0.579^b	2.65^b	1.187^b	4.5000	4
S7[a]	−0.028	0.711	0.902	4.61	2.438	3.9167^b	1
S8[a]	−0.030	0.741	0.911	4.79	2.583	3.7500^b	1
S9[a]	−0.030	0.716	0.931	5.30	2.955	4.1667^b	1
S10[a]	−0.030	0.736	0.933	5.50	3.116	3.9167^b	1
S11	0.097^b	0.489^b	0.139^b	0.30^b	0.024^b	3.8333^b	6

[a]Retained items.
[b]The deletion criterion is satisfied (top 6 items with lower or higher value, for 5 items would be retained); the discrimination parameter and the average information amount are based on Graded Response Model (an IRT model).

reach 0.7 or above. In another way, the scores are then compared by paired t-test. The closer the scores are, the more reliable the scale is.

(2) Split-half reliability

It is a measure of consistency between scale takers' performance on different halves (e.g., odd- and even-numbered items) of a scale. The correlation coefficient r of the two-part scores is calculated, and the formula for Spearman–Brown calculation of the semi-reliability is as following:

$$R = \frac{2r}{1+r} \tag{10-1}$$

(3) Internal consistency

Internal consistency reliability defines the consistency of the results delivered in a scale, ensuring that the various items measuring the different constructs deliver consistent scores. Internal consistency can be considered as the harmony level of multiple survey items. The Cronbach's α, as shown in Equation (10-2), is commonly used to evaluate the internal consistency. Generally speaking, the internal consistency of the scale could be considered to be good when the Cronbach's α reaches 0.7 or above.

$$\alpha = \frac{k}{k-1}\left(1 - \frac{\Sigma S_i^2}{S_T^2}\right) \tag{10-2}$$

in which, k is the number of items in the scale, S_i^2 represents the variance of the score of item i, and S_T^2 represents the variance of the total score of the scale.

2. Validity

Validity, also known as accuracy, is used to reflect the degree of proximity between the result of measurement and the real value. There are following three main indicators to evaluate the validity of the scale.

(1) Content validity

Content validity is also known as the logical validity. It refers to the extent to which a measure represents all facets of a given conceptual framework. A scale may lack content validity if the respondent's understanding and response are inconsistent with the designer's. Content validity of the scale is assessed by experts scoring. There is a correlation between content validity and construct validity, so the quantitative index of evaluating construct validity also indirectly reflects the content validity.

(2) Criterion-related validity

Criterion-related validity, also known as the criterion validity. It refers to the extent to which a measure is related to an outcome. It can be assessed by the correlation between the new scale and an existing scale, which is universally recognized as a standard measurement. The correlation coefficient of the two measured scores represents the standard validity.

(3) Contract validity

It is also called construct validity, which refers to whether the structure of the scale is consistent with the theoretical assumption. A scale may lack construct validity, if the internal components of the scale are inconsistent with the dimensions that designers intend to measure. The construct validity is mainly evaluated by confirmatory factor analysis (CFA) (see Chapter 27 for details). Comparative fit index (CFI) and other goodness of fit indexes are calculated to assess the extent of a specific factor model fit to the actual data. When CFI >0.9, it is considered that the fit is good. The construct validity can also be evaluated by means of exploratory factor analysis (see Chapter 24 for details). If the extracted common factors have a close logical relationship with the scale domains determined at the time of scale design, it will be considered that the scale has a good construct validity.

In the evaluation stage of the "Multidimensional Functional Health Scale for Older Adults," the Cronbach's α for the refined pilot scale was 0.928, greater than 0.7. It can be concluded that the internal consistency of the scale is good. As a result of the CFA, CFI $=$ 0.917. So the construct of the scale is fitted with the real data well. The scale has a good construct validity.

3. Responsiveness

The responsiveness refers to the ability of a scale to accurately detect change when it has occurred in different objects and at different times. It indicates the scale's sensitivity to change. The commonly used statistic of responsiveness is effect size. Generally speaking, effect size should be larger than 0.2. The effect size is smaller, medium, and larger when it is in the range of 0.2–0.5, 0.5–0.8, and 0.8 or above, respectively.

$$\text{Effect size} = \frac{\bar{X}_{\text{after}} - \bar{X}_{\text{before}}}{S_{\text{before}}}$$

In order to evaluate the responsiveness of WHOQOL-BREF, 627 inpatients with pneumonia were tested with the scale before and after having treatment for a period. The average score of the patients before treatment was 70.26, and the standard deviation was 7.26. The average score after treatment was 77.09, and the effect size was $(77.09 - 70.26)/7.26 = 0.941$. Paired t-test showed that $t = 15.04$, $P < 0.001$, so the difference was statistically significant. It can be concluded that WHOQOL-BREF could better detect the improvement of patients' quality of life after treatment.

Reliability, validity and responsiveness are called the psychometrical properties of scale. The psychometrical evaluation is essential in the scale development. In addition, the acceptability should also be evaluated. Acceptability can be assessed in terms of refusal rate, rates of missing responses, and administration time. Generally, the refusal rate should be equal or less than 30%, while the missing response rate should be less than 10%, and the average time to complete the survey should be no more than 30 minutes.

In biomedical research, except for the development of scale, sometimes there is a need to introduce the foreign mature scale. When introducing a foreign scale, we should follow the normalized procedure, which is translation — back translation — cultural adaptation — equivalence evaluation. Due to limited space, it is not elaborated here. Please refer to other books. Both the development and the introduction of the scale should meet the relevant requirements of the questionnaire.

10.5. Sampling survey research plan and quality control

10.5.1. *Sampling survey research plan*

Before carrying out an investigation, it is necessary to have a good and thorough protocol. Also, there is a need to develop a scientific and rigorous investigation plan. The sampling survey plan mainly includes three stages: preparation, sampling survey, data analysis, and result expression.

1. Preparation

In this stage, tasks includes determination of the topic based on the literature review, clarifying the objective of the survey, determination of the survey subject, sampling methods and survey indicators. Design of the questionnaire and finally, formation of the protocol are also accomplished in this stage.

2. Sampling survey

Firstly, a small sample size pre-survey is conducted to check whether the survey plan is defective and operable based on the protocol. Then the protocol is modified based on the pre-survey. Finally, the formal sampling survey is implemented based on the modified protocol.

3. Data analysis and result expression

In this stage, all the original data are checked again. Supplementary of missing data and elimination of wrong data are carried out as occasion required. After establishment of the database, the survey data are input accurately into the computer and followed with data locking. Finally, descriptive and inferred analyze are implemented, coming up with report writing.

10.5.2. *Quality control in sampling survey research*

A good protocol cannot guarantee the high quality of the investigation. It is necessary to ensure the quality through every stages of the research. Quality control should be carried out in the stage of field investigation, data collocation and result expression, and analysis.

1. Quality control in field investigation

Measures on quality control in field investigation include selection and training of investigators, pre-investigation, and perfection of the protocol before the investigation. In the process of investigation, measures such as data check on that day, problems resolution in time, etc. should also be taken to control survey errors, such as registration errors, response bias, etc.

2. Quality control in data cleaning, presentation, and statistical analysis

The integrity and correctness of data registration should be checked in the stage of data collocation, result expression, and statistical analysis to ensure no repetition or omission. Measures, such as double entry, should be implemented to ensure the accuracy of data entry. Appropriate statistical analysis methods should be selected to deal with survey data. The results should be interpreted reasonably and the reports or papers should be written according to certain requirements and formats.

In addition to the above quality control measures, all kinds of bias shall be controlled in the sampling survey. The common bias and control methods are shown in other chapters of this book.

10.6. Report writing

1. Report of sampling survey

In general, the report of sample survey should include the followings:

(1) Objective.
(2) Subject, sampling method, and survey indicators.
(3) Instrument. The reliability and validity of the scale should also be reported for scale.
(4) Main results: sample statistics, standard errors, and confidence intervals of the population parameters of primary outcomes.

Report for Example 10.4

Objective: To investigate the serum TC level in physical examination population.

Subject: Persons who underwent physical examination in the area

Sampling method: Simple random sampling

Survey indicator: Serum TC (mmol/L)

Instruments: Information of the participants were extracted from the physical examination database.

Main results: A total of 684 participants were investigated. The mean of serum TC was 4.75 mmol/L, and the standard deviation was 1.14 mmol/L. The standard error of the mean was 0.044 mmol/L, and the 95% confidence interval of the population mean was (4.66, 4.84) mmol/L.

2. Report of scale development

In addition to the contents of the survey, the report of scale development should include the steps in scale development.

Report of scale development for Example 10.13

Target group: The elderly

Dimensions of the scale: Ability of daily life, social relationships, physical health, mental health, economic resources, and cognitive function.

Construction of item pool: The pool contained 120 Likert-type items based on relevant research articles.

Development of initial scale: After several rounds of discussions, importance rating from 15 specialist and interviewing 50 elderly people, the initial scale was constructed with 60 items.

Pilot form scale survey and item selection: 539 elderly people were surveyed with the pilot form of the scale. Items were further selected through Cronbach's α and the other 5 methods. The pilot form of the scale was refined to 30 items (see Table 10.6 for further item selection of social relationship).

Refined pilot form scale survey and scale validation: 2032 elderly people (less than 5% overlap with the pilot sample) were interviewed using the refined scale. The Cronbach's α was 0.928, and CFI was 0.917 based on CFA. Due to good internal consistency and construct validity, the refined pilot form of the scale with 30 items could be taken as the final version.

10.7. Case discrimination

Case 10.1 A multi-stage stratified sampling was used to come up with a survey on the prevalence of diabetes among residents aged 20 or above nationwide. In the first stage, all the provinces were divided as the east, middle, and west according to the geographical areas, and a typical province was chosen from each of the three parts. In the second stage, 2 typical municipalities (counties) were chosen from each of the 3 selected provinces. In the third stage, 4 streets (townships) were extracted using simple random sampling in each of the 6 selected municipalities (counties). In the fourth stage, 11 streets (townships) were selected through a simple random sampling in each of the 24 selected communities (villages), with a total of 154 urban communities and 110 rural villages being selected. Finally, all residents aged 20 or above in the chosen community (village) were recruited. 54,240 persons were eventually included in the survey, while 47,325 of whom (18,976 men and 28,349 women) completed the survey. The overall response rate was 87.3%, 81.0% for men and 92.0% for women; 88.1% for urban residents and 82.7% for rural residents. After exclusion of the incomplete information, 46,239 respondents were included in the final analysis, among which there were 4485 residents suffering from diabetes. This resulted in a 9.7% prevalence rate of diabetes among the residents aged 20 or above in the country. The questions are: What is the deficiency of this study? How should it be improved?

Case 10.2 In order to investigate the prevalence of cervical cancer in adult women and its influencing factors, a researcher designed the questionnaire as follows:

The questionnaire on the prevalence and risk factors of cervical cancer in adult women
Instructions: omission.
A1. Gender: ① male ② female
A2. Date of birth: month: year
A3. Residence: ① town ② rural
A4. Occupation: ① company white-collar/enterprises and institution cadre ② service personnel ③ self-employed/ freelancers ④ farmer ⑤ worker ⑥ other (please specify)
A5. Educational level: ① primary school and below ② junior high school ③ senior high/secondary/technical school ④ college school or above
A6. Your average monthly income_______ (CNY)
A7. Your first sexual age (years): ① $\leq$18 ② 19~25 ③ 26~30 ④ $\geq$31
A8. Do you experience a sexual transmission of disease: ① yes ② no
A9. Have you ever heard of cervical cancer screening: ① yes ② no
A10. Have you ever been screened for cervical cancer before: ① yes ② no
A11. The infection of HPV (human papilloma virus) can cause cervical cancer or condyloma acuminatum? ① yes ② no ③ unclear

Try to make a comment on the questionnaire.

Case 10.3 A researcher developed a service quality evaluation scale for pension institutions based on the literature review, score by experts, etc. A pool of 192 items was generated firstly. Then the items were sorted and merged, and the items with lower score by experts were deleted. Finally, a pilot form of the scale consisting 37 items was developed. The pilot form of the scale was administrated in 153 persons. Exploratory factor analysis was used to further screen items based on the survey data. The refined pilot scale consisted of 29 items, which are divided into 5 dimensions: hardware facilities and environment, operation management, safety protection, humanistic care, and basic health according to the results of exploratory factor analysis. In order to assess the psychometrical properties, the refined pilot scale was administrated in 501 persons. The results of reliability evaluation showed that the Spearman–Brown was 0.830, and the Cronbach's α coefficient was 0.918. It was concluded that the refined scale has a good internal consistency. The CFA based on the 5 dimensions resulted in that the compare fitting superiority index (CFI) was 0.94. The results also showed that the structural validity of the refined scale was good. In summary, it can be concluded that the scale was reliable and valid, and could be used to evaluate the service quality for pension institutions. Try to make a comment on the development process of the scale.

10.8. Computer experiments

Experiment 10.1 Calculate the internal consistency reliability for Example 10.14 with SPSS software.

Experiment 10.2 Calculate the split-reliability for Examples 10.14 with SPSS software.

10.9. Frequently asked questions and summary

10.9.1. *Frequently asked questions*

1. In sampling survey study, should we choose stratified random sampling method as much as possible for its smallest sampling error?

The four basic probability sampling methods (simple random sampling, systematic sampling, stratified random sampling, and cluster sampling) have their own advantages and disadvantages respectively. Researchers should weigh the pros and cons, and choose the appropriate sampling method based on specific situations. Although the sampling error of stratified random sampling is the smallest, stratified random sampling may lose its meaning when the intra-strata variation is large and the inter-strata variation is small. Although the sampling error of cluster sampling is the largest, a fair number of researches use cluster sampling method for their advantages such as saving money and being easy to organize and control the investigation quality.

2. The difference between questionnaire and scale

Since the scale is a special form of questionnaire, questionnaires are classified as scale questionnaire and non-scale questionnaire. For simplicity, the non-scale questionnaire is called questionnaire. The differences between scale and questionnaire are as follows.

(1) From the view of theoretical framework, scale measures a certain characteristic of the respondent, such as health status. While questionnaire often measures multi characteristics of the respondents, such as lifestyle, chronic diseases.
(2) From the view of relationship between questions, there exists strong correlation between the questions of the scale, and a conceptual framework can explain the correlations. Whereas, the questions of the questionnaire may be independent each other, and each independent question often measures different characteristics.
(3) The type of questions and the way of scoring are different. The scale consists of closed-ended questions, and the questions in the questionnaire may be semi-closed or open-ended. The scoring is based on the domain (sub-scale) or the entire scale, while the questionnaire often counts the frequency or calculate the mean of each question independently.
(4) The scale is a standardized measurement tool that needs to be normatively developed. While there is no need to be so strict for questionnaire. The reliability and validity must be evaluated in

scale development process. Due to independence between questions and less normalization, it is difficult to evaluate the reliability and validity on the whole questionnaire. Generally, some questions are evaluated selectively based on the specific attribute of the question (correlation coefficient, rank correlation coefficient, contingency coefficient, coincidence rate of two answers, etc.).

3. How to get a closer to truth reply for sensitivity issues?

For sensitive issues, some measures should be taken necessary to dispel the worries of the respondents to reduce the response bias. In addition to collecting data anonymously, investigation technique on sensitive question such as randomized response technique (RRT) can reduce the response bias for sensitive issues. We are not intended to discuss it in depth for limited space, so it is not introduced here. Interested readers can read the related monograph.

4. Are there ethical issues in sample survey?

For investigation research, there is often contradiction between the researcher and the respondent. The researcher has the right to conduct research, but the respondent has the right of autonomy, privacy, and dignity. So there are ethical issues in sampling survey research. The personal information of the respondents should be protected during the research design and implementation phase.

10.9.2. *Summary*

1. The commonly used probability sampling methods include simple random sampling, systematic sampling, stratified random sampling and cluster sampling. Each of the four methods has advantages and disadvantages. In practical application, researchers should weigh the pros and cons, and choose the appropriate sampling method based on specific situations.
2. The commonly used probability sampling methods are listed in descending order by the sampling error as follows, cluster sampling, simple random sampling, systematic sampling, stratified random sampling. Confidence interval of population parameters should be calculated based on their own sampling error.

3. Questionnaire is the most important instrument for data collection in survey. It is mainly composed of a series of questions related to the research objectives. The questionnaire consists of a title, survey items (background data, research variables, verification items), coding, and instructions.
4. Scale is a special form of questionnaire. The development and evaluation of scale are more strictly than other questionnaires. The development process of scale includes three stages: the pilot form — the refined pilot form — the final form. Item selection needs to be based on professional knowledge as well as statistical methods. The evaluation of scale includes reliability, validity, and responsiveness evaluation. The validity evaluation includes criterion validity, content validity, and construct validity. The reliability evaluation includes test–retest reliability, split-half reliability, and internal consistency reliability.
5. Protocol and quality control measures should be developed before the investigation. It is necessary not only to ensure all stages of the investigation (preparation, sampling survey, data analysis, and result expression) going on wheel, but also to ensure that the various bias is minimized.

Think and Practice

I. Best Choice

1. To estimate the positive rate of the Schick test at a school, the researchers randomly selected 8 classes from 80 classes; then all of the students from the 8 selected classes were surveyed. Which sampling method was used in this study? ( )
   A. Simple random sampling B. Systematic sampling C. Stratified random sampling D. Cluster sampling E. Multistage sampling
2. Theoretically, under the same conditions, whose sampling error is the largest? ( )
   A. Simple random sampling B. Systematic sampling C. Stratified random sampling D. Cluster sampling E. Multistage sampling

3. Under the same conditions, which of the following is a measure of the consistency between the results of a test over time? ( )
   A. Content validity B. Construct validity C. Test–retest reliability D. internal reliability E. Split-half reliability
4. Which of the following is the measure of the extent to which an instrument represents all facets of a given conceptual framework? ( )
   A. Content validity B. Construct validity C. Test–retest reliability D. Internal reliability E. Split-half reliability
5. With regard to the design of the questionnaire, which of the following statements is inappropriate? ( )
   A. Each item should be specific and concrete. B. Methods of data analysis should be determined in advance. C. The survey items should be coincide with the investigation. D. A pre-survey with large sample size must be done firstly. E. None of necessary items is omitted, and none of unnecessary items is included.

II. Thinking Questions

1. Which sampling methods can be used to investigate the prevalence and its influencing factors of diabetes mellitus for elderly people aged 60 and over in a city? What are the advantages and limitations for each sampling method? Which survey items should be included in the questionnaire?
2. What are the principles for item writing in questionnaire development?
3. What is the scale development process? Which statistical methods can be used to select item in scale development?

III. Questions on Calculation

1. In order to estimate the average height of a 7-year-old boy in a certain area, the height data of 100 boys aged 7 were gathered from the physical examination database through simple random sampling. The mean of the height was 122.7 cm and the standard deviation was 4.5 cm. Try to estimate the sampling error and the 95% confidence interval of the population mean of height for the 7-year-old boys.

Table 10.7 Sampling survey results of the myopia prevalence survey for middle school students in a certain area

Grade	Number of students	Number of students investigated	Number of students with myopia	Prevalence myopia (%)
Freshmen	20,000	100	29	29
Second year students	20,000	100	35	35
Junior students	20,000	100	45	45
Total	60,000	300	99	33

Table 10.8 Sampling survey results of the blood pressure survey for the elderly aged of 60 and above

Building door	Number of the elderly investigated	Systolic pressure (mmHg)		Diastolic pressure (mmHg)	
		Mean	Standard deviation	Mean	Standard deviation
A	89	133	23.5	85	12.5
B	105	135	24.0	89	13.3
C	114	130	23.3	83	13.0
Total	308	132.6	23.6	85.6	13.2

2. To estimate the prevalence of myopia for middle school students in a certain area, the stratified random sampling by grade was used. The results of the survey were shown in Table 10.7. Try to estimate sampling error and the 95% confidence interval of the population prevalence of myopia.
3. With the elderly from the same building being considered as a sampling unit, cluster sampling was used to select the elderly in a study on blood pressure of the elderly aged 60 and above. The statistics were shown in Table 10.8. Try to estimate the sampling error and population mean of systolic and diastolic pressure for the elderly aged 60 and above.
4. A researcher measured the health status of 106 adult women with a scale consisting of 5 Likert items. The responses were shown in Table 10.9. Try to assess the internal consistency reliability.

Table 10.9 Responses of 106 healthy female adults on the scale

I1	I2	I3	I4	I5	I1	I2	I3	I4	I5
0	0	0	1	0	2	3	2	3	2
1	2	1	2	0	3	2	4	3	4
1	2	2	3	0	2	2	3	4	3
0	0	0	0	0	4	3	3	4	3
2	2	2	3	3	2	2	2	4	3
2	1	2	3	1	2	2	2	4	4
2	2	2	1	1	2	3	1	3	3
1	1	1	1	0	3	3	3	4	4
2	2	2	3	1	2	2	2	3	4
2	2	2	3	1	2	2	2	4	2
2	2	2	2	4	2	2	3	3	2
0	2	3	2	1	2	2	4	4	4
3	2	2	3	1	0	3	3	4	1
2	2	2	3	1	2	2	2	3	2
2	2	3	3	1	3	3	3	3	2
2	2	2	3	1	2	2	3	3	2
2	2	3	2	1	4	2	4	4	4
2	2	2	2	2	2	2	2	4	3
2	2	3	3	2	1	3	3	3	1
2	2	2	3	1	2	2	3	4	3
2	0	2	2	0	2	2	3	3	1
2	2	3	3	1	2	2	2	4	1
3	2	2	2	0	3	3	3	4	4
2	2	2	2	1	3	1	3	2	1
1	2	2	2	3	4	4	4	4	4
2	0	2	3	2	3	3	2	4	3
3	3	3	3	2	3	1	4	3	2
1	2	3	2	1	3	3	3	3	3
2	2	0	3	1	3	3	4	3	2
3	3	3	2	1	2	2	2	3	3
2	3	2	3	2	3	2	3	3	3
3	2	3	3	1	2	2	3	4	2
1	1	2	2	2	4	4	4	4	3
1	1	2	4	1	2	2	3	4	4
2	2	2	3	2	2	2	3	4	2
1	1	2	2	1	3	3	1	3	3
2	2	2	3	2	4	4	3	3	2
2	2	2	4	2	3	3	3	3	2
2	2	2	3	2	4	3	4	3	2

Table 10.9 (*Continued*)

I1	I2	I3	I4	I5	I1	I2	I3	I4	I5
2	2	2	3	4	3	2	3	4	2
3	2	2	2	1	3	1	4	3	2
2	2	2	4	1	3	2	4	2	3
2	2	2	3	2	3	3	4	4	4
3	2	3	3	2	4	4	4	4	4
2	2	2	4	2	4	2	3	4	4
2	2	2	3	1	4	4	4	3	3
2	3	0	1	3	4	3	4	4	2
2	3	4	2	4	4	2	3	4	4
2	3	3	2	1	4	4	4	3	3
0	1	2	2	1	2	3	4	4	3
3	2	3	2	1	4	4	4	4	4
3	2	3	3	2	4	2	3	4	4
2	2	2	4	2	4	4	4	3	3

Ya Fang, Yaofeng Han

CHAPTER 11

INTERVENTIONAL STUDY

In experiment studies, subjects were randomly assigned to several experimental groups. By comparing the effects of different experimental factors, one could determine whether the experimental factors affect the outcomes. The most fundamental difference between experimental and observational studies is whether the experimental factors are controlled by the investigators.

Before an experimental study is conducted, investigators should develop a comprehensive plan based on the study aim. Formulating a clearly stated study aim and developing a pragmatic plan is critical for the experiments to be conducted smoothly with minimal resources (staff input, cost, and time) and to ensure that the results are accurate, reliable, and relevant. Such a plan is often referred to as an experimental study design. This chapter will provide an introduction on the concepts, theories, and methods of experimental study design. Key contents include the concept of experimental study design, three elements, four principles, and types of experimental study design.

11.1. Concept of experimental study design

What is experimental design? Why designs an experiment? How to implement the experimental study design correctly? Beginners are eager to know, but there are no easy answers. Let us first look at a simple example, which may be helpful for beginners to gain a more comprehensive understanding of the aforementioned issues, and to build the necessary foundation for further study of this topic.

Example 11.1. An institute plans to examine the efficacy of "lipid A" in reducing blood lipids. Researchers use 40 mice as experimental subjects to investigate whether there is a statistical difference in efficacy of "lipid A" (using 20 mice) versus the well-known lipid-lowering drug "lovastatin" (using 20 mice) in lowering blood lipids. Low-density lipoprotein (LDL) is used as the primary measure to evaluate the efficacy of the two agents. How to implement this study?

Explanation: Based on preliminary experiments and previous experiences, the minimum number of mice required for each group is 20, with a total of 40 mice for the entire experiment. These mice are fed with a high-fat diet to establish a hyperlipidemia state (modeling). After successful modeling, LDL is higher than a certain value. Forty mice are then randomly divided into the "lipid A" group and the lovastatin group, and receive the assigned drugs for a period of time at the prescribed dose and usage. Changes in LDL values of each mouse, namely, the differences in LDL values prior to and after drug treatment, are measured. An appropriate statistical method is then applied to analyze the changes in LDL values in the two groups of mice to reach a conclusion whether the difference between the two groups is statistically significant. If the difference in efficacy is not statistically significant, we cannot conclude that the lipid-lowering effect is different between the new drug "lipid A" and lovastatin.

Arrangement and implementation of the aforementioned experiment represents a relatively complete example of "experimental study design and implementation process." It involves the following steps: (1) the selection of the study subjects (in this case, mice); (2) determination of the sample size (the appropriate sample size should be estimated according to the known conditions and design type, in this case, $N = 40$); (3) setting up an appropriate control group (in this case, lovastatin as a comparator); (4) determination of the experimental factor (in this case, types of drug, that is, "lipid A" and lovastatin); (5) deciding the experimental outcome (in this case, changes in the blood LDL to reflect the efficacy of the drugs); (6) scientific allocation of the study subjects, commonly a completely randomized method; (7) determining the appropriate type of experimental study (in this case, the subjects are randomly divided into two groups, known as completely random design). From these steps, three pillars can be extracted to construct an experimental study design: three elements (subjects, experimental factors, and experimental outcomes), four principles (randomization, control, repetition, and balance) and design types of an experimental study.

In social practice and human life, in order to understand and know nature, to develop and utilize nature rationally, observational studies only are not sufficient; and experimental studies are often needed. For example, clinicians want to understand "the clinical efficacy of a new surgical approach in treating myopia" and to determine whether this new modality can be used to replace traditional therapy; A researcher wants to explore the "sensitivity of three types of mice to impulse noise," and by studying the sensitivity of different species to noise, helps to identify some commonalities for humans. For these research issues of practical values, without correct experimental design, the researchers may fail to take into consideration all relevant factors, lose direction in the experimental process, or abandon the study halfway through the process. Therefore, the purpose and significance of a study design is to make rational arrangements for various experimental factors, to control and estimate the error size, and to achieve scientific rigor and accuracy with precision, and to reduce manpower, material resource use, and time.

Scientific design includes two parts: specialty design and statistical design. The latter mainly includes three categories: experimental design (non-clinical trial design), clinical trial design, and survey design. This chapter focuses on experimental design. The main contents of the experimental design are: how to follow three elements and four principles of the experimental design correctly, how to rationally select the type of experimental design for specific problems, and how to distinguish and avoid the errors that often occur in experimental design.

11.2. Three elements of experimental design

The three elements of experimental design were: subjects (i.e., experimental units), experimental factors, and experimental effects.

For example, to observe the clinical efficacy of several surgical methods in the treatment of myopia, patients with myopia are the subjects, surgical methods are experimental factors, and changes in the degree of diopter before and after treatment are the experimental effect; these three parts constitute the three indispensable elements of experimental design.

11.2.1. *Subjects*

Study subjects can be roughly divided into two categories according to their characteristics and attributes: living and non-living organisms. Animate objects can be roughly classified into humans and non-humans; human beings are often classified into patients and non-patients; non-humans are often classified into animals and plants. In addition, study subjects can also be ex vivo specimens or cells of the human body. If laryngeal cancer is studied in a clinic, a patient with laryngeal cancer is a "subject" of the experiment; if the cancer tissue section of the patient is used for the experiment, the test subject is described as a specimen. In this case, although the cancer tissue specimens of a patient can be cut into many sections, the number of experimental units is still the number of patients with laryngeal cancer.

To ensure homogeneity, both inclusion and exclusion criteria for the subjects must be specified prior to the experiment. For example, species, litter, sex, age, body weight, and pathological model should be considered in animal experiments. Furthermore, disease type, condition, course of disease, ethnicity, region, sex, body weight, health status, family history, and other general conditions, social factors (such as occupation, living condition, and economic situation) and psychological factors (such as positive and negative emotions) should also be considered in clinical studies.

Different attributes of experimental studies require selection of different types of subjects. The total number of subjects required in a complete experimental design is called the sample size. It is best to estimate the appropriate sample size according to the specific type. Too large a sample size will waste manpower and material resources, and result in an uncontrollable situation of non-experimental factors, whereas too small a sample size is not compatible with reliable conclusion.

11.2.2. *Experimental factors*

Experimental conditions that researchers hope to focus on are called experimental factors. For example, changes in white blood cell counts and platelet counts in mice are studied under different doses of γ-ray irradiation. In this experiment, γ-rays with different doses are called experimental factors, and the specific values of γ-rays in experiments (2 Gy, 4 Gy, 6 Gy, 8 Gy, etc.) are called different levels of γ-rays. In this study, the body weight and litter of mice may greatly influence the experimental results. Therefore, researchers should specify requirements for the body weight and litter of each group of mice before mice are irradiated, which allow the exclusion of these factors in subsequent statistical analysis so that the effects of experimental factors on the experimental results can be evaluated accurately. Body weight and litter of mice are not experimental factors in this case or rather they are confounding factors other than the experimental factors and are called non-experimental factors.

In general, many factors may affect the results of an experiment. It is impossible and unnecessary for researchers to study all the factors. In order to minimize the influence of subjects-specific factors on experimental results, it is necessary to identify and control for important non-experimental factors in the experimental design based on specialized knowledge and experimental conditions. These factors are called block factors. If the litter is selected as the block factor, different litters belong to different blocks. Due to the different methods of organizing and controlling experimental factors and block factors, various experimental design types have been generated. Specific experimental design types will be presented in Section 4 of this chapter.

11.2.3. *Experimental effect*

The experimental effect refers to the effect of experimental factors on the subjects, which is shown by observing the indicators.

Selection of an indicator is directly related to the success or failure of a study. Researchers should focus on the relevance, objectivity, accuracy, specificity, and sensitivity of the indicators.

11.2.3.1. *Relevance*

The primary requirement for selecting indicators is that indicators should be linked to the purpose of the study intrinsically; meanwhile, they should reflect the effects of the experimental factors accurately. For example, when observing the therapeutic effect of anti-hepatitis B virus drugs, investigators should select changes in DNA copy numbers of hepatitis B virus as the indicator instead of changes in transaminase levels to monitor the efficacy of an anti-hepatitis B virus drug.

11.2.3.2. *Objectivity*

Observed indicators are classified into objective indicators and subjective indicators by nature. When a hyperlipemia patient is treated with a hypolipidemic drug, the physician may pay attention to changes of these indicators such as triglyceride and cholesterol before and after treatment. These indicators are quantitative variables and are parts of objective indicators When evaluating the treatment effect of a psychotropic drug, changes of subjective feelings (such as tension, anxiety, etc.) before and after taking the drug are frequently considered as indicators, which are subjective indicators.

11.2.3.3. *Accuracy*

Objective indicators should be selected as much as possible when selecting indicators, which are required to possess accuracy and precision. Accuracy describes the degree of consistency between a measured value and the true value, which is highly related to systematic errors. Precision describes the degree of closeness between a measured value and the mean value of all measured values. Coefficient of variation, standard deviation, and variance are employed to indicate the precision of an experiment in statistics.

11.2.3.4. *Sensitivity and specificity*

Sensitivity refers to the ability of an indicator to identify true positives, and specificity refers to the ability of an indicator to identify true negatives. High sensitivity and specificity reflect high utility. For example, coronary angiography (CAG) has a high sensitivity and specificity for diagnosing coronary heart disease. Electrocardiography, though also used as a standard method for diagnosing coronary heart disease, is only regarded as an auxiliary indictor because of its lower sensitivity and specificity versus CAG.

11.3. Four principles of experimental design

What makes an experimental design scientifically sound? In addition to the aforementioned three elements of experimental design, the following four basic principles of experimental design should be strictly followed: control, randomization, replication, and balance.

11.3.1. *Control*

There can be no differentiation without comparison, and setting up a control group provides the basis for comparison. The magnitude of the effects of experimental and non-experimental factors on experimental effect can be appreciated by setting up a control group. Since multiple-factors influence the experimental results in a study, researchers can only study one or several experimental factors at a time. A reliable estimation of experimental effect can be made only when non-experimental factors are under the same conditions in the experimental group and the control group. Besides, as many diseases recover naturally, such as respiratory infections and oral ulcers, the true relationship between experimental factors and outcomes can be determined only when a control group is established in the study.

11.3.1.1. *Blank control*

No intervention is undertaken in the control group. Studies of this type examine the changes in study subjects during the course of the experiments. Blank control is generally used in animal experiments and is generally only applicable to comparative studies of chronic diseases.

11.3.1.2. *Standard control*

Well established classic treatment or standard treatment, or standard or normal reference values are used as the standard control. For example, a currently universally recognized drug of the same class is used as the standard control for comparison of the efficacy of a new drug.

11.3.1.3. *Self-control*

The intervention and control are applied to the same subjects. For example, to evaluate the efficacy of a drug for treating tinea manus and tinea pedis, if the patient suffers from the disease in both arms, the experimental drug can be used on one arm and the control drug can be used on the other arm. Then, the efficacy of the two drugs can be compared. Comparison of data before and after a certain treatment in clinics is also a self-control design.

11.3.1.4. *Mutual control*

Sometimes, a certain factor under investigation cannot take the zero level. For example, to explore the effect of reaction temperature on outcome in a chemical experiment, a series of experimental groups are tested under different temperature conditions, and each group serves as a comparative group for other groups in the experiment.

11.3.1.5. *Experimental control*

When an important non-experimental factor is present, the use of blank controls alone is not sufficient. It is necessary to set up an experimental group containing only the non-experimental factor that serves as an experimental control group. For example, to study the effect of a surgical method on the treatment of brain trauma, dogs with brain trauma are experimental subjects, the experimental group undergoes the surgical treatment, while the experimental control group only receives surgical suture for brain trauma.

11.3.1.6. *Placebo control*

To exclude psychological effects on the occurrence, development, and prognosis of disease, subjects in the control group are given a placebo without pharmacological activity. The purpose of placebo control is mainly to remove any bias caused by mental and psychological factors of the subjects. It should be noted that the placebo should be identical to the experimental drug in dosage, form, packaging, color, size, shape, and smell; otherwise, it will lead to loss of the placebo effect and failure of the experiment. In addition, placebo controls should be used only if there is no other valid drug treatment. Placebo is not necessarily a drug. For example, the use of sham electroacupuncture can be a placebo control in the study of efficacy of electroacupuncture.

In a study, multiple types of controls are often chosen to rule out the effects of important but non-experimental factors. For example, to study changes in peripheral blood leukocyte counts in mice irradiated at two different doses of γ-rays, four groups are designed: the blank control group, the sham group (regular fluorescent lamp irradiation), the irradiation group with γ-ray at dose 1 and the irradiation group with γ-ray at dose 2. Besides, the four groups are balanced in terms of other important but non-experimental factors such as body weight and litter. In the study, the blank group is established to reflect the state of mice without any exposure to irradiation; the sham group could present the effect of general illumination on mice, which is an experimental control group; two groups with different doses of irradiation constitute a pair of mutual control. If there is no sham group as the experimental control group, even though the difference in peripheral blood leukocyte count in mice after receiving different doses of γ-ray irradiation are statistically significant, it can only be explained that different doses of γ-ray have different influences on peripheral blood leukocyte. It is not clear whether the difference in peripheral blood leukocyte count is statistically significant between mice receiving gamma irradiation and mice receiving no gamma irradiation. Meanwhile, if there is no blank control group, investigators cannot determine the magnitude of effect of irradiation versus no irradiation on the experimental results.

In addition, the control group commonly refers to a level group in a study with a single factor multi-level design. That is, if the study has a multi-factor design, multiple control groups may be included to allow mutual controls for each experimental factor at each level.

11.3.2. *Randomization*

The purpose of randomization is to balance the distribution of all factors other than the one controlled by the investigators between the experimental and control groups. Randomization flows through the whole process of experiment design and implementation, and can be summarized into three aspects: (1) when sampling or grouping, each subject from a population should have an equal opportunity to be recruited into the sample to make sample representative. (2) Each subject in the sample has an equal opportunity to be assigned to any group to make the groups balanced and comparable. (3) The opportunity of being treated in any location of the sequence is the same that excludes the effects of intervention sequence.

Randomization reduces the impact of systematic errors. There are many ways to achieve randomization, such as drawing lots, using random number tables, and using computers to generate pseudo-random numbers.

11.3.3. *Repetition*

Repetition means that both the experimental group and the control group have an adequate number of experimental units, that is, an adequate sample size. This is due to the influences of variation among individuals that render different effects of the same treatment on different subjects, yielding different values of a parameter. The true effect will only be uncovered through repeating an experiment for a great number of times. Therefore, the principle of repetition should be followed in experimental studies.

The term "repetition" usually has three meanings in an experimental study, namely repeated experiments, repeated sampling, and repeated measurements. Repeated experiments refer to independent and repeated observations of m samples (or subjects) under the same experimental conditions, the purpose of which is to reduce experimental errors arising due to variation among individuals. Repeat sampling is the acquisition of multiple samples at the same time point from the same subject or the same specimen. The purpose of repeat sampling is to evaluate the distribution of a quantitative indicator in each subject or specimen. Repeated measurement refers to repeated measurement of indicators for the same sample (or subject) when some or all of the experimental conditions change regularly. This kind of repetition can be the best way to exclude the influence of variation among individuals on outcome and reflect comprehensive dynamic changes in indicators.

It must be noted that too large a sample size may waste manpower and material resources. Meanwhile, the confounding of non-experimental factors is difficult to control. If the sample size is too small, correct conclusions cannot be drawn. It is better to make a reasonable estimate of the sample size based on professional and statistical knowledge. Methods for estimating specific sample size are described in Chapter 15 of this book.

11.3.4. *Balance*

Balance indicates that non-experimental factors are balanced between the experimental group and the control group. In an experimental study, comparison between groups can be made only when non-experimental factors are well balanced between groups. For example, when comparing the effects of two drugs on lowering blood lipids, the subjects are animals with hyperlipidemia. If the randomization principle is not followed when allocating these subjects, one group is heavier in weight than the other group, and it is obviously inappropriate to compare the effects of the two drugs on blood lipids. If body weight has an effect on blood lipid levels and one group is higher in weight than the other group, body weight is an important non-experimental factor that is not comparable in the two groups, greatly jeopardizing the credibility of this study.

11.4. Types of experimental design

Study design type is a specific structure or method to arrange experimental factors and their different levels. According to the number of experimental factors, the number of levels, and whether each group is independent, the common types and characteristics of experimental design are presented as follows.

11.4.1. *Complete randomization design*

There is only one experimental factor in the experimental study, and the number of levels depends on the specific situation, and each group is independent of the other.

1. Single arm design
Assuming that the theoretical mean μ_0 of a certain indicator (generally a recognized value or a standard value) is known, a group of values of an indicator is obtained through experiments, and the purpose is to analyze whether the difference between the population mean estimated from the sample and the theoretical mean is statistically significant or not. That is the so-called single-group design.

Example 11.2. It is known that the mean birth weight of infants in China is 3300 g. A survey found that the mean birth weight of 100 live births was 2900 g at a maternity ward in a hospital located in a low-income area. Is the mean birth weight of full-term live births at the hospital lower than the national average? (Actual measurements are not provided.

Answer: In this example, the birth weight was measured in only one group (100 infants). The infants were not grouped according to any factors. The quantitative data is based on a single group design. Standard values or theoretical values (in the current example, 3300 g for the mean national birth weight) should be provided so that the hypothesis test can be tested.

2. Two-arm design

There are two different scenarios in a two-arm design. One scenario is that two samples are taken randomly from the same population that receives two different treatments. Another scenario is that two independent samples are taken from two populations that receive the same treatment.

For example, "A" is a class of drugs that raise white blood cell counts. There are two drugs, A1 and A2. All subjects are randomly divided into two groups to receive A1 and A2, respectively. Changes in white blood cell counts of each subject are recorded. In another example, to examine the influence of gender of the subjects on platelet counts, normal adults including males and females aged 18–60 years are sampled randomly in a certain area, and the number of platelets is observed.

3. Multi-arm design

When only one experimental factor is investigated and the level of the experimental factor is $k \geq 3$ in the experimental study, this kind of design is called "multi-arm design" or "single-factor multi-level design."

For example, 240 patients with hypertension were randomly assigned to three antihypertensive drug treatment groups, a certain quantitative indicator is measured post-treatments. The purpose of this study is to investigate whether there are statistically significant differences in the population means of the indicator among the three groups. In this experiment, there is only one experimental factor (antihypertensive drug) that has three levels (three types of drugs). This kind of design is also called multi-group design or single factor 3-level design.

11.4.2. *Matching design*

1. Paired design

Usually, the paired design is to firstly pair the subjects according to certain characteristics or conditions of the subjects, and then divide the two subjects from each pair into different treatment groups. This is called the heterologous paired design. If two individuals in each pair share the same source, it is called homologous paired design; otherwise, it is called paired design with similar conditions.

For example, there are 10 litters, and 2 mice are of the same sex in each litter. Two mice in each litter are randomly divided into the experimental group and the control group, and the value of an indicator is observed. The purpose of this study is to examine whether there are statistically significant differences between two different interventions. It is a homologous paired design. If 20 mice are matched into 10 pairs according to some important non-experimental factors, 2 mice in each pair are randomly assigned into the experimental group and the control group to receive different treatments. The value of an indicator is observed. The purpose of this study is to investigate whether the difference between the two treatments is statistically significant. It is a paired design with similar conditions. In a paired design with similar conditions, the non-experimental factors for matching are mainly a combination of one or more non-experimental factors that have a great influence on the experimental indicators, such as gender, age, and weight.

In fact, the self-controlled design is another paired design to observe two values from the same subject before and after treatment, two measurements from each individual are considered as a pair; therefore, n individuals can build n pairs. It is worth mentioning that caution should be exercised in studies with a self-controlled design, because the subject may sometimes have a tendency of "natural outcome or self-healing." If so, the effect of drug or treatment may be exaggerated.

2. Randomized block design

It is an extension of the paired design. All subjects are allocated into groups according to one or more important attributes (block factors, such as litter, weight, or age), k subjects (k is the number of levels of an experimental factor) with the closest condition are considered as subjects in the same block, subjects in each block are assigned to k groups randomly including the control group and the experimental group.

Table 11.1 Coronary plaque area in rabbits treated with four lipid-lowering drugs

	Plaque area (cm^2)			
Group by weight	Antamine	Drug A	Drug B	Drug C
1	0.000	0.283	0.114	0.094
2	0.009	0.196	0.146	0.131
3	0.003	0.217	0.158	0.065
4	0.001	0.236	0.159	0.087

Example 11.3. A research institute has developed three traditional Chinese medicines (A, B, and C) for lowering blood lipids, and it is proposed that the effects of the three medicines are compared with a standard lipid-lowering drug (antamine). Male rabbits are used as subjects, and randomized block design is performed with body weight as a block factor.

Design: Sixteen healthy male rabbits of the same strain are selected and divided into four groups according to weight, and four rabbits with the closest weight in each block are assigned randomly to receive any of the four drugs. Animals are sacrificed on day 45 and the atherosclerotic plaque size of the coronary arteries is observed. The data are shown in Table 11.1. The study is a randomized block design.

11.4.3. *Cross-over design*

When the experimental factors the researcher cares about have two levels (A and B), two levels are applied to each subject in succession: some subjects receive A firstly, and then B; the sequence of treatment is reversed in other subjects. It is called a cross-over design.

There are two ways to arrange experiments for cross-over design. The first one is "grouped crossover design": all 2n subjects are divided into two groups completely and a random method is applied to determine the order. One group receives treatment A and B in turn, and the other group receives treatment in the opposite order.

For example, the result of randomization is: one group take A firstly and then B, another group takes B firstly and then A.

The second is the "paired crossover design," which matches all $2n$ subjects into n pairs according to some important non-experimental factors, and uses a random method to determine the order of treatment. One in each pair receives treatment A and the other in the same pair receives treatment B.

Generally, it is better to use the second type of crossover design, but matching is not easy to implement.

It is worthy of caution that, since the two treatments are applied to the same subject in succession and the effects of the two treatments may be mixed, cross-over design is limited to research issues in which the effect of a treatment disappears in a short period. The appropriate length of the "wash-out period" should be determined in conjunction with this specific issue, and there should be a period of "blank" between before the two treatments in the same subject. If the experimental factor is two sphygmomanometers, the wash-out period can be very short; if the experimental factor is two drugs, a longer wash-out period may be required. In particular, cross design should be used with caution when it is difficult to restore the value of an indicator to the original level after drug use.

Example 11.4. An anesthesiologist studies the effect of eucerin on fluridine. Six rats are used for this experiment. All rats are injected intraperitoneally with fluridine 40 mL/kg and atropine sulfate 0.05 mL/kg. The rats are injected with a 0.5 mg/kg eucerin intraperitoneally 15 min after sleep. The same amount of saline is used as the control drug. The purpose of this study is to investigate the effect of eucerin on fluridine. The time of squatting and walking after taking the drug is used as an indicator. Please arrange this experiment with a cross-over design.

Design: Six rats are selected and divided into 3 pairs according to certain conditions. One rat in a pair is given a 15 min intraperitoneal injection of 0.5 mg/kg eucerin (T) after asleep. The other receives an equivalent volume of normal saline (C). The time of squatting and walking is observed. After 6 rats are completely awake 3 days later,

Table 11.2 Effect of eucerin 0.5 mg/kg (T) and normal saline (C) on fluridine

Rats		Drug code and time of squatting and walking (min)	
Pair	Order	First time	Second time
1	1	T(15)	C(27)
	2	C(31)	T(25)
2	1	T(17)	C(28)
	2	C(30)	T(14)
3	1	C(25)	T(18)
	2	T(5)	C(26)

the rats that have received eucerin previously take normal saline (C), the rats that have received normal saline (C) previously take eucerin. The time of squatting and walking is observed again. Experimental Arrangement and Results (The data in parentheses is "Time of squatting and walking," min) are shown in Table 11.2. The study has a paired crossover design.

11.4.4. *Factorial design*

When k ($k \geq 2$) experimental factors are involved in the experiment, all the levels of the k factors are combined. Let the number of combinations be m, there are m different experimental conditions. M experimental conditions are simultaneously implemented without order, and the influence of each factor on indicators is equal, and effects of the experimental factors and their interaction are analyzed. This design is called factorial design or full factor design.

The advantage of a factorial design is that it cannot only estimate the main effects of each experimental factor, but also estimate the interaction effects between the experimental factors. The disadvantage is that the required number of experimental groups will be large. The factorial design is not suitable when the experimental factors and their levels are large and each experiment takes a long time and costs substantially.

Example 11.5. There are two drugs, A and B, to reduce aminotransferase. In order to investigate whether the difference is statistically significant in transaminase reduction between hepatitis A and hepatitis B patients, it is proposed that 8 patients with either type of hepatitis are chosen as subjects, and a factorial design is selected.

Design: There are two factors in the design, each of which has two levels: hepatitis type (type A and type B) and drug type (drug A and drug B); there are $2 \times 2 = 4$ combinations between two factors: type A and drug A, type A and drug B, type B and drug A, type B and drug B, and it is necessary to set up 4 experimental groups.

Eight patients are randomly selected from the overall population of the two types of patients, and they are assigned to receive drug A or drug B randomly. There are 4 patients in each experimental group. The study has a two-factor two-level factorial design or a 2×2 factorial design. Arrangement and measurement of experimental factors and their levels are shown in Table 11.3.

11.4.5. *Repeated measures design*

The subjects are divided into several groups according to the experimental factors, and each group receives a specific treatment. Indicators are measured at several different time points repeatedly in the same subject (or sample); it is called repeated measures design. This design meets the characteristics of many medical experiments, so the frequency of application in medical research is rather high.

Table 11.3 Experimental results of two types of drugs in reducing transaminase in patients with hepatitis A and B

	Reduction of aminotransferase			
Drug	Hepatitis A		Hepatitis B	
A	100	85	65	75
	90	88	100	80
B	120	90	45	30
	110	100	50	40

Table 11.4 Effect of two drugs on frequencies in electromyography in rats at different time points

		Frequencies in electromyography (times per second)					
Drug	Rat	Time points (min): 0	5	10	30	90	180
Tetamine	1	8.5	5.5	5.0	4.5	3.5	4.5
	2	9.0	5.5	5.0	4.5	3.5	3.0
	3	8.5	7.0	5.5	5.0	4.5	5.0
	4	8.5	5.5	5.0	4.5	3.5	3.0
	5	8.5	6.0	5.5	5.0	4.0	6.5
	6	9.0	4.5	6.0	5.5	4.5	4.0
Ketamine	7	7.5	8.0	8.0	7.0	7.0	7.0
	8	7.5	8.0	8.0	7.0	7.0	7.5
	9	9.5	8.5	6.5	6.0	6.0	7.0
	10	9.0	9.0	8.5	8.0	7.5	8.0
	11	8.0	8.5	8.0	7.5	7.5	8.0
	12	8.5	8.0	8.0	7.0	6.5	7.0

Sometimes, indicators are obtained from different parts (or tissues) of the same individual at the same time point; this type of study also has repeated measures design.

Example 11.6. The effects of two drugs (tetamine (20 mg/kg) and ketamine (20 mg/kg)) on frequencies in electromyography in rats are studied. The experimental design and results are shown in Table 11.4. Please determine what type of experimental design the study has.

Answer: Drug type is one experimental factor for grouping. Twelve rats are randomly divided into two drug groups and receive different drug treatments. Frequencies in electromyography (times/s) of six rats in each drug group are observed repeatedly at six different time points. This experimental design is called repeated measurement design with two factors (drug and time point).

11.5. Report writing

Generally, report on experimental design includes the following aspects:

(1) Contents related to the subjects: how the subjects are selected (inclusion criteria and exclusion criteria), how the sample size is determined, and how the samples are taken (whether or not the randomization principle is followed).
(2) Contents related to experimental factors: what kind of treatment the subjects have received and how to exclude the influence of non-experimental factors.
(3) Indicators to be observed and how to collect the data.
(4) Content related to experimental design: What kind of experimental design is performed.

11.6. Case discrimination

Case 11.1 The investigators plan to examine the potential inhibitory effects on tumor growth and chemosensitization of the E1A gene in nude mice. Fifteen four-week-old nude mice are divided into three groups by "hand picking": the 5 mice picked by the investigators first were assigned to group A, 5 mice picked next were assigned to group B, and the 5 mice picked last were assigned to group C. Assuming that sex and weight of the nude mice could affect the experiment outcomes, please identify the key flaws in the experimental design and re-design the experiment to fix the problems.

Case 11.2 In order to observe the histopathological changes of the normal parotid gland in miniature pigs injected with methyl violet, 15 six-months old miniature pigs, including 9 males and 6 females. The parotid gland on one side is selected as the experimental group and the other side as the normal control group to eliminate the influence of variation among individuals and age on the experimental results. Fifteen pigs are randomly divided into 5 groups at 1 week, 2 weeks, 1 month, 3 months, and 6 months after methyl violet is injected, 3 pigs are in each group and 3 pigs are randomly injected with 0.6, 1.0, or 4.0 mL 1% methyl violet solution. Histopathological changes are observed. Please analyze the mistakes in the experimental design and show how it can be improved.

Case 11.3 An animal experiment is conducted to study the efficacy of a $\beta 2$ receptor agonist combined with hormone in the treatment of asthma. Animal models of asthma are established using Wistar rats. The effects of $\beta 2$ agonists and hormones alone and effects of the interaction between the two drugs are investigated. Investigators designed three groups as follows: the $\beta 2$ receptor agonist group, the hormone group, and the $\beta 2$ receptor agonist plus hormone group. Is the design reasonable?

11.7. Computer experiments (see electronic resources from exp11-1 to exp11-3)

Experiment 11.1 Generate random numbers by SPSS.

Learn how to use SPSS to generate random numbers and observe the influence of seed selection (the same seed will produce the same random numbers).

Experiment 11.2 Completely randomized grouping by SPSS.

In order to conduct a study on respiratory function, 50 normal subjects were required in both the experimental group and the control group. Assuming that 100 volunteers come to register and record their registration number (NUMBER). How to divide them into A and B groups randomly by SPSS?

Experiment 11.3 Stratified randomization by SPSS.

In a study on respiratory function, 50 normal subjects are required in both the experimental group and the control group. Assuming that 100 volunteers have signed up and their registration number (NUMBER) and gender (SEX) are recorded. Moreover, it is assumed that there are 50 men and 50 women. How to use SPSS to randomly divide them into two groups with gender stratification?

11.8. Frequently asked questions and summary

11.8.1. *Frequently asked questions*

1. Even though the experimental conditions meet the requirements of paired design, the researchers have adopted a completely random

design. What does it mean? If the experimental conditions do not meet requirements of paired design, the researcher must apply the paired design, what will it mean?

If the experimental conditions meet the requirements of paired design, and important non-experimental factors that affect the observations have been found, the subjects can be matched according to those non-experimental factors. If the researchers insisted on adopting a completely random design, which would increase the experimental error and lead to false negative results easily.

If the experimental conditions do not meet the requirements of paired design, and important non-experimental factors that have an impact on the observations cannot be found, and if the researcher insists on applying a paired design. Actually, in addition to the different levels of treatment factors, the subjects show great differences in other conditions. If the experimental data are analyzed using the paired design method, it may lead to false positive results.

2. The single factor design is simple and easy to implement. The randomization method can be used to balance the influence of other factors on the results of each group. Is it possible to ignore any other experimental designs with multiple factors?

In the experimental design, there are usually two types of factors: one is the experimental factor that the researcher cares about; the another is the factor that the researcher does not care about but objectively affects the value of the results, such as the block factor. When an experiment involves multiple experimental factors and the level of experimental factors is greater than or equal to 2, in each batch of experiments, if other experimental factors are controlled at specific levels during the study design, and only one experimental factor is allowed to assume different levels, that is, a single factor design is used instead of a multi-factor design, substantial amounts of experiments are required and the results are one-sided. If the individual effects of multiple experimental factors and the interaction among them are studied, usually a factorial design is preferred.

3. In experimental design, the establishment of control group is very important. In general, how many control groups should be established?

In experimental design, it is difficult to generalize about the number of control groups, which mainly depends on the purpose of a study and the number of experimental factors involved. (1) If it is a standard single factor design with multiple levels, only one control group should be set up. For example, a study is to examine whether there exist statistically significant differences in effects among small, medium, and large doses of a drug. When the efficacy of the drug is unknown, it is necessary to set up a blank control group, which is a single factor design with four levels. When the lowest dose of the drug is known to be effective, a blank control group can be ignored, the small, medium and large dose groups of the drug serve as mutual control groups, and the study has a single factor design with three levels. (2) In some practical problems, researchers may set up multiple control groups, such as a normal (or blank) control group, a model control group, and a positive control group, and other groups are experimental groups with different doses of the new drug. (3) If it is a standard multi-factor experimental design, all groups have their specific function; generally, each experimental factor is compared with each other like multi-factorial factorial design.

11.8.2. *Summary*

1. The key points of the "three elements" of experimental design are (1) Subjects: determination of the type of subject, quality standards and sample size; (2) Experimental factors: clarifying the experimental factors to be investigated and the corresponding levels, searching and confirming all important non-experimental factors that may affect indicators; (3) Evaluation indicators: find all kinds of indicators and confirm the primary and secondary outcomes which can be divided into "diagnostic indicators," "efficacy indicators," and "safety indicators"; determination of the time and time points of observations; determination of methods to record, store, and manage outcomes of the study.

2. The main elements of the "four principles" are (1) Randomization principle: The subjects are allocated strictly according to the randomization principle, and the most appropriate randomization should be implemented according to the specific condition, such as stratified randomization. (2) Control principle: A rational control group must be set up and usually be in the form of multiple control groups. (3) Repetition principle: Based on prior knowledge and limitation of the upper limit of the two types of error, appropriate sample size can be estimated. (4) Balance principle: In the whole process from the consideration of the "three elements" to the implementation of the three principles (randomization, control, and repetition), each step should be as balanced as possible to make all non-experimental factors to have the same influence across all groups.
3. The key points of "design type" are (1) To identify all the experimental factors and determine their levels and specific values; (2) To screen out the most important non-experimental factors as far as possible; (3) To clarify the professional requirements for specific experiments; (4) To choose the most appropriate design type based on the aforementioned three key points.

Think and Practice

I. Best Choice

1. The basic principle of experimental design is ( ).
   A. Randomization, control, repetition, balance B. Control, repetition, blinding, randomization C. Randomization, repetition, paired, control D. Randomization, repetition, blinding, control E. Randomization, control, homogeneity, repetition
2. The three basic elements of the experimental design are ( ).
   A. Experimental factors, experimental subjects, experimental sites B. Experimental subjects, researchers, experimental effects C. Experimental factors, experimental subjects, experimental effects D. Experimental factors, experimental effects, researchers E. Experimental objects, experimental factors, experimental sites

3. The essential feature of experimental design that differs from observational research design is ( ).
   A. The experimental design needs to set a comparison B. Experimental design requires random sampling C. Experimental design requires random allocation of experimental subjects D. Experimental design requires active intervention on the subject E. Experimental design requires estimation of sample size
4. In the following study design, no intervention was applied to the study subjects ( ).
   A. Group randomized trial B. Clinical trial C. Survey design D. Experimental design E. None of the above

II. Questions

1. What are the advantages and disadvantages of a crossover design?
2. A study plans to observe the antihypertensive effect of a new calcium antagonist compared with Norvasc (a marketed drug). When the patients are admitted to the hospital, mild cases are assigned to the experimental group and moderate and severe cases

Table 11.5 Effects of different drugs on delayed hypersensitivity in mice

Drug	Dose (g/kg)	Number of mice	Weight of swollen ear (mg)
Control	—	10	21.2 ± 2.7
Kidney reinforcing medicine	5	10	22.3 ± 3.5
Kidney reinforcing medicine	10	10	18.8 ± 3.1
Kidney reinforcing medicine	20	10	16.5 ± 2.4
Cyclophosphamide	0.025	10	11.2 ± 1.5
Cyclophosphamide + kidney reinforcing medicine	0.025 + 5	10	14.3 ± 2.9
Cyclophosphamide + kidney reinforcing medicine	0.025 + 10	10	18.6 ± 3.6
Cyclophosphamide + kidney reinforcing medicine	0.025 + 20	10	19.2 ± 3.4

Kidney reinforcing medicine is kidney-tonifying and life-prolonging capsules.

are assigned to the control group. The results show that the efficacy of the new drug is greater than that of the control drug. Do you think that the research design is correct? Why?

3. Someone considers the experimental design with data in Table 11.5 as a multiple group design. It is not correct to use Student's t-test for analysis. The type of the experimental design is not correctly estimated, resulting in misuse of analytical method. Which type do you think the design of this experiment belongs to? How should it be analyzed?

Changping Li

CHAPTER 12

CLINICAL TRIAL

A clinical trial is a study that examines the potential efficacy and defines safety profile of an intervention in the prevention, diagnosis and treatment of a specific disease under a set of strictly controlled conditions. It could be conducted in patients or in health volunteers. Clinical studies that examine drug absorption, distribution, metabolism, and excretion are also considered clinical trials.

The safety and efficacy of new drugs should be verified by clinical trials. As a result, clinical trials constitute a critical part in the research, development, and regulatory approval of new drugs. Key considerations in clinical trial design include: 1) allowing meaningful and reliable conclusions; 2) protecting the interests of study participants. To achieve such goals, investigators should follow a specific set of principles, procedures, and methodologies in conducting clinical trials.

In this chapter, we will use a virtual case to highlight the key issues in the design and data analysis in clinical trials:

A pharmaceutical company identified a drug candidate for hyperlipidemia. The agent was a plant-derived monomer referred to as Lipid A. Preclinical studies had established its lipid-lowering actions, mainly on low-density lipoprotein cholesterol (LDL-C). Experiments in animal models indicated mild gastrointestinal adverse reactions, mainly abdominal distension and diarrhea. The company planned to conduct a clinical trial as a part of the effort to obtain regulatory approval.

12.1. Preparing a clinical trial

12.1.1. *Regulatory requirements for initiating a clinical trial*

Prior to enrollment of the first study subject, the sponsor must apply for, and obtain approval from the state regulatory agencies. The proposed trial should meet the regulatory requirements in terms of trial organization and implementation. Table 12.1 shows the regulatory authorities and major relevant regulations in China, United States, European Union, and Japan.

For Lipid A to enter clinical trial, the sponsor should submit documents as specified by regulatory agencies and meet the minimum requirement set by laws and regulations, including but not limited to the Drug Administration Law of the People's Republic of China (2019) and Provisions for Drug Registration (2020).

12.1.2. *General principles*

The International Conference on Harmonization of Technical Requirements for the Registration of Pharmaceuticals for Human Use (ICH) has developed a set of guidelines for drug trials. ICH is a collaborative organization initiated by the United States, European Union, and Japanese government authorities and pharmaceutical companies based on the spirit of mutual equality. The major goal of ICH is to develop a set of recommendations on the procedural aspect of clinical research of drug safety, quality control and efficacy through scientific discussion and technical refinements. The efforts by ICH have been instrumental for drug trials conducted in a specific country/region to gain worldwide recognition and for use of regulatory purposes worldwide. Documents released by ICH, exemplified by the Good Clinical Practice (GCP), have been widely acknowledged and used worldwide.

The China "Good Clinical Practice for Drugs" was officially released and implemented by National Medical Products Administration (NMPA; previously referred to as China Food and Drug Administration or CFDA) in 2003. The revised version will be implemented in 2020. GCP provides comprehensive regulations for the standardization and normalization of clinical trials, including protocol design, organization and implementation, monitoring, auditing,

Table 12.1 Management authorities, specific regulatory authorities and major relevant regulations in China, United States, European Union and Japan

Regions	Management authorities	Specific regulatory authorities	Major regulations
China	National Medical Products Administration (NMPA)	Department of Drug Registration	Drug Administration Law of the People's Republic of China, 2019; Provisions for Drug Registration, 2020
United States	Food and Drug Administration (FDA)	Center for Drug Evaluation and Research (CDER)	Food, Drug and Cosmetic Act, 1938; Code of Federal Regulations (CFR) title 21
European Union	The European Agency for the Evaluation of Medicinal Products (EMEA)	The Committee for Proprietary Medicinal Products (CPMP)	Directive 65/65/European Economic Community (EEC), 1965
Japan	Ministry of Health and Welfare (MHW)	Central Pharmaceutical Affairs Council (CPAC) and the Pharmaceutical and Medical Device Evaluation Centre (PMDEC)	The Pharmaceutical Affairs Law, 1960

recording, analysis and reporting. In addition to GCP, NMPA has issued a number of more specific guidelines, including the Technical Guidance for Clinical Trial Data Management (2016), Biostatistical Principles for Drug Clinical Trials (2016) and Guidelines for Planning and Reporting of Drug Clinical Trial Data Management and Statistical Analysis (2016).

To register a trial in China, proposed clinical trials of Lipid A should meet the requirements set forth by the China GCP and other relevant guidelines.

12.1.3. *Ethical standards*

Clinical trials are conducted on human subjects with the ultimate goal of reducing patient suffering, promoting health of the population. Accordingly, clinical trials should be conducted within the norms of common ethics and moral standards. The rights and interests of trial participants should be protected. The Declaration of Helsinki is the most fundamental consensus statement with regards to the guidelines and methods of medical research using human subjects. Since the adoption by the 18th Congress of the World Medical Association in 1964, the Declaration has been widely recognized across the world, and revised several times, with the most recent revision in October 2013.

Chinese GCP requires drug clinical trials to comply with the principles of the Declaration of Helsinki and relevant ethical requirements. The rights and safety of participants are the primary factors to consider and should take precedence over the benefits to science and society. Ethical committee and informed consent are important means to protect participant rights/interests.

For a clinical trial of Lipid A to commence, the trial protocol should be approved by ethics committee. All study participants should sign informed consent form prior to enrollment.

12.1.4. *Phases of clinical trials*

Clinical trials can be divided into phases I, II, III, and IV. In most cases, phase I, II, and III trials should be completed prior to regulatory approval and eventual marketing. Phase IV trials are conducted after a drug enters the market.

Phase I trials include clinical tolerance trials and clinical pharmacokinetics trials. Preliminary data on clinical pharmacology and safety profiles obtained in phase I trials form the basis of dosage regimen in subsequent trials. In the majority of the cases, phase I trials are conducted in healthy volunteers.

Phase II trials provide preliminary evaluation of the potential efficacy of drug candidates against a specific disease condition (target indication). Safety is also examined, and particularly in cases where phase I trial is conducted in healthy volunteers. In addition to verifying efficacy, phase II trials provide information for optimal design of definitive phase III trial. Phase II trials could be based on a variety of designs, but typically take the form of randomized controlled trials (RCTs).

Phase III trials are designed to provide more definitive answers with regards to potential efficacy and safety profile of a test drug in the target population, and to allow regulatory agencies to balance the potential benefits versus risks and to for a decision of approval or disapproval. Phase III trials typically take the form of RCTs, with sufficient sample size.

Phase IV trials are post-marketing clinical studies to examine the effectiveness and adverse reactions of a test drug after the approval in a population that have received the approved agent based on physician prescription rather than in a population with highly homogeneous conditions in earlier phase clinical trials. The purpose of phase IV trials is to generate more understanding of the benefits in a real-world setting, to identify risks unforeseen in trials of earlier phases, and to develop strategies and methods to address newly emerged issues.

Bioequivalence trials evaluate the consistency between generic and brand-name drugs. These trials are designed to compare the bioavailability and pharmacokinetic parameters (including absorption, distribution, metabolism and clearance) between the two dosage forms containing the same active ingredient.

Based on these requirements, for Lipid A to apply for regulatory approval, the sponsor should complete phase I, II, and III trials. We will use the following scenario to discuss the principles of trial design:

Based on the safety profile obtained in phase I trial, the recommended dosage of Lipid A in subsequent trials was set at oral administration of 10–20 mg/time, one time/day. Phase II trial was designed to achieve two purposes: 1) to evaluate efficacy and safety of Lipid A using lovastatin, a widely used lipid-lowering agent, as a control; 2) to evaluate potential differences between 10 and 20 mg. The results of phase II trial showed comparable efficacy of Lipid A at 10 mg versus lovastatin. The phase II trial also indicated that in comparison to 10 mg, subjects taking 20 mg Lipid A had an increased rate of adverse events without further improvement in efficacy. A dosage of 10 mg was used in phase III trial.

12.1.5. *Site requirements*

Provisions for Drug Registration requires that "drug clinical trials should be carried out in drug clinical trial institutions that have the appropriate conditions and registered in accordance with regulations." Institutions that carry out drug clinical trials must be registered on the designated registering platform. Each institution includes a variable number of specialties with corresponding conditions. Detailed information is available from the "Drug Clinical Trial Institution Registering Management Information Platform".

If Lipid A is registered in China, it was necessary to select a registered drug clinical trial institution for clinical trials. The institutions should have conditions for clinical trials in regulation of blood lipids. Institutions should have Phase I clinical research qualifications when conducting Phase I clinical studies.

12.2. Design of clinical trials

12.2.1. *Principles of clinical trial design*

Clinical trials should follow the principles of control, randomization, replication, and balance. A general discussion of these 4 principles can be found in Chapter 11 ("Experiment Studies") of this book. Calculation of sample size based on replication principle is reviewed in Chapter 15, "Sample Size Estimation." This section only discusses special cases in clinical trials.

In addition to complete randomization and stratified randomization, other randomization methods commonly used in clinical trials include block randomization and stratified block randomization and adaptive randomization. In block randomization, subjects are first divided into blocks and random allocation is made of subjects within each block, which can reduce the impact of objective factors on estimation of efficacy, such as seasons and disease epidemics. Stratified block randomization is a method that combines stratified randomization with block randomization. In multi-center clinical trials, this method is generally recommended, considering center as a stratification factor. Adaptive randomization (e.g., minimization) is used to ensure balanced distribution of confounding factors that could result in major biases if not sufficiently balanced among study groups. However, its operation is complicated and its use is still controversial. In terms of implementation and organization of randomization, more and more studies use a central randomization system.

For scientific credibility, the sample size estimation must conform to statistical principles. Usually, a drop-out rate of not more than 20% should be considered.

According to the principle of experimental design, a valid and effective control drug should be selected in phase II and phase III clinical trials; moreover, the control drug had been listed in national standard drugs. The study of Lipid A selected lovastatin as the control drug, and stratified block randomization was applied with clinical trial center as a stratification factor. If influence of age and gender on outcome could not be ignored, they could also be considered as stratification factors. According to statistical calculations, phase II clinical trials required 90 subjects per group. Taking into account a drop-out rate equal to 25% (In order to facilitate explanation and processing, the drop-out rate is set larger here, the same below), each group of subjects was determined as 120 subjects and the total number of subjects was determined to be 360 subjects. Based on statistical calculation for phase III clinical trial, the treatment group and the control group required 270 subjects and 90 subjects, respectively. When considering a drop-out rate equal to 25%, 360 subjects in the treatment group and 120 subjects in the control group were required with a total of 480 subjects.

12.2.2. *Types of clinical trial design*

In clinical trial design, the choice of statistical design type is crucial because it determines estimation of sample size, research process and quality control. Common design types include parallel group design, crossover design, factorial design, and group sequential design. The first three types can be found in Chapter 11 "Experiment Studies." This section mainly describes the group sequential design, and we will also introduce pragmatic clinical trials (PCTs), basket trials and umbrella trials, which have emerged in recent years.

1. Group sequential design

Group sequential design divides the whole trial into several consecutive stages. The number of subjects in each stage is equal or different, but the proportion of subjects in the treatment group and the control group should be equal to the proportion in the total sample. After each stage is completed, the main variables (including efficacy and safety) are analyzed. If a positive conclusion is reached, this trial can be stopped; otherwise, it is continued. If the difference is still not statistically significant in the final phase, the trial should be terminated. Group sequential design is often applied in large clinical trials with long observation periods or an indefinite sample size. The advantage is that the conclusion can be drawn earlier when there is a difference between groups, therefore shortening the duration of the trial, which is consistent with ethical requirements and can decrease trial costs.

A series of interim analyses are conducted in group sequential design. Interim analysis refers to planned mid-term evaluation based on accumulated data before formal completion of the clinical trial, and efficacy and/or safety between groups are compared.

The purpose of interim analysis is to provide a support for decision making as to whether subsequent trials need to be continued or not. When interim analyses are completed, repletion of hypothesis test increases the rate of type I errors, so the test level needs to be adjusted to control the total type I error rate not exceeding a predetermined level (e.g., $\alpha = 0.05$). Commonly used adjustment methods for test level are Pocock method, O'Brien-Fleming method, and α spending function approach proposed by Lan and DeMets. The α spending function method combines the Pocock method and the O'Brien-Fleming method and has been widely applied to group sequential trials.

2. Pragmatic clinical trials

A Pragmatic clinical trial is a study that compares the treatment outcomes (including effectiveness, safety, cost, etc.) of different interventions in a real clinical setting. Pragmatic trials are different from traditional RCTs in terms of subjects, interventions, and outcomes. The main features are: inclusion criteria of subjects are broad and exclusion criteria are few. The subjects with different characteristics and different sources can be included to ensure the extrapolation of the research results. Both design and implementation of intervention are flexible, less limitations are made on investigator's professional skills; no longer follow-up are arranged except regular clinical observations, and outcome data can be obtained from other sources such as a health database. Generally, multiple outcomes are determined; moreover, it is emphasized to select variables with clinical significance for subjects as the primary outcomes. Reasonable deviation from the study protocol is permitted. Compliance of subjects is not measured and controlled. Statistical analysis is performed on all enrolled subjects according to established grouping plan, and no additional qualification is made on whether the subjects meet the protocol.

3. Basket trials and umbrella trials

Basket trials and umbrella trials are innovative trial design in cancer research.

A basket trial is a group of trials in which subjects have the same biomarker or genomic features, called a basket, and are treated with the same targeted drug. According to the site or pathological type of tumor, the trial is divided into different subtests to observe efficacy and safety. Basket trial is usually applied in early stage of drug development and is designed as a single-arm, and it is a proof-of-concept trial. Advantages of basket trials: providing molecularly targeted drugs for patients with different tumor types; suitable for studying biomarkers in rare tumors; small study cohort and easy implementation. Disadvantages: subjects in the same basket may have very different prognoses due to differences in tumor location and pathological type; reliability of results may be affected due to frequent use of historical controls; multiple testing issue may arise when performing subgroup analysis, which increases type I error rates. A description of the basket trial is shown in Figure 12.1(A).

The umbrella trial is also composed of a set of trials. Different from basket trials, it only includes subjects with the same disease type and divides subjects into multiple subgroups based on molecular markers. In each subgroup, subjects have the same target gene and take the same targeted drug. In different subgroups, the target genes of the subjects are different and the targeted drugs also differ. The term umbrella refers to all subjects with the same disease but in varying subgroups. Umbrella trial usually consists of two or three stages, and can be either single-arm or RCTs with two arms. Since all study subjects in umbrella trials share identical tumor type and disease stage, observed differences in efficacy could be more readily attributed to interaction between the active treatment and its molecular markers. Accordingly, prognostic homogeneity is higher in umbrella trials than in basket trials. Evaluation of efficacy of the drug can be more explicit. Its shortcomings include a large sample size, long duration of trial, and difficulty in implementation. A description of the umbrella trial is shown in Figure 12.1(B).

According to the aforementioned purpose of phase II and III clinical trials on Lipid A, parallel group design was more suitable for phase II trial in which subjects were assigned into three groups: Lipid A 10 mg/time, Lipid A 20 mg/time and the lovastatin group.

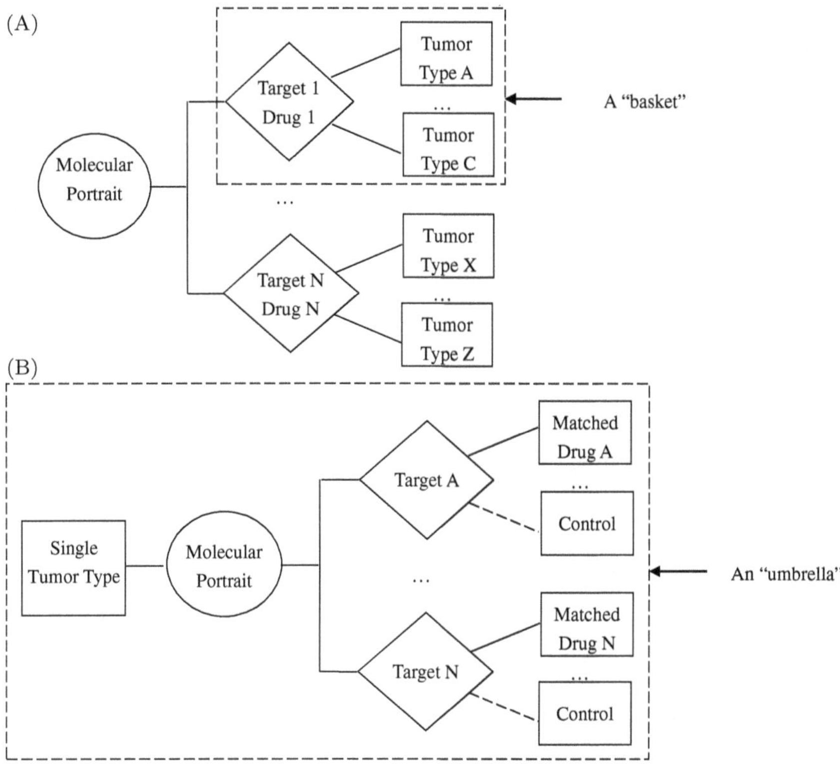

Figure 12.1 Schematic diagram of the basket trial (A) and the umbrella trial (B)

Phase III trial could employ group sequential trial and divide subjects into the Lipid A 10 mg/time group and the lovastatin group. Interim analysis was conducted at predefined time point using Lan and DeMets's α spending function.

12.2.3. *Multi-center clinical trials*

A multi-center clinical trial is a trial conducted by one or several principal investigators, and multiple research units work together and follow the same clinical study protocol. The institution with which the principal investigator is affiliated the leader institution.

Multi-center trials can rapidly enroll the required number of subjects, and the geographical range of the subjects is broad, the clinical conditions for the use of drug are extensive, and trial results are more representative.

Multi-center trials should be conducted under a unified organization and protocol. Multi-center trials require investigator from each center to clarify the purpose of the study and use the same experimental method. Investigator should be trained uniformly before the trial, and quality control should be carried out throughout the trial. If the primary outcome is susceptible to subjective factors, consistency test is required. If the results of the central laboratory test are different or the reference range is different, measures should be taken to achieve consistency, such as unified test by the central laboratory, or unified training for test methods and procedures, or regular consistency determination. These measures are of uttermost importance when laboratory outcomes are the primary outcomes. The proportion of subjects from different groups in each center should be approximately the same as the proportion of subjects in the total sample.

Assuming that phase II and III clinical trials on Lipid A were conducted in four hospitals (Beijing, Guangzhou, Shanghai, and Xi'an), and the hospital in Beijing was the leader unit. Trial protocol should be drafted by the principle investigator in Beijing, discussed (and revised if necessary) by all investigators in the four participating sites, and approved by the Ethics Committee of the leading site. Thereafter, the protocol was completed.

12.2.4. *Blindness and double-blind clinical trials*

Blinding is one of the important principles that clinical trials should follow. The main purpose of blinding is to reduce bias caused by subjective factors of both investigators and subjects. Blinding methods can be classified into single-blind and double-blind. Double blind refers to that both investigators (including the data analyst, etc.) and subjects do not know subject group when implementing the trial protocol. Single blind refers to that the investigator knows subject group while the subject does not know. A non-blinded trial is called an open-label study. If the conditions permit, a double-blind trial should be employed; if a double-blind trial is not feasible, a single-blind trial should be considered. Measures must be taken to control and minimize bias regardless of the blinding (or not). For instance, a central randomization system can be applied to manage the enrollment of subjects, and investigators assessing efficacy and safety are blinded as much as possible during the trial. If blinding is not applied, reasons and measures to minimize bias should be stated in the protocol.

From the perspective of medical ethics, a double-blind trial should set up an emergency letter for each blind number. The envelope is printed with the emergency letter of clinical trial of drug X, number of drugs and the unblinding rules in case of emergency. Emergency letter is sealed in an appropriate envelope and sent to each clinical trial center with the drug, and the letter will be collected after the end of the trial. The emergency letter should not be dismantled when it is not necessary. In an emergency, such as a serious adverse event, the investigator can dismantle it according to the procedure specified in the trial protocol. Once being read, the corresponding subject should be excluded from the trial and the investigator should record the reason for the discontinuation in the case report form (CRF). All emergency letters are collected along with CRF for a blind review after completion of the trial.

Blind review refers to checking and evaluating data in the database after completion of the trial (the conclusion of the last observation of the last subject) and before the first unblinding. A blind review report is required. Meanwhile, the database will also be locked.

After the database is locked, the first unblinding is performed to only unravel the groups (such as group A or group B) to which each subject belongs. The treatment group and the control group are not specified. Unblinding results are sent to biostatisticians for statistical analysis. After completion of statistical analysis, the second unblinding is performed to unravel the treatment group from group A and B.

In phase II and phase III clinical trials on Lipid A, if a double-blind method was applied, 10 mg Lipid A capsules, 20 mg Lipid A capsules and 20 mg lovastatin capsules should be made with the same appearance, and the above procedure for double-blind trial should be implemented. If the appearance, odor, or usage of Lipid A and lovastatin was not identical, a double-dummy technique could be used, which needed to prepare mimetic agents for both Lipid A and lovastatin.

12.2.5. *Clinical trial protocol*

The clinical trial protocol is a research plan that guides all investigators involved in clinical trials to initiate and implement a trial. It is also an important basis for statistical analysis after the trial. Therefore, the trial protocol is an official document for the declaration of new drugs. Moreover, it is a main factor for success of a new drug clinical trial. Trial protocol is typically a fairly large document. Taking phase II clinical trial for Lipid A as an example, the protocol contains information on items in the clinical trial as well as the main contents of certain items.

Common items in a trial protocol include the title page, summary of the protocol, research background, purpose, design, selection and withdrawal of subjects, therapeutic regimen, trial procedures, observation of adverse events, outcome measurements, data management, interim analysis, statistical analysis, quality control and assurance of trials, ethical requirements, data retention, references, signatures of principal investigator and study dates. A brief introduction to some of the major items of the protocol is presented below.

(1) Title page (not shown except for the title) A multi-center randomized double-blind phase II clinical trial to compare the efficacy and safety of Lipid A capsule with lovastatin capsule in the treatment of hyperlipidemia.
(2) Purpose: To evaluate the efficacy and safety of Lipid A, and to evaluate difference in clinical efficacy and safety of Lipid A 10 mg/time and 20 mg/time.

(3) Design

(1) Overall: a multi-center, randomized, double-blind, parallel control clinical trial design.
(2) Control design: a 1:1:1 parallel control design method was applied and the subjects were divided into the lovastatin group, the low-dose Lipid A group and the high-dose Lipid A group.
(3) Sample size: According to the preliminary results, the low-dose group, the high-dose group and the control group reduced LDL-C by 1.40, 1.59 and 1.38 mmol/L, respectively. Take $\alpha = 0.05$, $\beta = 0.2$, two-sided test, 90 subjects were required for each group based on statistical calculation. Considering a drop-out rate equal to 25%, the total number of subjects was determined to be 360, with 120 subjects in each group.
(4) Randomized allocation: stratified block randomization was used, and the appropriate block length was selected and stratification was done by hospitals. Given a random seed, the SAS 9.4 software was used to generate a random grouping scheme for 360 subjects, 90 subjects in each hospital, and the allocation proportion of each group was 30:30:30.
(5) Blinding and unblinding: According to the random coding table, the blinding work of the double-blind trial was completed, a two-stage blinding method was adopted. After subject enrollment was completed, two stage of unblinding were performed after the database was established and locked. Firstly, code of the corresponding group of each subject number was unblinded for statistical analysis. After statistical analysis was completed, the corresponding code of each treatment was revealed.

(4) Subject selection and withdrawal

(1) Diagnostic criteria (details omitted).
(2) Inclusion criteria: subjects who were diagnosed with hyperlipidemia, LDL-C >3.5 mmol/L, aged 18–65 years, signed

informed consent, and fertile women should have effective contraceptive measures.

(3) Exclusion criteria: dyslipidemia caused by other diseases; severe primary diseases such as diseases of the cardiovascular, liver, kidney and hematopoietic system, psychiatric patients; allergy; serum transaminase greater than 1.5 times the upper limit of normal reference values; pregnant or lactating women; those who had participated in clinical trials of other drugs in the preceding 3 months.

(4) Elimination criteria: those who had severely violated the inclusion criteria, those who had not used the drug after inclusion, and those who did not have any evaluable records were withdrawn from the trial.

(5) Conditions and steps for withdrawal from the trial

Withdrawal decided by investigators: subjects suffering from certain complications or specific physiological changes, and who were not suitable to continue the trial. Subjects with poor compliance, or the use of the drug did not reach 80% of prescribed amount or exceeded 120% of the prescribed dosage. Subjects with unmasked blinding or emergency unblinding in the trial; subjects taking drugs banned in the protocol.

Withdrawal decided by subjects: According to informed consent, a subject had the right to withdraw from the trial at any time, or a subject did not explicitly withdraw from the trial but no longer accepted medication and observation, which subjects to loss to follow-up (or drop-out). Reason for withdrawal should be known as much as possible and recorded. For subjects withdrawn from the trial, records should be retained for a comprehensive analysis of efficacy and adverse reactions.

(6) Conditions for discontinuation: The trial should be discontinued if serious safety problems occurred during the trial or if the drug treatment was found to be too poor or even invalid.

(5) Therapeutic regimen

(1) Test drug (contents omitted).
(2) Treatment: A low-dose group of Lipid A 10 mg/time, 1 time/day; A high-dose group of Lipid A 20 mg/time, 1 time/day; the lovastatin group of 20 mg/time, 1 time/day.
(3) Duration: 6 weeks.
(4) Concomitant medication: All Chinese and Western medicines for treating hyperlipidemia are prohibited during the trial.

(6) Outcome measurements

(1) Efficacy
Primary outcome: LDL-C.
Secondary outcomes: TC, TG, HDL, hemorheology, and clinical symptoms.
(2) Safety
Adverse events; routine blood and urine chemistries, electrocardiogram, liver and kidney function.

12.2.6. *Case report form*

The case report form is a very important research material in clinical trials. The CRF was defined in ICH6 as "Case Report Form (CRF): A printed, optical, or electronic document designed to record all of the protocol required information to be reported to the sponsor on each trial subject." Chinese GCP defined it as: "a paper or electronic document designed in accordance with the requirements of the trial protocol and used to report to the sponsor to record relevant information about the subjects."

Quality of CRF is a direct reflection of the level of clinical research. After a trial protocol is determined, quality of filling the CRF is key to the success of the trial; it is also an important basis for statistical analysis, summary and approval of the trial.

There is no uniform format for CRF, but certain principles should be followed. For example, CRF should fully reflect the outcome measurements required in the trial protocol; CRF entries should be in the form of choices as much as possible. Each CRF page should have the investigator's signature and date. Values of the same outcome at different time points cannot be filled in the same CRF page. The CRF should not contain any information that reveals personal identity of the study subjects, including name, address, and any other original medical records (such as lab reports).

The main content of CRF includes title page, filling guide, inclusion and exclusion criteria, baseline information, vital signs and physical examination, efficacy evaluation, laboratory tests, adverse events, concomitant medication, drug delivery and recycling records, and study summaries, etc.

12.3. Data management and statistical analysis of clinical trials

12.3.1. *Data management*

Data management of clinical trial refers to the whole process of data input, encoding, verification, query and correction, database locking and data archiving of research data via computer and network technology. The data management should follow relevant regulations and guidelines formulated by drug regulatory authority, and it should comply with the standard operating procedures (SOPs) established by the institution or department, and it should also comply with the trial protocol.

(1) Key persons involved in data management

The main persons in data management include sponsor, investigator, monitor, and data manager. The sponsor is the ultimate person responsible for quality of clinical data, and takes overall responsibility for data quality and authenticity. The investigator is responsible for follow-up and observation of subjects to fill in CRF completely and truthfully. The investigator should ensure that the data on CRF are derived from source data on the subject's medical record. The monitor is responsible for checking authenticity and reliability of CRF filled out by the investigator, and communicating the data. The monitor serves as the bridge between the sponsor and the investigator, and the investigator and the data manager. The data manager is the main worker of data management.

(2) Plan and report of data management

Key documents in data management include data management plan (DMP) and data management report (DMR). When the drug is listed for registration, the regulatory agency regards the DMP and DMR as important documents and the basis for evaluation of a trial. DMP is a dynamic document drafted by data manager based on trial protocol, which specifies and records data management tasks of a specific clinical trial in detail and comprehensively, including personnel roles, work contents, and operational specifications. DMR is a summary of data management process drafted by the data manager after completion of clinical trials. It is an important presentation of the execution process of data management, operation specification and management quality.

(3) The main contents of data management

The main content of data management includes establishment of data collection and management system, CRF and database design, data import and entry, data verification and query, medical coding, external data management, blinding audit, database locking, data export and transfer, archiving data and data management documents, etc.

Data acquisition can be done using paper CRF or electronic data capture (EDC) systems. The EDC system is a computer network-based technology for collection of trial data. The clinical data is directly collected and transmitted in electronic form through the organic combination of software, hardware, SOP and staffing. With the improvement of regulatory requirements and the advancement of related technologies, EDC systems are gradually replacing paper CRF, and will be the main means of clinical trial data collection in the future.

In addition to dataset name, the database should contain the names, types, and specific rules of the variables. Once the database is created, testing and validation should be conducted on the database. The content of database testing should include database design, data entry interface, data entry, data storage, regular calculation for derived variables, consistency in data format between export data and input data, generation of data queries, and audit trails when data is updated, etc.

Acceptable forms of data delivery include: fax, mail by postal office, courier service with tracking systems, on-line submission, and personal delivery. The data receiving process should be documented, including CRF number, handover date, handover personnel, signature and remarks, etc.

Before data verification, a detailed data validation plan (DVP) should be developed, which will describe the contents, methods and requirements of verification for each data field and each data point. Data verification should be carried out in a blinding state. The main contents include verification of the following: trial completion, inclusion/exclusion criteria, missing values, logical consistency, outliers, time windows, concomitant medications, and adverse events. Generated queries after data verification are sent to the clinical monitor or investigator via a data query form (DQF). After the investigator responds to the queries, the data manager modifies the data based on the returned response.

Medical coding is the process of matching the description of adverse events, medical diagnosis, concomitant medication, past medication and previous medical history collected from CRF with the terms in the standard dictionary. Widely used standard dictionaries are MedDRA (medical dictionary for regulatory activities), WHO ART (WHO adverse reaction terminology), and WHO DD (WHO drug dictionary).

External data refers to data provided by other suppliers (such as central laboratories) that are collected based on the trial protocol but obtained outside the research unit. It includes laboratory data, pharmacokinetics/pharmacodynamics data, and biomarker data. Data manager should develop a detailed protocol of data transfer that specifies the technical requirements for the structure, content, transmission method, transmission time, and workflow of external data. External data is usually transmitted using an electronic file and should be checked for consistency and accuracy.

Blind review can be checked in the previous section. It should be emphasized that blinding audits should be conducted regardless of whether the clinical trial is open-label or blinded.

Database lock is a key step in the clinical trial process. It prohibits database editing in order to prevent unintentional or unauthorized changes to the database document. The process and time of database locking should be clearly documented and completed by the sponsor, principal investigator, data managers, biostatisticians, and relevant personnel who maintain blind codes. Blind trials cannot be unblinded until the database is locked. Locking and unlocking should be strictly controlled and the necessary unlocking and re-locking procedures should be recorded in detail.

The file format, exported content (database, variable name, and variable value coding), submission program and transmission medium for data export and transmission should be specified. The trial data and documents formed during the data management process need to be completely preserved, and period of retention should be implemented according to specific requirements of the regulations.

12.3.2. *Statistical analysis*

Statistical analysis of clinical trials should comply with not only statistical principles and methods but also requirements of relevant regulations and guidelines. Biostatisticians should participate in the entire process of the clinical trial. Prior to the enrollment, biostatisticians should be an important part in the development and revision of trial protocol and the design of CRF. Biostatisticians should be responsible for sample size estimation, randomization of the study subjects, development of data analysis plan, statistical analysis of trial results and drafting statistical analysis report. Biostatisticians should also assist principal investigators to draft summary report upon trial completion. Biostatistician involved in the study should ensure accuracy of statistical methods, analysis results and terminology in the trial protocol, CRF and summary report.

(1) Type of statistical test

In most cases, hypothesis test employs difference test, the purpose of which is to infer whether difference between drugs is statistically significant. In clinical trials, in addition to difference test, superiority testing, equivalence testing, and non-inferiority testing are often used.

Superiority test is used to infer whether the efficacy of a test drug is superior to the control drug. It can be divided into two types: statistical superiority and clinical superiority. A superiority margin should be provided in clinical superiority test. The superiority test is a one-sided test. When the difference is statistically significant, it can be concluded that the test drug is superior to the control drug.

Equivalence test is used to infer whether the difference in efficacy between the test drug and the control drug falls within a certain range that is clinically acceptable. The clinically acceptable range is defined by two equivalence margins, which are called margin of superior side and margin of inferior side. The two margin values can be unequal, but in practice, they are equal generally. In the equivalence test, two one-sided tests (TOST) are conducted at the same time. Only when both tests are statistically significant, the conclusion that the test drug and the control drug are equivalent can be drawn.

Non-inferiority test is used to infer whether the difference in efficacy between the test drug and the control drug is not less than a clinically acceptable range, which is determined by a non-inferiority margin. The non-inferiority test is a one-sided test. When the difference is statistically significant, it can be concluded that the test drug is not inferior to the control drug.

In the above three tests, determination of the margin is very important and should be clarified at the design stage. The margin can be determined based on prior professional knowledge and experience, such as difference in blood pressure can be 5 mmHg, difference in cholesterol can be 20 mg/dL. When it is difficult to determine, 1/5 to 1/2 standard deviation or 1/10 to 1/5 of the mean of the control group can be the margin when comparing the means of two groups. For comparison of two rates, values below 15% or a threshold value of 1/5 of the sample rate of the control group are recommended.

(2) Statistical analysis set

In statistical analysis, which subjects should be included or excluded is the first question to be considered, which is also a categorization of analytic sets. When defining statistical dataset, bias should be minimized as much as possible; meanwhile, increase in type I error should be controlled. Generally, statistical analysis sets include a full analysis set, per protocol set and safety set.

Intention to treat (ITT) means that all randomized subjects are evaluated and analyzed based on allocated group regardless of compliance with the plan. It preserves the original randomization and avoids bias caused by destruction of randomization. Analysis sets based on this principle are ITT analysis sets. However, implementation of the ITT in practice is difficult, so it is just a principle. Therefore, the concept of full analysis set is proposed in the ICH E9 statistical analysis guidelines.

The full analysis set (FAS) refers to a collection of subjects as close as possible to the ITT principle, which implies the least number of subjects are removed from all randomized subjects using the most rational method. Excluded subjects include those who seriously violate the trial protocol, those who do not take the investigational drug, and those who have no data after randomization.

The per protocol set (PPS), also known as effective subjects, effective sample and evaluable subjects, is a subset of subjects who comply with the protocol more strictly in the FAS. PPS refers to study subjects who completed the trial as assigned upon randomization, including minimal dosing, assessment of the baseline information and primary outcome measures at planned time point(s), and no major protocol violation. Examples include: subjects who decide to withdraw after achieving desired responses, those who decide to withdraw since the expected response was not achieved but have completed minimal dosing and available primary outcome measures prior to withdrawal. If subjects receive more than 130% the dose of the investigational drug, or take concomitant drugs with synergistic effect on the investigational drug, or violate the inclusion/exclusion criteria, or take the test drug but in the control group, these subjects should be excluded from the PPS.

The safety set (SS) should include these subjects who have received at least one treatment after randomization and have at least one safety assessment for safety and tolerability assessment.

The FAS includes randomized subjects as much as possible, which can reduce bias, but the results are more conservative and closer to the real scenario. The PPS reflects scientific consistency of the trial protocol better, but may exaggerate the efficacy. If the violation of protocol by a subject is related to treatment factor, a serious bias will be introduced. If too many subjects are excluded from the PPS, efficacy of the entire trial will be affected. In confirmatory trials, both the FAS and PPS should be analyzed. If conclusions from the two datasets are consistent, the results are reliable; if they are inconsistent, the differences should be discussed and explained. In a superiority test, the FAS is generally used as the main analysis set because its results are conservative; however, in an equivalent or non-inferiority test, the results from the FAS may not be conservative.

(3) Statistical analysis plan and report

Statistical analysis plan (SAP) and statistical analysis report (SAR) are the main documents of statistical analysis. They need to be submitted to the regulatory authorities as application materials for drug evaluation and registration. The SAP should be drafted by a statistical professional who requires a comprehensive and detailed presentation of analytical methods and expression of trial data, as well as an explanation of expected analysis results. The SAR is a report of the statistical analysis of trial data according to the SAP. It is an important way to present results of a clinical trial and provides an important basis for writing clinical study reports. The main contents of SAP include overview of the study, evaluation outcomes, analysis datasets, analysis software and analysis methods, and templates of tables and graphics for expected results. The SAR should supplement the statistical analysis results and statistical conclusions based on the SAP.

(4) Main contents of statistical analysis

The main contents of statistical analysis of clinical trials include description of distribution of subjects, analysis of compliance, analysis of baseline comparability, analysis of efficacy and safety, and analysis of concomitant drugs. Statistical analysis software and methods should be recognized around the world. According to the attributes of outcomes, the type of design, the preconditions of data and analysis purposes, the corresponding statistical analysis methods are determined. Hypothesis testing should clearly indicate whether the analysis is one- or two-sided. If a one-sided test is used, relevant reason should be stated. The test level for one-sided test is often chosen to be half of the two-sided test.

Description of study subjects must include: the number of screened subjects, the number of excluded subjects and the reasons, the number of subjects randomized, and the number of dropout in each dataset. A list is employed to describe the details of the dropout and exclusion. In addition to contexts and tables, distribution of subjects should be described in a form of a flow chart.

In compliance analysis, definition of compliance in the trial protocol should be used to clarify the status of each subject in the trial. A list describes the details of these subjects with poor compliance and compares the incidence of poor adherence between groups.

For demographic data, past history, family history, history of drug allergy, and baseline of efficacy outcomes, statistical description is generally used for comparability analysis. Hypothesis test should be performed for baseline when necessary. Analysis of baseline comparability employs the FAS.

For primary and secondary efficacy outcomes, in addition to statistical descriptions, interval estimation and hypothesis test should be performed according to pre-determined statistical analysis methods. The main results include baseline characteristics, outcome measures at preset time points and changes over time, as well as the description statistics, confidence interval, test statistics, and P value of group differences. Efficacy comparison should be analyzed simultaneously for the FAS and the PPS. If the primary outcome is a quantitative variable, it is usually necessary to include a baseline value as a covariate, to consider the effect of treatment and center, and to adopt multiple linear regression. If the primary outcome is a qualitative variable, logistic regression is appropriate.

Safety outcomes include adverse events and adverse reactions, laboratory tests, vital signs, physical examinations, and other specific tests (such as electrocardiograms, imaging examination). In safety analysis, adverse events and adverse reactions should be classified and summarized, and the incidences of adverse events and adverse reactions are calculated and compared between groups. A list is used to present the details of each adverse event in each subject. For laboratory tests, vital signs, physical examination, electrocardiogram and other safety-related tests, in addition to descriptive statistics, their changes before and after treatment are usually described in a cross-tabulation, and hypothesis tests are performed if necessary. If some outcomes are normal before treatment but become abnormal after treatment with clinically significant changes, or if some outcomes, which are abnormal before treatment become worsened post treatment, these outcomes should be followed up until they change to normal or return to pre-treatment levels. Meanwhile, investigators should report adverse events, and determine the relationship between abnormal changes and drugs. Safety analysis adopts the SS.

The analysis method of concomitant drug is similar to that of adverse event. It is necessary to summarize the use of concomitant drugs, calculate the incidence of use of concomitant drugs and compare it between groups. A list is used to describe the details of each concomitant drug for each subject.

In statistical analysis of trial data, other specific issues that need attention include manipulation of missing data and outliers, data transformation, analysis of covariates, center effects, multiplicity issues and subgroup analysis. The manipulation of missing values is described in Chapter 16, "Missing Data."

12.3.3. *Clinical study report*

Clinical study report (CSR) is a summary document that reflects the design and implementation of clinical trials, and analysis and evaluation of results. It is an important basis for correctly evaluating whether the drug has clinical practical value, and it is also an important technical material required for drug registration. Report writers should have professional morality and legal responsibility. In order to make a reasonable evaluation of the efficacy and safety of the drug, a CSR should focus on explanation of the trial results, complete description of the trial design, trial management, and trial process, which can clarify the scientific basis of conclusions.

According to the registration requirements of the NMPA, the CSR should include at least the following seven aspects: report cover, signature page, table of contents, abbreviations, ethics issues, summary and body of the report. The latter is the core part and should proceed in form of introduction, the objective of the trial, methods, results, discussion and conclusions. Methods usually should introduce overall design, randomization, blinding method, research object, control method and its basis, treatment process, efficacy outcomes and evaluation method, safety outcomes and evaluation methods, quality control and assurance, data management, statistical analysis and others. Results should include analysis of subjects, efficacy analysis and safety analysis.

For detailed requirements for the preparation of a CSR, please refer to the "Technical Guidelines for The Structure and Content of Chemical Drug Clinical Trial Reports" (2005) and "Principles for Writing Clinical Trial Summary Reports of Traditional Chinese Medicines and Natural Medicines" (2005) issued by the NMPA.

12.4. Report writing

When reporting the results of statistical analysis of clinical trials, the main content should include:

(1) Distribution of subjects.
(2) Results of analysis of baseline characteristics.

(3) Results of efficacy analysis.
(4) Results of safety analysis.
(5) Statistical conclusions.

Taking the phase III clinical trial of Lipid A as an example, a brief report on the results of statistical analysis is given in the form of a written statement.

A total of 480 subjects were enrolled in the phase III clinical trial of Lipid A. 453 completed the trial and 27 dropped out. The treatment group consisted of 360 subjects, and 341 completed the trial and 19 dropped out. 120 subjects were included in the control group, and among them, 112 completed the trial and eight dropped out.

At baseline, there was no statistically significant difference in age, gender, and past history between the treatment and control group. The baseline characteristics of the two groups were balanced.

At the end of the study, the primary outcome LDL-C of the treatment and the control group decreased by 1.33 ± 0.68 and 1.25 ± 0.52 respectively, and there was no statistically significant difference between the two groups by analysis of variance. There were no statistically significant differences between the two groups on the secondary outcomes, except TG, which was slightly better in the treatment group than that in the control group.

The incidences of adverse events in the treatment and control group were 14% and 12% respectively, and there was no statistically significant difference between the two groups by Chi-square test.

In summary, except the secondary efficacy outcome TG, there were no statistically significant differences on the outcomes for efficacy and safety between Lipid A and lovastatin. It could not be considered yet that the two drugs were different in efficacy and safety.

12.5. Case discrimination

Case 12.1 A pharmaceutical company had developed a new drug for the treatment of diabetes, and planned to conduct a phase II clinical trial in comparison with metformin. The new drug had a special odor and could not be made into the same dosage form as metformin. Some investigators believed that the double-blind method could not be applied for this trial. How should we deal with this issue?

Case 12.2 In a randomized, double-blind, parallel control of positive drugs, multi-center clinical trial, the difference between the two groups was not statistically significant (P = 0.8270), and the investigators concluded that the test drug and the positive control drug were of clinical equivalence in efficacy. Was this conclusion correct?

Case 12.3 A statistician used a mixed-effect model for repeated measurements (MMRM) to analyze the main efficacy based on the FAS. Another statistician thought that his method was wrong; because the last observation carried forward (LOCF) method was not applied to impute the missing value of the main outcome. How to evaluate their practices or opinions?

12.6. Computer experiments (see electronic resources exp12.1 to exp12.2)

Experiment 12.1 Three hundred sixty subjects were equally assigned by block randomization into a positive drug control group, a low-dose test drug group, and a high-dose test drug group. The length of block was 6. Please implement the grouping process using the SPSS software.

Learn to use SPSS to complete block randomization.

Experiment 12.2 A clinical trial was conducted in four hospitals. Four hundred eighty subjects were grouped into the treatment group and the control group according to the stratified block randomization. The ratio of the treatment group to the control group was 3:1, the length of block was 8, and the stratification factor was hospital. Please implement the allocation process through SPSS software.

Learn to use SPSS to complete stratified block randomization.

12.7. Frequently asked questions and summary

12.7.1. *Frequently asked questions*

(1) How to select suitable evaluation outcomes when conducting clinical trials?

Selection of evaluation outcomes is a core issue of clinical trials. Based on clear determination of purpose of clinical trials, the most appropriate evaluation outcomes should be selected based on clinical knowledge. Generally, there is only one primary outcome, which is easy to quantify, highly objective and reproducible. There may be more than one secondary outcome, but do not have too many secondary outcomes. Global assessment variable and the surrogate variable should be selected with sufficient caution. It is forbidden to use numerous outcomes as the primary outcomes when the purpose of trial is not clear.

(2) What is the difference between adverse events and adverse reactions?

Adverse events refer to adverse medical events that occur during the process of a clinical trial. The causal relationship between adverse events and investigational drug is not necessary. Adverse reactions are unintended harmful reactions that are causally related to drug use during clinical trials. Adverse events that are causally related to drug use are adverse reactions, and adverse reactions are only a part of adverse events.

(3) What is the center effect? How to deal with the existing center effects?

Center effect refers to different treatment effects between centers resulting from differences in baseline characteristics, medical levels and others between centers in a clinical trial. When there is a center effect, but no significant interaction between center and the treatment factor, statistical model should include main effect of center but do not include interaction term between the center and the treatment factor. When both center effect and interaction between center and treatment factor are present, if directions of difference in effect between the treatment group and the control group in each center are the same, a suitable statistical model is essential to estimate the treatment effect and results should be interpreted with great caution. If the direction of difference in any center is different from that of other centers, a reasonable explanation should be provided and the clinical trial should be re-run. When the number of centers is large, or the number of subjects per center is small, there is no need to consider the impact of center effect on study outcomes.

12.7.2. *Summary*

(1) Clinical trial should comply with relevant legal regulations and ethical requirements, and should be implemented in phases in registered clinical trial institutions in accordance with specific technical guidelines.
(2) Clinical trial design should follow the principles of control, randomization, replication and balance. Common design types include parallel design, cross-over design, factorial design and group sequential design. In trial, particular attention should be paid to implementation of blinding method and scientific formulation of clinical trial plan and the CRF.
(3) Data management of clinical trials covers the entire process from establishment of data collection and management systems to archiving of data and data management documents; it involves sponsors, investigators, auditors and data managers. The main documents are the DMP and DMR.
(4) Trial data analysis shall be conducted in distinct datasets, and 3 special types of tests are commonly used. The main contents of statistical analysis include description of distribution of subjects, compliance analysis, analysis of baseline comparability, efficacy and safety analysis, and concomitant drug analysis. The main documents for statistical analysis are the SAP and SAR.

Think and Practice

I. Best Choice

1. In a clinical trial to evaluate preventive efficacy of influenza vaccine, what was the more appropriate randomized method ( ).
A. Simple randomization B. Stratified randomization C. Block randomization D. Stratified block randomization E. Cluster randomization

2. The commonly used design in clinical trials did not include ( ).
   A. Factorial design B. Orthogonal design C. Cross-over design D. Parallel group design E. Group sequential design
3. In clinical trials, it would be considered as poor compliance, if the dosage subjects took is greater than ( ).
   A. 110% B. 115% C. 120% D. 125% E. 130%
4. In accordance with relevant guidelines, test level for non-inferiority tests should be ( ).
   A. 0.0125 B. 0.025 C. 0.05 D. 0.10 E. 0.15

II. Questions for Reflection

1. What is a multi-center clinical trial? What are the advantages of multi-center clinical trials and the issues that need attention?
2. What are the main contents of data management of a clinical trial? What are the audit trails and access control of data management system?
3. What are the analysis datasets commonly used in clinical trials? Where are they applied?

III. Questions on Calculation

1. In a clinical trial of group sequential design, an interim analysis was planned, and the total number of analyses was 2. Please use the O'Brien-Fleming method according to the formula:

$$z_{iK} = \frac{c_K\sqrt{K}}{\sqrt{i}}$$

(K was the total number of analyses; i was the ith analysis; c_K was a constant value corresponding to the total number of analyses K, $c_2 = 1.978$; z_{iK} followed standard normal distribution).

Calculate the nominal test level (two sides) in each analysis.

References

[1] Thorpe, KE, Zwarenstein, M, Oxman, AD, *et al.* A pragmatic-explanatory continuum indicator summary (PRECIS): a tool to help trial designers. *J Clin Epidemiol.* 2009; 62: 464–475. doi:10.1016/j.jclinepi.2008.12.011

[2] Deng, W, He, J. *Design and Statistical Analysis of Clinical Trials.* Beijing: People's Medical Publishing House; 2012.
[3] National Medical Products Administration (NMPA). *Technical Guidance for Clinical Trial Data Management.* Beijing; 2016.
[4] National Medical Products Administration (NMPA). *Biostatistical Principles for Drug Clinical Trials.* Beijing; 2016.
[5] Renfro, LA, Mandrekar, SJ. Definitions and statistical properties of master protocols for personalized medicine in oncology. *Journal of Biopharmaceutical Statistics.* 2018; 28: 217–228. doi:10.1080/10543406.2017.1372778
[6] Renfro, LA, Sargent, DJ. Statistical controversies in clinical research: basket trials, umbrella trials, and other master protocols: a review and examples. *Annals of Oncology.* 2017; 28: 34–43. doi:10.1093/annonc/mdw413

Weiwei Liu

CHAPTER 13

OBSERVATIONAL COMPARATIVE EFFECTIVENESS RESEARCH

Observational studies are widely applied in medical practice to observe and describe the distribution of diseases and health conditions among populations, and to explore the relationships between exposures and diseases by objectively performing field research and recording data while no interventions (treatments) are provided. Traditional observational studies include cross-sectional, case–control, and cohort studies. These studies are bolstered with the development of registration data and claims records. Methods based on such data have received increasing attention.

13.1. Proposal of comparative effectiveness research

Due to the presence of confounders, observational studies are usually characterized as having a weaker quality of evidence than randomized controlled trials. However, more and more research has indicated that well-designed observational studies can provide valuable information about the intervention effects, with their quality of evidence being as good as that of randomized controlled trials. The following examples show some conditions in which a comparative effectiveness research design is particularly appropriate for observational studies:

(1) When large-scale studies are needed

Although multiple treatment guidelines recommend the use of systemic corticosteroids for flare-ups of chronic obstructive pulmonary disease, the optimal dose and route of administration have not yet been well defined. Data from an observational study of 84,621 patients conducted at 414 U.S. hospitals in 2006 and 2007 demonstrated that physicians were more likely to administer high-dose intravenous systemic corticosteroids (average 600mg/day) than low-dose oral corticosteroids (average 60mg/day) in such cases. Notably, 92% of all patients were initially treated with intravenous systemic corticosteroids, whereas the remaining 8% received oral corticosteroids. The death rates and adverse event frequencies were 1.4% and 10.9% in the intravenously treated patients and 1.0% and 10.3% in the orally treated patients, respectively. When confounders were adjusted by propensity-matched analysis (the method is introduced later in this chapter), the treatment effects of the two therapies were found to be quite similar; however, the risk of side effects, length of stay, and cost of treatment were lower in the orally treated group(JAMA, 2010; 303: 2359-67). To evaluate these findings in a randomized trial, the trial would have to be very large, with approximately 30,000 patients in the two groups combined (JAMA,2010;303:2409-10).

(2) When a randomized controlled trial cannot be performed

Patients usually show poor compliance with the use of inhaled steroids, which are considered as the gold standard for treating asthma. An insurer-requested observational study conducted in the U.S. using administrative claims data on approximately 51,168 patients who have at least one record between September 2003 and August 2005 evaluated the clinical, economic, and treatment effects on patients to explore the association between asthma medications and outcomes. The researchers concluded that although inhaled corticosteroids were associated with a lower risk of inpatient admissions and emergency department visits, patients taking oral medications were significantly more likely to adhere to their treatment regimen. Even when the investigators controlled the severity of disease, patients taking oral medications derived greater benefit from treatment than those taking inhaled medications. Based on the study, the insurance company decided to continue its favorable reimbursement level for the oral medication. However, differences in treatment adherence will influence outcomes if the randomized trial is unable to realize blind (Mayo Clinic Proceedings, 2009; 84: 675–84).

(3) When the intervention implementers are different

Implantable cardioverter defibrillators for patients at risk of sudden cardiac death can be implanted by physicians with a range of training from accredited electrophysiology fellowships to less formal training programs. A study of physician certification and outcomes in 111,293 patients showed that patients had a higher rate of procedural complications when the devices were implanted by thoracic surgeons or cardiologists who were not electrophysiologists than when the devices were implanted by electrophysiologists. Furthermore, among 35,841 patients who met the standard criteria for the use of defibrillators with cardiac resynchronization therapy, patients were more likely to receive the indicated resynchronization device when their defibrillators were implanted by an electrophysiologist, i.e., electrophysiologists were more likely to implant the appropriate type of device than non-electrophysiologist cardiologists. In randomized trials, once the providers themselves influence outcomes, they must balance the groups during the design stage; however, such adjustment can make the design more difficult and even infeasible in some clinical practices.

13.2. Useful techniques in observational comparative effectiveness research

With the development of social informatization, the accumulation and continuous improvement of medical information have provided unprecedented convenience for the comparative study of effects based on real-world data. Issues on how to reasonably use these observational data to compare the effects of different treatments and interventions deserve exploration. This section introduces some techniques that can be used to improve the comparability of group data when randomized controlled trials are not available and non-random or observational studies are used.

13.2.1. *Propensity score*

In an analysis based on clinical records, because clinicians may prefer certain treatment options (for example, clinicians may intend to administer new treatment to patients who have severer clinical conditions), it may be difficult to observe the real effects of interventions because of the imbalance of basic information and disease severity between different groups. Methods commonly used to deal with potential confounders include stratification and adjustment. In recent years, researchers have proposed that propensity score matching be applied to balance the influence of confounders between different groups.

Example 13.1. To explore the effects of two surgical methods, A and B, on the survival time of lung cancer patients, researchers collected data (data13-1) of 902 patients, including 562 patients who underwent A surgery (group = 0) and 340 patients who underwent B surgery (group = 1). The investigators collected information on gender (male = 1, female = 2), age (years), education level (primary school or below = 1, secondary school = 2, college or above = 3), pathological features (small cell carcinoma = 1, squamous cell carcinoma = 2, adenocarcinoma = 3), tumor stage (stage I = 1, stage II = 2, stage III = 3), survival time (months), survival outcomes (censor = 0, death = 1), and other information.

As in practice, doctors usually choose a surgical method based on the actual conditions of the patient while do not randomize them into different (here two) surgical method groups, the distribution of covariates between groups may not be balanced. Therefore, the propensity score matching method was used to balance the covariates between the two groups.

A propensity score represents the probability of individuals' entering surgery group B rather than group A under the condition of observable covariants. Logistic regression or discriminant analysis can be used to calculate the propensity score. In this case, the surgical method was used as the dependent variable, and five variables (gender, age, education level, pathological features, and tumor stage) were used as independent variables (observable covariants) to construct the logistic regression model and calculate the propensity score.

$$Ln\left(\frac{P}{1-P}\right) = \beta_0 + \beta_1 X_1 + \beta_2 X_2 + \cdots + \beta_k X_k$$

P denotes the probability of participants entering group B, and X_k is the kth possible confounders; β is the corresponding regression coefficient. By constructing the above model and estimating the parameters, the estimation of each β_i can be obtained. The propensity score of the ith individual can be obtained by substituting the X_is with observations of the individual:

$$PS_i = \frac{e^{\beta_0 + \beta_1 X_1 + \beta_2 X_2 + \cdots + \beta_k X_k}}{1 + e^{\beta_0 + \beta_1 X_1 + \beta_2 X_2 + \cdots + \beta_k X_k}}$$

The propensity score is a number between 0 and 1, which comprehensively reflects the influence of several observable covariants on the treatment allocation. Computing the propensity score is also a way of reducing dimensions: reducing a multi-dimensional feature of several observable covariants to a one-dimensional feature of the propensity score. Based on the propensity score, data can be further analyzed by matching or adjustment.

1. Matching

After obtaining propensity scores for all individuals, each one in the intervention group can be matched to one (or more) appropriate subject(s) in the control group. Several types of matching methods are available. Commonly used methods include nearest-neighbor matching, radius matching, kernel matching, and local linear matching. Here we only introduce two of them.

Nearest-neighbor matching: This is one of the most commonly used methods of matching. Each intervention group is matched with the control group based on the principle of the closest propensity score. Based on the order of the propensity score from low to high, individuals are selected from the intervention group, and all individuals from the control group with scores closest to the scores of the individuals from the intervention group are identified. If more than one individual are identified, one is randomly selected. Each intervention can also have more than one matched controls, by selecting n individuals (usually $n < 5$) with the closest scores from the control group. During matching, both with and without replacement can be adopted. With replacement means that the same individual in the control group can be used as the matching object of multiple individuals of the intervention group at the same time, while without replacement means that an individual in the control group can only be matched once. The nearest-neighbor matching method is simple and easy to understand, however, when there is a great difference in the propensity scores between the two groups, it will lead to poor matching.

Radius matching: Also known as "caliper matching", this method is used to set the clamp value on the basis of the nearest neighbor matching method, i.e., only individuals having difference of propensity scores within the range of the clamp value can be matched. The radius matching method also allows for replacement as mentioned above. The radius matching method solves the problem of far distances between the two individuals in the nearest neighbor matching, but it may lead to exclusion of data as some individuals may fall outside the range of clamp values and be eliminated, resulting in sampling bias.

Because not every individual in the intervention group can find a "matching object" in the control group, after the completion of matching, the number of individuals in the intervention and control groups must be reduced. However, the two groups should be close to each other after matching. A t-test or χ^2 test can be used to compare the difference in characteristics and propensity scores between the two groups. However, in recent years, it has been recommended to measure the balance of matched samples by calculating the standardized difference (SD). For continuous variables, the SD is calculated as follows:

$$d = \frac{100|\overline{X}_T - \overline{X}_C|}{\sqrt{\frac{S_T^2 + S_C^2}{2}}}$$

Where $\overline{X}_T$ and $\overline{X}_C$ represent the mean of the variables to be tested in the intervention and control groups, respectively, and S_T^2 and S_C^2 represent the variance of the variables to be tested in the treatment and control groups, respectively. For discrete variables, the SDs are calculated as follows:

$$d = \frac{100|\hat{p}_T - \hat{p}_C|}{\sqrt{\frac{\hat{p}_T(1-\hat{p}_T)+\hat{p}_C(1-\hat{p}_C)}{2}}}$$

Where $\hat{p}_T$ and $\hat{p}_C$ represent the positive rates of the variables to be tested in the treatment and control groups, respectively. The size of the normalized difference is not affected by the sample size; therefore, it can better measure the balance between the two groups after matching. It was generally believed that an SD greater than 10% indicates an imbalance in covariates between the two groups. If there is no balance between the two groups, the reasons for the difference need to be studied and the matching method needs to be adjusted until a balance between the two groups is reached. None of the above matching methods are absolutely superior to the others; therefore, several attempts can be made to choose a preferable matching method.

The above example elaborates the use of the caliper matching method, in which the clamp value was set to 0.03 using the 1:1 matching without replacement, and finally, 276 pairs were matched successfully. The SD was then used to evaluate the balance between the two groups. It was found that all covariates between the two groups reached balance after matching (SD < 0.1). The results are shown in Table 13.1. Subsequently, survival analysis of the matched data (276 cases of surgery A and 276 of surgery B) revealed that there was a lower risk of mortality in surgery B group than in surgery A group [$HR = 0.389$,95% $CI = (0.287, 0.527)$, see results in Table 13.2].

The application of propensity score matching should pay attention to the following aspects:

First, the propensity score construction should include as many variables as possible that may affect the outcome. If important variables are missing, the estimation of the intervention effect will be inaccurate. However, in practice, it is often impossible to verify

Table 13.1 Balance comparison of covariates of the two groups before and after matching

	Before matching			After matching		
	A surgery	B surgery	*SD*	A surgery	B surgery	*SD*
Sample size (%)	562 (62.3)	340 (37.7)		276 (50)	276 (50)	
Gender (%)			0.357			0.023
Male	419 (68)	197 (32)		179 (49.6)	182 (50.4)	
Female	143 (50)	143 (50)		97 (50.8)	94 (49.2)	
Age,mean ± SD	50.62 ± 10.35	60.71 ± 10.51	0.297	60.11 ± 9.97	59.67 ± 10.39	0.017
Education level			0.132			0.039
Primary school or below	168 (62.9)	99 (37.1)		79 (50.3)	78 (49.7)	
Middle school	202 (61.4)	127 (38.6)		94 (48.7)	99 (51.3)	
College or above	192 (62.7)	114 (37.3)		103 (51)	99 (49)	
Pathological type (%)			0.244			0.066
1	177 (69.1)	79 (30.9)		72 (48)	78 (52)	
2	275 (57.1)	207 (42.9)		151 (50)	151 (50)	
3	110 (67.1)	54 (32.9)		53 (53)	47 (47)	
Tumor stage (%)			0.609			0.037
1	190 (47.1)	213 (52.9)		149 (49.7)	151 (50.3)	
2	136 (71.6)	54 (28.4)		56 (51.9)	52 (48.1)	
3	236 (76.4)	73 (23.6)		71 (49.3)	73 (50.7)	

Table 13.2 Estimation of the effects of two surgical methods on the survival of lung cancer patients

	b	*SE*	*P*	*HR*	95%*CI*
Propensity score matching ($N = 552$)	−0.944	0.155	<0.001	0.389	(0.287, 0.527)
Propensity score weighting ($N = 902$)	−0.863	0.081	<0.001	0.422	(0.360, 0.494)

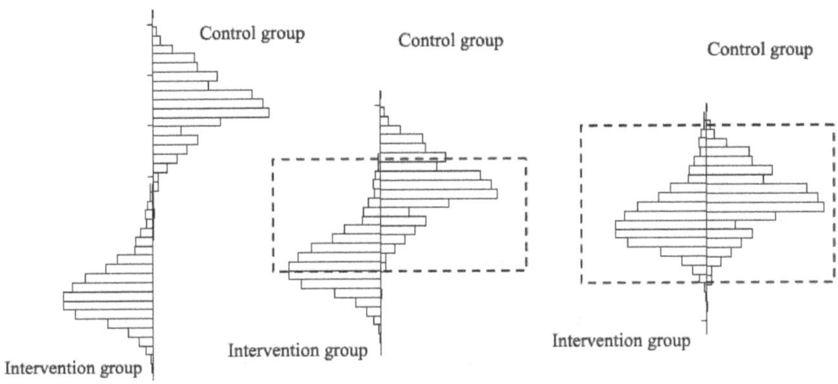

(a) No overlap (b) Partial overlap (c) Complete overlap

Figure 13.1 Distribution of propensity scores

whether this condition is met. Therefore, researchers should have in-depth understanding of which variables may be affected by the study outcome and include as many baseline survey variables as possible.

Second, there should be enough overlap between the two groups to find a large overlapping area for the propensity score distribution before applying the matching method. During the matching process, the observed data that are not in the overlapping area of propensity score distribution would be eliminated, resulting in the loss of that information. Figure 13.1 shows three distributions: in case a, there was no overlap in the propensity score distribution between the two groups, and individuals could not be matched; in case b, the distribution of the two groups partially overlapped, and the individuals in the box could find their matching objects, but the individuals outside the box may not be matched; in case c, the distribution of the two groups overlapped completely, and most individuals could be matched.

Third, propensity score matching will exclude unmatched data, so a large sample size is usually required. Meanwhile, because the data involved in the analysis may no longer represent the population, the results might be biased. An analysis on the characteristics of the excluded data would help to understand and explain the potential bias of the results.

Fourth, the requirements for matching is crucial: strict requirements would lead to better results of matching, but the sample size would be small; conversely, if the requirements are loose, the balance between the groups will be poor after matching even if the sample size is large.

2. Propensity score weighting

Propensity score weighting is an individual-based standardization method, and its principle is similar to those of the traditional standardization methods. Propensity scores are calculated and then used to estimate the statistical weights for each individual. Applying these weights to the study subjects creates an artificial population. In this artificial population, all observed covariates tend to be balanced between the two groups and are similar to those of a target standard population.

In practice, a popularly used method is the inverse probability of treatment weighting (IPTW). Using the entire study (total) population as the standard population, the inverse probability of treatment weight (w) is defined as follows:

$$w_i = \frac{Z_i}{PS_i} + \frac{1 - Z_i}{1 - PS_i},$$

Where Zi denotes treatment assignment with $Z = 1$ denoting the treatment group and $Z = 0$ denoting the control group. PS is the estimated propensity score. In general, a subject's weight is equal to the inverse of the propensity score if the subject is from the treatment group or the inverse of 1 minus the propensity score (1-PS) if the subject is from the control group. In Example 13.1, the fourth subject belonged to the surgery A group with $Z = 1$.Its PS value was 0.6301, and the weight was $w = 1/0.630 + 0 = 1.5870$. The sixth subject belonged to the surgery B group with $Z = 0$.Its PS value was 0.6127, and the weight was $w = 0 + 1/(1 - 0.6127) = 2.582$. Propensity score weighting may result in a very large weight if the treated subjects have a very low propensity score or the control subject has a propensity score close to one. To address extreme weights, we can use a stabilizing weight, which is equal to the product of the inverse probability of treatment weight and the marginal probability of receiving the treatment. Another option is to use a truncated weight, in which each of the weights that exceed a specified threshold are set to that threshold.

Methods of assessing covariate balance in a weighted sample are similar to those in a propensity score-matched sample. A weighted sample was subjected to survival analysis, and the results are reported in Table 13.2. The results indicate that surgery B was associated with a lower risk of death than surgery A [$HR = 0.389$, 95% $CI = (0.287, 0.527)$]. Compared with propensity score matching, a key advantage of propensity score weighting is that it does not reduce sample size and all sample information can be used. However, propensity score weighting is sensitive to model specification. Propensity score stratification is an alternative approach to matching and weighting. In practice, we can choose an appropriate approach from matching, stratification, and weighting using propensity scores to reduce or eliminate the effects of confounding variables based on the research objectives and data characteristics.

13.2.2. *Instrumental variable method*

1. Concept of instrumental variable

In an analysis based on clinical registration data, results are inevitably affected by various biases and confounders, leading to an over- or under-estimation of the effect size. For example, in a study comparing effects of different treatments for coronary heart disease, patients with more serious illness tend to undergo more expensive surgical treatments, such as angioplasty and bypass surgery, and also tend to have higher risks of subsequent heart disease and mortality. Therefore, compared with patients receiving conservative treatment, those undergoing surgical treatment have a higher risk of adverse events because of a more severe underlying illness, which, if not accounted, would lead to an underestimation of the conservative treatment effect. Conversely, in other situations, relatively healthy patients tend to choose surgery, and studies directly comparing different treatment effects may also be biased by confounding due to differential baseline health status between the groups. Therefore, even well-designed observational studies cannot completely rule out biases.

To reduce such biases, although we may control for confounding factors using the above-mentioned methods, such as matching and statistical adjustment, a wide variety of confounding factors need to be identified first. Next, the confounding factors can be adjusted using statistical approaches only if accurate information about them is collected. However, in reality, confounding factors often cannot be fully identified. The reasons are as follows: (1) the types of confounding factors cannot be fully identified. For any exposure–outcome associations, confounding factors that are already known may only be a small part of total confounders. (2) For a particular exposure variable, the information collected often cannot be completely accurate. Therefore, the issue of residual confounding cannot be ruled out in observational studies. Traditional analysis based on observational data fails to account for residual confounding, and thus, other methods such as instrumental variable (IV) analysis are warranted to handle this problem.

The IV method is commonly used in economics and has recently started being used in medical studies to analyze causal associations between medical treatments and health effects. Investigators can obtain an IV from observational data. It must be directly related to the treatment used in patients *per se* and not to the study outcome. Using an IV, patients can be randomly assigned to different

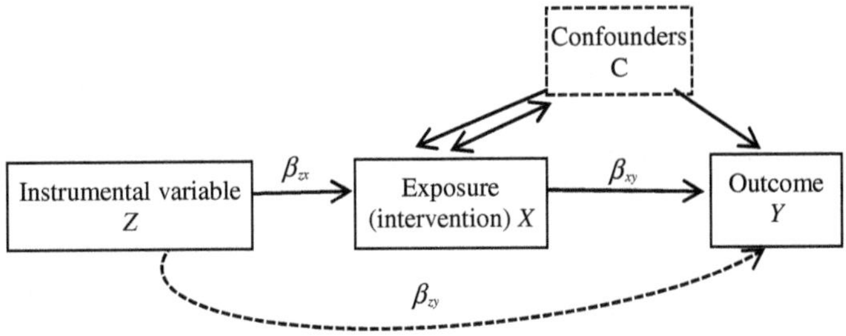

Figure 13.2 Illustration of an instrumental variable

treatment groups. An effective IV needs to meet the following three assumptions (please refer to Figure 13.2):

First, the IV Z should be statistically strongly associated with the exposure (or intervention) variable X. In this premise, Z becomes a valid IV of X, and this assumption is probably the easiest to meet among the three assumptions. Second, the IV Z must be independent of various confounding factors C, i.e., there must be no correlation between Z and C. This assumption is difficult to meet in a traditional IV analysis because most of the study variables are affected by factors that also influence the disease occurrence, progression, or prognosis, including disease severity, health status, lifestyle, and socioeconomic status. Therefore, it is difficult to find a study variable that remains unaffected by the above-mentioned factors. Third, the effect of the IV Z on outcome Y must only through its effects on the exposure (or intervention) variable X.

Example 13.2. A study comparing the effects of intensive treatment (i.e., angioplasty or bypass surgery) versus non-intensive treatment on mortality in elderly patients with acute myocardial infarction (MI) using Medicare claims data (please refer to Figure 13.3). The data showed that patients who lived away from the treatment hospital were less likely to choose intensive treatment, whereas those who lived near the treatment hospital tended to choose intensive treatment. No difference was observed in the health status between patients who lived away from and those who lived near the treatment

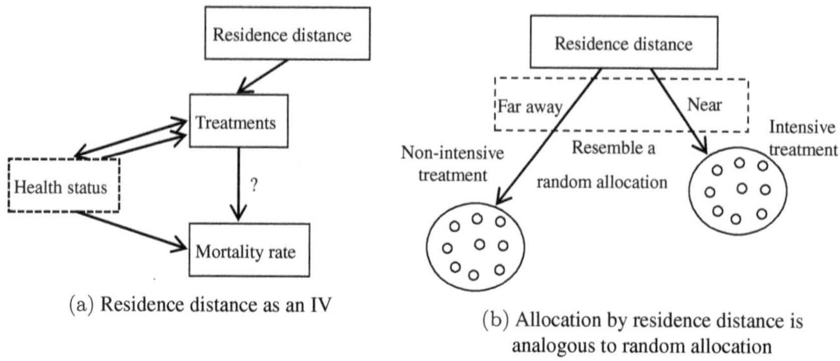

Figure 13.3 Illustration of an instrumental variable using residence distance as an example

hospital because the distance of residence was related only to the choice of treatments and not to the health status. In this case, the distance of residence was used as an IV for treatment types in the study, considering that it may satisfy the three abovementioned assumptions. First, there was a strong association between the distance of residence and choice of treatment. Second, there was no association between the distance of residence and potential confounding factors such as disease severity and health status. Third, the distance of residence *per se* could not affect the mortality risk in patients with MI and only played a role through affecting the choice of different treatments. Data analysis using the IV method showed that the mortality risk was slightly lower in the intensive treatment group (i.e., including patients who lived near) than in the non-intensive treatment group, but this difference was statistically significant only on the first day of admission. No difference was observed between the two groups in terms of long-term mortality risks, suggesting that the intensive treatment of elderly patients with acute MI had limited effects on mortality (JAMA, 1994; 272: 859-66).

As mentioned above, because of ethical issues, randomized controlled trials are not always applicable and ethical in determining and comparing different treatment effects. Thus, IV analysis incorporating observational data serves as a more effective method for dealing with residual confounding. The results of IV analysis are often comparable with those of randomized controls trials. Regarding the abovementioned example using Medicare claims data and IV analysis, patients who lived away from the treatment hospital tended to choose non-intensive treatment (as if they were randomly assigned to the non-intensive treatment arm), whereas those who lived near tended to choose intensive treatment (as if they were randomly assigned to the intensive treatment arm).

2. Instrumental variable regression method

In the above example, we used two-stage least squares (2SLS) regression for IV analysis. First, we regressed the types of treatments on differential residence distance and computed the predictors of the types of treatment based on residence distance. We then performed second regression for the association between the predicted values and mortality to obtain estimated effects of different treatments on the risks of death in patients with MI. In case of a valid IV, comparison of the results from a traditional regression model with those from an IV regression revealed that estimates obtained from IV regression generally tended to be closer to the true value. Thus, the IV method is often considered to be superior to the conventional least squares method, proving the existence of a valid IV. Currently, there are some statistical software programs that provide tools for conducting IV analysis using 2SLS, such as Stata, SAS, and R.

Example 13.3. The use of selective COX-2inhibitors (COX-2s) and non-selective non-steroidal anti-inflammatory drugs (NSAIDs) is often accompanied by a range of potential adverse effects, including effects on blood vessels and the gastrointestinal tract. To date, there is no convincing evidence to support the recommendation of these two drug types. To compare the effects of these two drug types on gastrointestinal complications (GCs), a researcher collected treatment data of 56,898 patients from medical records. Of these patients, 15,386 used COX-2s and 41,512 used non-selective NSAIDs. Data on physicians' prescription preferences (non-selective NSAIDs = 0, COX-2s = 1), patients' gender (female = 0, male = 1), age ($<$70 years = 0, $\geq$70 years = 1), previous history of coronary

Table 13.3 Comparison of the balance of covariates between COX-2s and non-selective NSAIDs groups

	COX-2s	*non-selective NSAIDs*	*P* value
Number of cases(%)	15,386 (27)	41,512 (73)	
Gender(%)			<0.001
Male	5,170 (33.6)	17,850 (43.0)	
Female	10,216 (66.4)	23,662 (57.0)	
Age(years)			<0.001
<70 years	7,047 (45.8)	23,662 (57.0)	
≥70 years	8,339 (54.2)	17,850 (43.0)	
Previous history of coronary heart disease			<0.001
No	13,524 (87.9)	37,029 (89.2)	
Yes	1,862 (12.1)	4,483 (10.8)	

heart disease (no = 0, yes = 1), and GC outcomes (not occurred = 0, occurred = 1) were collected.

As physicians often prescribe drugs according to the patients' actual condition, some covariates between the two groups of patients (those who used COX-2s and those who used non-selective NSAIDs) may affect the prognosis or the occurrence of adverse effects (please refer to Table 13.3). As prescription preferences *per se* were not related to other patient characteristics, prescription preferences were used as an IV for drug use to eliminate potential confounding effects. An IV analysis showed that compared with the patients using non-selective NSAIDs, those using COX-2s had a lower risk of GCs[$\beta = -1.31$, 95% $CI = (-2.42, -0.20)$]; however, the traditional least squares regression showed no difference in the effect on GCs. The results are shown in Table 13.4.

3. Limitations and progress of the IV method

The biggest concern with the IV method lies in the difficulty in identifying credible IVs that meet the three above-mentioned assumptions for IV analysis. Using uncredited IVs may lead to biased estimates. A common bias in IV analysis is the weak IV bias, which refers to the bias caused by a weak association between the IV and the exposure (or intervention) variable. A weak IV bias tends to bias the results

Table 13.4 Comparison of parameter estimation between conventional least squares and 2SLS regression models

	Number of GC events (COX-2s/non-selective NSAIDs)	β value #	95% *CI*
Conventional least squares	501/240	−0.06	(−0.26, 0.14)
Two-stage least squares	363/205	−1.31	(−2.42, −0.20)

#: The non-selective NSAID group is used as the reference group;
*: F-statistic = 864.44; Partial $R^2 = 0.08$.

of IV analysis towards the results of traditional regression analysis. When using 2SLS regression to conduct IV analysis, an $F-$statistic value in the first stage can be obtained from the regression model. It is generally considered that an IV is acceptable (i.e., not weak) when the $F-$statistic value is at least 10. Another method to determine the existence of a weak IV bias is using a partial R^2 (Shea's partial R-squared) value, i.e., regressing the exposure (or intervention) variable on the selected IV in the first stage to obtain the proportion of variance in the exposure (or intervention) variable that can be explained by the IV. A partial R^2 of not less than 0.03 is often preferably required. A weak IV bias generally cannot be improved using statistical models. Efforts to find better IVs are needed.

Another problem with the IV method is that even if there is a strong statistical association between the IV Z and the exposure (or intervention) variable X, it is difficult to completely rule out the effects of confounding factors on the outcome. For example, in the above analysis using Medicare claims data, if the residence distance Z is related to the socio-economic status (i.e., patients who lived near the hospital also had higher income and better medical service than those who lived far), the effects of treatments on mortality may also be influenced by the socio-economic status. If this is the case, the second and third assumptions of IV analysis cannot be met, which would lead to a biased estimate.

Mendelian randomization is another IV method. In 2003, G. Davey Smith first proposed the concept of Mendelian randomization in a conference of the *International Journal of Epidemiology.*

Basically, Mendelian randomization is a subtype of IV analysis that uses one or a group of single nucleotide polymorphisms (SNPs) as IV(s) for a phenotype (i.e., an exposure variable) to identify causal associations between modifiable environmental factors and disease outcomes or health status in observational studies. Owing to the rapid development in modern gene sequencing technology, information on the phenotype-related SNPs can now be accurately obtained. Information misclassification bias that often occurs during the data collection process can be substantially reduced. In addition, because the SNPs that determine differential phenotypes follow Mendel's second law (the law of independent assortment), the genetic variants are expected to be independent of each other. Moreover, these genetic variants are determined at conception, and the process of their acquisition is similar to the random assignment of interventions in randomized controlled trials. The genetic variants are not affected by any environmental exposure or lifestyle factor after birth. Thus, by analyzing the association among SNPs, related phenotypes, and health outcomes of interest, we can obtain unbiased estimate of the causal association between phenotypes and outcomes. Causal inferences that cannot be confirmed in traditional intervention studies due to ethical issues can now be obtained using Mendelian randomization. A large number of Mendelian randomization studies have been conducted since 2003, indicating that the value of this method in medical research is gradually being realized.

13.3. Report writing

Result reporting of propensity score matching should include (1) baseline characteristics of subjects after matching; (2) covariate balance after matching; and (3) estimation of treatment effect, including point estimation, 95% CIs, and$P$ value. In Example 13.2, result reporting should include the following information:

After propensity score matching, a total of 276 pairs of data were included in analysis. (Describe the characteristics of the paired samples). All baseline characteristics were balanced between the two groups ($SD < 0.1$).

After matching, the Cox regression model showed that surgery B was associated with a lower risk of death than surgery A [HR = 0.389, 95% CI = (0.287, 0.527)].

Result reporting of IV analysis should include (1) an IV; (2) assumption of IV analysis; (3) test level α of IV and treatment effects, including point estimation, 95% CIs, and P value. In Example 13.3, result reporting should include the following information:

Physician's prescription preference was a valid IV for comparing the effect of exposure to COX-2s with that of exposure to non-selective NSAIDs on GCs (the first-stage F-statistic value = 864.44). Conventional multivariable regression revealed no protective effect caused by COX-2s (β = −0.06; 95% CI: −0.26 to 0.14). However, the proposed IV method attributed a protective effect to exposure to COX-2s (β = −1.31; 95% CI: −2.42 to −0.20).

13.4. Case discrimination

Case 13.1 One research aimed to compare the mortality and risk of cardiovascular disease due to different insulin secretagogues and metformin in type 2 diabetes patients with or without previous myocardial infarction (MI). Due to the huge cost and great variety of insulin secretagogues, it is unrealistic to conduct a large-sample RCT. Every Denmark resident has a unique, permanent registration number, which is linked with various domestic registrations. The registration data used in the study included the National Prescription Registry of Danish (recorded information of all medication prescriptions since 1995), the National Patient Registry (record of all primary diagnoses of hospitalizations at discharge since 1978), and the National Causes of Death Register (record of information about causes of death). All individuals aged 20 years and above who initiated single-agent treatment with an insulin secretagogue or metformin between 1997 and 2006 were included in the study, whereas those treated with insulin alone or with the combination of multiple drugs were excluded. A total of 107,806 patients with type 2 diabetes were included and were followed up for up to 9 years (median, 3.3 years).

Table 13.5 Comparison of basic information and comorbidity of type 2 diabetes patients (without MI) who accepted treatment with metformin or insulin secretagogues

	Metformin	Glimepiride	Gliclazide	Glibenclamide	Glipizide	Tolbutamide	Repaglinide
N (%)	43,340 (54.3)	36,313 (37.0)	5,926 (6.0)	12,495 (12.7)	6,965 (6.1)	5,335 (5.4)	2,513 (2.6)
Age (years)	52.5 ± 14.0	60.9 ± 13.3	60.0 ± 13.2	63.2 ± 13.7	63.0 ± 13.5	64.4 ± 13.5	57.9 ± 12.6
Men (%)	50.9	55.3	56.5	54.4	54.1	53.8	56.0
Treatment duration (years)	1.76 ± 1.58	2.11 ± 1.75	2.10 ± 1.75	2.35 ± 2.08	2.35 ± 2.08	2.36 ± 2.13	1.97 ± 1.76
Congestive heart failure (%)	1.1	2.5	1.6	2.4	2.4	2.6	0.7
Cardiac dysrhythmia (%)	1.6	3.2	2.1	3.0	3.2	2.8	1.5
Peripheral vascular disease (%)	0.3	0.6	0.5	0.7	0.9	0.9	0.6
Cerebrovascular disease (%)	1.6	2.8	1.4	2.9	2.8	3.3	1.2
Chronic pulmonary disease (%)	1.5	2.6	1.6	2.4	2.8	2.6	1.2

The results of data stratification according to the presence of MI indicated the correlation between the use of insulin secretagogues (glimepiride, glibenclamide, glipizide, gliclazide, tolbutamide, and repaglinide) or metformin and the outcomes (all-cause mortality and cardiovascular mortality). However, the baseline characteristics (age, gender, treatment duration, etc.), comorbidity, and combined use of cardiovascular medication were not comparable across groups (partly listed in Figure 30.1). These factors potentially confounded the correlation between the drug and the outcomes.

Therefore, the researcher used propensity score matching to control for confounders between the two groups. In developing a logistic model, the treatment (an insulin secretagogue or metformin) was defined as the dependent variable; then stepwise approach was adopted to select independent variables from potential confounders in baseline characteristics. Then the logistic equation was built, and the propensity score was then calculated for each subject. The nearest neighbor matching method was used to match data. A t−test or χ^2 test was used to evaluate the balance between the two groups. Adjusted factors remained unbalanced after matching, and Cox regression analysis further indicated the inferiority of six insulin secretagogues to metformin in preventing all-cause mortality and cardiovascular death.

1. Did the researcher use the propensity score matching method correctly? How?
2. If imbalance remained after matching, what methods could have been used to improve the results of matching?
3. If a key variable in the propensity score model had missing data and it then affected the sample size after matching, can the researcher delete it? If not, how can the problem be solved?

Case 13.2 To compare the effects of two hypoglycemic agents A and B on the reduction of fasting glucose level in patients with type 2 diabetes, a researcher collected information on the following seven indicators from 31 patients with type 2 diabetes: fasting blood glucose level (Y, mmol/l), drug type (X_1; 1 = A, 2 = B), gender

Table 13.6 Parameter estimation of multiple linear regression models*

	Unstandardized coefficients			
Variable	B	Std. Error	t	P
(Intercept)	0.726	1.377	0.527	0.598
Drug type#	1.031	0.384	2.686	0.007
Education	0.427	0.261	1.634	0.102
Age	0.026	0.015	1.713	0.087
Income	−0.171	0.199	−0.861	1.611
Gender	0.092	0.246	0.372	0.71

#: Drug A is used as the reference group; *: F statistic = 22.84; Partial $R^2 = 0.48$

(X_2; 0 = female, 1 = male), age (X_3; years), education (X_4; 1 = primary school, 2 = secondary school, 3 = university or above), annual income (X_5; RMB; 1 =< 10,000, 2 = 10,000–15,000, 3 => 15,000), and physicians' prescription preferences (IV; 1 = Drug A, 2 = Drug B).The researcher conducted IV analysis using physicians' prescription preferences as an IV for the use of two drugs. The results are shown in Table 13.6.

The results of IV analysis showed that patients who used drug B had significantly higher fasting glucose levels than those who used drug A ($P < 0.05$). Please take the F-statistic value and the partial R^2 value into account and explain whether the "physicians' prescription preferences" can be used as an IV for the use of these two drugs.

13.5. Computer Experiments (See electronic resources Experiment 13.1 to Experiment 13.2)

Experiment 13.1 Propensity score matching Propensity score matching was used to study the impact of two surgical methods A and B on the survival time of patients with lung cancer.

Experiment 13.2 Instrumental variable method An IV analysis was used to determine the causal association between alanine aminotransferase levels and serum low-density lipoprotein cholesterol levels.

13.6. Frequently asked questions and summary

13.6.1. *Frequently asked questions*

1. Which variables should be included in the propensity score model?

A common approach is to include all variables potentially related to the outcome in the propensity score model. Some simulation and practice studies have been conducted to address this problem. In one study, based on the relationships between covariates, treatment assignment, and outcome, all possible variables were divided into four sets: variables related to both treatment allocation and outcome, variables related to neither outcome nor treatment allocation, variables related to treatment allocation but not outcome, and variables related to outcome but not treatment allocation. Researchers compared the variance and bias of treatment effect estimates using different combinations of variables to construct a propensity score model. The results indicated that the optimal model comprised all variables related to outcome regardless of whether they were related to treatment allocation. In addition, variables related to outcome but not treatment allocation in the propensity score model would reduce the variance of treatment effect estimates with no increase in the bias, whereas variables related to treatment allocation but not outcome in the propensity score model would increase the variance of treatment effect estimates without decreasing the bias. Thus, a recommended approach to construct a propensity score model is to include all variables potentially related to the outcome in the model. In practice, researchers can construct the propensity score model based on baseline variables and professional knowledge. However, the use of stepwise variable selection to construct the model is not a good idea because the variables related to outcome but not treatment allocation would be deleted.

2. How to choose a valid IV?

As mentioned above, a valid IV should meet the abovementioned three assumptions (please refer to 13.4.2). The first assumption is easier to meet, and the second assumption, i.e., the IV should not be related to any confounding factor, is often difficult to meet. The third assumption, i.e., the "exclusion restriction" criterion, can only be tested using the exclusion method. For example, if it is observed that the IV can also affect the outcome through other pathways, the "exclusion restriction" assumption is violated. The selection of IVs requires a comprehensive consideration of previous studies, research experience, pathogenic mechanisms, and data accuracy and should also take into account the specific circumstances of the population under study. As in the previous example of Medicare claims data, which used the residence distance as an IV, the residence distance in the study population may not be related to other socioeconomic factors and personal health status, but in some other populations, the residence distance may be associated with income, which is one of the socio-economic factors that affect disease prognosis. In the latter case, the residence distance would not be a valid IV.

3. Why is a traditional randomized controlled trial an effective application of the IV method?

Traditional randomized controlled trials meet the three assumptions of the IV method: (1) results of random allocation are directly related to the treatment allocation; (2) randomization obviously will not be affected by common confounding factors such as the health status, disease severity, medical service, and socioeconomic position; and (3) random allocation *per se* cannot affect disease outcomes. Random allocation can affect outcomes only through the corresponding treatments. Therefore, traditional randomized controlled trials are effective applications of the IV method in medical research.

13.6.2. *Summary*

Comparative effectiveness research focuses on obtaining evidence of the effectiveness of different treatments or interventions in the real world to guide medical practice. The design of comparative effectiveness research is not limited to randomized controlled trials or other interventional studies but encourages the full use of existing medical registration data and the use of appropriate analytical techniques for non-randomized controlled trials or observational studies. The propensity score and IV method introduced in this chapter are analysis methods based on the data of non-randomized controlled design. The purpose of these methods is to reduce the effects of selection or confounding bias in the process of treatment effect estimation. However, because these methods are based on existing real-world data, it is also necessary to evaluate the suitability and possible bias of the methods from a comprehensive and multi-angle perspective to obtain a better reflection of the real-world law as far as possible.

Think and Practice

I. Best Choice

1. Which of the following is a misstatement about propensity score matching?
   A. Propensity score matching can control unmeasured confounding. B. The most common method is nearest neighbor matching. C. Caliper matching may produce sampling bias. D. Propensity score plays an objective role in dimensionality reduction. E. Even if no statistical significance is shown in the hypothesis testing results of baseline comparison between groups, we cannot draw the definite conclusion that matching improves the baseline covariate balance between groups.
2. Which of the following is not a condition that must be met as a valid instrumental variable?
   A. Direct relation to exposure variables B. Direct relation to outcome variables C. Indirect relation to outcome variables D. Indirect relation to confounding factors E. Direct relation to confounding factors

II. Questions

1. Why was hypothesis testing not a good choice to assess baseline balance in matched samples?
2. If differences remained after matching using the nearest neighbor matching method, how could the problem be solved?
3. Recently, some researchers have used genetic variants as instrumental variables to conduct medical research. Please explain why genetic variants can be used as instrumental variables.

References

[1] Ellis, P. *Research on the Comparative Effectiveness of Medical Treatments: Issues and Options for an Expanded Federal role.* Congress of the US, Congressional Budget Office; 2007.
[2] Gertler, PJ, Martinez, S, Premand, P, *et al. Impact Evaluation in Practice.* Washington, DC: The World Bank; 2011.
[3] Austin, PC, Grootendorst, P, Anderson, GM. A comparison of the ability of different propensity score models to balance measured variables between treated and untreated subjects: a Monte Carlo study. *Stat Med.* 2007; 26: 734–753. https://doi.org/10.1002/sim.2580
[4] McClellan, M, McNeil, BJ, Newhouse, JP. Does more intensive treatment of acute myocardial infarction in the elderly reduce mortality:analysis using instrumental variables.*JAMA*. 1994; 272(11): 859–866. https://doi.org/10.1001/jama.1994.03520110039026
[5] Pearl, J. *Causality: Models, Reasoning, and Inference.* Cambridge: MIT Press; 2000.

Jing Gu, Lin Xu

CHAPTER 14

DIAGNOSTIC TEST

In medical study, both clinical diagnosis and population screening require the application of kind of test methods so as to make a diagnosis or screening conclusion, which are commonly referred to as diagnostic test or screening test. The methods to find and create better diagnostic or screening tests are important directions for medical study. It is very necessary to make further study for them about their research, design, and analysis.

14.1. Test design and data format

Individuals in such studies should be patients or non-patients diagnosed with "reference standard" or "the gold standard." The so-called "reference standard" or "gold standard" refers to the diagnosis based on biopsy, surgical findings, pathological or autopsy, X-ray, CT, long-term follow-up, and other convincing examination results.

14.1.1. *Format of the data*

Suppose we have a sample with case and control groups taking respectively from patients and non-patients diagnosed through gold standard method. And each of the group has more than 20 observations (Youden, 1950). Now we want to judge the characteristic of another diagnostic method to evaluate the presence of disease compared with the gold standard. Then we should usually arrange the data in a fourfold table (Table 14.1) to express the relationship between two methods.

Table 14.1 Four-grid table of diagnostic test data

	Gold standard (D)		
Diagnosis (T)	Case (D_+)	Control (D_-)	Total
Positive (T_+)	True positive (A)	False positive (B)	$A+B$
Negative (T_-)	False negative (C)	True negative (D)	$C+D$
Total	$A+C$	$B+D$	N

14.1.2. *Design of diagnostic test*

The diagnostic test generally goes through the following four steps: selecting gold standard, collecting study subjects, determining the diagnostic threshold (cut-off value), obtaining the evaluation index and method, and carrying out the evaluation.

1. To select gold standard

Gold standard is the reliable, acknowledged diagnostic method that can correctly distinguish disease case from control.

Gold standard could usually be pathological diagnosis (biopsy and autopsy), surgical exploration, or specific imaging diagnosis. For example, coronary angiography is the gold standard used for the diagnosis of coronary heart disease (CHD). Some comprehensive diagnostic standards issued by medical authorities could also be taken as gold standard in the case of no specific diagnostic methods. For some chronically progressed and non-self-limited diseases, the gold standard may be too risky to make correct diagnosis. Fortunately, syndromes of the disease may become clear during months or years of follow-up, so the disease may be diagnosed effectively. And then the results of follow-up for these diseases may also serve as the gold standard.

Why do we need to make a relevant study about diagnostic tests while there is already a standard diagnosis?

Some of the gold standards, such as HIV and HBsAg antibody testing, are simple, safe, and cheap. But usually most of the standard diagnoses noted above are complex, dangerous with invasion. At the same time, the simple and relatively safe methods are more accessible to clinicians and patients than those dangerous, expensive and tedious diagnoses (even the accuracy is higher), especially at the beginning of acknowledging the methods. However, it must be noted that the diagnostic method could only be used clinically if we understand the possibility of misclassification and the acceptable and low level of misclassification.

2. To collect study subjects

The study subjects for diagnostic tests should consist of two groups. One is the case with disease, the other is the control without disease. Both the case and control were diagnosed through gold standard. The so-called "disease-free" patients mean the subjects don't have the target disease diagnosed through gold standard diagnosis, rather than the completely disease-free people.

When collecting subjects, it should be noted that the representativeness of subjects will have direct effect on the generalization and popularization of screening or diagnostic tests.

In order to ensure the clinical value of the diagnostic test, we should pay more attention to the choice of the case group. This group should include various types of cases: such as typical and untypical cases; early, middle, and late cases; mild, moderate, and severe cases and those with or without complication; etc.

Attention should be paid to the control group. The subjects with some disease except the target one confirmed by gold standard, but easily confused with it should be considered firstly so as to clarify the diagnosis value of the study methods. These control subjects may have the same or similar symptoms or signs as the cases studied. However, it's difficult to make correct clinical diagnosis and misdiagnosis might occur to them. The normal people without disease are usually exclusive from the control group.

The study methods may have representative and differential diagnostic value only if the involving subjects are qualified to the requirements.

3. To determine the diagnostic threshold (cut-off value)

A cut-off point is defined as the point at which a diagnostic test is positive or negative. Typically, individuals whose test values are greater (or less) than the diagnostic threshold are considered sick or abnormal.

4. To choose the index, determine the methods and make evaluation

The evaluation should be based on authenticity, reliability, and good performance. Validity refers to the degree of conformity between the measured and the actual value. It is the ability to distinguish patients from normal people correctly. Reliability refers to the degree of stability of the same results obtained through repeated tests under identical conditions. The predictive value (PV), or diagnostic value, is the value of the results. Refer to the second section for the specific evaluation indicators and methods.

14.2. Common evaluation indexes of diagnostic tests

Example 14.1 To investigate the effect of myocardial perfusion imaging (ECT) in the diagnosis of angina type CHD. ECT was performed on 134 positive patients with coronary angiography and 38 negative patients (gold standard). The results were shown in Table 14.2. Please choose the appropriate indexes to evaluate the diagnosis value of ECT.

14.2.1. *Index of validity evaluation*

The indexes for evaluating the validity of the test include sensitivity, specificity, false positive rate (FPR), false negative rate (FNR), Youden's index, and crude agreement rate.

Table 14.2 Results of ECT myocardial perfusion imaging and coronary angiography among 172 subjects

	Coronary angiography		
ECT	+ (Case group)	− (Control group)	Total
+	116 (A)	6 (B)	122 ($A+B$)
−	18 (C)	32 (D)	50 ($C+D$)
Total	134 ($A+C$)	38 ($B+D$)	172 (N)

1. Sensitivity (*Sen*): Sensitivity also called the true positive rate (*TPR*), is the proportion of samples that are genuinely positive that give a positive result using the test in question. For example, a test that correctly identifies all positive samples is very sensitive.

$$Sen = P(T_+|D_+) = \frac{A}{A+C} = TPR \tag{14-1}$$

According to the binomial distribution, the standard error is

$$SE_{sen} = \sqrt{\frac{Sen(1-Sen)}{(A+C)}} = \sqrt{\frac{A \times C}{(A+C)^3}}$$

In this case, $TPR = Sen = \frac{116}{134} = 0.8657$, namely the TPR was 86.57%, that is, 86.57% patients with CHD were diagnosed as positive by ECT myocardial perfusion imaging.

$$SE_{sen} = \sqrt{\frac{0.8657(1-0.8657)}{134}} = 0.0295 = 2.95\%$$

Sensitivity is associated only with the case group and reflects the ability of diagnostic tests to detect cases.

2. Specificity (*Spe*): Specificity called the true negative rate (*TNR*), is the proportion of samples that test negative using the test in question that are genuinely negative. For example, a test that identifies all healthy people as being negative for a particular illness is very specific.

$$Spe = P(T_-|D_-) = \frac{D}{B+D} \tag{14-2}$$

According to the binomial distribution, the standard error is

$$\mathrm{SE}_{spe} = \sqrt{\frac{Spe(1-Spe)}{B+D}} = \sqrt{\frac{B \times D}{(B+D)^3}}$$

In this case,

$$Spe = \frac{32}{38} = 0.8421,$$

$$\mathrm{SE}_{spe} = \sqrt{\frac{0.8421(1-0.8421)}{38}} = 0.0592 = 5.92\%$$

Specificity was associated only with the control group and reflected the ability of diagnostic tests to exclude non-cases.

3. *FPR*, also known as misdiagnosis rate, measures the probability of being wrongly diagnosed as positive in non-cases diagnosed by gold standard. Among the 14.1 cases, the misdiagnosis rate was determined through the following equation

$$\alpha = 1 - Spe = \frac{B}{B + D} = 1 - 0.8421 = 0.1579$$

4. *FNR*, also known as the rate of missed diagnosis, measures the proportion of negatives that are correctly identified as positive. Among the 14.1 cases, the missed diagnosis was determined through the following equation

$$\beta = 1 - Sen = \frac{C}{A + C} = 1 - 0.8657 = 0.1343$$

The relationship between sensitivity, specificity, missed diagnosis rate and misdiagnosis rate can be shown in Figure 14.1. In this figure, the intersection point between the vertical line and the horizontal axis is the cut-off point, which is the critical point defining the diagnosis as positive and negative.

The range of sensitivity and specificity value is between $(0, 1)$. The closer the value is to 1, the greater the diagnostic value will be. When comparing two diagnostic tests, it may appear that

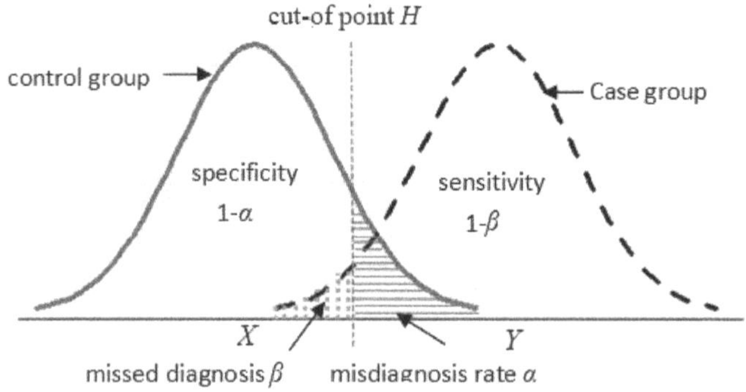

Figure 14.1 The diagram of sensitivity, specificity, missed diagnosis rate, and misdiagnosis rate

one diagnostic test has higher sensitivity and lower specificity, while the other diagnostic test has lower sensitivity and higher specificity. So it is impossible to judge which diagnostic test is better. Therefore, some people put forward diagnostic test evaluation indicators that combine sensitivity and specificity, such as Youden's index, positive likelihood ratio (PLR), and negative likelihood ratio (NLR).

5. Youden's index: It is the sum of sensitivity and specificity minus 1, that is, the difference between TPR and FPR.

$$YI = Sen + Spe - 1 = TPR - FPR \qquad (14\text{-}3)$$

$$SE_J = \sqrt{\frac{Sen(1 - Sen)}{A + C} + \frac{Spe(1 - Spe)}{B + D}}$$
$$= \sqrt{\frac{A \times C}{(A + C)^3} + \frac{B \times D}{(B + D)^3}}$$

In Case 14.1, $YI = 0.8657 + 0.8421 - 1 = 0.7078$, the Youden's index is 0.7078; Its standard error is:

$$SE_J = \sqrt{\frac{0.8657(1 - 0.8657)}{134} + \frac{0.8421(1 - 0.8421)}{38}} = 0.0661$$

The value range of Youden's index is between $(0, 1)$, and the closer the value is to 1, the better the diagnostic accuracy.

6. Crude agreement rate (CAR): also known as accuracy, is the percentage of the number of true positive and true negative cases detected in the test. In Case 14.1, the crude consistency rate was

$$CAR = \frac{A + D}{A + B + C + D} = \frac{116 + 32}{172} = 0.8605.$$

14.2.2. *Index of reliability evaluation*

The test reliability was evaluated by the following indicators: coefficient of variation, coincidence rate, Kappa value, etc.

1. Coefficient of variance is used as a reliability index for quantitative test.

2. Coincidence rate is used to evaluate the reliability of qualitative-measured test. It is the proportion of coincident numbers of the tests.
3. Kappa coefficient is used to assess the reliability agreement of two diagnostic or screening tests.

14.2.3. *Index of performance evaluation*

The performance of a test could be evaluated through predictive value (PV) and likelihood ratio (LR).

1. PV: it represents the probability that the test results are judged correctly and reflects the actual clinical significance of the test results. It also includes positive PV and negative PV.

① Positive PV: it measures the proportion of the number of people whose test results are predicted to be positive, denoted as PV_+. Please note the result $PV_+ = A/(A+B) = 116/122 = 0.9508$ is wrong (why is that? please think about) based on the data in Table 14.2. In order to use the Bayes formula to calculate PV_+ based on the similar design as Table 14.2, we need to know the prevalence in the population in advance.

$$PV_+ = P(D_+|T_+) = \frac{P(T_+|D_+)P(D_+)}{P(T_+|D_+)P(D_+) + P(T_+|D_-)P(D_-)}$$

plug the sensitivity and specificity into the above equation, we get

$$\begin{aligned} PV_+ &= \frac{P_0 \cdot Sen}{P_0 \cdot Sen + (1 - Spe)(1 - P_0)} \\ &= \left(1 + \frac{(1 - Spe)(1 - P_0)}{P_0 \cdot Sen}\right)^{-1} \end{aligned} \tag{14-4}$$

P_0 is the prevalence of a disease in the population.

When the sensitivity and specificity are constant, the positive prediction value is greater while the prevalence is larger.

In this case, $Sen = 0.8657$, $Spe = 0.8421$, If the prevalence of CHD in the total population is $P_0 = 0.0005$, according to the previous study, then the positive PV of this test is

$$PV_+ = \left(1 + \frac{(1-0.8421)(1-0.0005)}{0.8657 \times 0.0005}\right)^{-1} = \frac{1}{366} \approx 0.0027$$

In other words, when the ECT myocardial perfusion imaging method was used to diagnose the entire population, only one of the approximately 366 positive subjects was patient with CHD, which indicated the PV of this method.

If the prevalence expands to $P_0 = 0.2$, we get $PV_+ = 0.5782 = 57.82\%$.

② Negative PV: it measures the percentage of people whose test results were predicted to be negative, who were actually negative.

$$\begin{aligned} PV_- = P(D_-|T_-) &= \frac{P(T_-|D_-)P(D_-)}{P(T_-|D_-)P(D_-) + P(T_-|D_+)P(D_+)} \\ &= \frac{Spe(1-P_0)}{Spe(1-P_0) + (1-Sen)P_0} = \left(1 + \frac{(1-Sen)P_0}{Spe(1-P_0)}\right)^{-1} \end{aligned} \tag{14-5}$$

When the sensitivity and specificity are constant, the negative PV is smaller while the prevalence is larger.

Plug $Sen = 0.8657$ and $Spe = 0.8421$ into the above equation,

$$PV_- = \left(1 + \frac{(1-0.8657) \times 0.0005}{0.8421 \times (1-0.0005)}\right)^{-1} = \frac{9999}{10,000} = 0.9999$$

Of the approximately 10,000 tested negative, 9999 were not CHD and only one was CHD, indicating the PV of the method in the negative results.

If $P_0 = 0.2$, $PV_- = 0.9617 = 96.17\%$, the negative PV does not lower significantly.

Only when $P_1 = (A+C)/N$ in the sample is equal to $P_0 = P(D_+)$ in the population, Formulas (14-4) and (14-5) can be simplified to

$$PV_+ = \frac{A}{A+B} \quad PV_- = \frac{D}{C+D} \tag{14-6}$$

In this case, the PV is $PV_+ = \frac{116}{122} = 0.9508$ according to Equation (14-6).

This result is quite different from the calculation result of Equation (14-5). Because the prevalence that $P_1 = (A + C)/N = (116 + 18)/172 = 0.7791$ in this sample is not equal to the overall prevalence $P_0 = 0.0005$. So Formulas (14-4) and (14-5) should be used to calculate the PV instead of Formula (14-6).

In other words, if the case and control group are not sampled from two subgroups of confirmed patients and non-patients, but a random sample from the population and divided into case and control group according to their health conditions, the prevalence $P_1 = (A + C)/N$ in the sample can be used to replace population prevalence $P_0 = P(D_+)$. If and only if this is the case, Equation (14-6) can be established; otherwise, only Equations (14-4) and (14-5) could be used.

The values of PV+ and PV− are generally between $(0, 1)$. For the same population prevalence, the closer the values are to 1, the higher the diagnostic value of the test is.

2. Likelihood ratio (LR): it measures the ratio of the probability of the occurrence of a certain test result in patients to the probability of the occurrence of the test result in non-patients. It also includes positive PLR and NLR.

① PLR: it is the ratio of the TPR and the FPR of the test results, indicating the number of times of the positive rate of some test results in non-patients.

$$LR_+ = \frac{TPR}{FPR} = \frac{Sen}{1 - Sen} \qquad (14\text{-}7)$$

In this case $LR_+ = \frac{0.8659}{1-0.8421} = 5.48$

The value range of LR_+ is $(0, \infty)$, the larger the value is, the stronger the ability of detection method to prove the disease is. Since it involves logarithmic transformation, the standard error formula is too complicated to be written here.

② NLR: It is the ratio of FNR to TNR, indicating the times of the probability of negative test results in non-patients.

$$LR_{-} = \frac{1 - TPR}{1 - FPR} = \frac{1 - Sen}{Spe} \tag{14-8}$$

In this case $LR_{-} = \frac{1-0.8657}{0.8421} = 0.1593$

The value range of LR_{-} is $(0, \infty)$, the smaller the value is, the better the ability of the test to rule out disease is.

14.3. ROC analysis of diagnostic or screening tests

Although the Youden index, positive (or negative) LR, positive (or negative) PV and other indicators listed above make comprehensive use of the information of TPR and FPR, these indicators are all related to the selection of diagnostic threshold values. The normal threshold value has an immense impact on the diagnostic result. As shown in Figure 14.1, if H is the critical value, the red shade indicates the number of misdiagnoses, the green shade indicates the number of missed diagnoses; if the number of patients missed diagnosis is to be reduced, the number of misdiagnosis will increase if the X value is taken as the critical value. If the number of misdiagnoses is to be reduced and Y value is taken as the critical value, the number of missed diagnoses will increase greatly. Therefore, it is critical to maintain a suitable threshold according to the profession. For example, different diagnostic thresholds will result in different TPR and FPR for the same test method. In order to evaluate the diagnostic value of test methods more comprehensively, various possible diagnostic bounds must be considered.

The ROC curve, short for the Receiver Operating Characteristic receiver operating characteristic curve or relative operating characteristic curve, has been widely used to evaluate the performance of medical diagnostic tests, multiple pairs of TPR and FPR values were obtained by changing the diagnostic boundary. The ROC curve was drawn with FPR as the abscissa and TPR as the ordinate, and the area under the ROC curve was calculated to reflect the performance of the diagnostic or screening test.

The point nearest the top left corner is generally considered a good threshold, which is used to distinguish normal value from the abnormal. The sensitivity and specificity of the point were relatively high, and the sum of misdiagnosis and missed diagnosis cases is small.

The data for ROC curve can be roughly divided into two forms: continuous data and orderly categorized data. Continuous data are often used in some quantitative tests, while ordered data are more commonly used in medical imaging related diagnosis or psychological evaluation. Different from the routine evaluation index of diagnostic test, ROC allows transforming the continuous data into more than two categories. So it could be widely used in the performance evaluation.

ROC curve analysis includes two steps. First, ROC curve drawing. According to the professional knowledge, the results of the disease group and the control group were analyzed to determine the upper and lower limits of the determination values, the class interval, and the cut-off points. The cumulative frequency distribution table was listed according to the selected class interval. The sensitivity, specificity, and FPR (1-specificity) of all cut-off points were calculated, respectively. Taking the sensitivity as the ordinate to represent TPR and (1-specificity) as the abscissa to represent FPR, ROC curve was drawn. Second, ROC curve evaluation statistics calculation. Area under the curve (AUC) was between 0.5 and 1.0.The closer it is to 1, the better the diagnostic result is; there is a lower accuracy when AUC ranged from 0.5 to 0.7. There is median accuracy when AUC ranged from 0.7 to 0.9. When the value of AUC was above 0.9, the diagnosis result had higher accuracy. When AUC equal to 0.5, it is equivalent to "throwing coins," and there is no diagnostic value. When AUC less than 0.5, it does not match the real situation and it rarely occurs in practice.

Table 14.3 Test results of 100 breast cancer patients and 200 normal people

BMI cutoff value (kg/m^2)	Breast cancer patients ($n = 100$)		Normal people ($n = 200$)				
	True positive	False negative	False positive	True negative	Sensitivity	Specificity	False positive rate
18	100	0	200	0	1.00	0.000	1.000
20	100	0	198	2	1.00	0.010	0.990
22	99	1	177	23	0.99	0.115	0.885
24	95	5	117	83	0.95	0.415	0.585
26	85	15	80	120	0.85	0.600	0.400
28	66	34	53	147	0.66	0.735	0.265
30	47	53	27	173	0.47	0.865	0.135
32	34	66	17	183	0.34	0.915	0.085
34	21	79	14	186	0.21	0.930	0.070
36	17	83	6	194	0.17	0.970	0.030
38	7	93	4	196	0.07	0.980	0.020
40	1	99	1	199	0.01	0.995	0.005

14.3.1. *ROC analysis of continuous data*

Example 14.2 To verify the role of body mass index (BMI) in screening for breast cancer, 100 cases of breast cancer patients and 200 normal people were selected for comparison. These people aged between 30 and 80 years old were diagnosed with the gold standard of pathology. The data obtained were shown in Table 14.3.

Within the range of the measured BMI of the subjects, a cut-off point was taken for every $2\,kg/m^2$, the cumulative number of cases of breast cancer patients and normal people was counted, and the corresponding sensitivity and specificity were calculated, as shown in Table 14.3. With sensitivity as the ordinate and (1-specificity) as the abscissa, the ROC curve of BMI screening for breast cancer was plotted by connecting the points of each stage and (0,0) and (1,1) points, as shown in Figure 14.2.

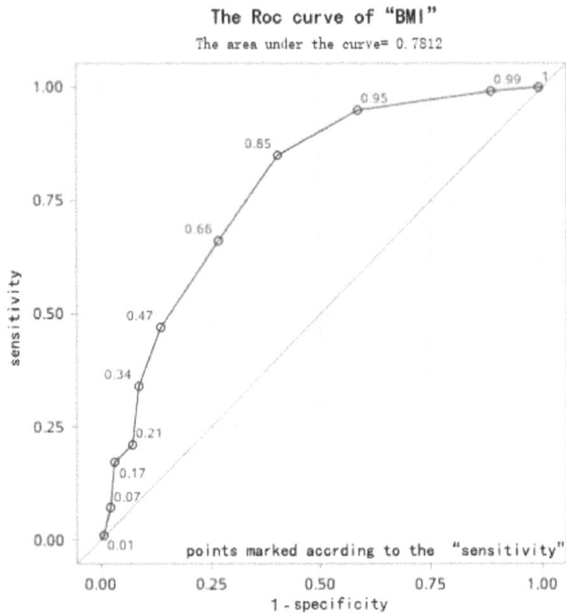

Figure 14.2 ROC curve of BMI screening for breast cancer

14.3.2. *ROC analysis of classified data*

Example 14.3 In one study, the researchers analyzed 97 consecutive patients using parathyroid CT as a diagnostic test. According to the results of CT, the researchers divided the patients into five grades of 1–5 according to the patients' parathyroid gland lesions. Grade 1 is the complete absence of parathyroid lesions, grade 2 is the probable absence of parathyroid lesions, grade 3 is the probable presence of parathyroid lesions, grade 4 is suspected parathyroid lesions, and grade 5 is the confirmed parathyroid lesions. The correlation between CT diagnosis and actual parathyroid lesions of these 97 patients was shown in Table 14.4.

For the five-level classification data, it is arranged from the largest to the smallest in terms of level. The previous four classifications were respectively chosen as the diagnostic boundary value, and those with a value greater than or equal to the diagnostic boundary value were positive, while those with a value less than the diagnostic

Table 14.4 Correlation between CT diagnosis and actual parathyroid lesions among 97 patients

	CT diagnosis					
Surgical results	1	2	3	4	5	Total
Sick	18	1	2	9	40	70
Non-sick	23	1	2	0	1	27

boundary value were negative. So four cross-tables can be listed as the following table.

	CT diagnosis	
Surgical results	Case group	Control group
+	40	30
−	1	26

	CT diagnosis	
Surgical results	Case group	Control group
+	49	21
−	1	26

	CT diagnosis	
Surgical results	Case group	Control group
+	51	19
−	3	24

	CT diagnosis	
Surgical results	Case group	Control group
+	52	18
−	4	23

The operating point of ROC curve corresponding to each four-grid table was shown in Table 14.5, and the corresponding ROC curve was shown in Figure 14.3.

14.3.3. *Calculation of area under ROC curve*

The area under the ROC curve (A_Z) is the probability that the anomaly group observation value is larger than the normal group observation value, and its value ranges from 0.5 to 1.0. The AUC

Table 14.5 FPR and TPR values of different diagnostic thresholds

	CT diagnosis			
Surgical results	5	4	3	2
FPR	0.0370	0.0370	0.1111	0.1481
TPR	0.5714	0.7000	0.7286	0.7429

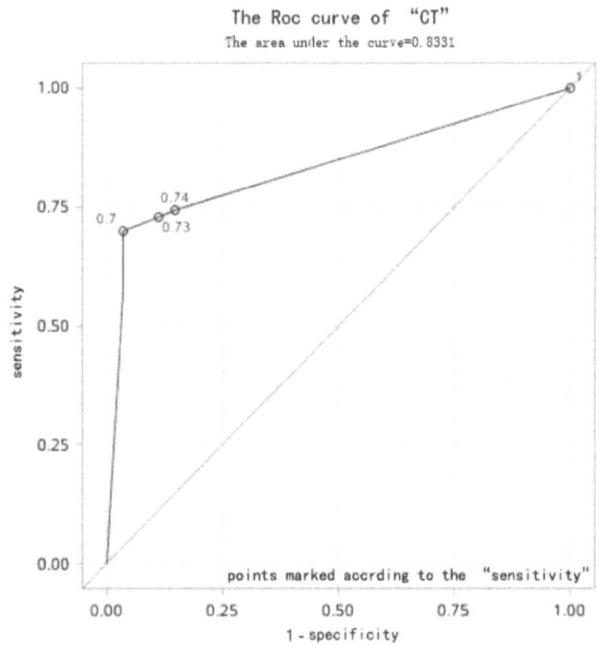

Figure 14.3 ROC curve of CT diagnosis

was 1, which is an ideal diagnosis, that is, the indicator can completely correctly distinguish the "sick" and "non-sick" population, and the sensitivity and specificity are both up to 100%. At this time, the ROC curve is composed of the left vertical coordinate and the top of the graph. The ROC curve of a test indicator with no judgment ability is the diagonal line between the coordinate points of the lower left corner (0,0) and the coordinate points of the upper right corner (1,1). At this time, the AUC is 0.5, which has no diagnostic value and is equivalent to the diagnosis by coin toss.

The method to estimate the area under the ROC curve is the trapezoidal principle calculation method, which is connecting two adjacent truncation points on the ROC curve and drawing the vertical line of the abscissa based on the two points. The sum of the trapezoid areas between all adjacent truncation points can be used as an approximate estimate of the area under the ROC curve. When there are more cut-off points, the curve becomes smoother, and the estimated area is to closer the real value. With fewer cutoff points, the estimated area is lower than the real value.

At present, the most commonly used methods for calculating AUC and standard error include binormal model parameter method, Hanley and McNeil non-parametric method, Delong, Delong, and Clarke–Pearson non-parametric method, etc. In which, Hanley and McNeil non-parametric method (Hanley and McNeil, 1983) is simple and easy to understand. But In practice, we can use statistical software to calculate the area under the ROC curve and conduct statistical test.

14.4. Report writing

The following results of diagnostic tests should be reported:

(1) Reliable evaluation indicators, such as sensitivity, specificity, Youden's index, etc.
(2) Beneficial evaluation indicators, such as positive PV and negative PV, etc.
(3) ROC analysis of diagnostic or screening tests.

Example 14.1 is reported as follows:

To investigate the effect of ECT myocardial perfusion imaging in the diagnostic of CHD with angina pectoris. ECT examination was performed on 134 patients and 38 negative patients confirmed by coronary angiography (gold standard). The sensitivity and specificity of ECT were 86.57% and 84.21%, respectively, with Youden's index 0.7078. The positive and negative PVs were 0.0027 and 0.9999, respectively. ECT could provide good sensitivity and specificity for the diagnosis of CHD with angina pectoris.

Regarding ROC analysis results, taking Example 14.2 as an example, the report is as follows:

To verify the efficiency of BMI in screening breast cancer, 100 breast cancer patients and 200 normal people diagnosed with pathology (gold standard) were recruited with age of 30–80 years old. According to the measurement of BMI, cut-off points were taken every $2\,\mathrm{kg/m^2}$, and the corresponding sensitivity and specificity were calculated. ROC curve was made as shown in Figure 14.2. The AUC is 0.7812, which is greater than 0.5, indicating that BMI has some value in screening breast cancer.

14.5. Case discrimination

Example 14.1. To evaluate the screening value of peripheral blood glucose for gestational diabetes. In 220 cases of late pregnancy women without serious medical complications during prenatal examination, venous blood glucose >7.8 mmol/L was taken as the positive group by traditional diagnostic test method. The critical value of peripheral blood glucose screening was determined by ROC curve method to be 9.1 mmol/L. Results show that among the 43 patients with positive venous blood glucose, 36 patients with positive peripheral blood glucose screening had a sensitivity of 84%(36/43). And then among 177 patients with negative venous blood glucose, 165 patients had negative peripheral blood glucose, with a specificity of 94%(165/177). Please consider: is it reasonable to use the authenticity evaluation index in this study? Are sensitivity and specificity calculated correctly?

14.6. Computer experiments (See electronic resources exp14-1 to exp14-4)

Experiment 14.1: SPSS20.0 was used to analyze the data of Example 1.1

Master the basic principles of diagnostic test and learn to use SPSS to calculate Kappa consistency coefficient.

Experiment 14.2: SPSS20.0 was used to analyze the data of Example 14.2

Learn to draw ROC curve with SPSS and calculate the AUC.

Experiment 14.3: SPSS20.0 was used to analyze the data of Example 14.3

Based on Example 14.3, know well the method of drawing ROC curve by SPSS.

Experiment 14.4: SPSS20.0 was used to analyze the data of example 14.1.

To further master the method of calculating Kappa value with SPSS, and to know well the meaning of Kappa consistency coefficient.

14.7. Frequently asked questions and summary

14.7.1. *Frequently asked questions*

1. Should the diagnostic test follow the randomization principle? How should the comparison be chosen?

Answer: Diagnostic test is a clinical test to evaluate diagnostic methods, so it should follow the three principles of control, repetition, and randomization.

In diagnostic tests, control can be divided into "standard" control and non-standard control. The former refers to the most accurate and authoritative method currently used in clinical practice or the standards formulated by the industry. The latter means that the control method is not enough to become the "gold standard." The evaluation methods of the two control designs are quite different. This chapter mainly describes the comparison of gold standards.

2. When the diagnosis result is a continuous variable, how to deal with it?

Answer: Diagnostic results generally adopt the dichotomous form. If it is a continuous variable, grade variable, or multi-classification variable, the conversion of dichotomous variable is required firstly. Although this can lose some information, there is no better method or no operable method at present. If the diagnosis results need subjective evaluation by doctors, such as image quality, blind evaluation design is very important.

14.7.2. *Summary*

1. The design of diagnostic tests usually requires the following steps: (1) determining the gold standard; (2) selecting research objects; (3) determining the diagnostic critical value (truncation value); (4) determining evaluation index, evaluation method and conducting the evaluation.
2. To evaluate a diagnostic test, we usually use the evaluation index of validity, reliability and performance. indexes of validity include sensitivity, specificity, FPR, FNR, Youden's index, crude coincidence rate, etc. Index of reliability include coefficient of variation, coincidence rate, Kappa coefficient, etc. Index of performance include positive PV, negative PV, PLR, NLR, etc.
3. The main application of ROC curve is as following (1) to easily find out the disease screening ability of any cut-off point, (2) to select the best diagnostic cut-off value, (3) to compare the disease screening ability of two or more different diagnostic tests. When comparing the performance of two or more diagnostic tests for the same disease, the ROC curve of two tests can be drawn into the same coordinate system to visually identify the advantages and disadvantages. The diagnostic test performs better when the curve is closer to the left top. The area under the ROC curve (AUC) of each test can also be calculated separately for comparison. The test with the largest AUC has the best diagnostic value.

Think and Practice

I. Best Choice

1. The purpose of the screening test is ( ).
   A. to diagnose suspected patients B. to evaluate the specificity of the screening tests C. to evaluate the sensitivity of the screening tests D. to prevent missed diagnosis in screening

population E. to screen suspected patients or high-risk groups of a certain disease from apparently healthy people

2. Authenticity indicators used for the diagnostic tests are ( ).
   A. sensitivity, specificity, reliability B. specificity, positive predictive value, repeatability C. sensitivity, specificity, Jordan index D. false positive rate, sensitivity, variation E. false positive rate, Youden index, consistency
3. Which statement about the evaluation index of diagnostic is correct? ( )
   A. The higher the sensitivity, the lower the missed diagnosis rate B. The higher the sensitivity, the lower the misdiagnosis rate C. The higher the specificity, the lower the missed diagnosis rate D. The higher the sensitivity, the higher prediction value E. The higher the specificity, the higher the misdiagnosis rate
4. The missed diagnosis means ( ).
   A. Diagnosis test is positive when the subject has the target disease B. Diagnosis test is negative when the subject has the target disease C. Diagnosis test is negative when the subject has not the target disease D. Diagnosis test is positive when the subject has not the target disease E. The subject does have the target disease when diagnosis test is positive
5. The following indicators that directly affect the diagnostic test positive predictive value index is ( ).
   A. Prevalence rate B. Case fatality rate C. Incidence rate D. Mortality rate E. Attack rate
6. Which statement about likelihood ratio is incorrect? ( )
   A. Likelihood ratio is divided into positive likelihood ratio and negative likelihood ratio. B. The greater the positive likelihood ratio, the higher the diagnostic value. C. Both positive and negative likelihood ratios are used to illustrate the reliability of test results. D. The greater the negative likelihood ratio, the higher the diagnostic value. E. None of the above statements is correct.
7. Which one is not an indicator of evaluating diagnostic test? ( )
   A. Coincidence rate B. Relative risk C. Predicted value D. Likelihood ratio E. Kappa value

8. What factors are those that affect the reliability of diagnostic test? ( )
   A. Subjects' individual variation, observer variation, and hospital environment variation. B. Subjects' individual variation, living environment variation and test method variation. C. Subjects' individual variation, observer variation and test method variation. D. Hospital environment variation, observer variation and test method variation. E. Hospital environment variation, living environment variation, and test method variation.
9. In the blood sugar screening work, if the abnormal standard of a blood sugar test method is set to over 130 mg/100 mL and over 160 mg/100 mL, respectively, this means ( ).
   A. The false negative rate of the test is higher when the former standard is adopted B. The sensitivity of the test is higher when the former standard is adopted C. The specificity of the test is higher when the former standard is adopted D. The Youden index of the test is higher when the former standard is adopted E. The accuracy of test diagnosis of diabetes is higher when the former standard is adopted
10. Which statement is correct? ( )
    A. Sensitivity is also called as true positive rate. B. Sensitivity is also called as true negative rate. C. Sensitivity is also called as false positive rate. D. Sensitivity is also called as false negative rate. E. Sensitivity is also called as coincidence rate.
11. Which of the following statements about ROC curve is correct? ( )
    A. The larger the area under the curve, the smaller the specificity and sensitivity to disease diagnosis. B. The smaller the area under the curve, the smaller the specificity and sensitivity to disease diagnosis. C. The larger the area under the curve, the greater the specificity but the smaller the sensitivity to disease diagnosis. D. The larger the area under the curve, the smaller the specificity but the larger the sensitivity to disease diagnosis. E. The largest the area under the curve, the best combination of specificity and sensitivity to disease diagnosis.

12. The abscissa and ordinate of ROC curve represent respectively ( ).
    A. TNR, TPR B. FNR, FPR C. FPR, TPR D. FPR, FNR
    E. FNR, TNR

II. Short-answer questions

1. What conditions do the research subjects need to meet when evaluating the value of a diagnostic test?
2. Prostate specific antigen (PSA) was measured in 1000 men over 60 years old. Among all of the population, 70 prostate cancer patients had abnormal PSA, and 90 non-patients had abnormal PSA. Can you use the data to calculate the positive PV of PSA test for prostate cancer screening for the population?

III. Question on Calculation

1. A cervical cancer screening test was applied to 800 women, among whom 400 people had been confirmed as cervical cancer cases diagnosed through biopsy and 400 people controls without disease. The test results showed 100 of cases and 50 of controls were positive. According to the data, please calculate the sensitivity, specificity, positive PV, negative PV, positive likelihood ratio, negative likelihood ratio, and Youden's index of this screening test.

Suzhen Wang, Fuyan Shi

CHAPTER 15

SAMPLE SIZE ESTIMATION

There is an unavoidable part of study design for both survey and experiment, which is to determine the number of subjects, commonly referred as sample size estimation. This chapter introduces the basic concepts of sample size estimation, common conditions for which sample size estimation is applicable, preconditions, and application examples of sample size estimation.

15.1. Basic concepts

15.1.1. *Two implications of sample size*

Sample size usually includes two implications: firstly, the number of observation units or subjects involved in the entire research project, it can be expressed by N; secondly, the entire research project needs to be divided into several research groups, the number of observation units or subjects in each group, it can be expressed by n (assuming equal sample size of each group). Normally, we should not only pay attention to the size of N, but also to the size of n. Please point out what N and n are respectively in the following examples.

In order to observe the histopathological changes of the normal parotid gland after the injection of methyl violet into a miniature pig, a researcher selected 15 Chinese miniature pigs at 6-month old with a weight of 20–25 kg, 9 males and 6 females. In each animal, one side of parotid gland was chosen as the experimental side, and the other side as the normal control, to eliminate the influence of individual differences and aging on the experimental results. 15 animals were randomly divided into 5 groups according to 1 week, 2 weeks, 1 month, 3 months, and 6 months after injection of methyl violet. Each group had 3 animals (they were randomly injected with 1% methyl violet solution 0.6, 1.0, and 4.0 mL, respectively). Then the histopathological changes were observed.

In this study, 15 miniature pigs were used, that is $N = 15$. At first glance, the number of "15" is not too small. But it is not difficult to find that there are two experimental factors involved in this project. The first factor is the action time of methyl violet, which has "1 week, 2 weeks, 1 month, 3 months, and 6 months" 5 levels; the second factor is the dose of methyl violet, which has "0.6, 1.0, and 4.0 mL" 3 levels. The total combination of these two factors at each level has a total of 15 cases, each of which constituted a special experimental condition with only one animal in each condition, that is, the sample size of each group $n = 1$, violates the "repetition principle" in the experimental design. Because the phenomena of biomedical research often have variability, the change rule of random phenomena can be revealed correctly only when multiple repeated experiments are carried out independently under the same experimental conditions. Obviously, the conclusion of this study is not convincing.

So how many animals should each group use? Strictly speaking, it is necessary to calculate the sample size with corresponding formula, according to the information provided by the pre-experiment or literature, combined with the accuracy of the experiment required by the researchers, and based on the type of experimental design to be adopted. Generally, when it is not convenient to use the formula to calculate, if for small animal experiment (convenient source, not too expensive), the appropriate quantity of animals in each group should be no less than 10; if for larger animal experiment, the appropriate quantity of animals in each group should be no less than 5. The term "each group" here refers to each individual group determined by the independent experimental conditions in the experiment. For example, In such case, it refers to the experimental group formed by a specific action time and a specific dose of methyl violet, with a total of 15 groups.

15.1.2. *Significance of determining sample size*

Correctly determining sample size is an important part of experimental design. When estimating sample size, two tendencies should be paid attention to avoid. One is unilateral pursuit of increasing sample size, believing that the more sample size the better and even putting forward that "mass observation" is an important principle for determining sample size. As a result, it not only waste manpower, material resources, and time, but may also introduce more confounding factors, and have adverse impact on the results of the study. The other is to ignore the importance of ensuring adequate sample size, which makes the sample size too small and the power $(1 - \beta)$ too low, resulting in the failure to detect the original differences in the overall population and the emergence of false negative results, which is a particularly noteworthy problem in current medical research.

In medical research design, the sample size should be estimated according to the design type, the nature of the outcome variables and the research purpose with the aid of appropriate formulas. Different design types require different sample sizes. This chapter only introduces several commonly used sample size estimation methods and application examples, and how to estimate sample size in more cases, please refer to the relevant literature.

15.1.3. *Conditions to determine sample size*

One question that statisticians are often asked is "I want to show that a new treatment is better than the old one. How many patients should I choose?" This question often makes statisticians unable to answer, because it is necessary to have some basic information in order to make a reasonable estimate of the required sample size. For example, in experimental design, if the observed results are quantitative data and mean values are to be tested by hypothesis, the following information is needed:

1. Significance level

The probability α of type I (false positive) errors allowed in this experiment is stipulated beforehand, and it is usually stipulated

$\alpha = 0.05$. At the same time, the unilateral test or bilateral test should be clearly specified. The smaller setting of α, the larger sample size required; the sample size of bilateral test is larger than that of unilateral test.

2. Power

Prescribe the power $(1-\beta)$ required for this experiment, or the probability β of allowing type II (false negative) errors. The greater the power required, the larger the sample size required. During scientific research design, the power should be no less than 0.75; otherwise the test results may not reflect the real difference between the overall parameters.

3. Information about population

When comparing the differences between the two population means or probabilities, it should be known how large the difference δ between the population parameters and the population standard deviation σ may be. Usually, people obtain such information by consulting materials, learning from experience of predecessors or conducting preliminary experiments.

Sometimes it is difficult for researchers to obtain the information of the total parameters, which can be replaced by the difference value that is considered meaningful in professionally (clinically), such as the difference value of the average diastolic blood pressure $\geq$0.69 kPa (5 mmHg), the average difference value of white blood cells 0.5×10^9/L (500/mm^3), etc. Others also advocate estimating the difference value between the population means with a standard deviation of 0.25 or 0.50 times. Of course, it can also be artificially stipulated according to the experimental purposes, such as stipulating that the effective probability of the new drug in the experiment must exceed 30% of the effective probability of the standard drug before it can be popularized.

15.1.4. *Estimation of power*

As mentioned before, power is determined by the probability β of type II error, that is, efficacy $= 1 - \beta$. When the "negative" result of hypothesis test appears ($P > 0.05$), it is necessary to input current sample size value into the calculation formula, calculate whether the power is low, so as to analyze the correctness of hypothesis test "negative" conclusion. When the conclusion of hypothesis test is "negative" ($P > 0.05$), the standard normal deviation Z_β corresponding to the probability β of type II error can be calculated by using the formula under certain hypothesis conditions. Then the area under the standard normal distribution curve can be checked to determine the value of power $(1 - \beta)$.

$$\text{Power} = 1 - \beta = \Phi(Z_\beta)$$

In which, $\Phi(Z_\beta)$ is the area under the left curve of Z_β value.

If the power is low, it represents that the sample size of the experiment is insufficient; it should further increase the sample size and continue the experiment.

15.2. Sample size estimation when comparing the mean values of quantitative data

15.2.1. *Single group and paired design t-test*

1. Information needed to be provided

In such case, the information required includes the mean difference value δ, sample standard deviation S(or S_d), the probability α of allowing type I error, and the probability β of allowing type II error.

2. Calculation formula

If a unilateral t-test is made, then

$$n = \left[\frac{(t_\alpha + t_\beta)S}{\delta}\right]^2 \tag{15-1}$$

If a bilateral t-test is performed, then

$$n = \left[\frac{(t_{\alpha/2} + t_\beta)S}{\delta}\right]^2 \tag{15-2}$$

The above formulas are used to t-test of single group data. If paired design or crossover design, S in the formula is replaced by the standard deviation S_d of the difference of each pair observed objects, and n is the number of observed pairs.

$t_{\alpha/2}$ and t_β in the above formulas are related to sample size, so iteration is needed in calculation (see the Example).

3. Example

Example 15.1. In silicosis patients treated with a certain drug, the average amount of silica excretion increased by about 15 mg/L, and the standard deviation was about 25 mg/L. If $\alpha = 0.05$ (unilateral), $\beta = 0.10$, how many patients should be observed to draw a conclusion that there is a statistically significant difference in the amount of silica excretion before and after medication?

Answer: This case is paired design. Because the amount of silicon excretion in urine will not decrease after treatment, unilateral test can be performed.

Let $S = S_d$,

Input $\delta = 15$, $S_d = 25$, $t_{\alpha(\infty)} = t_{0.05(\infty)} = 1.645$, $t_{\beta(\infty)} = t_{0.10(\infty)} = 1.282$ into Example 15.1 formula, and get

$$n_1 = \left[\frac{(t_\alpha + t_\beta)S}{\delta}\right]^2 = \left[\frac{(1.645 + 1.282) \times 25}{15}\right]^2 = 23.798 \approx 24$$

Input $\delta = 15$, $S_d = 25$, $t_{\alpha(23)} = t_{0.05(23)} = 1.714$, $t_{\beta(23)} = t_{0.10(23)} = 1.319$ into Example 15.1 formula, and get

$$n_2 = \left[\frac{(t_\alpha + t_\beta)S}{\delta}\right]^2 = \left[\frac{(1.714 + 1.319) \times 25}{15}\right]^2 = 25.553 \approx 26$$

Input $\delta = 15$, $S_d = 25$, $t_{\alpha(25)} = t_{0.05(25)} = 1.708$, $t_{\beta(25)} = t_{0.10(25)} = 1.316$ into Example 15.1 formula, and get

$$n_3 = \left[\frac{(t_\alpha + t_\beta)S}{\delta}\right]^2 = \left[\frac{(1.708 + 1.316) \times 25}{15}\right]^2 = 25.402 \approx 26$$

Therefore, taking $n = 26$, that is, 26 pairs of patients need to be observed before the conclusion that the urinary silicon excretion before and after taking medicine is statistically significant.

The required sample size can also be obtained by looking up table.

Since $\alpha = 0.05$ (unilateral), $\beta = 0.10$, $\delta = 15$, $S_d = 25$, $\frac{\delta}{\sigma} \approx \frac{\delta}{S_d} = 0.60$ and the sample size obtained by looking up table (attached Table C14) is $n = 26$, it is very consistent with the calculated results.

15.2.2. *Group design t-test*

1. Information needed to be provided

In such case, it needs to provide the difference δ between the two population means, the standard deviation S of merging two samples, the distribution ratio q_1 and q_2 of sample size in the two groups, $q_1 + q_2 = 1$, and the probability α of allowing type I error and β of allowing type II error.

2. Calculation formula

If a unilateral t-test is made, then

$$N = \frac{(q_1^{-1} + q_2^{-1})(t_\alpha + t_\beta)^2 S^2}{\delta^2} \tag{15-3}$$

If a bilateral t-test is performed, then

$$N = \frac{(q_1^{-1} + q_2^{-1})(t_{\alpha/2} + t_\beta)^2 S^2}{\delta^2} \tag{15-4}$$

When the two groups have the same sample size, $q_1 = q_2 = 0.5$, $(0.5)^{-1} + (0.5)^{-1} = 4$, Equations (15-3) and (15-4) are simplified to:

If a unilateral t-test is made, then

$$N = \frac{4(t_\alpha + t_\beta)^2 S^2}{\delta^2} \tag{15-5}$$

If a bilateral t-test is performed, then

$$N = \frac{4(t_{\alpha/2} + t_\beta)^2 S^2}{\delta^2} \tag{15-6}$$

Note: N in Equations (15-3)∼(15-6) is the total content of samples in both groups. Generally, the number of cases in two groups is expected to be equal. Because when n is determined and the number of cases in the two groups is equal, the power is great and the calculation is simple. However, two conditions should be met for such design: First, each additional object added will cost the same amount for both groups; second, it is not too difficult to find the same number of subjects. If either of these conditions is not met, the sample size of the two groups should or must be unequal. However, if sample size is not equal, in both groups, the smaller sample size must be slightly more than 1/4 of the total sample size N when the two samples are equal.

3. Example

Example 15.2. One researcher intends to analyze the difference in serum testosterone levels (ng%) between patients with hirsutism and normal people. From the previous research data, the difference $\delta = 10$ of the average serum testosterone content was estimated, the standard deviation was 13.33; take $\alpha = 0.05$, $\beta = 0.10$. If there are fewer patients with hirsutism, it is intended to investigate patients and healthy people in a ratio of 1:4. How many hirsutism patients and healthy people should be observed in the formal study?

Answer: Set hypertrichosis group as Group 1, normal people group as Group 2, perform bilateral t-test. Suppose $S_c = 13.33$, since it is intended to survey patients and healthy people on a ratio of 1:4. So $q_1 = \frac{1}{1+4} = \frac{1}{5}$, $q_2 = 1 - q_1 = \frac{4}{5}$, and $\delta = 10$, $\alpha = 0.05$, $\beta = 0.10$, then $t_{\alpha/2(\infty)} = t_{0.05/2(\infty)} = 1.960$, $t_{\beta(\infty)} = t_{0.10(\infty)} = 1.282$.

Input above data into Formula (15-4), and then get:

$$\begin{aligned} N^{(1)} &= \frac{(q_1^{-1} + q_2^{-1})(t_{\alpha/2} + t_\beta)^2 S^2}{\delta^2} \\ &= \frac{\left[\left(\frac{1}{5}\right)^{-1} + \left(\frac{4}{5}\right)^{-1}\right] \times (1.960 + 1.282)^2 \times (13.33)^2}{10^2} \\ &= 116.7 \approx 117 \end{aligned}$$

So, $n_1^{(1)} = q_1 N^{(1)} = \frac{1}{5} \times 117 = 23.4 \approx 24$, $n_2^{(1)} = 4n_1^{(1)} = 4 \times 24 = 96$

Then with free degree $df = n_1^{(1)} + n_2^{(1)} - 2 = 24 + 96 - 2 = 118$

Find t value from the boundary table $t_{0.05/2(118)} = 1.980$, $t_{0.10(118)} = 1.289$, Input into Formula (15-4), and get

$$N^{(2)} = \frac{(q_1^{-1} + q_2^{-1})(t_{\alpha/2} + t_\beta)^2 S^2}{\delta^2}$$
$$= \frac{\left[\left(\frac{1}{5}\right)^{-1} + \left(\frac{4}{5}\right)^{-1}\right] \times (1.980 + 1.289)^2 \times (13.33)^2}{10^2}$$
$$= 118.7 \approx 119$$

Then, $n_1^{(2)} = q_1 N^{(2)} = \frac{1}{5} \times 119 = 23.8 \approx 24 = n_1^{(1)}$, $n_2^{(2)} = 4n_1^{(2)} = 4 \times 24 = 96 = n_2^{(1)}$.

Therefore, take $n_1 = 24$, $n_2 = 96$, $N = 24 + 96 = 120$, that is, if the sample size is 1:4, 24 patients and 96 normal persons should be investigated.

Example 15.3. In an animal antitussive experiment, a comparison was made between Chinese herbal compound I and compound II that delayed the onset of cough in mice. In the preliminary experiment, the mean of compound I and compound II was 31.67s and 44.00s, respectively, and the standard deviation was about 25s. Therefore, suppose $\delta = 44.00 - 31.67 = 12.33$s and set the standard deviations of the two groups equal, into 25s. Let $\alpha = 0.05$ (bilateral), $\beta = 0.10$. How many mice do we need to use to draw a conclusion that the difference between the two groups is statistically significant?

Answer: Input $\delta = 12.33$, $S = 25$, $t_{\alpha/2(\infty)} = t_{0.05/2(\infty)} = 1.960$, $t_{\beta(\infty)} = t_{0.10(\infty)} = 1.282$ into Formula (15-6), get

$$N^{(1)} = \frac{4 \times (t_{\alpha/2} + t_\beta)^2 S^2}{\delta^2} = \frac{4 \times (1.960 + 1.282)^2 \times 25^2}{12.33^2}$$
$$= 172.8 \approx 173$$

Then with free degree $df = N^{(1)} - 2 = 173 - 2 = 171$, $\delta = 12.33$, $S = 25$, $t_{\alpha/2(\infty)} = t_{0.05/2(171)} = 1.960$, $t_{\beta(\infty)} = t_{0.10(171)} = 1.282$ input into Formula (15-6), get $N^{(2)} = N^{(1)} = 173$, so get $N = 173$, that is, total 173 mice are needed in the two groups, with 87 mice in each group.

Sample size can also be obtained by looking up the table. Since $\alpha = 0.05$(bilateral), $\beta = 0.10$, $\delta = 12.33$, $S = 25$, $\frac{\delta}{\sigma} \approx \frac{\sigma}{S} = \frac{12.33}{25} = 0.4932 \approx 0.50$, Check the attached Table C17 and get the sample size $n = 86$, this is close to the calculated result.

15.2.3. *Multi-group design F-test*

1. Information needed to be provided

In such case, the mean number of each group μ_i, standard deviation S, group numbers k, probability of type I error α and probability of type II error β should be provided.

2. Calculation formula

$$n = \frac{\lambda}{\Delta} \tag{15-7}$$

In which,

$$\Delta = \frac{1}{\sigma^2} \sum_{i=1}^{k} (\mu_i - \mu_0)^2 \tag{15-8}$$

Note: Bilateral test, and assume that the sample size of each group is equal, that is, n represents the required sample size of each group. μ_0 represents the average of each group's mean number μ_i

Check Table 15.1 and get λ value:

3. Example

Example 15.4. Four drugs were used to treat hypertension. The average number of systolic blood pressure lowered by four drugs was known to be $\mu_1 = 8.25$, $\mu_2 = 11.75$, $\mu_3 = 12$, $\mu_4 = 13$, respectively. The standard deviation of reducing systolic blood pressure for each drug was 3.5. Take $\alpha = 0.05$, $\beta = 0.10$, bilateral test, how many samples do we need to prepare?

Table 15.1 λ value table of multi-group mean design

$1-\beta$	$1-\beta=0.80$		$1-\beta=0.90$	
k	$\alpha=0.01$	$\alpha=0.05$	$\alpha=0.01$	$\alpha=0.05$
2	11.68	7.85	14.88	10.51
3	13.80	9.64	17.43	12.66
4	15.46	10.91	19.25	14.18
5	16.75	11.94	20.74	15.41
6	17.87	12.83	22.03	16.47
7	18.88	13.63	23.19	17.42
8	19.79	14.36	24.24	18.29
9	20.64	15.03	25.22	19.09
10	21.43	15.65	26.13	19.83
11	22.18	16.25	26.99	20.54
12	22.89	16.81	27.80	21.20
13	23.57	17.34	28.58	21.84
14	24.22	17.85	29.32	22.44
15	24.84	18.34	30.04	23.03
16	25.44	18.82	30.73	23.59
17	26.02	19.27	31.39	24.13
18	26.58	19.71	32.04	24.65
19	27.12	20.14	32.66	25.16
20	27.65	20.56	33.27	25.66

Answer: $\sigma = 3.5$, input average number of each group μ_i into Formula (15-7):

$$\mu_0 = \frac{\mu_1+\mu_2+\mu_3+\mu_4}{4} = \frac{8.25+11.75+12+13}{4} = 11.25$$

$$\begin{aligned}\Delta &= \frac{1}{\sigma^2}\sum_{i=1}^{k}(\mu_i-\mu_0)^2 \\ &= \frac{1}{3.5^2}\times[(8.25-11.25)^2+(11.75-11.25)^2 \\ &\qquad +(12-11.25)^2+(13-11.25)^2] \\ &= 1.0510\end{aligned}$$

$\alpha = 0.05$, $k = 4$, $\beta = 0.10$, check Table 15.1 get: $\lambda = 14.18$, input it into Formula (15-8)

$$n = \frac{\lambda}{\Delta} = \frac{14.18}{1.051} \approx 14$$

Therefore, at least 14 patients were required for each group.

15.3. Sample size estimation when comparing qualitative sample frequency

15.3.1. *Single group and paired design χ^2-test*

1. Information needed to be provided

In such case, it needs to provide 4 basic data in the four-grid table, probability α of type I errors and probability β of type II errors.

2. Calculation formula

Suppose the paired χ^2-test is applied to the following paired four-grid table data:

		Second check	
		+	−
First Check	+	a	b
	−	c	d

Let $\pi_{\pm} = \frac{b}{a+b}$, $\pi_{\mp} = \frac{c}{a+c}$, $\pi_c = \frac{\pi_{\pm}+\pi_{\mp}}{2}$,
Then the number of sample pairs required is:

$$n = \left[\frac{Z_{\alpha/2}\sqrt{2\pi_c} + Z_{\beta}\sqrt{\frac{2\pi_{\mp}\pi_{\pm}}{\pi_c}}}{\pi_{\mp} - \pi_{\pm}}\right]^2 \tag{15-9}$$

3. Example

Example 15.5. A certain strain was inoculated into two kinds of media, A and B. The results of the preliminary experiment are as follows: The probability of A-positive B-negative is approximate to

$\pi_{\pm} = 0.04$, and the probability of A-negative B-positive is approximate to $\pi_{\mp} = 0.24$. Suppose $\alpha = 0.05$ (bilateral), $\beta = 0.10$, how many pairs of samples should be used in the formal experiment?

Answer: Input $\pi_{\pm} = 0.04$, $\pi_{\mp} = 0.24$, $\pi_c = (0.04 + 0.24)/2 = 0.14$, $Z_{0.05/2} = 1.960$, $Z_{0.10} = 1.282$ into Formula (15-9), get

$$n = \left[\frac{1.960\sqrt{2 \times 0.14} + 1.282 \times \sqrt{\frac{2\times 0.24\times 0.04}{0.14}}}{0.24 - 0.04}\right]^2 = 57.146$$

Therefore, 58 pairs are required.

15.3.2. *Group design Z-test*

1. Information needed to be provided

In such case, it needs to provide the estimates of the two population probabilities p_1 and p_2, the ratio of two sample sizes c (assuming $c = n_2/n_1$), the probability of type I errors α and the probability of type II errors β.

2. Calculation formula

Since $c = n_2/n_1$, that is, $n_2 = cn_1$, then the calculation format of n_1 is as below:

Unilateral test:

$$n_1 = \frac{\left[Z_\alpha\sqrt{\frac{p(1-p)(1+c)}{c}} + Z_\beta\sqrt{p_1(1-p_1) + \frac{p_2(1-p_2)}{c}}\right]^2}{(p_1 - p_2)^2} \tag{15-10}$$

Bilateral Test:

$$n_1 = \frac{\left[Z_{\alpha/2}\sqrt{\frac{p(1-p)(1+c)}{c}} + Z_\beta\sqrt{p_1(1-p_1) + \frac{p_2(1-p_2)}{c}}\right]^2}{(p_1 - p_2)^2} \tag{15-11}$$

In which $p = \frac{p_1+cp_2}{c+1}$, n_2 can get by calculating cn_1.

3. Example

Example 15.6. To study the therapeutic effect of two kinds of antibiotics (one of which is the control drug) on an infectious disease. Preliminary experiments showed that the effective rate of the experimental drug was 80% and that of the control drug was 60%. A formal clinical trial will be conducted. How many patients should be observed in each group (assuming a bilateral test)?

Answer: In such case $p_1 = 0.8$, $p_2 = 0.6$, $p = \frac{0.8+0.6}{2} = 0.7$, suppose $\alpha = 0.05$, $\beta = 0.10$, $Z_{0.05/2} = 1.960$, $Z_{0.10} = 1.282$, taking $c = 1$, input into Formula (15-11), get:

$$n_1 = \frac{\left[1.960\sqrt{\frac{0.7\times(1-0.7)\times(1+1)}{1}} + 1.282\sqrt{0.8\times(1-0.8) + \frac{0.6\times(1-0.6)}{1}}\right]^2}{(0.8-0.6)^2}$$

$$= 108.27$$

$$\approx 109$$

$$n_2 = n_1 = 109$$

Therefore, 109 patients need to be observed in each group.

15.4. Sample size estimation in simple linear correlation analysis

1. Information needed to be provided

In such case, it is necessary to provide estimates of the population correlation coefficient ρ, probability α of type I errors and probability β of type II errors.

2. Calculation formula

$$\text{Unilateral test}: n = 4\left[\frac{Z_\alpha + Z_\beta}{\ln\left(\frac{1+\rho}{1-\rho}\right)}\right]^2 + 3 \qquad (15\text{-}12)$$

$$\text{Bilateral test}: n = 4\left[\frac{Z_{\alpha/2} + Z_\beta}{\ln\left(\frac{1+\rho}{1-\rho}\right)}\right]^2 + 3 \qquad (15\text{-}13)$$

3. Example

Example 15.7. It is estimated that the population correlation coefficient is about $\rho = 0.70$. Suppose $\alpha = 0.05$, $\beta = 0.10$, what is the sample size required testing the correlation coefficient in a formal study?

Answer: Since $\rho = 0.70 > 0$, unilateral test should be used. Input $\rho = 0.70$, $Z_{0.05} = 1.645$, $Z_{0.10} = 1.282$ into Formula (15-12), get

$$n = 4\left[\frac{1.645 + 1.282}{\ln\left(\frac{1+0.70}{1-0.70}\right)}\right]^2 + 3 = 14.390$$

Taking $n = 15$, that is to say it needs 15 cases.

15.5. Sample size estimation in multivariate analysis

In real applications, statistical analysis is not only an univariate analysis of quantitative or qualitative data comparisons between groups, but also a multivariable analysis of data. When the sample size is sufficient for univariate analysis, it does not mean that the sample size is sufficient for multivariate analysis. Therefore, in real practice, it is necessary to combine univariate and multivariate analysis to estimate the sample size needed in the study.

15.5.1. *Sample size estimation for multiple linear regression*

1. Information needed to be provided

In such case, it needs to provide the expected correlation coefficient ρ between the expected dependent variable Y and the variable X_1 to be tested, the determinant coefficient $\rho^2_{1|2,3,\ldots,p}$ of the multiple regression of to be tested variable X_1 with respect to the other $(p-1)$ independent variables $X_2, X_3, \ldots, X_p$, the probability α of allowing type I errors and the probability β of making type II errors.

2. Calculation formula

$$n_1 = 4\left[\frac{Z_{\alpha/2}+Z_\beta}{\ln\left(\frac{1+\rho}{1-\rho}\right)}\right]^2 + 3 \tag{15-14}$$

$$n_p = \frac{n_1}{1-\rho^2_{1|2,3,\ldots,p}} \tag{15-15}$$

In which, n_1 is the sample size required for simple linear regression of dependent variable X_1 and n_p is the sample size required for multiple linear regression of dependent variable p.

3. Example

Example 15.8. A cardiac surgeon wanted to study the relationship between serum homocysteine (HCY) and atherosclerosis. The platelet burden index (PBI), which represents the degree of atherosclerosis, is planned as a dependent variable. In addition to serum HCY, there are six control factors including age, sex, plasma folic acid level, and vitamin B6, vitamin B12 and serum cholesterol. According to the previous literature, the correlation coefficient between PBI and HCY is about 0.35; through the pre-survey of small samples, HCY makes multiple linear regressions for the other six control factors, and the determination coefficient is about 0.12. According to the above design, the multiple linear regression of PBI on HCY and other six control factors was carried out. The significance level was 0.05 on both sides, and the power was 90%. How many samples were needed at least?

Answer: Given $\alpha = 0.05$(bilateral), $\beta = 0.10$, $\rho = 0.35$, $Z_{0.05/2} = 1.96$, $Z_{0.10} = 1.28$, $\rho^2_{1|2,3,\ldots,7} = 0.12$ input into Formulas (15-14) and (15-15), get

$$\ln\left(\frac{1+\rho}{1-\rho}\right) = \ln\left(\frac{1+0.35}{1-0.35}\right) = 0.7309$$

$$n_1 = 4\times\left(\frac{1.96+1.28}{0.7309}\right)^2 + 3 \approx 81$$

$$n_p = \frac{81}{1-0.12^2} \approx 92$$

It can be seen from above that at least 92 cases of the above multiple linear regression are required.

15.5.2. *Logistic regression sample size estimation*

1. Sample size estimation for an independent variable X

(1) Information needed to be provided

In such case, it is necessary to provide the probability P of the occurrence of the event under the condition of taking the mean of X, the expected detected effect size $\ln(OR)$, the probability α of allowable type I errors and the probability β of type II errors.

(2) Calculation formula

If the independent variable X is a continuous variable obeying normal distribution, then the sample size is:

$$n = \frac{(Z_{(\alpha/2)} + Z_{\beta})^2}{P(1-P)\ln(OR)^2} \tag{15-16}$$

If the independent variable X is a binary variable ($X = 0$ or $X = 1$), the sample size is:

$$n = \frac{\left[Z_{(\alpha/2)}\sqrt{\frac{P_{总}(1-P_{总})}{B}} + Z_{\beta}\sqrt{P_1(1-P_1) + \frac{P_2(1-P_2)(1-B)}{B}}\right]^2}{(P_1-P_2)^2(1-B)} \tag{15-17}$$

where, B is the proportion of the number of individuals corresponding to $X = 1$ in the total number of individuals; P_1 is the occurrence frequency of events corresponding to $X = 0$, P_2 is the occurrence frequency of events corresponding to samples corresponding to $X = 1$, and $P_{总}$ is the total occurrence rate $P_{总} = (1-B)P_1 + BP_2$.

2. Sample size estimation for multiple independent variables $X_1, X_2, \ldots, X_p$

Firstly, an independent variable of main interest (assuming X_1 is selected) is determined from $X_1, X_2, \ldots, X_p$, and the sample size n is estimated when an independent variable X_1 is selected. Then, according to the determination coefficient $\rho^2_{1|2,3,\ldots,p}$ obtained by multiple regression of variable X_1 for other $(p-1)$ independent variables, the probability α of allowable type I error and the probability β of type II error, the sample size N required for p independent variables is calculated according to Formula (15-18).

$$N = \frac{n}{1-\rho^2_{1|2,3,\ldots,p}} \tag{15-18}$$

3. Example

Example 15.9. Clinicopathological factors may influence the prognosis of patients with colorectal cancer. A researcher collected data of 158 patients with colorectal cancer who underwent surgical treatment, including sex (X_1), age (X_2), histological classification (X_3), tumor size (X_4), Dure's stage (X_5), lymphatic infiltration (X_6), vascular infiltration (X_7), and 5-year survival status (Y). In such case, vascular infiltration (X_7) was determined as the main independent variable of interest. Please estimate the sample size. The data are summarized in Table 15.2.

Calculate sample Size n based on Formula (15-17)

Suppose $\alpha = 0.05$ (Bilateral), $\beta = 0.20$ (Unilateral), calculate:

$$B = \frac{31+3}{158} = 0.2152 \quad P_1 = \frac{54}{70+54} = 0.4355$$

$$P_2 = \frac{3}{31+3} = 0.0882$$

$$P_{总} = (1-0.2152) \times 0.4355 + 0.2152 \times 0.0882 = 0.3608$$

Table 15.2 Five-year survival of patients with or without vascular infiltration of colorectal cancer

Vascular invasion (X_7)	Sample size	Death ($Y=1$)	Survival ($Y=0$)
Without ($X_7=0$)	124	70	54
With ($X_7=1$)	34	31	3
Total	158	101	57

When $\alpha = 0.05$, $Z_{\alpha/2} = 1.96$; $\beta = 0.20$, $Z_\beta = 0.8416$, input B, P_1, P_2, $P_{总}$, $Z_{\alpha/2}$, Z_β into Formula (15-17), obtain estimated sample size $n \approx 74$.

After calculation, $\rho^2_{7|2,3,\ldots,6} = 0.0732$. Sample size required for calculating 7 independent variables based on Formula (15-18) is:

$$N = \frac{74}{1 - 0.0732} \approx 80$$

15.5.3. *Sample size estimation for Cox regression analysis*

1. Information needed to be provided

It is necessary to provide the incidence of end-point events P at the end of the study, the determination coefficient R^2 when the main effect variable X_1 is used for regression analysis of other co-variables, the variance σ^2 of X_1, the logarithmic risk ratio $\ln HR$ of X_1, the allowable probability α of type I error and the probability β of type II error.

2. Calculation formula

$$n = \frac{(Z_{\alpha/2} + Z_\beta)^2}{P(1 - R^2)\sigma^2(\ln HR)^2} \tag{15-19a}$$

Or the number of deaths reached

$$nP = \frac{(Z_{\alpha/2} + Z_\beta)^2}{(1 - R^2)\sigma^2(\ln HR)^2} \tag{15-19b}$$

(Source: Hsieh and Lavori, 2000)

3. Example

Example 15.10. A clinical trial is planned to compare the efficacy of a new drug with that of a standard drug in the treatment of lung cancer. Assuming that the mortality rate $P = 70\%$ at the end of the study, the standard deviation of the variable "taking drugs" is 0.8, the logarithmic risk ratio is 0.5 (i.e., the death risk of standard drugs is $e^{0.5} = 1.65$ times of that new drugs), and the determination coefficient of "taking drugs" is estimated to be 0.30 for regression analysis of other covariates. How many lung cancer patients need to be observed according to the significance level of 0.05 and the power of 0.90?

Answer: Given $\alpha = 0.05$, $Z_{\alpha/2} = 1.96$; $\beta = 0.10$, $Z_\beta = 1.282$; $P = 0.70$; $R^2 = 0.30$; $\sigma = 0.80$; $\ln HR = 0.5$, input them into Formula (15-19a) and get:

$$n = \frac{(1.96 + 1.282)^2}{0.70 \times (1 - 0.30) \times 0.8^2 \times (0.5)^2} \approx 135$$

$$nP = \frac{(1.96 + 1.282)^2}{(1 - 0.30) \times 0.8^2 \times (0.5)^2} \approx 95$$

Therefore, it is necessary to observe at least 135 lung cancer patients, or at least 95 deaths.

15.6. Sample size estimation in sample survey design

Here only introduces the estimation method of sample size in the design of one-stage sampling survey. When designing a sample survey under complex conditions, the estimation method of sample size should refer to the relevant literature.

15.6.1. *Sample size estimation of simple random sampling and systematic sampling*

1. Information needed to be provided

For simple random sampling or strict systematic sampling, the information required includes the size of the population N, the estimated value P of the population probability, the maximum allowable error δ of the estimated value and the true value of the population probability, and the required confidence $(1 - \alpha)$.

2. Calculation formula

$$n = \frac{Z_{\alpha/2}^2 P(1 - P)N}{\delta^2(N - 1) + Z_{\alpha/2}^2 P(1 - P)} \quad (15\text{-}20a)$$

For an infinite population,

$$n = \frac{Z_{\alpha/2}^2 P(1 - P)}{\delta^2} \quad (15\text{-}20b)$$

3. Example

Example 15.11. From 4000 children living in a certain area, 50 children were randomly selected for preliminary investigation, and 30 children were found to have ascaris. It is now proposed to investigate the overall probability of children with ascariasis in this area through simple random sampling, the maximum allowable error between the estimated value and the true value should not exceed 95%, and the confidence level should be 95%. How large should the sample size be?

Answer: Given $N = 4000$, $P = \frac{30}{50} = 0.60$, $\alpha = 0.05$, $Z_{\alpha/2} = 1.96$, $\delta = 0.05$, input them into Formula (15-20), get:

$$n = \frac{1.96^2 \times 0.60 \times (1 - 0.60) \times 4000}{0.05^2 \times (4000 - 1) + 1.96^2 \times 0.60 \times 0.40} = 337.74 \approx 338$$

At least 338 children should be selected for ascaris test.

15.6.2. *Sample size estimation in stratified random sampling*

1. Information needed to be provided

In such case, the information to be provided includes the population size N, the number of layers L, the size of each layer (sub-population) N_i ($i = 1, 2, 3, \ldots, L$, the same below), probability estimator P_i of each layer (sub-population), proportion of samples of each layer (sub-population) W_i, maximum allowable error δ of estimated population probability and truth value, and confidence degree $1 - \alpha$ required.

2. Calculation formula

When $N_i \gg n_i$, it calculated as below:

$$n = \frac{Z_\alpha^2 \sum \frac{N_i^2 P_i (1-P)_i}{W_i}}{N^2\delta^2 + Z_{\alpha/2}^2 \sum N_i P_i (1 - P)_i} \tag{15-21}$$

If the number of individuals extracted from each layer is the same, then $W_i = 1/L$; If the number of individuals extracted from each layer is proportional to the total number of individuals in each layer, then $W_i = N_i/N$. At this point, if $N_i \gg n_i$, Formula (15-19) can be simplified as

$$n = \frac{Z^2_{\alpha/2}\sum\frac{N_iP_i(1-P)_i}{W_i}}{N^2\delta^2} \tag{15-22}$$

3. Example

Example 15.12. City A, B, and C has 2000, 3000, and 5000 families available for investigation respectively, as shown in Table 15.3. Samples are to be distributed proportionally. With 95% confidence, families with one or more stillbirths in the last 5 years were surveyed. It is estimated that the incidence of stillborn families in the three cities is 0.10, 0.15, and 0.20, respectively. When the difference between the estimate and the truth value is not more than ±3%, how large the sample size should be taken by each city?

Answer: Given $\alpha = 1 - 95\% = 0.05$, then $Z_{\alpha/2} = 1.96$. Due to proportional distribution of samples, $W_1 = 2000/10,000 = 0.2$, $W_2 = 0.3$, $W_3 = 0.5$. After calculation, get:

$$\sum N_iP_i = 1650, \quad \sum N_iP_i(1-P)_i = 1362.5$$

$$\sum\frac{N_i^2P_i(1-P_i)}{W_i} = 13,625,000, \quad \delta = 0.03$$

Input them into Formula (15-21), get:

$$n = \frac{1.96^2 \times 13,625,000}{10,000^2 \times (0.03)^2 + 1.96^2 \times 1362.5} = 549.61$$

Table 15.3 Sample distribution ratio

City	Number of families N_i	Stillbirths rate P_i	Distribution ratio W_i (%)
A	2000	0.10	20.0
B	3000	0.15	30.0
C	5000	0.20	50.0
Total	10,000		100.0

Therefore, a total of 550 families are needed as test units: City A should select $550 \times 0.2 = 110$ families; City B should select $550 \times 0.3 = 165$ families; City C should select $550 \times 0.5 = 275$ families.

15.6.3. *Sample size estimation of cluster sampling*

1. Information needed to be provided

In such case, the confidence coefficient $1 - \alpha$, allowable error δ, and total variance S^2 need to be provided.

2. Calculation formula

Let k groups be randomly selected from an infinite population or a finite population with K groups. The i group contains N_i individuals, $\bar{N}$ is the average number of individuals per group, p_i (or $\bar{x}_i$) is the sample frequency (or sample mean) of the i group, and p (or $\bar{x}$) is the total sample frequency (or total sample mean). The formula for calculating the number of sample groups G to be extracted is (15-23) in Table 15.5.

$$G = \frac{Z_{\alpha/2}^2 S^2}{\delta^2} \tag{15-23}$$

Among them, S^2 is the estimate of the total variance. For qualitative data, when there is an infinite population,

$$S^2 = \frac{\sum \left[\frac{N_i}{\bar{N}}(p_i - p)\right]^2}{k - 1} \tag{15-24a}$$

In a finite population,

$$S^2 = \frac{\left(1 - \frac{k}{K}\right) \sum \left[\frac{N_i}{\bar{N}}(p_i - p)\right]^2}{k - 1} \tag{15-24b}$$

For quantitative data, whether the population is finite or not, all should be:

$$S^2 = \frac{\sum \left[\frac{N_i}{\bar{N}}(\overline{x_i} - \bar{x})\right]^2}{k - 1} \tag{15-24c}$$

It can be seen from Formula (15-23) that the number of groups taken by cluster sampling is mainly related to the variance S^2 of the data. As can be seen from the calculation formula of S^2, its size mainly depends on the difference in the properties of each group. If there is an obvious difference in properties between groups in the population and S^2 is large, more groups need to be extracted. On the contrary, if groups have similar properties and S^2 is small, it is not necessary to extract too many groups.

3. Example

Example 15.13. A city plans to investigate the prevalence of tuberculosis by cluster sampling in 450 committees. 5 committees were randomly selected to obtain variance S^2. The results are shown in Table 15.4. The allowable error is 0.05%, $\alpha = 0.05$. How many committees should be investigated?

Answer: According to the question, in order to estimate the overall probability from the sample frequency, first calculate the values in Table 15.4, and then use the variance calculation Formula (15-24b) to calculate the variance of the qualitative data, and get

$$S^2 = \left(1 - \frac{k}{K}\right) \frac{\sum \left[\frac{N_i}{N}(p_i - p)\right]^2}{(k-1)}$$
$$= \left(1 - \frac{5}{450}\right) \times \frac{0.00000487}{5-1} = 0.00000120$$

Table 15.4 Variance calculation of qualitative data in cluster sampling

Committees	People N_i	Number of patients c_i	Sick rate p_i (%)	$p_i - p$ (%)	$\frac{N_i}{N}$	$\left[\frac{N_i}{N}(p_i - p)\right]^2$
A	1512	7	0.4630	−0.0729	1.0949	0.00000064
B	1437	10	0.6959	0.1601	1.0406	0.00000277
C	1026	5	0.4873	−0.0485	0.7429	0.00000013
D	1732	10	0.5774	0.0415	1.2542	0.00000027
E	1198	5	0.4174	−0.1185	0.8675	0.00000106
Total	6905	37	0.5358	—	—	0.00000487

With $\delta = 0.05\%$, $\alpha = 0.05$, check from table and get $Z_{\alpha/2} = Z_{0.05/2} = 1.96$, input relevant numbers into Formula (15-23) and get

$$G = \frac{(1.96)^2 \times 0.00000120}{(0.0005)^2} = 18.44$$

Therefore, about 19 committees should be randomly selected, 5 committees have been investigated, and 14 more need to be investigated.

By the way, if you want to compare two groups through cluster sampling, the sample size calculation formula is similar to the previous one, but only expressed in the number of groups, as shown in Table 15.5.

Example 15.14. Five years ago, a city conducted a census of the prevalence of tuberculosis. After 5 years of tuberculosis prevention and control, we want to know whether the current prevalence rate has declined. Using a cluster sampling method, specified $\delta = 0.1\%$ (i.e., if the prevalence of tuberculosis decreased by 0.1%, the difference can be found), $\alpha = 0.05$, $\beta = 0.05$, in order to obtain the standard deviation, a sample of 5 committees was sampled, and the results are shown in Table 15.4 of Example 15.13. How many committees should be sampled?

Table 15.5 The formula for calculating sample size (group number *G*) in cluster sampling

Investigation target	Unilateral or bilateral	Calculation formula	
Estimating population from samples	—	$G = \frac{Z_{\alpha/2}^2 S^2}{\delta^2}$	(15.23)
Comparison with a particular population	Unilateral	$G = \frac{(Z_\alpha + Z_\beta)^2 S^2}{\delta^2}$	(15.25)
	Bilateral	$G = \frac{(Z_{\alpha/2} + Z_\beta)^2 S^2}{\delta^2}$	(15.26)
Comparison of two samples	Unilateral	$G_1 = G_2 = \frac{2(Z_\alpha + Z_\beta)^2 S^2}{\delta^2}$	(15.27)
	Bilateral	$G_1 = G_2 = \frac{2(Z_{\alpha/2} + Z_\beta)^2 S^2}{\delta^2}$	(15.28)

Answer: According to the question, this example is the comparison between the unilateral sample frequency and the overall probability, check from table and get $Z_\alpha = Z_0.05 = 1.645$, $Z_\beta = Z_{0.05} = 1.645$, input relevant data into Formula (15-25), get:

$$G = \frac{(Z_\alpha + Z_\beta)^2 S^2}{\delta^2} = \frac{(1.645 + 1.645)^2 \times 0.00000120}{(0.001)^2} \approx 13$$

That is, 13 committees should be randomly selected (5 committees have been checked and 8 more committees should be checked).

Example 15.15. In order to investigate the difference of tuberculosis prevalence between cities A and B, cluster sampling method is adopted. It is hoped that when the difference of tuberculosis prevalence between the two cities is 0.2% (i.e., $\delta = 0.2\%$), the difference can be detected. Stipulating $\alpha = 0.05$, $\beta = 0.05$ and assuming $S^2 = 0.0120$ (same as Example 15.13), how many committees should be sampled in each city?

Answer: According to the meaning of the question, this example is a comparison of the frequency of two samples on both sides, and the relevant data is substituted into Formula (15-28) to get

$$\begin{aligned} G_1 = G_2 &= \frac{2(Z_{\alpha/2} + Z_\beta)^2 S^2}{\delta^2} \\ &= \frac{2 \times (1.96 + 1.645)^2 \times 0.00000120}{(0.002)^2} \approx 7.8 \end{aligned}$$

That is, each of the 2 cities needs to check 8 committees.

15.7. Result report

To report the estimation results of sample size scientifically and reasonably, one of the most basic principles is to specify under what circumstances the sample size or power is estimated, how the specific values of each parameter are selected, through which (or some) formulas to calculate or look up the table, and how many samples are finally calculated or looked up. The specific values of each parameter can refer to the pre-experimental results and relevant literature data.

Below, two examples are given to illustrate the reporting method of sample size estimation results.

Example 15.15. The following is the Chinese and English report on the sample size estimation of group design of Example 15.13.

为估计成组设计的样本含量，假设根据预实验结果，$\delta = 12.33$，$S = 25$，取 $\alpha = 0.05$，$\beta = 0.10$，$t_{\alpha/2(\infty)} = t_{0.05/2(\infty)} = 1.960$（双侧），$t_{\beta(\infty)} = t_{0.10(\infty)} = 1.282$，计算得所需要的样本含量为 173 例。

To estimate the sample size of the two-group design, according to pilot experiment, $\delta = 12.33$, $S = 25$, given $\alpha = 0.05$, $\beta = 0.10$, $t_{\alpha/2(\infty)} = t_{0.05/2(\infty)} = 1.960$ (two-sided), $t_{\beta(\infty)} = t_{0.10(\infty)} = 1.282$, the sample size can be estimated to be 173.

Example 15.16. A researcher wants to study the factors influencing the prognosis of a certain malignant tumor. For example, the main variable of interest to the researcher is X_1. The following is the English and Chinese report on the estimation of the multivariate analysis sample size.

本研究中主要感兴趣的变量为 X_1，预估计其对数风 险比 $\ln HR = 1$，研究结束时死亡率 即终点事件发生率 $P = 74\%$，X_1 的标准差 $\sigma = 0.3$，对 X_1 和其他协变量做多重线性回归的 $R^2 = 0.2$。已知 $\alpha = 0.05$，$\beta = 0.10$，$Z_{\alpha/2} = 1.96$，$Z_\beta = 0.842$，计算得所需要的样本含量为 135 例。

The variable of primary interest in this study is X_1, for which the log hazard ratio estimate is 1 ($\ln HR = 1$) and the standard error is 0.3($\sigma = 0.3$). The mortality (end incidence) when the study terminates is 74% ($P = 74\%$). The square of the correlation (R^2) between X_1 and other independent variables in the multiple linear regression is 0.2. Given $\alpha = 0.05$, $\beta = 0.10$, $Z_{\alpha/2} = 1.96$, $Z_\beta = 0.842$, the sample size can be calculated to be 135.

15.8. Case analysis

Case 15.1 The average effective time of a drug was originally 6 hours, but now the formula has been improved, which is said to be extended to 7 hours. To verify this, a research group observed 25 patients with the disease, but the results were negative ($P > 0.05$), that is, the average effective time could not be considered to extend to 7 hours. Sample standard deviation $S = 2$ is known. Are the conclusions of this study reliable? How to improve the reliability of research conclusions?

Case 15.2 A study on the prevention of colds with vitamin C was conducted. The researcher randomly selected two groups of 30 healthy people. One group took vitamin C and the other group took placebo to compare the frequency of colds in a given period of time. As a result, 6 people in the placebo group had a cold and 3 people in the vitamin group had a cold. There was no significant difference in the level of $\alpha = 0.05$. How do you evaluate this conclusion?

15.9. Computer experiment

Experiment 15.1 When other factors remain unchanged, the relationship between sample size, the overall parameter difference, unilateral and bilateral test

Data file: Data 15.1.xls

Experiment purpose: To understand: (1) When other factors remain unchanged, in order to achieve the same power, the larger the difference between the population parameters, the smaller the sample size required; (2) When other factors remain unchanged, the sample size required for bilateral test is larger than that for unilateral test.

Operation steps: Change the difference of population parameters δ, population standard deviation σ and type I error probability α in Excel program, and observe the change of sample size.

Experimental results: (1) When other factors remain unchanged, the sample size required decreases when the difference value of the

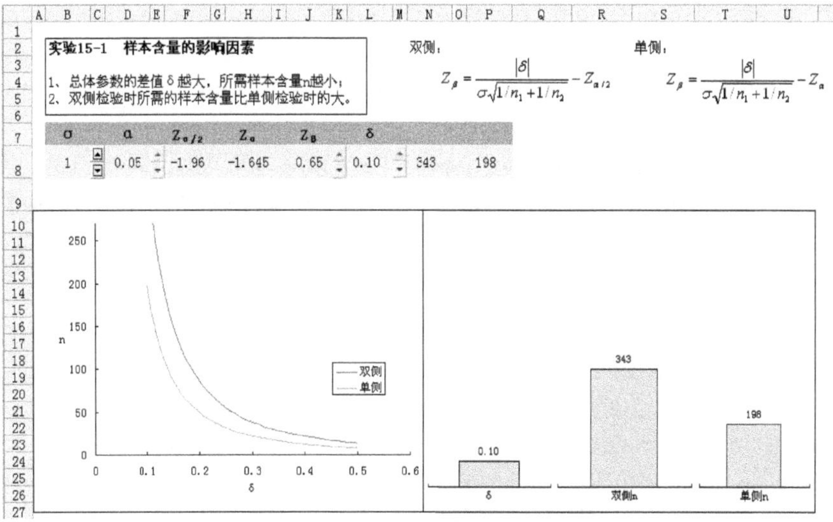

Figure 15.1 Influencing factors of sample size

population parameters δ increased, while the sample size required increases when the population parameters δ decreased (see the bar graph on the right). (2) No matter the line graph on the left or the bar graph on the right and how other conditions change, the sample size required by bilateral test is always larger than that of unilateral test. (3) When the population standard deviation σ is large and the type I error α is small, the sample size required is large (Figure 15.1).

Experiment 15.2 Estimation of sample size

Data file: Data 15.2.xls

Experiment purpose: By inputting the known conditions that determine the sample size, the calculation of various sample sizes listed above can be realized.

Operation steps: In this Excel file, there are 8 Excel worksheets, each of which completes a type of the calculation of sample size. Eight worksheets are implemented respectively: 1. Quantitative data single group and paired design; 2. Quantitative data group design;

3. Qualitative data paired design; 4. Qualitative data group design; 5. Simple linear correlation analysis; 6. Simple random sampling and systematic sampling; 7. Stratified random sampling; 8. Sample size estimation of cluster sampling.

In Excel worksheet, the required sample size estimation can be obtained by inputting the known conditions that determine the sample size, such as probability α of type I error, power $(1-\beta)$, difference δ of the population parameters, and population standard deviation σ.

Experimental results: The following is an example of sample size estimation designed by group design of quantitative data to observe the estimated results of sample size. On the right side of "please enter known conditions," enter the values of significance level, power, mean difference, variation index and proportion (blue), and on the right side of "required sample size" below, the single and bilateral estimated sample size of Group 1, Group 2 and total can be obtained (Figure 15.2).

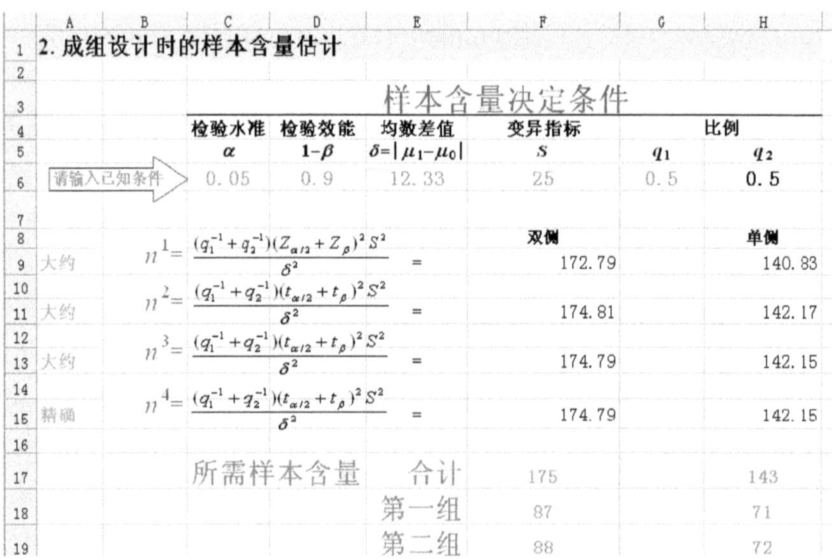

Figure 15.2 Sample size estimation for group design of quantitative data

Experiment 15.3 Sample size estimation for multivariate analysis

Data file: Data 15.3.sav

Experiment purpose: Calculate the sample size of Example 15.16 by operating SPSS.

Answer: Given $Z_{\alpha/2} = 1.96$, $Z_\beta = 0.842$, $P = 0.74$, $R^2 = 0.2$, $\sigma = 0.3$, $\ln HR = 1$, the formula for calculating sample size is: $n = \frac{(Z_{\alpha/2}+Z_\beta)^2}{P(1-R^2)\sigma^2(\ln HR)^2}$

Operation steps: In the SPSS operator interface, click Transform → Compute Variable → Target Variable: n → Numeric Expression: input formula → get result $n = 134.06 \approx 135$. Therefore, at least 135 samples are needed.

15.10. Frequently asked questions and summary

15.10.1. *Frequently asked questions*

1. If I want to show whether a new drug or therapy is better than a conventional drug or therapy, what sample size should I use?

This is a question that quite a few researchers often ask before they do their research work, but it cannot be answered. Because it requires a lot of information to estimate the sample size, first of all, it is necessary to know what type of study was conducted. The sample size calculation formulas used in the experimental design, clinical trial design, and investigation design are not completely the same. Second, even the experimental design involves the complexity of the proposed problem. Third, some basic information corresponding to the proposed problem should be given. There is no scientific basis for estimating sample size in a vacuum, so it is meaningless.

2. When the sample size is small, the conclusion is not credible. Is the conclusion credible when the sample size is very large?

Not always! It depends on the complexity of the problem to be solved and the quality of control over important non-experimental factors. If the experimental study involves multi-factor and multi-level design, even though the total sample size is very large, the number of subjects assigned to each group is very small, so the conclusion is still not credible; if the experimental study involves single-factor and multi-level design, because the impact of many important non-experimental factors on each level group is very uneven, the results are doubtful and even very wrong though the sample size of each group is very large.

3. Is there any way to minimize the probability of false positives and false negatives in a scientific study at the same time?

A better approach is to improve the quality of the statistical research design and the quality control level of the research process, and at the same time, let each group have enough sample size and make good balance between groups.

4. I don't want to demonstrate the difference between the efficacy of the two drugs, but rather to show that the two drugs have the same effect, so that one cheaper drug can replace the other more expensive drug. At this time, how should the sample size be considered?

At this time, the study is called "equivalence trail," which should be estimated according to the corresponding sample size estimation formula of such test. Please refer to the relevant monographs.

15.10.2. *Summary*

This chapter describes the concept of sample size in research design, the significance of determining sample size and power, and the information needed. It also focuses on the sample size estimation methods of population mean estimation, population probability estimation, single group design, paired design, group design, simple linear correlation analysis, multiple linear regression, logistic regression, and Cox regression, and provides calculation formulas and application instance. At the same time, some cases and computer experiments are presented for readers to analyze and observe.

The estimation of sample size is an important part of research design, which must be paid enough attention to. The key to correctly estimating sample size is to correctly select the formula of estimating sample size according to the type of design and some known conditions to obtain convincing estimating results. In the "method" section of the research paper, besides reporting sample size, the basis for estimating sample size must also be reported.

Think and Practice

I. Best Choice

1. Which of the following statements is correct ( )
   A. Because the sampling error decreases with the increase of sample size, it is always considered that the larger the sample size, the better. B. When other conditions are fixed, the smaller the allowable error is, the larger the sample size is needed. C. The more repeated experiments, the more objective facts of chance variation can be reflected, thus eliminating the influence of non-treatment factors. D. The error of cluster sampling is the smallest, that of systematic sampling is the second, and that of stratified sampling is the largest. E. A good experimental design can eliminate random errors
2. The purpose of estimating sample size is to ( ) under a certain accuracy and power
   A. determine more observational units B. determine the minimum number of observation units C. determine the number of effective observation units D. determine the number of random observation units E. determine the exact number of observation units
3. The calculation formula of the sample size required for the comparison of two sample rates is ( )
   A. $n = \left[\frac{(Z_\alpha + Z_\beta)\sigma}{\delta}\right]^2$ B. $n = 2 \times \left[\frac{(Z_\alpha + Z_\beta)\sigma}{\delta}\right]^2$
   C. $N = \left[\frac{(Z_\alpha + Z_\beta)\sigma}{\delta}\right]^2$ D. $n = \frac{2p(1-p)(Z_\alpha + Z_\beta)^2}{(p_1 - p_2)^2}$
   E. $n = \frac{\left[Z_\alpha\sqrt{2\bar{p}} + Z_\beta\sqrt{2(p_1 - p)(p_2 - p)/\bar{p}}\right]^2}{(p_1 - p_2)}$

4. Which of the following is a non-probability sampling method ( ).
   A. Simple random sampling B. Systematic random sampling C. stratified random sampling D. cluster sampling E. Snowball Sampling
5. Stratified sampling requires that the population be stratified. In order to reduce sampling errors, it requires ( ).
   A. individual differences within layers are small, while interlayer differences are large. B. individual differences within layers are large, while interlayer differences are small. C. individual differences within layers are small, while interlayer differences are small. D. both individual and interlayer differences are large. E. layered completely randomly.
6. The following Cox proportional risk regression model was used to estimate the sample size

$$n = \frac{(Z_{\alpha/2} + Z_\beta)^2}{P(1 - R^2)\sigma^2(\ln HR)^2}$$

   It can be seen that, assuming a major independent variable is taken as the outcome variable, the multiple correlation coefficients between this independent variable and all other independent variables are calculated. Among the following possible multiple correlation coefficient values, the largest estimated result of the sample size is ( ).
   A. 0.05 B. 0.2 C. 0.4 D. 0.6 E. 0.8

II. Questions for Reflection

1. What is the basis for determining the sample size?
2. What is the significance of rechecking the sample size when the hypothesis test result is "negative" ($P > 0.05$)?

III. Questions on Calculation

1. It is said that the average normal temperature of an ethnic group is higher than 37°C. In order to verify it, a sampling survey is planned. If the average temperature is higher than 0.1°C

in general, it cannot be ignored. The standard deviation of known normal human body temperature is about 0.2°C. Then, in order to control the probability of type I and II errors in $\alpha = 0.05$ and $\beta = 0.05$, please estimate the sample size.

2. A person decides to take sample size $n = 25$ artificially without estimating before conducting the abovementioned investigation. Is this sample size adequate?
3. In order to compare the dissolution rates of the two kinds of tablets, it was decided to randomly select 10 tablets and determine the dissolution amount in 5 minutes, and then they were tested based on level $\alpha = 0.05$ and $\beta = 0.10$. According to the preliminary experiment, the variability of the two kinds of tablets is the same, the standard deviation is about 6 units, and the difference between the mean is about 6 units. Whether the sample size of the study is adequate?
4. The internal medicine departments of A and B hospitals randomly investigated 30 inpatients, in which 20 of whom were satisfied with the medical services in A hospital, and 23 of whom were satisfied in B hospital. After statistical test, it cannot be considered the satisfaction rate of internal medicine inpatients in the two hospitals is unequal. If you want to examine whether the satisfaction rates of internal medicine inpatient in two hospitals differ by more than 10%, at least how many patients should be investigated in each hospital?
5. In the above sample, satisfaction rates are respectively $20/30 = 67\%$ and $23/30 = 77\%$, with a difference of 10%, which seems to be not a small difference. However, the statistical test cannot reject the assumption that the overall satisfaction rates are equal. If both the number of respondents and the number of people satisfied are 10 times of the current number, the satisfaction rate of the sample is still 67% and 77%, respectively; at that time the statistical test can reject the assumption that the overall satisfaction rate is equal. How to explain this phenomenon? What can we learn from the above phenomenon?
6. The double-blind experiment results of lowering blood pressure of patients with myocardial infarction with a certain drug are as

Table 15.6 Systolic pressure (kPa) after treatment in two groups of patients with myocardial infarction

Medicine	n	$\bar{x}$	s
Experimental medicine	15	14.4	1.6
Controlled	15	15.3	1.6

Table 15.7 The relationship between chemotherapeutic remission and concurrent infection in patients with acute leukemia

Remission after chemotherapy	n	Frequency of infection (%)	P
Remission	17	88.2	>0.05
Non-remission	27	70.3	

follows (see Table 15.6). If the test result $t = 1.54$, $0.1 < P < 0.2$, it is considered that the drug is ineffective in lowering blood pressure, is this conclusion reliable?

7. The relationship between remission of chemotherapy and concurrent infection in acute leukemia patients was observed. According to the test results (see Table 15.7) $P > 0.05$, there was no significant difference between the two groups. Assuming that it is meaningful when the infection rates of the two groups differ by more than 0.30. And $\alpha = 0.05$ and $\beta = 0.05$, is the sample size sufficient?
8. A researcher plans to conduct a clinical trial to compare the effect of a new treatment and traditional treatment on delaying local infection in burn patients. Assuming the incidence of delaying effect at the end of the study is $P = 65\%$, the standard deviation of the treatment is 0.7, and the logarithmic risk ratio is 2, the estimated determination coefficient of regression analysis of the

treatment method for other covariates is 0.40. Then, how many burn patients need to be observed according to the significance level of 0.05 and the power of 0.80?

Chun Hao, Jinyue Li, Minghui Zhang

CHAPTER 16

MISSING DATA

Missing data is a common problem in medical research. If not handled, it will cause information loss and bias. Many reasons can result in missing data. In medical research, the common reasons can be summarized as the following:

1. Data did not collect during the study, such as the dropout of subjects in the clinical trial; Omission of information in the survey or no response from the respondents.
2. Data were collected, but not available: such as obvious input error or logic error.

In statistical analysis, the imputation of missing data is very important. In this chapter, common missing data imputation methods are introduced.

16.1. Patterns of missing data

Example 16.1: To evaluate the efficacy of electroacupuncture on severe chronic constipation, a multi-center randomized controlled clinical trial was conducted in China. Subjects who met the inclusion and exclusion criteria were randomly assigned to the electroacupuncture group (EA) and the sham electroacupuncture group (SA). The screening period was 2 weeks before randomization, with 8 weeks of treatment and 12 weeks of follow-up. The primary efficacy outcome was the change from baseline of weekly complete spontaneous bowel movements (CSBMs) during weeks 1–8. The first 199 cases were selected, among 177 subjects who completed the trial, and 22 subjects stopped the clinical study earlier (12 cases were lost to follow-up, 5 cases withdrew from the trial due to adverse events, and 5 cases withdrew by themselves). Please compare the primary outcome in the two groups. The data were shown in the Table 16.1.

In the example, weekly CSBMs of 22 cases were missing due to the earlier stop of clinical study, and the missing data need to be imputed before further statistical analysis. At first, we need to explore the patterns of missing data, describes which data in the data set are observed and which data are missing. It is helpful to explore the relationship between different variables and find a better solution to the missing data. In general, the patterns of missing data can be classified into two types:

1. Monotone missing pattern

As is shown in the Figure 16.1(a), a matrix can be obtained after proper row and column transformation on the data set y, which presents a pattern of missing hierarchy: when the elements y_i in the matrix are missing, the elements y_p are also missing for any $p \geq i$. This pattern is most common in longitudinal clinical study. For example, if a subject drops off at a certain time point, the data behind the time point are missing. Besides, in a questionnaire survey, if the subject stops earlier or discontinued, the missing data is monotone missing pattern.

2. Arbitrary missing pattern

As is shown in Figure 16.1(b), missing data is caused by accidental reason and has no certain rules. The missing data which were caused by non-response for the questionnaire is always follow arbitrary missing pattern.

Example

To summarize the missing data of weekly CSBMs from baseline to week 8 (w0–w8) and explore the missing data pattern. Table 16.2 shows that the missing data conformed to the monotone missing

Table 16.1 Weekly CSBMs during the 8-week treatment period ($\overline{x} \pm s$)

Group	W0	W1	W2	W3	W4	W5	W6	W7	W8
EA	0.77 ± 0.84	0.66 ± 0.86	0.87 ± 1.02	2.35 ± 1.82	2.35 ± 1.90	2.57 ± 1.93	2.71 ± 2.03	2.79 ± 2.09	3.23 ± 2.18
SA	0.78 ± 0.71	0.76 ± 0.78	0.79 ± 0.85	1.79 ± 1.75	1.93 ± 1.95	1.92 ± 2.00	1.86 ± 1.88	2.00 ± 1.89	1.99 ± 1.88
n_a	98	98	98	95	94	93	92	92	90
n_b	101	101	101	92	92	91	90	87	87
Total	199	199	199	187	186	184	182	179	177

*W0 was the baseline, and w1–w8 were week 1–week8, respectively

	y_1	y_2	y_3	y_4	y_5
1	x	x	x	x	x
2	x	x	x	x	.
3	x	x	x	.	.
4	x	x	.	.	.
…	…	…	…	…	…
n	x	.	.	.	.

(a) Monotone missing pattern

	y_1	y_2	y_3	y_4	y_5
1	x	.	x	.	x
2	.	x	x	x	.
3	x	x	.	x	x
4	x	x	x	x	.
…	…	…	…	…	…
n	x	.	x	x	.

(b) Arbitrary missing pattern

Figure 16.1 Data missing patterns **X means observed data; ".'' means missing data**

Table 16.2 Missing data patterns at baseline and 1–8 weeks of CSBMs

		Week										
Pattern	Baseline	1	2	3	4	5	6	7	8	EA	SA	In total
1	√	√	√	√	√	√	√	√	√	90 (91.8%)	87 (86.1%)	177
2	√	√	√	√	√	√	√	√	×	2 (2.0%)	0 (0.0%)	2
3	√	√	√	√	√	√	√	×	×	0 (0.0%)	3 (3.0%)	3
4	√	√	√	√	√	√	×	×	×	1 (1.0%)	1 (1.0%)	2
5	√	√	√	√	√	×	×	×	×	1 (1.0%)	1 (1.0%)	2
6	√	√	√	√	×	×	×	×	×	1 (1.0%)	0 (0.0%)	1
7	√	√	√	×	×	×	×	×	×	3 (3.1%)	9 (8.9%)	12
8	√	√	×	×	×	×	×	×	×	0 (0.0%)	0 (0.0%)	0
9	√	×	×	×	×	×	×	×	×	0 (0.0%)	0 (0.0%)	0

√ observed data × missing data

pattern, and there was no significance between the two groups by Fisher's exact test ($P = 0.088$).

16.2. The mechanism of missing data

The mechanism of missing data is used to describe as the relationship between missing data and other variables in the dataset and to explore the missing reason.

Different scholars classified the missing data mechanism differently. The mechanism of missing data was classified three type, which was more common and proposed by Little and Rubin in 1976: Missing Completely at Random (MCAR), Missing at Random (MAR) and Not Missing at Random (NMAR).

1. Missing Completely at Random: whether it is missing or not, the target variable y has no relationship with the observed data. In other words, the observed data and the unobserved data are mutually independent. For example, laboratory test results are missed due to the loss of blood sample; the loss of follow-up in clinical trials, and so on.

   MCAR can be expressed as:

   $$\Pr(R_i \mid \mathrm{Y}_i) = \Pr(R_i) \tag{16-1}$$

   i means subjects and j means variables, if $R_{i,j} = 1$, $\mathrm{Y}_{i,j}$ was observed, which means no data were missed; If $\mathrm{R}_{i,j} = 0$, $\mathrm{Y}_{i,j}$ was not observed, which means data were missed.

   In this case, both the observed data and the unobserved data are a random sample of all the data. Therefore, to directly analyze the observed data without concerning missing data will not cause bias, and this method is called the complete data analysis method. Most of the current statistical software defaults to this analysis method. However, MCAR is rare in practice.
2. Missing at Random: Whether the target variable y is missing or not is only related to the observed data and has nothing to do with the unobserved data. For example, in a clinical trial, all subjects are taken a physical examine, and if indicators meet certain criteria, hospitalization is required. In this case, hospitalization depends on the observed data and has nothing to do with the unobserved data. According to whether the data is observed or not, Y_i can be divided into observed data (Y_{obs}) and unobserved data (Y_{mis}). For MAR, it can be expressed as:

   $$\Pr(R_i \mid Y_i) = \Pr(R_i \mid Y_{obs}) \tag{16-2}$$

   In other words, under MAR assumption, the distribution of missing data (i.e., unobserved data) is the same as that of observed data, which is the theory base we use to handle missing data.

Under MAR, missing data is no longer a random sample of all the data. It will bring bias to directly analyze the complete data.

3. Not Missing at Random: The missing of the target variable y is related to itself, whether it is observed or not. NMAR can be expressed as:

$$\Pr(R_i \mid Y_i) \neq \Pr(R_i \mid Y_{obs}) \tag{16-3}$$

NMAR is common in practice but difficult to deal with. For example, no responses to sensitive questions in the questionnaire.

The mechanism of missing data is different, so are the applicable statistical processing methods. This chapter will briefly introduce common methods to deal with missing data.

16.3. Processing methods of missing data

Different mechanisms of missing data are processed differently. For MCAR, missing data can be ignored, that is, missing data cannot be handled and complete observed data can be directly analyzed, which default for popular statistical analysis software. For NMAR, the processing of missing data will be complicated. At present, most statistical methods assume that the mechanism of missing data is MAR, and the methods introduced in this chapter are mainly for MAR.

Processing for missing data can be classified three types: direct inference, imputation, and re-sampling. In this chapter, we will emphases on imputation method, which is to give each missing datum several substitute values, called imputation values. According to the number of imputation values, imputation methods can be classified as Single Imputation (SI) and Multiple Imputation (MI).

1. Single imputation: One imputation value is given to each missing datum. The basic principle is to provide a predicted distribution for the imputation values based on the observed data, and then impute the missing data with the average value of its predicted distribution or extract a value from it. A "complete data set" is obtained and analyzed.

Common single imputation methods include:

Mean imputation: for the missing data of each variable, the mean of all observed data of the variable is used to impute. Mean imputation is simple, but the variance is underestimated after imputation.

Stratified mean imputation: before imputation, covariates information is applied to stratify the whole population to make the features of each stratum as close or similar as possible. Then in each strata, the mean of the observed data is used to impute the missing data of this strata. The stratified mean imputation is more precise than the single mean imputation, but it still underestimated variance after imputation.

Regression value imputation: besides the single missing pattern, the regression model between the dependent variable y and the independent variable x is established, and then the predicted value of regression is used as the imputation value, which is commonly used.

Last Observation Carried Forward (LOCF): this method is widely used in longitudinal studies. If a subject drops out of a trial, the last observed data will be used for all subsequent missing values. In a clinical trial of hypertension drug, a subject lost follow-up at visit 3, the systolic and diastolic blood pressure of this and subsequent visits, can be replaced by the values at visit 2.

In addition, in clinical trials, there are other imputation methods, such as the worst observation carried forward and the baseline observation carried forward, which are similar as LOCF.

Example 16.2, using LOCF to impute the missing data of Example 16.1 and analyze the change from baseline of average weekly CSBMs at 8 weeks treatment by covariance analysis, set center as the fixed effect, the baseline CSBM was covariate. The analysis results are shown in Table 16.3.

As can be seen from Table 16.3 and Table 16.4, the results of covariance analysis after LOCF showed that there was statistical significant difference in the change from baseline of average weekly CSBMs at 8 weeks between the two groups, and the adjusted difference between groups was 1.207, 95% CI was (0.646, 1.767).

2. Multiple imputation: every missing value is imputed with m values, so as to obtain m "completed" data sets. Then, the "completed" data

Table 16.3 The change from baseline of average weekly CSBMs at 8 weeks treatment with LOCF

The sources	Type III sum of squares	df	Mean square	F	Sig.
Corrected model	191.949	4	47.987	11.963	0.000
Intercept	37.284	1	37.284	9.294	0.003
Group	1.848	1	1.848	0.461	0.498
Center	40.938	1	40.938	10.205	0.002
CSBMs baseline	75.272	1	75.272	18.764	0.000
Group*center	3.980	1	3.980	0.992	0.320
Error	778.222	194	4.011		
Total	1515.750	199			

Table 16.4 Estimation values for the change from baseline of average weekly CSBMs at 8 weeks treatment with LOCF

			95% *CI*	
Group	Mean	*SE*	Lower limit	Upper limit
EA	2.274	0.202	1.875	2.673
SA	1.067	0.199	0.674	1.460
EA-SA*	1.207	0.284	0.646	1.767

*$P < 0.001$

set after imputation is analyzed separately, and the m estimations obtained are synthesized to use for the statistical inference, as is shown in Figure 16.2. Considering the uncertainty of missing values, MI method has been widely accepted and applied.

(1) Basic steps of MI

MI are generally carried out in three steps:

1) Imputation: Imputed the missing data set m times to produce m "completed data set"; The hypothesis of MI on the mechanism of missing data is MAR, and the data conform to multivariate normal distribution. According to the assumption of MAR and Formula 16-2,

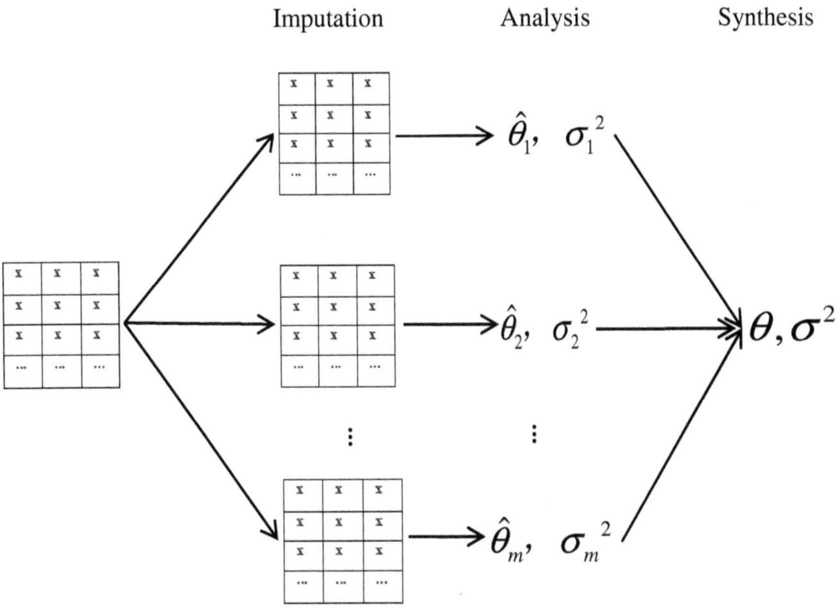

Figure 16.2 Multiple imputation procedure

it can be concluded that:

$$\Pr(Y, R = 0) = \Pr(Y, R = 1) \tag{16-4}$$

Therefore, the imputation values for missing data can be generated based on the distribution of the observed data $Y^{(1)}$, $Y^{(2)}, \ldots, Y^{(k)}$.

Different missing patterns have different MI methods.

For the monotone missing pattern, propensity score method or regression methods based on the multivariate normal distribution can be used. And the following variables should be included in the model to generate the imputation values as far as possible: (1) critical variables in the analysis;(2) predictive covariates of critical variables; (3) predictive covariates of missing data. Some researchers suggest including as many covariates as possible that may influence the target variables.

Parametric regression method: Constructing a fitting model for each variable with missing data. Considering the missing data is monotone missing pattern, the non-missing variables are regarded as covariates. Then, based on the constructed model, the new regression model is calculated and used to impute the missing values for the target variable.

Propensity score method: calculate a propensity score for each missing variable in the model, indicating the missing probability of the variable. Then all the observations were grouped according to the propensity score and then imputed with the approximate Bayesian bootstrap method. However, compared with the parametric regression method, the propensity score method does not consider the correlation between variables, only focuses on the covariance between variables, so this method is not appropriate in the case of correlation between variables.

If the missing data follow to arbitrary missing pattern, the MCMC method based on the multivariate normal distribution should be adopted. Because monotone missing pattern is a special case of the arbitrary missing pattern, MCMC can also be applied. For arbitrary missing pattern, we can directly impute the data set by MCMC to obtain a completed dataset, or impute the missing data to the monotone missing pattern firstly, and then impute the missing data based on the monotonic missing pattern.

The existing statistical analysis software includes the above three methods, and we can choose the appropriated method according to the missing data pattern.

2) Analysis: analyze each complete data set after imputation. For example, separately analyze m data sets after imputation with t test.

3) Synthesis: With m imputations, m different sets of the point and variance estimates for a parameter θ. Suppose $\hat{\theta}_i$ and $\hat{\sigma}_i^2$ are the point and variance estimates from the ith imputed data set, $i = 1, 2, \ldots, m$. Then the synthesized point estimate for θ is the average of the m complete-data estimates:

$$\hat{\theta} = \frac{1}{m} \sum_{i=1}^{m} \hat{\theta}_i \tag{16-5}$$

The synthesized variance is composed of two parts: the between-imputation variance,

$$\sigma_B^2 = \frac{1}{m-1}\sum_{i=1}^{m}(\hat{\theta}_i - \hat{\theta})^2 \tag{16-6}$$

and the within-imputation variance, which is the average of the m complete-data estimates,

$$\sigma_w^2 = \frac{1}{m}\sum_{i=1}^{m}\hat{\theta}_i^2 \tag{16-7}$$

Therefore, the total variance is:

$$\sigma_T^2 = \sigma_w^2 + \left(1 + \frac{1}{m}\right)\sigma_B^2 \tag{16-8}$$

Example 16.3 To impute the missing data of Example 16.1 by MI, and compare the change from baseline of average weekly CSBMs at 8 weeks between the two groups.

(1) Imputation: Suppose the missing data mechanism of CSBMs is MAR and conform to the monotone missing pattern (Example 16.1), parameter regression method was used to impute the missing data. According to the characteristics of CSBMs, the following variables were included in the regression model: baseline CSBMs, weekly CSBMs, age, gender, use of rescue medications. Set $m = 5$, that is, a total of 5 "complete" data sets were generated after imputation.
(2) Analysis: five complete-data sets after imputation were analyzed with the analysis of covariance, and the change from baseline of average weekly CSBMs at 8 weeks was set as dependent variable, center as the fixed effect and the baseline CSBM as covariate. The estimates for 5 complete-data after imputation are shown in Table 16.5.
(3) Synthesis: the synthesized results of 5 imputed data sets are shown in Table 16.6. The imputation numbers 1–5 respectively

Table 16.5 Summary of the estimates for 5 complete-data after imputation

Imputation No.	Sources	Type III sum of squares	*df*	MS	F	P
The original data	Corrected model	229.482	6	38.247	9.778	0.000
	intercept	597.261	1	597.261	152.699	0.000
	baseline	90.315	1	90.315	23.090	0.000
	group	80.726	1	80.726	20.639	0.000
	center	46.529	2	23.264	5.948	0.003
	Group* center	16.394	2	8.197	2.096	0.126
	Error	664.933	170	3.911		
	Total	1487.500	177			
1	Corrected model	211.970	6	35.328	8.483	0.000
	intercept	705.670	1	705.670	169.447	0.000
	baseline	95.802	1	95.802	23.004	0.000
	group	55.073	1	55.073	13.224	0.000
	center	49.894	2	24.947	5.990	0.003
	Group*center	16.768	2	8.384	2.013	0.136
	error	799.592	192	4.165		
	Total	1740.178	199			
5	Corrected model	214.957	6	35.826	8.905	0.000
	intercept	710.476	1	710.476	176.587	0.000
	baseline	107.172	1	107.172	26.637	0.000
	group	54.256	1	54.256	13.485	0.000
	center	43.080	2	21.540	5.354	0.005
	Group*center	13.574	2	6.787	1.687	0.188
	error	772.488	192	4.023		
	Total	1695.041	199			

Note: The results of the No. 2, 3, 4 imputation data sets are omitted

represented the estimates of 5 complete-data sets after imputation, and the combined results were the combined estimates of 5 complete-data sets after imputation, that is, the change from baseline of average weekly CSBMs at 8 weeks in EA group was 2.506 (95%CI, 2.096 to 2.917), and 1.404 (95%*CI*, 1.003 to 1.805) in SA group. The difference between two groups was 1.102.

4) Sensitivity analysis

MI is based on the assumption that the missing data conform to MAR, that is, the distribution of missing data is the same as that

Table 16.6 Estimates of the change from baseline of average weekly CSBMs at 8 weeks

Imputation No.	Group	Means	95% *CI* Lower limit	95% *CI* Upper limit
Original data	EA	2.577	2.158	2.995
	SA	1.212	0.792	1.632
1	EA	2.510	2.098	2.921
	SA	1.450	1.049	1.851
2	EA	2.452	2.054	2.851
	SA	1.420	1.031	1.809
3	EA	2.563	2.162	2.964
	SA	1.396	1.005	1.787
4	EA	2.532	2.142	2.923
	SA	1.332	0.951	1.713
5	EA	2.474	2.070	2.879
	SA	1.423	1.028	1.817
Combined	EA	2.506	2.096	2.917
	SA	1.404	1.003	1.805

Table 16.7 The differences of the change from baseline of average weekly CSBMs at 8 weeks between two groups

Imputation No.	(I) group	(J) group	Difference (i–j)	*P*	95% CI Lower limit	95% CI Upper limit
Original data	EA	SA	1.365	0.000	0.772	1.958
1	EA	SA	1.060	0.000	0.485	1.635
2	EA	SA	1.032	0.000	0.475	1.589
3	EA	SA	1.167	0.000	0.607	1.727
4	EA	SA	1.200	0.000	0.655	1.746
5	EA	SA	1.052	0.000	0.487	1.617
Combined	EA	SA	1.102			

of the observed data. However, since the missing data cannot be observed, it is impossible to verify the assumption of MAR. Therefore, sensitivity analysis is needed to validate whether the MI results based on MAR are consistent with that departure from MAR.

The National Research Council recommends that sensitivity analysis should be conducted for MI results based on MAR and must be reported.

Pattern mixture Model was a recommended method for sensitivity analysis of MI (Little 1993; Molenberghs and Kenward 2007) and it was recommended by some high-impact journals.

The basic steps of the pattern mixture model are the same as those of the MI, including imputation, analysis, and synthesis. The difference is that the distribution of which the imputation values are generated is different.

(1) Imputation: Under the NMAR assumption, the distribution of the missing data is different from that of the observed data, that is, $\Pr(Y, R = 0) \neq \Pr(Y, R = 1)$, the imputation values cannot be generated based on the distribution of observed data.

In a clinical trial, assume that R is a response indicator whose element is 0 or 1, depending on whether Y is missed or observed, and G is the group, with G = 1 as the treatment group and G = 0 as the control group. Y represents the value of the indicator variable at a visit. When Y is not fully observed, under the MAR assumption,

$$\Pr(Y \mid G = 0, R = 0) = \Pr(Y \mid G = 0, R = 1) \tag{16-9}$$

and

$$\Pr(Y \mid G = 1, R = 0) = \Pr(Y \mid G = 1, R = 1) \tag{16-10}$$

under the NMAR assumption,

$$\Pr(Y \mid G = 0, R = 0) \neq \Pr(Y \mid G = 0, R = 1) \tag{16-11}$$

and

$$\Pr(Y \mid G = 0, R = 0) \neq \Pr(Y \mid G = 0, R = 1) \tag{16-12}$$

Therefore, under the NMAR assumption, we can specify the set of observations that are used to derive the imputation model:

The first method: creating control-based pattern imputation, that is:

$$\Pr(Y \mid G = 1, R = 0) = \Pr(Y \mid G = 0, R = 1) \tag{16-13}$$

The second method: adjusting imputed values by adding a sensitivity parameter δ that is not 0 to the imputation model, that is

$$\Pr(Y = y + \delta \,|\, G = 1, R = 0) = \Pr(Y = y \,|\, G = 1, R = 1) \quad (16\text{-}14)$$

δ is the means difference of the observed data and the missing data, which is generally determined by discussing with clinical researchers and considering professional knowledge. The larger is the δ value, the greater is the difference between the distribution of missing data and observed data. δ is close to or beyond the critical value. When the MI results based on MAR are consistent with those obtained based on NMAR, it suggests the assumption of MAR is reliable. On the contrary, it indicates that the assumption of MAR is problematic, and the MI analysis results under this assumption are not reliable.

Other steps and setting of the sensitivity analysis are the same as MI.

(2) Analysis and synthesis: the same as MI.

Example 16.4 Conduct sensitivity analysis under NMAR assumption for the MI results of Example16.3.

(1) Imputation

Using the same imputation model and covariates as Example 16.3 to create the imputation values derived from the distribution of observed data in the control group. Set a parameter δ to adjust imputed values. For patients with severe chronic constipation, it was not common that weekly CSBMs was 8 times a week. Therefore, δ was set 8. Considering the variability of CSBMs, δ was set $(-8, 8)$.

(2) Analysis and synthesis

The imputed data set were analyzed and combined by the same method as that of Example 16.3. The results are showed in Table 16.8.

As can be seen from Table 16.8 and Figure 16.3, in the most extreme case, the missing data was imputed based on the distribution of observed data in the control group, and when the value of δ was

Table 16.8 Between-group differences of estimated values and 95% CI based on NMAR assumption and different δ

δ	Differences between groups	Lower limit of 95% *CI*	Upper limit of 95% *CI*
−8	0.73	0.31	1.15
−6	0.71	0.30	1.11
−4	0.68	0.29	1.06
−2	0.61	0.27	0.96
0	0.52	1.19	0.84
2	0.42	0.08	0.77
4	0.37	0.01	0.74
6	0.34	0.05	0.74
8	0.33	0.07	0.73

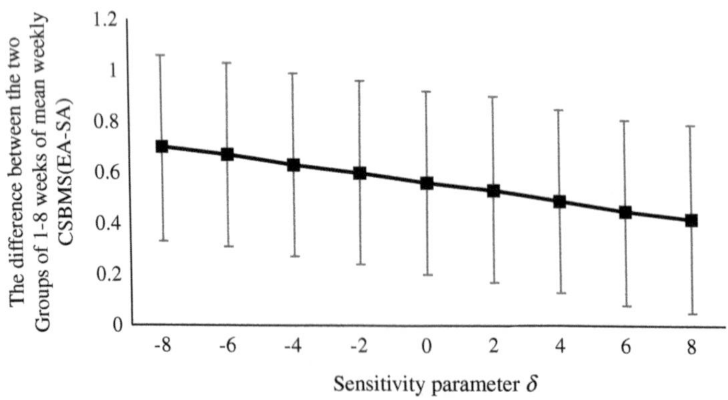

Figure 16.3 The between-group differences of 1–8 weeks of mean weekly CSBMs departed from MAR assumption

8, the difference of weekly CSBMs between the two groups was 0.42 (95%*CI*, 0.05 to 0.79), and consistent with the MI results under the MAR assumption (Example 16.3). It showed that the results of MI was reliable.

16.4. Report writing

The results report of missing data processing should include: ① Patterns and mechanisms of missing data; ② Missing data processing methods, such as LOCF or MI. When MI is used, the imputed target variables and the methods to generate the imputation values should be reported in detail. If the parametric regression method or propensity method is used, the specific variables in the model and number of data sets imputed should be given; ③ Statistical analysis methods and results after imputation; ④ Sensitivity analysis methods, parameters and results. The reports of MI examples in this chapter were:

For missing data of the primary outcome, we used MI for weekly CSBMs during weeks 1–8. We assumed the data were MAR and were monotone missing pattern, and the missing data were imputed week by week. The following variables were included in the imputation models: baseline CSBMs, weekly CSBMs, age, sex, and rescue medicine used. Five imputed datasets were created. After MI, each of the five MI datasets were analyzed by the general linear model. The overall estimates were calculated using Rubin's rules. After MI, the estimate of the primary outcome was 2.506 (95%*CI*, 2.096 to 2.917) in the EA group and 1.404 (95%*CI*, 1.003 to 1.805) in the SA group (between-group difference, 1.102, $P < 0.001$).

The sensitivity analysis with a pattern-mixture model assessed whether the change from baseline in mean weekly CSBMs over weeks 1–8 was robust to departure from MAR. The analysis was conducted by adding a constant δ $(-8, 8)$ as a sensitivity parameter to the estimated treatment effect for the primary outcome. In addition, we specified the observations in the SA group to derive the imputed values and construct the imputation model. When δ was 8 and the imputed values were derived from the SA group, the estimated between-group differences of the change from baseline in mean weekly CSBMs was 0.83 (95%*CI*, 0.67 to 0.99). Under this strong assumption about the departure from MAR, the conclusion of the primary outcome was not change and the results under the MAR assumption were valid.

16.5. Case discrimination

Case 16.1 In a randomized controlled clinical trial of acupuncture on obesity, a total of 60 subjects were included and randomly assigned to the treatment group and the control group. There were five times treatment per week, and lasted 12 weeks. At the end of the study, a total of 51 subjects completed the trial, seven subjects were lost to follow-up, and two subjects withdrew by themselves. After analyzing the weight changes of 51 subjects before and after treatment, the researchers concluded that acupuncture was effective for obesity ($P < 0.001$). Whether the conclusion was correct and provided the reasons.

16.6. Computer experiments

Experiment 16.1 Conduct MI analysis of the missing data of Example 16.1 with SPSS software

To explore the missing data pattern and conduct MI for the missing data of primary outcome under the MAR assumption, then compare the difference between the two groups using a general linear model.

Experiment 16.2 Conduct the sensitivity analysis for the MI results of Example 16.1 with R software

The sensitivity analysis of Example 16.1 was carried out to verify the reliability of the MI results departure from the MAR assumption.

16.7. Frequently asked questions and summary

16.7.1. *Frequently asked questions*

1. How much imputation times were needed in the MI procedure?

Usually, three to five times are sufficient. For variables with a missing information was about 50%, high relative efficiency can be achieved after 5 times imputation. However, in recent years, some researchers suggested that the number of imputation should be 20–100. We suggest that it should be started from five times and gradually increased to about 20 times. When the analysis results are close each other, the one with fewer imputation times is as the final results.

2. How to determine the missing data mechanism?

The following methods can be used: explore the observed factors that can explain the missing variables and analyze whether there is a difference of these factors between the observed data and the missing data. If there is a difference, it may be not MAR; if there is no difference, it may be MAR. Therefore, the potential factors, which can result in missing data, should be considered as far as possible in the design phase, and these factors should be included in the model to generate the imputation values in the MI procedure.

16.7.2. *Summary*

1. In clinical trials, missing data should be prevented at first. Missing data should be reduced as much as possible by reasonable design and strict quality control during the study.
2. In actual clinical trials, MCAR is really rare. Therefore, missing data should be processed to avoid bias.
3. The processing of missing data usually includes: analyzing missing data pattern, missing data mechanism, data imputation and sensitivity analysis. Different missing data mechanisms have different imputation methods. The widely accepted methods are LOCF and MI based on MAR assumption.
4. After the imputation of missing data, sensitivity analysis should be carried out to verify the reliability of the analysis results under the assumption of MAR.

Think and Practice

I. Questions for Reflection

1. How to set a reasonable δ value in the sensitivity analysis of MI?
2. What are the advantages and disadvantages of single imputation and MI?

II. Questions on Calculation

For Example 16.1, the quality of life was measured with PAC-QOL at baseline, 4 weeks, and 8 weeks after treatment, as is shown in data16-1.Please impute the missing data with MI, and analyze the changes from baseline of PAC-QOL at 8 weeks by covariance analysis (considering baseline value of PAC-QOL as covariable), and conduct sensitivity analysis for the results of MI.

References

[1] Yan, C. *Data Management in Clinical Research.* 2011.
[2] Liu, Z, Yan, S, Wu, J, *et al.* Acupuncture for chronic severe functional constipation: A randomized trial. *[J]. Ann Intern Med.* 2016; 165(11): 761–769. doi:10.7326/M15-3118
[3] Molenberghs, G, Fitzmaurice, G, Kenward, MG, *et al.* Handbook of Missing Data Methodology. Handbooks of Modern Statistical Methods, 2014.

Shiyan Yan

CHAPTER 17

STATISTICAL REPORTING GUIDELINES FOR MEDICAL PAPERS

In this chapter, we introduce international guidelines that should be followed when reporting statistical designs, methods, results and conclusions in medical papers, including the consolidated standards of reporting trials (CONSORT) for randomized controlled clinical trials, the strengthening the reporting of observational studies in epidemiology (STROBE) for observational studies, the standards for reporting diagnostic accuracy studies (STARD) for diagnostic accuracy studies, and the preferred reporting items for systematic reviews and meta-analyses (PRISMA) for systematic reviews and meta-analyses. The main components of these guidelines are flow diagrams and checklists. The standard use of statistical symbols is also introduced in this chapter.

17.1. Aims and implications of standardizing the reporting guidelines

Medical research papers are usually evaluated in terms of novelty, scientific nature and practicality, and among them, the scientific nature is mainly reflected in the statistics-related research design, data analysis and statistical inference. In medical papers published at home and abroad, statistical errors and deficiencies are very common, and defects in reporting were among the most crucial issues.

The standardization of statistical reporting improves the quality of medical research papers, which is also the aim of these guidelines. In addition, because the research design is specified in relevant guidelines, learning norms in reporting can also help researchers to design, implement, analyze, infer, and write articles more accurately, thereby enhancing the design and regulating the writing. Eventually, the scientific nature of medical research papers can be better displayed.

Similarly, the knowledge of relevant norms in reporting can also help medical journal editors, reviewers, and readers to understand the research design, data analysis, results, and inferences in a paper more scientifically and comprehensively, and even enable them to question or verify the data reported. As the use of evidence-based medicine increases, meta-analysis has been recognized as a reliable tool for clinical decision-making. However, the reliability of conclusions in a meta-analysis is greatly influenced by the quality of papers included. Therefore, regulation of statistical reporting is also crucial in reanalysis research such as meta-analysis.

17.2. Recommendations from the international committee of medical journal editors

In 1988, the International Committee of Medical Journal Editors (ICMJE), for the first time, added statistical report-related items to the *Uniform Requirements for Manuscripts Submitted to Biomedical Journals* (URM). In 2004, the Committee specified requirements for different types of medical research designs, for example, randomized controlled trials (RCTs) should report in line with the CONSORT statement. Information other than that related to reporting can also be found on the CONSORT website (www.consort-statement.org). Since the gradual expansion of URM scope, the guideline was later renamed as *Recommendations for the Conduct, Reporting, Editing, and Publication of Scholarly Work in Medical Journals.* In the recommendation released in December 2017, the following requirements have been listed.

Reporting guidelines have been developed for different study designs. Examples include the CONSORT statement for RCTs (www.consort-statement.org), the STROBE statement for observational studies (http://strobe-statement.org/), the PRISMA statement for systematic reviews and meta-analyses (http://prisma-state ment.org/), and the STARD statement for diagnostic accuracy studies (www.stard-statement.org/). Journals are encouraged to ask authors to follow these guidelines because they help authors describe the study in enough details for it to be evaluated by editors, reviewers, readers, and other researchers evaluating the medical literature. Authors of review manuscripts are encouraged to describe the methods used for locating, selecting, extracting, and synthesizing data, and such is mandatory for systematic reviews. The EQUATOR Network (www.equator-network.org/home/) and the NLM's Research Reporting Guidelines and Initiatives (www.nlm.nih.gov/services/res earch_report_guide.html) provide resources for reporting guidelines.

17.3. Reporting guidelines for RCT papers — The CONSORT statement and extensions

The lack of adequate reporting fueled the development of the original CONSORT statement in 1996, which describes the evidence-based minimum requirements for reporting RCTs. Its latest version was released in 2010, and its major components are a flow diagram (Figure 17.1) and a 25-item checklist (Table 17.1).

The document *Explanation and Elaboration* provided on the website provides essential explanations on all of the items mentioned in the statement. The checklist should be examined together with the document, as is suggested. Moreover, the CONSORT website provides different extensions of the CONSORT statement for different study designs, interventions, and data types. For example, exclusive extensions are provided for the following study designs: cluster trials, non-inferiority and equivalence trials, pragmatic trials, N-of-1 trials, pilot and feasibility trials, and within person

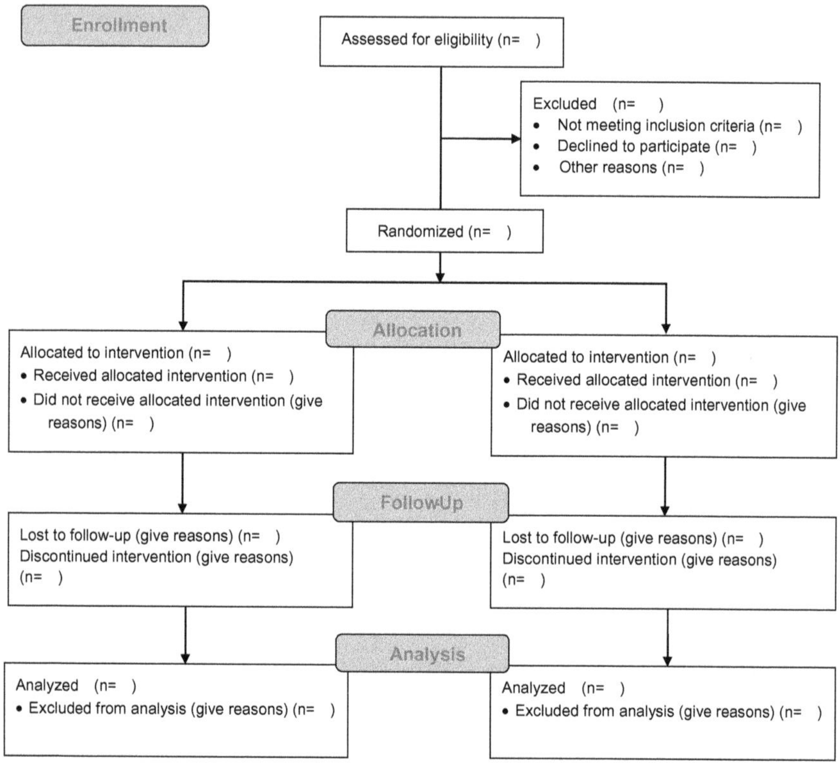

Figure 17.1 CONSORT 2010 flow diagram

trials; for the following interventions: herbal medicinal interventions, non-pharmacological treatment interventions, acupuncture interventions, and Chinese herbal medicine formulas; and for different data types: CONSORT-PRO(patients-reported outcomes), adverse reactions, abstracts etc.

17.4. Statistical reporting guidelines for observational studies — The STROBE statement

In epidemiology research, cohort studies, case-control studies, and cross-sectional studies are categorized as observational studies, which also face the problems of incomplete statistical reporting. Therefore, the STROBE group developed the STROBE statement taking the CONSORT statement as a reference. The main component of

Table 17.1 CONSORT 2010 checklist of information to be included when reporting a RCT

Section/Topic	Item No.	Checklist item	Reported on page No.
Title and abstract			
	1a	Identification as a randomized trial in the title	
	1b	Structured summary of trial design, methods, results, and conclusions (for specific guidance see CONSORT for abstracts)	
Introduction			
Background and objectives	2a	Scientific background and explanation of rationale	
	2b	Specific objectives or hypotheses	
Methods			
Trial design	3a	Description of trial design (such as parallel, factorial) including allocation ratio	
	3b	Important changes to methods after trial commencement (such as eligibility criteria), with reasons	
Participants	4a	Eligibility criteria for participants	
	4b	Settings and locations where the data were collected	
Interventions	5	The interventions for each group with sufficient details to allow replication, including how and when they were actually administered	
Outcomes	6a	Completely defined pre-specified primary and secondary outcome measures, including how and when they were assessed	
	6b	Any changes to trial outcomes after the trial commenced, with reasons	
Sample size	7a	How sample size was determined	
	7b	When applicable, explanation of any interim analyses and stopping guidelines	

(*Continued*)

Table 17.1 (*Continued*)

Section/Topic	Item No.	Checklist item	Reported on page No.
Randomization			
Sequence generation	8a	Method used to generate the random allocation sequence	
	8b	Type of randomization; details of any restriction (such as blocking and block size)	
Allocation concealment mechanism	9	Mechanism used to implement the random allocation sequence (such as sequentially numbered containers), describing any steps taken to conceal the sequence until interventions were assigned	
Implementation	10	Who generated the random allocation sequence, who enrolled participants, and who assigned participants to interventions	
Blinding	11a	If done, who was blinded after assignment to interventions (e.g., participants, care providers, those assessing outcomes) and how	
	11b	If relevant, description of the similarity of interventions	
Statistical methods	12a	Statistical methods used to compare groups for primary and secondary outcomes	
	12b	Methods for additional analyses, such as subgroup analyses and adjusted analyses	
Results			
Participant flow (a diagram is strongly recommended)	13a	For each group, the numbers of participants who were randomly assigned, received intended treatment, and were analyzed for the primary outcome	
	13b	For each group, losses and exclusions after randomization, together with reasons	
Recruitment	14a	Dates defining the periods of recruitment and follow-up	
	14b	Why the trial ended or was stopped	
Baseline data	15	A table showing baseline demographic and clinical characteristics for each group	

Table 17.1 (*Continued*)

Section/Topic	Item No.	Checklist item	Reported on page No.
Numbers analyzed	16	For each group, number of participants (denominator) included in each analysis and whether the analysis was by original assigned groups	
Outcomes and estimation	17a	For each primary and secondary outcome, results for each group, and the estimated effect size and its precision (such as 95% confidence interval)	
	17b	For binary outcomes, presentation of both absolute and relative effect sizes is recommended	
Ancillary analyses	18	Results of any other analyses performed, including subgroup analyses and adjusted analyses, distinguishing pre-specified from exploratory	
Harms	19	All important harms or unintended effects in each group (for specific guidance see CONSORT for harms)	
Discussion			
Limitations	20	Trial limitations, addressing sources of potential bias, imprecision, and, if relevant, multiplicity of analyses	
Generalizability	21	Generalizability (external validity, applicability) of the trial findings	
Interpretation	22	Interpretation consistent with results, balancing benefits and harms, and considering other relevant evidence	
Other information			
Registration	23	Registration number and name of trial registry	
Protocol	24	Where the full trial protocol can be accessed, if available	
Funding	25	Sources of funding and other support (such as supply of drugs), role of funders	

[a]We strongly recommend reading this statement in conjunction with the CONSORT 2010 Explanation and Elaboration for important clarifications on all the items. If relevant, we also recommend reading CONSORT extensions for cluster randomized trials, non-inferiority and equivalence trials, non-pharmacological treatments, herbal interventions, and pragmatic trials. Additional extensions are forthcoming: for those and for up to date references relevant to this checklist, see www.consort-statement.org.

STROBE is a 22-item checklist, 18 items of which are listed for all three types of observational studies and four items for exclusive use in a certain type of study. The STROBE initiative also published a document for explanation and elaboration, which is suggested to be used together with the checklist. The STROBE checklist (version 4, 2004) is presented in Table 17.2 (strobe-statement.org/).

17.5. Standards for reporting diagnostic accuracy studies

Diagnostic accuracy studies can assess the ability of one or more medical diagnostic tests to correctly divide subjects into target groups based on, for example, the presence of illness, the stage of illness, therapeutic effects, adverse events, or prognosis. The ability of medical diagnostic methods to correctly classify patients is usually concluded by comparing with the diagnostic results of a gold standard. The STARD statement was developed to contribute to completeness and transparency in the reporting of diagnostic accuracy studies (2015 edition, Table 17.3).

17.6. Preferred reporting items for systematic reviews and meta-analyses

The international standards for improving the reporting quality of systematic reviews and meta-analyses were based on the results of the Quality of Reporting of Meta-analysis (QUOROM) statement and then refined into the PRISMA statement. Its main components are a 27-item checklist (Table 17.4) and a flowchart (Figure 17.2), accompanied by a document with explanation and elaboration.

17.7. Statistical terms and common symbols

Statistical terms and their abbreviations should be used correctly. Medical papers should not use statistical terms for ordinary meanings. For example, "random" is a standard sampling or grouping

Table 17.2 STROBE statement — Checklist of items that should be included in reports of observational studies

	Item No.	Recommendation
Title and abstract		
	1	(a) Indicate the study's design with a commonly used term in the title or the abstract (b) Provide in the abstract an informative and balanced summary of what was done and what was found
Introduction		
Background/ rationale	2	Explain the scientific background and rationale for the investigation being reported
Objectives	3	State specific objectives, including any pre-specified hypotheses
Methods		
Study design	4	Present key elements of study design early in the paper
Setting	5	Describe the setting, locations, and relevant dates, including periods of recruitment, exposure, follow-up, and data collection
Participants	6	(a) Cohort study — Give the eligibility criteria, and the sources and methods of selection of participants. Describe methods of follow-up Case-control study — Give the eligibility criteria, and the sources and methods of case ascertainment and control selection. Give the rationale for the choice of cases and controls Cross-sectional study — Give the eligibility criteria, and the sources and methods of selection of participants (b) Cohort study — For matched studies, give matching criteria and number of exposed and unexposed Case-control study — For matched studies, give matching criteria and the number of controls per case
Variables	7	Clearly define all outcomes, exposures, predictors, potential confounders, and effect modifiers. Give diagnostic criteria, if applicable

(*Continued*)

Table 17.2 (*Continued*)

	Item No.	Recommendation
Data sources/ measurement	8[a]	For each variable of interest, give sources of data and details of methods of assessment (measurement). Describe comparability of assessment methods if there is more than one group
Bias	9	Describe any efforts to address potential sources of bias
Study size	10	Explain how the study size was arrived at
Quantitative variables	11	Explain how quantitative variables were handled in the analyses. If applicable, describe which groupings were chosen and why
Statistical methods	12	(a) Describe all statistical methods, including those used to control for confounding (b) Describe any methods used to examine subgroups and interactions (c) Explain how missing data were addressed (d) Cohort study — If applicable, explain how loss to follow-up was addressed Case-control study — If applicable, explain how matching of cases and controls was addressed Cross-sectional study — If applicable, describe analytical methods taking account of sampling strategy (e) Describe any sensitivity analyses
Results		
Participants	13[a]	(a) Report numbers of individuals at each stage of study — e.g., numbers potentially eligible, examined for eligibility, confirmed eligible, included in the study, completing follow-up, and analyzed (b) Give reasons for non-participation at each stage (c) Consider use of a flow diagram
Descriptive data	14[a]	(a) Give characteristics of study participants (e.g., demographic, clinical, social) and information on exposures and potential confounders (b) Indicate number of participants with missing data for each variable of interest (c) Cohort study — Summarize follow-up time (e.g., average and total amount)

Table 17.2 (*Continued*)

	Item No.	Recommendation
Outcome data	15[a]	Cohort study — Report numbers of outcome events or summary measures over time Case-control study — Report numbers in each exposure category, or summary measures of exposure Cross-sectional study — Report numbers of outcome events or summary measures
Main results	16	(a) Give unadjusted estimates and, if applicable, confounder-adjusted estimates and their precision (e.g., 95% confidence interval). Make clear which confounders were adjusted and why they were included (b) Report category boundaries when continuous variables were categorized (c) If relevant, consider translating estimates of relative risk into absolute risk for a meaningful time period
Other analyses	17	Report other analyses done — e.g., analyses of subgroups and interactions, and sensitivity analyses
Discussion		
Key results	18	Summarize the key results with reference to study objectives
Limitations	19	Discuss the limitations of the study, taking into account sources of potential bias or imprecision. Discuss both direction and magnitude of any potential bias
Interpretation	20	Give a cautious overall interpretation of results considering objectives, limitations, multiplicity of analyses, results from similar studies, and other relevant evidence
Generalizability	21	Discuss the generalizability (external validity) of the study results
Other information		
Funding	22	Give the source of funding and the role of the funders for the present study and, if applicable, for the original study on which the present article is based

[a]Give information separately for cases and controls in case-control studies and, if applicable, for exposed and unexposed groups in cohort and cross-sectional studies.

Table 17.3 STARD 2015 checklist

Section and topic	No	Item	Reported on page #
Title or abstract			
	1	Identification as a study of diagnostic accuracy using at least one measure of accuracy (such as sensitivity, specificity, predictive values, or AUC)	
Abstract			
	2	Structured summary of study design, methods, results, and conclusions (for specific guidance, see STARD for Abstracts)	
Introduction			
	3	Scientific and clinical background, including the intended use and clinical role of the index test	
	4	Study objectives and hypotheses	
Methods			
Study design	5	Whether data collection was planned before the index test and reference standard were performed (prospective study) or after (retrospective study)	
Participants	6	Eligibility criteria	
	7	On what basis potentially eligible participants were identified (such as symptoms, results from previous tests, inclusion in registry)	
	8	Where and when potentially eligible participants were identified (setting, location and dates)	
	9	Whether participants formed a consecutive, random or convenience series	

Table 17.3 (*Continued*)

Section and topic	No	Item	Reported on page #
Test methods	10a	Index test, in sufficient detail to allow replication	
	10b	Reference standard, in sufficient detail to allow replication	
	11	Rationale for choosing the reference standard (if alternatives exist)	
	12a	Definition of and rationale for test positivity cut-offs or result categories of the index test, distinguishing pre-specified from exploratory	
	12b	Definition of and rationale for test positivity cut-offs or result categories of the reference standard, distinguishing pre-specified from exploratory	
	13a	Whether clinical information and reference standard results were available to the performers/readers of the index test	
	13b	Whether clinical information and index test results were available to the assessors of the reference standard	
Analysis	14	Methods for estimating or comparing measures of diagnostic accuracy	
	15	How indeterminate index test or reference standard results were handled	
	16	How missing data on the index test and reference standard were handled	
	17	Any analyses of variability in diagnostic accuracy, distinguishing pre-specified from exploratory	
	18	Intended sample size and how it was determined	
Results			
Participants	19	Flow of participants, using a diagram	
	20	Baseline demographic and clinical characteristics of participants	
	21a	Distribution of severity of disease in those with the target condition	
	21b	Distribution of alternative diagnoses in those without the target condition	
	22	Time interval and any clinical interventions between index test and reference standard	

(*Continued*)

Table 17.3 (*Continued*)

Section and topic	No	Item	Reported on page #
Test results	23	Cross tabulation of the index test results (or their distribution) by the results of the reference standard	
	24	Estimates of diagnostic accuracy and their precision (such as 95% confidence intervals)	
	25	Any adverse events from performing the index test or the reference standard	
Discussion			
	26	Study limitations, including sources of potential bias, statistical uncertainty, and generalizability	
	27	Implications for practice, including the intended use and clinical role of the index test	
Other information			
	28	Registration number and name of registry	
	29	Where the full study protocol can be accessed	
	30	Sources of funding and other support; role of funders	

Table 17.4 PRISMA 2009 checklist

Section/Topic	Item	Checklist item	Reported on page #
TITLE			
Title	1	Identify the report as a systematic review, meta-analysis, or both.	
ABSTRACT			
Structured summary	2	Provide a structured summary including, as applicable: background; objectives; data sources; study eligibility criteria, participants, and interventions; study appraisal and synthesis methods; results; limitations; conclusions and implications of key findings; systematic review registration number.	
INTRODUCTION			
Rationale	3	Describe the rationale for the review in the context of what is already known.	
Objectives	4	Provide an explicit statement of questions being addressed with reference to participants, interventions, comparisons, outcomes, and study design (PICOS).	
METHODS			
Protocol and registration	5	Indicate if a review protocol exists, if and where it can be accessed (e.g., Web address), and, if available, provide registration information including registration number.	
Eligibility criteria	6	Specify study characteristics (e.g., PICOS, length of follow-up) and report characteristics (e.g., years considered, language, publication status) used as criteria for eligibility, giving rationale.	
Information sources	7	Describe all information sources (e.g., databases with dates of coverage, contact with study authors to identify additional studies) in the search and date last searched.	

(*Continued*)

Table 17.4 (*Continued*)

Section/Topic	Item	Checklist item	Reported on page #
Search	8	Present full electronic search strategy for at least one database, including any limits used, such that it could be repeated.	
Study selection	9	State the process for selecting studies (i.e., screening, eligibility, included in systematic review, and, if applicable, included in the meta-analysis).	
Data collection process	10	Describe the method of data extraction from reports (e.g., piloted forms, independently, in duplicate) and any processes for obtaining and confirming data from investigators.	
Data items	11	List and define all variables for which data were sought (e.g., PICOS, funding sources) and any assumptions and simplifications made.	
Risk of bias in individual studies	12	Describe the methods used for assessing risk of bias of individual studies (including specification of whether this was done at the study or outcome level), and how this information is to be used in any data synthesis.	
Summary measures	13	State the principal summary measures (e.g., risk ratio, difference in means).	
Synthesis of results	14	Describe the methods of handling data and combining results of studies, if done, including measures of consistency (e.g., I^2) for each meta-analysis.	
Risk of bias across studies	15	Specify any assessment of risk of bias that may affect the cumulative evidence (e.g., publication bias, selective reporting within studies).	
Additional analyses	16	Describe methods of additional analyses (e.g., sensitivity or subgroup analyses, meta-regression), if done, indicating which were pre-specified.	
RESULTS			
Study selection	17	Give numbers of studies screened, assessed for eligibility, and included in the review, with reasons for exclusions at each stage, ideally with a flow diagram.	

Table 17.4 (*Continued*)

Section/Topic	Item	Checklist item	Reported on page #
Study characteristics	18	For each study, present characteristics for which data were extracted (e.g., study size, PICOS, follow-up period) and provide the citations.	
Risk of bias within studies	19	Present data on risk of bias of each study and, if available, any outcome level assessment (see item 12).	
Results of individual studies	20	For all outcomes considered (benefits or harms), present, for each study: (a) simple summary data for each intervention group (b) effect estimates and confidence intervals, ideally with a forest plot.	
Synthesis of results	21	Present results of each meta-analysis done, including confidence intervals and measures of heterogeneity.	
Risk of bias across studies	22	Present results of any assessment of risk of bias across studies (see Item 15).	
Additional analysis	23	Give results of additional analyses, if done (e.g., sensitivity or subgroup analyses, meta-regression [see Item 16]).	
DISCUSSION			
Summary of evidence	24	Summarize the main findings including the strength of evidence for each main outcome; consider their relevance to key groups (e.g., healthcare providers, users, and policymakers).	
Limitations	25	Discuss limitations at study and outcome level (e.g., risk of bias), and at review-level (e.g., incomplete retrieval of identified research, reporting bias).	
Conclusions	26	Provide a general interpretation of the results in the context of other evidence, and implications for future research.	
FUNDING			
Funding	27	Describe sources of funding for the systematic review and other support (e.g., supply of data); role of funders for the systematic review.	

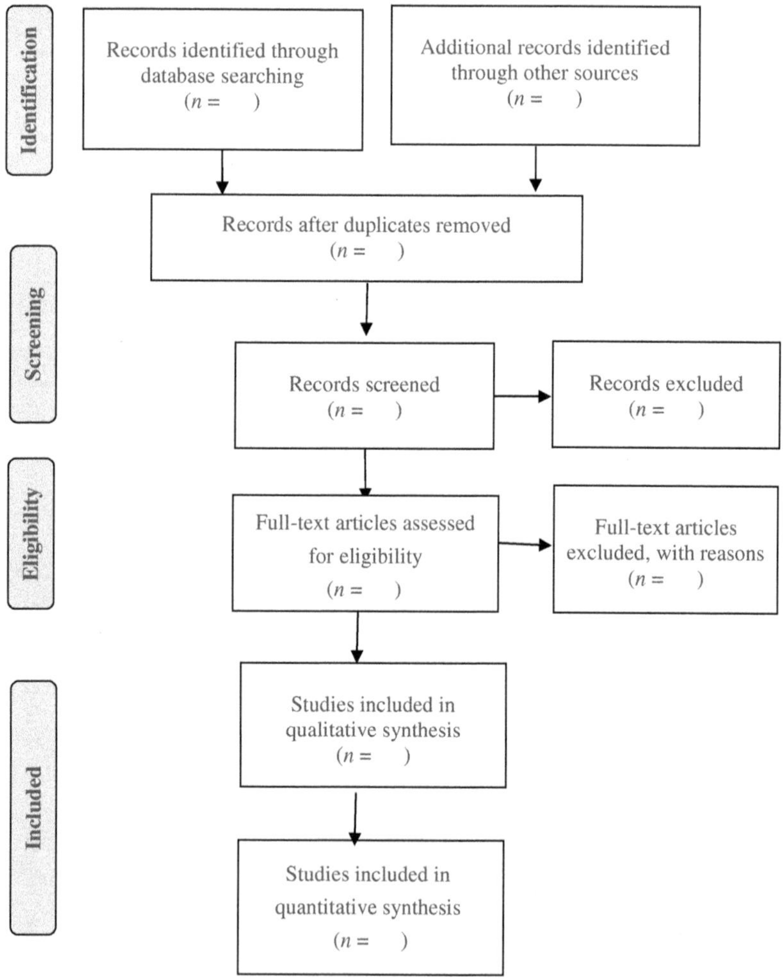

Figure 17.2 PRISMA 2009 flow diagram

method, which should not be used to mean "optional." "Normal distribution" is a bell-shaped distribution that satisfies special mathematics requirements; it's incorrect to refer to all bell-shaped distributions as normal distribution. "Correlation" refers to the statistical term for the degree of closeness between two variables, which cannot be confused with "relation." Some non-statistical subjective words, such as "good tolerance," should be used only for qualitative summary and not to characterize the measurement results.

Statistical symbols are generally the italicized forms of single Latin or Greek alphabetical symbols, representing the parameters, probability functions, or variables. For example, the use of uppercase italics such as N represents the population size, $P(A)$ represents the probability of an event A, and S^2 represents the sample variance (as a vector). Further, the variable values are mostly denoted in lowercase italics and represent the sample statistics, such as $\bar{X}$, s (as a specific value), n, r, α, and p. A decorative plus can be used in the lower right corner to add a note, such as n_1, n_{control}, and r_{xy}; it is commonly used in formulas and charts. The symbols for statistical software output were often abbreviated in terms, so for convenience, they have now been converted to statistical symbols for use in formulas and charts. China published the national standards for statistical vocabulary and symbols (replacing the standards set in 1993) based on ISO 3534-1:2006, which was required to be implemented in 2010. The commonly used statistical symbols are listed in Table 17.5 for reference.

In medical papers, the expression "$a \pm b$" is common, but it has many meanings and the exact meaning should be clarified to avoid ambiguity. In general, if it appears in a table, it must state its specific meaning, such as $\bar{X} \pm S$ or $\bar{X} \pm S_{\bar{X}}$, in the upper right corner of the table or in the table note section. In the text, the expression "average age of $a \pm b$ years" is common but incorrect. The same variable can have only one meaning in the same sample; therefore, the above expression should be revised to "average age of a $(S = b)$ years."

17.8. Results reporting

The reporting requirements for the statistical content of medical papers are closely related to the type of research design. Each type of paper has a different set of requirements. Please refer to the relevant format and requirements when writing a paper. Table 17.6 is an example of a report extracted from CONSORT.

Table 17.5 Common statistical symbols

Symbols	Technical terms	Symbols	Technical terms
$X, Y \ldots$	Random variable	$x, y \ldots$	Observed value of the variable
$P(A)$	Probability of an event A	p	Probability
$F(X)$	Distribution function	$f(X)$	Probability density function
$F, t, \chi^2 \ldots$	Distribution variables or numeric values such as $F, t, \chi^2 \ldots$	$Z(z)$	Standard normal variable (variable value)
$N(n)$	Population size (sample size)	ν	Degrees of freedom, *df*
$\bar{X}$	Arithmetic mean of the sample (variable)	$\bar{x}$	Arithmetic mean of the sample (value)
$E(X), \mu$	Expectation of the random variable X	X_p	p-Quartile of the random variable X
R	Range of the sample	k	Dimension
σ^2	Population variance	$S^2(s^2)$	Sample variance (specific value)
$\sigma_{\hat{\theta}}$	Standard error of the mean	$\sigma_{\bar{X}}$	Standard error of the mean
α	Significance level, probability of type I error	β	Probability of type II error
ρ	Population correlation coefficient	r	Sample correlation coefficient
$\hat{\theta}$	Estimate of the parameter θ	$\hat{Y}$	Estimate of the statistic Y (e.g., in regression analysis)

17.9. Case analysis

Case 17.1 Paper entitled "Small-dose contrast agent and feasibility study of special position in 320-slice CT angiography." The text was as follows (the introduction, discussion, and literature have been omitted). Please find the deficiencies or errors in the statistical report.

Table 17.6 Example of an RCT report

Report item	Example for reporting
Purpose and hypothesis	In the current study, we tested the hypothesis that a policy of active management of nulliparous labor would 1. reduce the rate of cesarean delivery; 2. reduce the rate of prolonged labor; and 3. not influence maternal satisfaction with the birth experience.
Test design	This was a multicenter, stratified (into groups of 6–11-year-old and 12–17-year-old children, with unbalanced randomization [2:1]), double-blind, placebo-controlled, parallel-group study conducted in the United States (41 sites).
Background and location of data collection	The study was conducted at the antiretroviral therapy clinic of Queen Elizabeth Central Hospital in Blantyre, Malawi from January 2006 to April 2007. Blantyre is the major commercial city of Malawi, with a population of 1 000 000 and an estimated HIV prevalence of 27% in adults in 2004.
Outcome indicator	The primary endpoint with respect to efficacy in psoriasis was the proportion of patients achieving a 75% improvement in psoriasis activity from baseline to 12 weeks as measured by the psoriasis area and severity index (PASI). Additional analyses were performed to determine the percentage change in PASI scores and improvement in target psoriasis lesions.
Sample size	To detect a reduction of 3 days (SD, 5 days) in post-operative hospital stay (PHS), based on the study of Lobo *et al.* with a two-sided significance level of 5% and a power of 80%, a sample size of 50 patients per group was considered as necessary, given an anticipated dropout rate of 10%. To recruit this number of patients, a 12-month inclusion period was anticipated.
Generation of random sequences	Independent pharmacists dispensed active or placebo inhalers in accordance with a computer-generated randomization list.
Restriction of random methods	Randomization sequence was created using Stata 9.0 statistical software and was stratified by center with a 1:1 allocation using random block sizes of 2, 4, and 6.
Allocation concealment mechanism	Doxycycline and placebo were in capsule form and identical in appearance. They were pre-packed in bottles and consecutively numbered for each woman according to the randomization schedule. Each woman was assigned an order number and received the capsules in the corresponding pre-packed bottle.

(*Continued*)

Table 17.6 (*Continued*)

Report item	Example for reporting
Random implementation	Determination of whether a patient would be treated by streptomycin and bed rest (S case) or by bed rest alone (C case) was made by reference to a statistical series based on random sampling numbers drawn up for each sex at each center by Professor Bradford Hill; the details of the series were unknown to all of the investigators and the coordinator. After acceptance of a patient by the panel and before admission to the streptomycin center, the appropriate numbered envelope was opened at the central office; the card inside specified whether the patient was to be an S or a C case. This information was then given to the medical officer of the center.
Blinding	Blinding and equipoise were strictly maintained by emphasizing to intervention staff and participants that each diet adheres to healthy principles and that each of them is advocated by certain experts to be superior for long-term weight-loss. Except for the interventionists (dieticians and behavioral psychologists), investigators and staff were kept blind to diet assignment of the participants. The trial adhered to established procedures to maintain separation between staff that took outcome measurements and staff that delivered the intervention. Staff members who obtained outcome measurements were not informed of the diet group assignment. Intervention staff, dieticians, and behavioral psychologists who delivered the intervention did not take outcome measurements. All investigators, staff, and participants were kept masked to outcome measurements and trial results.
Statistical methods	The primary endpoint was change in body weight during the 20 weeks of the study in the intention-to-treat population. Secondary efficacy endpoints included change in the waist circumference, systolic and diastolic blood pressure, and prevalence of metabolic syndrome. We used analysis of covariance (ANCOVA) for analyzing the primary endpoint and the secondary endpoints waist circumference, blood pressure, and patient-reported outcome scores; this was supplemented by a repeated measures analysis. The ANCOVA model included treatment, country, and sex as fixed effects and body weight at randomization as a covariate. We aimed to assess whether data provided the evidence of superiority of each liraglutide dose over placebo (primary objective) and orlistat (secondary objective).

Table 17.6 (*Continued*)

Report item	Example for reporting
Cases included in the analysis	One patient in the alendronate group was lost to follow-up; thus, data from 31 patients were available for the intention-to-treat analysis. Five patients were considered protocol violators. Consequently, 26 patients remained for the per-protocol analyses.
Endings and estimates	[Table(s) or Figure(s) are strongly recommended. In addition to measured values of outcome, differences or ratios and their estimated effects, such as RR and its 95% CI, are needed.]
Auxiliary analysis	Based on a study that suggested that perioperative β-blocker efficacy might vary across baseline risk, we pre-specified our primary subgroup analysis according to the revised cardiac risk index scoring system. We also pre-specified secondary subgroup analyses based on sex, type of surgery, and use of an epidural or spinal anesthetic. For all subgroup analyses, we used Cox proportional hazard models that incorporated tests for interactions, and the results were designated to be significant at $P < 0.05$. Figure 3 shows the results of our pre-specified subgroup analyses and indicates consistency of effects. Our subgroup analyses were underpowered to detect the modest differences in subgroup effects that one might expect to detect if there was a true subgroup effect.
Scope of application	As the intervention was implemented for both sexes, all ages, all types of sports, and at different levels of sports, the results indicated that the entire range of athletes, from young elite to intermediate and recreational senior athletes, would benefit from using the presented training program for the prevention of ankle sprain recurrence. By including non-medically treated and medically treated athletes, we covered a broad spectrum of injury severity, which suggests that the presented training program can be implemented for treating all athletes. Furthermore, as it is reasonable to assume that ankle sprains not related to sports are comparable to those related to sports, the program could benefit the general population.

1. Background information

Sixty patients with carotid plaque who underwent carotid artery angiography, dissection, stenosis, or occlusion in the neurology department from June 2016 to October 2017 were randomly divided into G1 and G2 groups (30 cases in each group). The G1 group included 24 males and 6 females aged 45–78 years. Their mean age and body weight were 52 ± 12.3 years and 60.72 ± 6.85 kg, respectively. The G1 group... Exclusion criteria... The G1 group was a regular body group, and the G2 group was a special body group. Regular position... Special position...

1.1. Subjective evaluation

Subjective evaluation of VR, CPR, and MIP image quality of carotid artery was performed using the double-blind method by two senior radiologists with experience in the diagnosis of vascular diseases. A consistency analysis was performed by two senior radiologists, and the result was subject to agreement. The rating criteria were as follows...

1.2. Statistical analysis

The vertebral artery and ... CT values of measured arteries were expressed as mean ± standard deviation ($\bar{x} \pm s$), and t-test was used for comparison between the two groups. First, the age, body weight, and CT values of each artery of patients were tested for normality, and only the data that followed normal distribution were then subjected to two independent sample t-tests. The data analysis was performed using SPSS 19.0.

2. Results

2.1. Participant characteristics

All 60 patients successfully completed the examination without any adverse reaction or contrast agent extravasation. The G1 group included 24 males and 6 females aged 45–78 years. Their mean age and body weight were 52 ± 12.3 years and 65.72 ± 6.85 kg, respectively. The G2 group... No significant difference was observed in age, body weight, and contrast agent dosage (42.82 ± 6.78 mL vs. 38.72 ± 9.12 mL) between the two groups ($P > 0.05$).

2.2. Subjective evaluation of images

The carotid CTA images of both the G1 and G2 patients could meet diagnostic needs. In the G1 group, the subjective image quality was rated 1 point in 18 cases, 2 points in 10 cases, and 3 points in 2 cases. In the G2 group, the image quality was rated 1 point in 3 cases, 2 points in 7 cases, and 3 points in 20 cases [Figure 3 (omitted)]. The difference in the subjective scores between the G1 and G2 groups was statistically significant (1.5 ± 0.81 vs. 3.93 ± 0.59, $P < 0.05$).

2.3. Comparison of transluminal CT values of each artery between the G1 and G2 groups (see Table 17.7 for details)

Table 17.7 Comparison of CT values of each artery between the two groups ($\bar{\chi} \pm$ s, HU)

Group	Aortic arch	Left common carotid artery	Right common carotid artery	Left internal carotid artery	....
G1	389.33 ± 36.84	360.72 ± 38.44	362.88 ± 33.18	344.65 ± 33.68	
G2	379.64 ± 39.33	387.32 ± 42.17	379.32 ± 43.31	348.62 ± 42.95	
P value	>0.05	>0.05	>0.05	>0.05	

17.10. Computer experiment (see electronic data Exp 17-1 for details)

Experiment 17.1 Please use EXCEL to verify the t value and the exact P value for the data table.

17.11. Frequently asked questions and summary

17.11.1. *Frequently asked questions*

In some publications, the reporting form for the mean and standard deviation is "$a \pm b$," for example, 35 ± 2 mm. When the upper and lower deviations are not equal, write them in the right upper and lower corners, respectively, for example, $35^{+2}_{-1}{}^\circ$C.

The meaning of "deviation" in the editorial publishing tutorial differs from that of the "deviation" of statistics. The former refers to the accuracy or controllable range of instrument measurement, which is the systematic error, and the latter is the deviation of a batch of samples caused by a sampling error, which may be "standard deviation" or "standard error." There are many meanings of the $a \pm b$ expression in medical papers, most of which are "$\bar{X} \pm S$" and a few of them are "$\bar{X} \pm S_{\bar{X}}$." Occasionally, the 95% reference range is expressed as "$\bar{X} \pm 1.96S$," etc., indicating that there are very few systematic deviations; thus, the meaning of the data on both sides of "$\pm$" must be explained. In general, if all data forms are identical in the table, the meaning of the $a \pm b$ form, such as $\bar{X} \pm S$, can be added in the upper right corner of the table. However, in the manuscript text, the description of age as, for example, 35 ± 10 years ($\bar{X} \pm S$) is not as concise and appropriate as "average age of 35 ($S = 10$) years."

17.11.2. *Summary*

This chapter first introduced the purpose and function of statistical reporting in a standard medical paper and then introduced the general statistical requirements of medical papers and the ICMJE recommendations on writing medical paper statistics. The chapter focused on several related standards, namely the CONSORT statement and individual extensions for RCTs, the STROBE statement for observational studies, the STARD statement for diagnostic accuracy studies, and the PRISMA statement for systematic reviews and meta-analyses. Subsequently, the national standards for statistical symbols were introduced. Finally, some specific examples of statistical report projects and case studies were provided. Please pay attention to the common problems.

Think and Practice

1. Please indicate errors or deficiencies in the following common expressions and explain the reasons and correct them.
   (1) We studied 53 patients with thyroid cancer admitted to our hospital from 2004 to 2006, including 30 males and 23 females

with an average age of 55 ± 12 years, according to TNM classification.

(2) The t-test revealed a very obvious difference in the number of white blood cells between the drug group and the drug-free group ($t = 2.85$, $P < 0.001$). This finding indicated that the number of white blood cells can be increased by medication.

(3) We compared plasmin activities between nine patients with severe hepatitis and eight patients with liver cancer. Analysis of variance revealed no significant difference between the two groups ($P = 0.09$), indicating that the plasmin activities in patients with hepatitis and liver cancer were consistent.

(4) We compared the blood glucose, insulin, and cholesterol levels among patients with normal blood glucose levels, impaired glucose tolerance, and type 2 diabetes. Analysis of variance revealed significant differences in the blood glucose, insulin, and cholesterol levels among the three groups ($P < 0.05$), and the prevalence of fatty liver in the three groups also showed an increasing trend. The results of chi-square test demonstrated that the prevalence of fatty liver was positively correlated with the blood glucose, insulin, and cholesterol levels ($P < 0.05$).

(5) Some studies investigated 1000 inpatients. The results showed that of the 1000 patients, 55 had cerebral hemorrhage and 45 had cerebral ischemia, indicating that the incidence of cerebral hemorrhage in the hospital was 5.5% and that of cerebral ischemia was 4.5%, which was much higher than the 0.7% incidence reported in the literature.

2. Please use Excel to design a template for calculating the P value of chi-square test.

Jing Gu, Qinghai Liu, Jiqian Fang

Part III

Frequently Used Powerful Statistical Methods

CHAPTER 18

ANALYSIS OF VARIANCE FOR COMPLICATED DESIGNS

Completely randomized design conceptually belongs to one-factor design, which is insufficient to consider multiple factors in real-life studies. When two or more factors are involved, a more complex design should be used based on specific aims of the research. In Chapter 12, principles of some more complex designs were introduced, including randomized block design, crossover design, factorial design, and repeated measurement design. In this chapter, we will illustrate the analysis of variance (ANOVA) using data from studies with these designs.

18.1. ANOVA for randomized block design

Example 18.1. To compare the effects of five types of disinfectants (A, B, C, D, E) on inhibiting bacteria, four species of bacteria were cultivated in five dishes under the same condition. The dishes were then randomly treated with one of the disinfectants. The diameter of inhibition zone was measured as an indicator of effect. The experimental results are shown in Table 18.1. Please analyze whether there is any difference in the antibacterial effects among the five kinds of disinfectants.

Example 18.1 is an experiment with randomized block design (RBD). The block factor (Bacteria) has four levels (E. coli, Pseudomonas, Staphylococcus, Shigella dysenteriae) while the treatment

Table 18.1 Antibacterial experiment results of five kinds of disinfectant — Inhibition zone diameter (mm)

	Bacteria					
Disinfectants	E.coli	Pseudomonas	Staphylococcus	Shigella dysenteriae	$\sum_{j=1}^{b} x_{ij}$	$\bar{X}_{i\cdot}$
A	15	11	25	20	71	17.75
B	17	12	28	17	74	18.50
C	15	14	25	19	73	18.25
D	14	13	30	13	70	17.50
E	12	9	20	11	52	13.00
$\sum_{i=1}^{k} x_{ij}$	73	59	128	80	340 $\left(\sum_{i=1}^{k}\sum_{j=1}^{b} x_{ij}\right)$	
$\bar{X}_{\cdot j}$	14.60	11.80	25.60	16.00		17.00 ($\bar{X}$)

factor (Disinfectants) has five levels (A, B, C, D, E). Each strain of the bacterium was cultured in five dishes under the same conditions, which formed a block; hence, there were four blocks for the four strains of bacteria. Then, five culture dishes of the same block were randomly assigned to five treatment groups of A, B, C, D, and E. In the analysis of variance, the total variability can be decomposed into three parts: the variability between the five treatment groups of the disinfectant, the variability between the four blocks of the bacterial strains, and the variability of random error.

18.1.1. *Decomposition of the sum of squares and degrees of freedom*

To easily explain this design with the formulas and denotations, the observations from the randomized block design can be organized as presented in Table 18.2, where the observation of the subject of the jth block in the ith treatment group is denoted by $x_{ij}(i = 1, 2, \ldots k; j = 1, 2, \ldots b)$. The total number of observations is denoted by N where $N = bk$.

Table 18.2 Experiment results of randomized block design

Treatment groups	Blocks							
	1	2	$\cdots$	j	$\cdots$	b	$\sum_{j=1}^{b} x_{ij}$	$\bar{X}_{i\cdot}$
1	x_{11}	x_{12}	$\cdots$	x_{1j}		x_{1b}	$\sum_{j=1}^{b} x_{1j}$	$\bar{X}_{1\cdot}$
2	x_{21}	x_{22}	$\cdots$	x_{2j}		x_{2b}	$\sum_{j=1}^{b} x_{2j}$	$\bar{X}_{2\cdot}$
$\cdots$	$\cdots$	$\cdots$	$\cdots$	$\cdots$	$\cdots$	$\cdots$	$\cdots$	$\cdots$
i	x_{i1}	x_{i2}		x_{ij}		x_{ib}	$\sum_{j=1}^{b} x_{ij}$	$\bar{X}_{i\cdot}$
$\cdots$	$\cdots$	$\cdots$	$\cdots$	$\cdots$	$\cdots$	$\cdots$	$\cdots$	$\cdots$
k	x_{k1}	x_{k2}	$\cdots$	x_{kj}	$\cdots$	x_{kb}	$\sum_{j=1}^{b} x_{kj}$	$\bar{X}_{k\cdot}$
$\sum_{i=1}^{k} x_{ij}$	$\sum_{i=1}^{k} x_{i1}$	$\sum_{i=1}^{k} x_{i2}$	$\cdots$	$\sum_{i=1}^{k} x_{ij}$	$\cdots$	$\sum_{i=1}^{k} x_{ib}$	$\sum_{i=1}^{k}\sum_{j=1}^{b} x_{ij}$	—
$\bar{X}_{\cdot j}$	$\bar{X}_{\cdot 1}$	$\bar{X}_{\cdot 2}$	$\cdots$	$\bar{X}_{\cdot j}$	$\cdots$	$\bar{X}_{\cdot b}$	—	$\bar{X}$

The overall mean, mean of the ith treatment group, and mean of the jth block are respectively shown as:

$$\bar{X} = \frac{\sum_{i=1}^{k}\sum_{j=1}^{b} x_{ij}}{N}, \quad \bar{X}_i = \frac{\sum_{j=1}^{b} x_{ij}}{b}, \quad \bar{X}_j = \frac{\sum_{i=1}^{k} x_{ij}}{k}$$

The deviation from the overall mean of each observation, $x_{ij} - \bar{X}$, can be decomposed as follows

$$x_{ij} - \bar{X} = (\bar{X}_{i.} - \bar{X}) + (\bar{X}_{.j} - \bar{X}) + (x_{ij} - \bar{X}_{.j} - \bar{X}_{i.} + \bar{X}) \quad (18\text{-}1)$$

Summing the squared deviations from the mean of all individual observations, we get:

$$\sum_{i=1}^{k}\sum_{j=1}^{b}(x_{ij} - \bar{X})^2 = \sum_{i=1}^{k} b(\bar{X}_{i.} - \bar{X})^2 + \sum_{j=1}^{b} k(\bar{X}_{.j} - \bar{X})^2 + \sum_{i=1}^{k}\sum_{j=1}^{b}(x_{ij} - \bar{X}_{i.} - \bar{X}_{.j} + \bar{X})^2 \quad (18\text{-}2)$$

The left side of the formula (18-2) is the total sum of squares denoted by SS_{Total}, and the three terms on the right-hand side are denoted by $SS_{\text{Treatment}}$, SS_{Block} and SS_{Error}, respectively. Thus, equation (18-2) can be expressed as

$$SS_{\text{Total}} = SS_{\text{Treatment}} + SS_{\text{Block}} + SS_{\text{Error}} \quad (18\text{-}3)$$

The corresponding degrees of freedom are as follows:

$$\begin{aligned} v_{\text{Total}} &= N - 1, v_{\text{Treatment}} = k - 1, v_{\text{Block}} = b - 1, \\ v_{\text{Error}} &= (k-1)(b-1) \\ v_{\text{Total}} &= v_{\text{Treatment}} + v_{\text{Block}} + v_{\text{Error}} \end{aligned} \quad (18\text{-}4)$$

The null hypothesis and the alternative hypothesis to test whether the experimental effects of k treatment groups being equal are as follows:

H_0: $\mu_{1\cdot} = \mu_{2\cdot} = \cdots = \mu_{k\cdot}$ (There is no treatment effect),
H_1: At least two of the k group means are not the same (There is treatment effect).

Table 18.3 Formula for ANOVA of randomized block design data

Variation	SS	ν	MS	F
Total	$\sum_{i=1}^{k}\sum_{j=1}^{b}(X_{ij}-\bar{X})^2$	$N-1$		
Treatment	$\sum_{i=1}^{k} b(\bar{X}_{i\cdot}-\bar{X})^2$	$k-1$	$\frac{SS_{\text{Treatment}}}{\nu_{\text{Treatment}}}$	$\frac{MS_{\text{Treatment}}}{MS_{\text{Error}}}$
Block	$\sum_{j=1}^{b} k(\bar{X}_{\cdot j}-\bar{X})^2$	$b-1$	$\frac{SS_{\text{Block}}}{\nu_{\text{Block}}}$	$\frac{MS_{\text{Block}}}{MS_{\text{Error}}}$
Error	$SS_{\text{Total}}-SS_{\text{Treatment}}-SS_{\text{Block}}$	$(k-1)(b-1)$	$\frac{SS_{\text{Error}}}{\nu_{\text{Error}}}$	

Under H_0, the differences among treatment groups can be attributed to the sampling error. Then, the mean square of between-treatment-groups, $MS_{\text{Treatment}}$, is the unbiased estimator of population variance σ^2, that is, its expected value $E(MS_{\text{Treatment}}) = \sigma^2$. Therefore, $MS_{\text{Treatment}}/MS_{\text{Error}}$ should follow $F_{k-1,(k-1)(b-1)}$ distribution, and $F = MS_{\text{Treatment}}/MS_{\text{Error}}$ can be treated as the test statistic.

Similarly, the F test can also be used to determine whether the population mean among the blocks are equal i.e. there is no block effect, with the test statistic defined as $F = MS_{\text{Block}}/MS_{\text{Error}}$. The corresponding ANOVA for the randomized block design is shown in Table 18.3.

18.1.2. *Solution*

The following is the complete process of ANOVA for the data of Example 18.1.

H_{10}: $\mu_{1\cdot} = \mu_{2\cdot} = \mu_{3\cdot} = \mu_{4\cdot} = \mu_{5\cdot}$, The population means of the inhibition zone diameters for the five treatment groups are all equal (the antibacterial effects of the five disinfectants are the same).

H_{11}: At least one pair of the population means of the five treatment groups are not equal.

Table 18.4 The results of ANOVA for the data of Example 18.1

Variation	SS	ν	MS	F	P
Total	684.00	19			
Treatment	82.50	4	20.63	3.95	0.029
Block	538.80	3	179.60	34.37	<0.001
Error	62.70	12	5.23		

H_{20}: $\mu_{\cdot 1} = \mu_{\cdot 2} = \mu_{\cdot 3} = \mu_{\cdot 4}$, The population means of the inhibition zone diameters for the four blocks are all equal (four strains of bacteria are identically sensitive to any disinfectant).

H_{21}: At least one pair of the population means of the four blocks are not equal.

The significant levels of the two pairs of hypotheses above are both set as $\alpha = 0.05$.

The calculation was conducted according to formulas presented in Table 18.3, and the results are shown in Table 18.4. For the test on the treatment factor, we get $P = 0.029$, which means that H_{10} should be rejected and H_{11} can be accepted under the significance level of 0.05. The conclusion was that the antibacterial effects of five kinds of disinfectants were not all the same. For the test on block factor, the P value was less than 0.001, so that H_{20} was rejected and H_{21} was accepted. The conclusion was that the four strains of bacteria were not all equally sensitive to the same disinfectant.

18.1.3. *Homogeneity test of variance*

The residual plots can be used to visualize whether the data of randomized block design satisfy the prerequisites of ANOVA. Based on formula 18-1, the residual of the observation $x_{ij}$is

$$e_{ij} = x_{ij} - \bar{X}_{i.} - \bar{X}_{.j} + \bar{X}_{ij} \qquad (18\text{-}5)$$

Residuals of the observations in Table 18.1 are displayed in Table 18.5. The scatter plots of residuals with treatment groups, blocks, and individual predicted values are displayed in Figures 18.1

Table 18.5 Residuals of bacteriostatic test results of five disinfectants (mm)

	Bacteria			
Disinfectants	E.coli	Pseudomonas	Staphylococcus	Shigella dysenteriae
A	−0.35	−1.55	−1.35	3.25
B	0.90	−1.30	0.90	−0.50
C	−0.85	0.95	−1.85	1.75
D	−1.10	0.70	3.90	−3.50
E	1.40	1.20	−1.60	−1.00

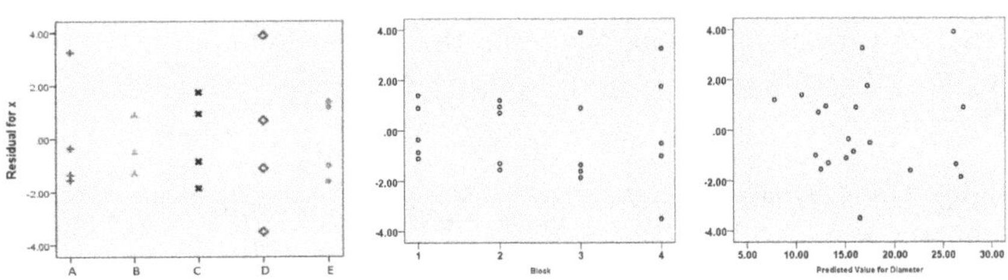

(A) Treatments (B) Blocks (C) Predicted values

Figure 18.1 Residual plots for the data in Example 18.1 (Y axis: Residual: X axis: (A)-Treatment, (B)-Block, (C)-Predicted values)

(A), (B) and (C). These plots showed that all the residuals were symmetrically distributed around 0, and there were no outliers. It means that there is no evidence to suggest that the data violated the assumptions of normality of distribution and homoscedasticity.

The method of residual plots can be used for data with other types of design to test normality and homoscedasticity. It will be omitted in the following sections of this chapter. Also, please refer to Chapter 6 for the procedure of post hoc comparisons of pair wise population means between multiple groups.

18.2. ANOVA for two-Stage crossover design

Example 18.2. Cyclosporine is a potent immunosuppressive agent widely used after organ transplantation to suppress the body's immunological response and prevent rejection of an organ. To study the pharmacokinetic parameters and bioequivalence of two kinds of cyclosporine microemulsion oral solution for healthy humans, an experiment with a two-stage crossover design was conducted. Twenty volunteers ordered by weight were randomly divided into two equal groups. Participants in Group A were assigned to orally take the test solution 500mg in the first phase and take the reference solution 500mg in the second phase after a washout period of one week. Participants in Group B were assigned to take the two kinds of solutions with the inverse order in the two phases. The area under the curve (AUC) of blood concentration-time was measured as the indicator of effect. The experimental data are displayed in Table 18.6.

The various means for Example 18.2 are as follows:

Overall mean: $$\bar{X} = \frac{\sum x}{2n} = \frac{648.94}{40} = 16.2235$$

Mean of treatment, T (test solution): $$\bar{X}_{\mathrm{T}} = \frac{\sum (x_i)_{\mathrm{T}}}{n} = \frac{324.48}{20} = 16.2240$$

Mean of control, C (reference solution): $$\bar{X}_{\mathrm{C}} = \frac{\sum (x_i)_{\mathrm{C}}}{n} = \frac{324.46}{20} = 16.2230$$

Mean of phase I: $$\bar{X}_{\mathrm{I}} = \frac{\sum (x_i)_{\mathrm{I}}}{n} = \frac{333.83}{20} = 16.6915$$

Mean of phase II: $$\bar{X}_{\mathrm{II}} = \frac{\sum (x_i)_{\mathrm{II}}}{n} = \frac{315.11}{20} = 15.7555$$

Means of each participant: Omitted for simplicity

18.2.1. *Decomposition of the sum of squares and degrees of freedom*

In the analysis of variance, the total variation can be decomposed into between-treatment-group variation, between-stage variation, between-individual variation, and random error.

The three pairs of hypotheses to be tested are for treatment, stage, and individuals, respectively.

H_{10}: $\mu_{\mathrm{T}} = \mu_{\mathrm{C}}$
H_{11}: $\mu_{\mathrm{T}} \neq \mu_{\mathrm{C}}$

Table 18.6 AUC ($\mu g \cdot h \cdot ml^{-1}$) of 20 subjects after taking test solution (T) and reference solution (C) of cyclosporine microemulsion in a two-stage crossover designed experiment

	Group A (Order: T → C)				Group B (Order: C → T)		
Subjects	Phase I	Phase II	Total	Subjects	Phase I	Phase II	Total
1	T 17.54	C 17.17	34.71	3	C 20.97	T 19.61	40.58
2	T 15.88	C 14.31	30.19	5	C 19.94	T 22.14	42.08
4	T 18.51	C 21.56	40.07	7	C 17.57	T 17.49	35.06
6	T 16.41	C 13.18	29.59	9	C 13.94	T 13.49	27.43
8	T 15.87	C 15.15	31.02	10	C 15.29	T 16.19	31.48
12	T 16.11	C 15.14	31.25	11	C 15.81	T 15.78	31.59
15	T 14.09	C 16.22	30.31	13	C 17.42	T 15.95	33.37
16	T 15.95	C 13.93	29.88	14	C 15.92	T 14.43	30.35
18	T 15.29	C 11.97	27.26	17	C 17.00	T 14.02	31.02
19	T 16.46	C 14.11	30.57	20	C 17.86	T 13.27	31.13
Summation of the Column	T 162.11	C 152.74	314.85		C 171.72	T 162.37	334.09
Summation within Treatment group	$\sum_{i=1}^{20}(x_i)_{\rm T} = 162.11 + 162.37 = 324.48$				$\sum_{i=1}^{20}(x_i)_{\rm C} = 152.74 + 171.72 = 324.46$		
Summation within Phase	$\sum_{i=1}^{20}(x_i)_{\rm I} = 162.11 + 171.72 = 333.83$				$\sum_{i=1}^{20}(x_i)_{\rm II} = 152.74 + 162.37 = 315.11$		

**Note*: 1. AUC is the area under the blood concentration-time curve; 2.T is test preparation, C is reference preparation; 3. References: (1) Jianchang He, Enfu Feng, Qing Zhang, *et al.* [Study on bioequivalence of cyclosporine microemulsion oral solution in healthy volunteers], Pham Care & Res. 2009;9(2):137–139; (2) Yuanjie Jia, Liangping Hu, Dehe Cheng. [Statistical analysis for quantitative data with crossover design and SAS solutions]. Pham Care & Res. 2012;12(3):172–174.

H_{20}: $\mu_{\mathrm{I}} = \mu_{\mathrm{II}}$
H_{21}: $\mu_{\mathrm{I}} \neq \mu_{\mathrm{II}}$
H_{30}: $\mu_1 = \mu_2 = \mu_3 = \cdots = \mu_{20}$
H_{31}: At least two individuals had different means of AUC
$\alpha = 0.05$.

The measurement of the subject $i(i = 1, 2, 3, \ldots n)$ in phase p $(p = 1, 2)$ is denoted as x_{ip}, and the number of levels of the treatment factor is denoted as $k(k = 1, 2)$. The sum of squared deviation from the mean and degrees of freedom of each part in the analysis of variance are:

$$SS_{\text{Total}} = \sum_{i=1}^{n}\sum_{p=1}^{2}\left(x_{ip} - \bar{X}\right)^2, \nu_{\text{Total}} = N - 1 = 2n - 1 \quad (18\text{-}6)$$

$$SS_{\text{Treatment}} = \sum_{k=1}^{2}\sum_{i=1}^{n}\left(\bar{X}_k - \bar{X}\right)^2 = \sum_{k=1}^{2} n\left(\bar{X}_k - \bar{X}\right)^2,$$
$$\nu_{\text{Treatment}} = 2 - 1 = 1 \quad (18\text{-}7)$$

$$SS_{\text{Phase}} = \sum_{p=1}^{2}\sum_{i=1}^{n}\left(\bar{X}_p - \bar{X}\right)^2 = \sum_{p=1}^{2} n\left(\bar{X}_p - \bar{X}\right)^2,$$
$$\nu_{\text{Phase}} = 2 - 1 = 1 \quad (18\text{-}8)$$

$$SS_{\text{Individual}} = \sum_{i=1}^{n}\sum_{p=1}^{2}\left(\bar{X}_i - \bar{X}\right)^2 = \sum_{i=1}^{n} 2\left(\bar{X}_i - \bar{X}\right)^2,$$
$$\nu_{\text{Individual}} = n - 1 \quad (18\text{-}9)$$

$$SS_{\text{Error}} = SS_{\text{Total}} - SS_{\text{Treatment}} - SS_{\text{Phase}} - SS_{\text{Individual}},$$
$$\nu_{\text{Error}} = \nu_{\text{Total}} - \nu_{\text{Treatment}} - \nu_{\text{Phase}} - \nu_{\text{Individual}} = n-2 \quad (18\text{-}10)$$

18.2.2. *ANOVA results of Example 18.2*

The ANOVA results of Example 18.2 are displayed in Table 18.7. It indicates that the means of AUC of the two solutions had no statistically significant difference ($P = 0.998$) under the significant

Table 18.7 The ANOVA results from the data of Example 18.2

Variation	SS	ν	MS	F	P
Total	207.084	39			
Treatment	0.00001	1	0.00001	0.000	0.998
Phase	8.761	1	8.761	4.293	0.053
Individual	161.585	19	8.504	4.167	0.002
Error	36.738	18	2.041		

level of 0.05. The difference of means between the two experimental phases was also not statistically significant ($P = 0.053$). However, the difference in the means of individual participants was statistically significant ($P = 0.002$).

Furthermore, since the 20 subjects were divided into two groups with different experimental sequences, the variability among individuals can be further decomposed into two parts — variability between-sequence (between groups A and B) and variability of residual effect from individuals. The null hypothesis of the two population means of two sequence groups being equally can be tested by an F-statistic, the ratio of the between-sequence mean square and residual mean square.

The measurement of the ith subject ($i = 1, 2, 3, \ldots n_g$), in the gth group($g = 1, 2$), in the pth phase is denoted as x_{gip}, and the mean of $2n_g$ measurements of n_g subjects in the gth group is written as

$$\bar{X}_g = \frac{1}{2n_g} \sum_{i=1}^{n_g} \sum_{p=1}^{2} x_{gip} \tag{18-11}$$

In this example, $\bar{X}_A = 314.85/20 = 15.7425, \bar{X}_B = 334.09/20 = 16.7045$. The sum of squares of deviation from mean and degrees of freedom between sequences (between groups) are:

$$SS_{\text{sequence}} = \sum_{g=1}^{2} \sum_{i=1}^{n_g} \sum_{p=1}^{2} (\bar{X}_g - \bar{X})^2 = \sum_{g=1}^{2} \left[2n_g \left(\bar{X}_g - \bar{X}\right)^2\right],$$

$$\nu_{\text{sequence}} = 2 - 1 = 1 \tag{18-12}$$

Table 18.8 The ANOVA results for the experimental sequence in Example 18.2

Variation	SS	ν	MS	F	P
Total individual	161.585	19			
Between-sequence	9.254	1	9.254	1.093	0.310
Residual	152.331	18	8.463		

The sum of squares and degrees of freedom of the residual effects between individuals are:

$$SS_{\text{residual}} = SS_{\text{individual}} - SS_{\text{sequence}},$$

$$\nu_{\text{residual}} = \nu_{\text{individual}} - \nu_{\text{sequence}} = n - 2 \qquad (18\text{-}13)$$

From formulas (18-12) and (18-13), the results of testing the effect of sequences are displayed in Table 18.8. There was no significant difference between the two sequences groups ($P = 0.310$).

18.3. ANOVA for factorial design

The following is an example of a study with 2×2 factorial design to illustrate the ANOVA for factorial designed data.

Example 18.3. A doctor studied the cholesterol-lowering effects of two newly developed drugs, A and B, on patients with hypercholesterolemia, to determine if there was an interaction between them. Twenty patients with hypercholesterolemia were recruited according to the predetermined inclusion criteria and randomly divided into four groups, with 5 patients in each group. Participants in Group 1 were the control group where neither drug A nor B was used. Participants in Group 2 were treated with drug A only. Participants in Group 3 were treated with drug B only. Participants in Group 4 were treated with both drugs A and B. For ethical reasons, all patients in the four groups were instructed to stay on a reasonable diet by professional practitioners during the entire process of the study. Before the beginning of the experiment and after one course of treatment, the blood cholesterol level of each patient was measured, and the

Table 18.9 Reduction in cholesterol (mmol/L) after treatment in patients with hypercholesterolemia*

Drug B	Not used (B_1)		Used (B_2)		
Drug A	Not used (A_1)	Used (A_2)	Not used (A_1)	Used (A_2)	Total
	0.8565	1.1365	1.1532	1.7862	
	0.7352	1.1025	0.9918	2.0123	
	0.9357	1.4213	1.2121	2.3242	
	1.2698	1.1876	0.9857	1.9892	
	0.9217	1.1564	0.8832	2.0012	
Sum of column	4.7189	6.0043	5.2260	10.1131	26.0623 (ΣX)
Sum of A_1 or A_2	$\sum(x)_{A_1} = 4.7189 + 5.2260 = 9.9449$		$\sum(x)_{A_2} = 6.0043 + 10.1131 = 16.1174$		
Sum of B_1 or B_2	$\sum(x)_{B_1} = 4.7189 + 6.0043 = 10.7232$		$\sum(x)_{B_2} = 5.2260 + 10.1131 = 15.3391$		

*The data are from: Li H. Statistical analysis of the data factorial experiment designed. The Journal of Evidence-Based Medicine. 2005;5(1):35-38.

amount of cholesterol reduction (mmol/L) after treatment was used as an indicator of effects. The data are shown in Table 18.9, where the A_1 means Drug A being not used and A_2 means Drug A being used, and B_1 and B_2 correspondingly means Drug B being not used and used.

18.3.1. *Decomposition of effects and variation of factorial design*

Example 18.3 is a 2×2 factorial design. Both factors A and B have two levels, so four combinations are formed. The corresponding population means are shown in Table 18.10.

The different combinations of the parameters μ_0, α, β and γ in Table 18.10 represent the population means corresponding to the four groups formed by the two levels of factor A and B. It can be seen from the table that when$\gamma = 0$, the differences of the population means between the two groups of A_2 and A_1 are equal (both equal to α) regardless of the level of B. Similarly, the differences of the population means between the groups of B_2 and B_1 are also equal

Table 18.10 Denotations of population means for four combinations of 2 × 2 factorial design

Factor A	Factor B: Level 1 (B_1)	Factor B: Level 2 (B_2)	The difference between the population means of B_2 and B_1
Level 1(A_1)	μ_0	$\mu_0 + \beta$	β
Level 2(A_2)	$\mu_0 + \alpha$	$\mu_0 + \alpha + \beta + \gamma$	$\beta + \gamma$
The difference between the population means of A_2 and A_1	α	$\alpha + \gamma$	γ

(both equal to β) regardless of the level of A. In such case, there is no interaction between factors A and B.

Inversely, if $\gamma \neq 0$, the differences of the population means between the groups A_2 and A_1 are different while B is equal to B_1 and B_2, which are α and $\alpha + \gamma$, respectively. That is, the effects of A vary depending on the levels of B. Similarly, the differences of the population means between the groups B_2 and B_1 are different while A is equal to A_1 and A_2, which are β and $\beta + \gamma$, respectively. That is, the effects of B vary depending on the levels of A. In such a case, the difference in the effects of one factor when the other factor taking different values, γ, reflects the interaction of two factors.

The parameter α in the table is the individual effect of factor A at B_1, and β is the individual effect of factor B at A_1. If $\gamma = 0, \alpha$ and β reflect the main effects of factor A and factor B, respectively. Otherwise, if$\gamma \neq 0$, the main effects of factor A can be considered as the average effects of factor A at the two levels of factor B, that is $\bar{E}_A = \frac{1}{2}(\alpha + \alpha + \gamma) = \alpha + \frac{\gamma}{2}$. Similarly, the main effect of factor B is $\bar{E}_B = \beta + \frac{\gamma}{2}$.

The purpose of the experiment of Example 18.3 was to demonstrate whether there was an interaction between drug A and drug B, and whether the main effects of A and B were zero. It is noteworthy that we would be unable to ascertain whether α or β is equal to zero if $\gamma \neq 0$, which means we would not be able to determine whether A or B, when used alone, is effective. Therefore, the effects of A should be analyzed separately for the two situations of using B or not, and vice versa.

The null hypotheses of Example 18.3 include:

H_{10}: $\gamma = 0$ (There was no interaction between factors A and B);
H_{20}: $\mu_{A_1} = \mu_{A_2}$ (The population means of two levels of factor A were equal);
H_{30}: $\mu_{B_1} = \mu_{B_2}$ (The population means of two levels of factor B were equal);

The significance levels of the three hypotheses tests were all set at $\alpha = 0.05$.

The sample means and the sample standard deviations of the groups as outlined in Example 18.3 are displayed in Table 18.11. As can be seen from the table, the estimated values of α, β and γ are 0.2571, 0.1014, and 0.7203, respectively.

Decomposition of variation: The individual measurement value x_{abi} in the factorial designed data indicates the ith observation at the level a of factor A and level b of factor B, and the number of observations in the corresponding group is denoted as n_{ab}. The total number of observations is denoted as N. The number of levels of factor A is written as p, and the number of levels of factor B is q. This implies that $a = 1, 2, \ldots p$; $b = 1, 2, \ldots q$; and the total number of groups $G = pq$. Evidently, in the 2×2 factorial design study, $p = 2$, $q = 2$, $G = 4$.

For simplicity, the symbols and formulae for the number of observations and the sample means of each group are listed in Table 18.12.

Table 18.11 The sample means ($\bar{X}$, mmol/L) of four groups in Example 18.3

	Drug B		
Drug A	Not used (B_1)	Used(B_2)	Effect size of drug B
Not used (A_1)	0.9438	1.0452	0.1014 ($\hat{\beta}$)
Used (A_2)	1.2009	2.0226	0.8217 ($\hat{\beta} + \hat{\gamma}$)
Effect size of drug A	0.2571 ($\hat{\alpha}$)	0.9774 ($\hat{\alpha} + \hat{\gamma}$)	0.7203 ($\hat{\gamma}$)

Table 18.12 The number of observations and the sample means for $p \times q$ factorial design data

Group	Number of observations	Sample mean
Level a of factor A combined level b of factor B	n_{ab}	$\bar{X}_{ab} = \frac{\sum_{i=1}^{n_{ab}} x_{abi}}{n_{ab}}$
Level a of factor A $(a = 1, 2, \ldots p)$	$n_{a\cdot} = \sum_{b=1}^{q} n_{ab}$	$\bar{X}_{a\cdot} = \frac{\sum_{b=1}^{q}\sum_{i=1}^{n_{ab}} x_{abi}}{\sum_{b=1}^{q} n_{ab}}$
Level b of factor B $(b = 1, 2, \ldots q)$	$n_{\cdot b} = \sum_{a=1}^{p} n_{ab}$	$\bar{X}_{\cdot b} = \frac{\sum_{a=1}^{p}\sum_{i=1}^{n_{ab}} x_{abi}}{\sum_{a=1}^{p} n_{ab}}$
Total	$N = \sum_{b=1}^{q}\sum_{a=1}^{p} n_{ab}$	$\bar{X} = \frac{\sum_{a=1}^{p}\sum_{b=1}^{q}\sum_{i=1}^{n_{ab}} x_{abi}}{\sum_{a=1}^{p}\sum_{b=1}^{q} n_{ab}}$

When conducting ANOVA for the factorial design, the total sum of squares of deviation from mean can be decomposed into four components: the main effects of factor A, the main effects of factor B, the interaction effects between factors A and B, and the random error. The degrees of freedom can also be decomposed correspondingly. The formulae are shown as follows:

$$SS_{\text{Total}} = \sum_{a=1}^{p}\sum_{b=1}^{q}\sum_{i=1}^{n_{ab}} (X_{abi} - \bar{X})^2, \quad \nu_{\text{Total}} = N - 1 \qquad (18\text{-}14)$$

$$SS_A = \sum_{a=1}^{p} n_{a\cdot}(\bar{X}_{a\cdot} - \bar{X})^2, \quad \nu_A = p - 1 \qquad (18\text{-}15)$$

$$SS_B = \sum_{b=1}^{q} n_{\cdot b}(\bar{X}_{\cdot b} - \bar{X})^2, \quad \nu_B = q - 1 \qquad (18\text{-}16)$$

$$SS_{A\times B} = \sum_{a=1}^{p}\sum_{b=1}^{q} n_{ab}(\bar{X}_{ab} - \bar{X}_{a\cdot} - \bar{X}_{\cdot b} + \bar{X})^2,$$

$$\nu_{A\times B} = (p-1)(q-1) \qquad (18\text{-}17)$$

$$SS_{\text{Error}} = \sum_{a=1}^{p}\sum_{b=1}^{q}\sum_{i=1}^{n_{ab}}(X_{abi} - \bar{X}_{ab})^2$$

$$\nu_{\text{Error}} = \sum_{a=1}^{p}\sum_{b=1}^{q}(n_{ab} - 1) = N - pq \tag{18-18}$$

The relationship of the above sum of squares of deviation from mean and degrees of freedom can be expressed as:

$$SS_{\text{Total}} = SS_A + SS_B + SS_{A\times B} + SS_{\text{Error}}$$

$$\nu_{\text{Total}} = \nu_A + \nu_B + \nu_{A\times B} + \nu_{\text{Error}}$$

Also, similar to completely random design, between-group variability, $SS_{\text{Treatment}} = \sum_{b=1}^{q}\sum_{a=1}^{p} n_{ab}(\bar{X}_{ab} - \bar{X})^2$, represents the deviation of a group mean from the overall mean that due to the difference of effects from different treatments. It comprehensively reflects the main effects and interaction effects of factor A and factor B. Therefore, $SS_{\text{Treatment}}$ is equal to the sum of SS_A, SS_B and $SS_{A\times B}$. The relationship can be written as:

$$SS_{\text{Treatment}} = \sum_{b=1}^{q}\sum_{a=1}^{p} n_{ab}(\bar{X}_{ab} - \bar{X})^2 = SS_A + SS_B + SS_{A\times B},$$

$$\nu_{\text{Treatment}} = G - 1 = pq - 1 \tag{18-19}$$

The sums of squares divided by their corresponding degrees of freedom in formula (18-15) $\sim$ (18-18) will generate mean squares MS_A, MS_B, MS_{AB} and MS_{Error}. Then, the test statistics F_A, F_B and F_{AB} can be obtained from the ratios of MS_A, MS_B, MS_{AB} to MS_{Error} respectively. The details are displayed in an ANOVA table (Table 18.13).

18.3.2. *The calculation and inference of Example 18.3*

The ANOVA results of Example 18.3 are shown in Table 18.14. It demonstrates that the interaction term between A and B was statistically significant ($P < 0.001$), indicating that drugs A and B would affect each other's effect when they are used simultaneously.

Table 18.13 ANOVA table of data from a two-factor factorial design

Source of variation	SS	ν	MS	F
Total	SS_{Total}	ν_{Total}		
Main effects of factor A	SS_A	ν_A	SS_A/ν_A	MS_A/MS_{Error}
Main effects of factor B	SS_B	ν_B	SS_B/ν_B	MS_B/MS_{Error}
Interactions of A and B	$SS_{A\times B}$	$\nu_{A\times B}$	$SS_{A\times B}/\nu_{A\times B}$	$MS_{A\times B}/MS_{\text{Error}}$
Error	SS_{Error}	ν_{Error}	$SS_{\text{Error}}/\nu_{\text{Error}}$	

Table 18.14 The ANOVA results for 2 × 2 factorial design in Example 18.3

Source of variation	SS	ν	MS	F	P
Total	4.062	19			
Main effects of factor A	1.905	1	1.905	68.77	<0.001
Main effects of factor B	1.065	1	1.065	38.46	<0.001
Interaction effects of A and B	0.649	1	0.649	23.42	<0.001
Error	0.443	16	0.028		

Meanwhile, tests for the main effects of A ($P < 0.001$) and the main effects of B ($P < 0.001$) were both statistically significant.

From Table 18.11, the estimate of the effect size of drug A without drug B, $\hat{\alpha}$, was 0.2571, and the estimate of the effect size of drug B without drug A, $\hat{\beta}$, was 0.1014. Compared with the case of not using B, the effect of A increased by0.7203 ($\hat{\gamma}$) from 0.2571 to 0.9774 if B was used simultaneously, which indicated that there was a synergistic effect (positive interaction effect) between A and B. The increment of 0.7203 was the estimated value of the interaction effect, $\hat{\gamma}$. We can demonstrate that $\hat{\alpha}, \hat{\beta}$ and $\hat{\gamma}$ were statistically different from zero.

The results of this study are shown in Figure 18.2. The endpoint on the left side of the dotted line segment is the sample mean of observations without using any drug (Group 1), and the right endpoint of the dotted line is the mean of using A alone (Group 2). The slope of the dotted line is not equal to 0, indicating that drug A may be effective when used alone. The left endpoint of the solid line is the mean of using B alone(Group 3), and its right endpoint is the

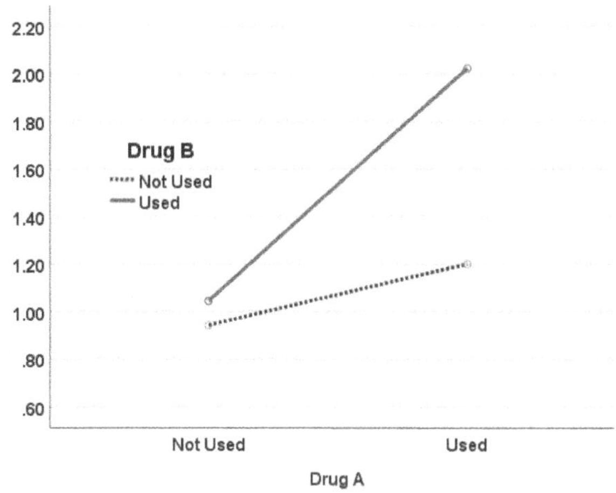

Figure 18.2 Line segments with group means from 2 × 2 factorial design data of Example 18.3

mean of using both A and B (Group 4). The solid line is steeper than the dotted line, indicating that the effect of drug A, when used with drug B, is stronger than when it was used alone. In other words, the fact that the two lines are not parallel shows that the interaction effect exists between the two factors.

18.4. ANOVA for repeated measurements

Repeated measurement design is a strategy involving multiple measurements for each subject. In such studies, the subjects are their own controls because the model assesses how a subject responds to all of the treatments. The simplest type of repeated measurement is single-group repeated measurement data, which means all the subjects belong to one group. Its objective is to find whether the mean of the measurements varies with time or experimental conditions. More typically, subjects are divided into different groups in repeated measurement design, which means other factors should be considered besides time or experimental conditions. The aims of multi-grouped repeated measurement data include testing whether the difference of mean values between time points for each group and between groups for each time point are significant, and comparing the changing trends over time of means among groups. The repeated measurement analysis of variance is illustrated by the following Example 18.4.

Example 18.4. In a nutritional experiment, 16 rats of the same species and with similar age in months were randomly divided into two equal-size groups, which were fed by two different kinds of feedstuff. They were weighted periodically and their weight gains for every two weeks were recorded at four consecutive time points (Table 18.15). We need to compare the effect of these two kinds of feedstuff on weight gains.

It is a typical example of repeated measurement data with the treatment (feedstuff) of two levels (A and B) and the repeated factor of four levels. Figure 18.3 illustrates the changing trend of the data. The objective is to test if the average weight gains between the

Table 18.15 Weight gains (gram) in every two weeks for 16 rats feed by two kinds of feedstuff

			Weight gains in every two weeks			
Group	No.	Feedstuff	1st	2nd	3rd	4th
1	1	A	33	40	31	25
1	2	A	25	34	33	31
1	3	A	38	33	29	35
1	4	A	25	36	27	30
1	5	A	24	32	29	32
1	6	A	32	33	36	31
1	7	A	28	35	28	24
1	8	A	16	20	35	32
2	9	B	17	22	30	38
2	10	B	19	23	23	33
2	11	B	16	24	32	39
2	12	B	17	25	33	34
2	13	B	21	24	29	28
2	14	B	18	25	25	36
2	15	B	23	26	33	37
2	16	B	30	37	32	26

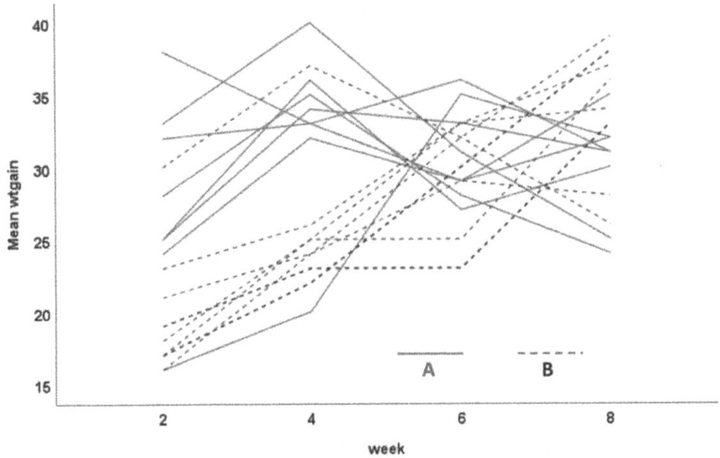

Figure 18.3 The trend of weight gains (grams) at four consecutive two-week periods

two groups at each period are different and whether there exists an interaction effect between treatment and time.

18.4.1. *Prerequisite assumption of the ANOVA for repeated measurements data*

In repeated measures ANOVA, the total effects can be decomposed into between-subject effects and within-subject effects. Between-subject effects are attributed to the variation between treatment groups and between-subject residual variation. Within-subject effects are attributed to the effects of repeated factor, the interactions between treatment effects and repeated effects, and repeated measurement error. The difference in treatment groups can be tested by conventional ANOVA since individuals are independent from one another. However, for within-subjects effects, the correlation between repeated measurements of the same subjects, and the structure of the covariance matrix should be examined at first. If the variances of measurement difference between any two repeated measures, $Y_{t_i} - Y_{t_j}, i \neq j$, are equal, then we say the covariance matrix of repeated measurements is spherical, which can be tested with sample data by Mauchly's sphericity test. When the null hypothesis of spherical assumption is not rejected, F statistic can be used. Nevertheless, if the assumption of sphericity is violated, the numerator and denominator degrees of freedom of the test statistic, F, should be adjusted for the within-subject effects. The method of adjusting for degrees of freedom is to multiply the original degrees by an adjustment factor, $\varepsilon(0 < \varepsilon \leq 1)$. The smaller value of ε reflects the stronger correlation between repeated measures. The methods to estimate ε includes Greenhouse-Geisserepsilon, Huynh-Feldtepsilon, Lower-bound epsilon, and so on, which can be obtained using SPSS software.

18.4.2. *Variation decomposition in ANOVA for repeated measures data*

The data of Example 18.4 are from a study using a completely randomized design with one treatment factor. The treatment has two levels, and the repeated measurement factor has four levels. Table 18.16 displays the denotations of the population mean at each time point for any group.

Three possible pairs of hypotheses for this data are as follows:

H_{10}: $\mu_{11} - \mu_{21} = \mu_{12} - \mu_{22} = \mu_{13} - \mu_{23} = \mu_{14} - \mu_{24}$ (There is no interaction between treatment effects and time effects)

H_{11}: Not all of $\mu_{11} - \mu_{21}$, $\mu_{12} - \mu_{22}$, $\mu_{13} - \mu_{23}$, and $\mu_{14} - \mu_{24}$ are equal (There is some interaction between treatment and time effects)

H_{20}: $\mu_{1\cdot} = \mu_{2\cdot}$ (The main effect of the treatment is zero)

Table 18.16 The denotations of the population mean at each time point for any group in Example 18.4

	Time points				
Group	t_1	t_2	t_3	t_4	General
1	μ_{11}	μ_{12}	μ_{13}	μ_{14}	$\mu_{1\cdot}$
2	μ_{21}	μ_{22}	μ_{23}	μ_{24}	$\mu_{2\cdot}$
General	$\mu_{\cdot 1}$	$\mu_{\cdot 2}$	$\mu_{\cdot 3}$	$\mu_{\cdot 4}$	μ (Total)

H_{21}: $\mu_{1\cdot} \neq \mu_{2\cdot}$ (The main effect of the treatment is not zero)
H_{30}: $\mu_{\cdot 1} = \mu_{\cdot 2} = \mu_{\cdot 3} = \mu_{\cdot 4}$(The main effects of time is zero)
H_{31}: Not all of $\mu_{\cdot 1}$, $\mu_{\cdot 2}$, $\mu_{\cdot 3}$ and $\mu_{\cdot 4}$ are equal (The main effects of time is not zero)

The significance levels are all set as $\alpha = 0.05$.

When there is no interaction between treatment and time effects, we focus on the following two aspects: (1) whether the mean value of each group is equal (or, if the main effect of treatment is zero), and (2) if the mean value at each time point is equal (or, if the main effect of time is zero). Conversely, when the interaction between treatment and time exists, the mean differences between groups at different time points are not all equal. Therefore, even if the main effect of the treatment is not significantly different from zero, it doesn't mean that the mean values of any two groups are always equal at any time point. Similarly, zero main effect of time doesn't mean that the mean values of all time points are always equal for any group. That is, when there is an interaction between treatment and time effects, the results of ANOVA for main effects make little sense. Instead, we should compare the means between groups at each time point and test whether the mean values of all time points are equal for a given group.

Denoting the measurement at time point t of the ith subject in the treatment group g as x_{git}, ($g = 1, 2, \ldots G$; $i = 1, 2, \ldots n_g$; $t = 1, 2, \ldots T$, $N = \sum_{g=1}^{G} n_g$), the variations of the repeated data with complete random design can be decomposed as follows:

$$SS_{\text{Total}} = \sum_{g=1}^{G} \sum_{i=1}^{n_g} \sum_{t=1}^{T} \left(x_{git} - \bar{X}\right)^2,$$

$$\nu_{\text{Total}} = NT - 1 \tag{18-20}$$

$$SS_{\text{Between-subject}} = \sum_{g=1}^{G} \sum_{i=1}^{n_g} T\left(\bar{X}_{i\cdot} - \bar{X}\right)^2,$$

$$\nu_{\text{Between-subject}} = N - 1 \tag{18-21}$$

$$SS_{\text{Treatment}} = \sum_{g=1}^{G} n_g T(\bar{X}_g - \bar{X})^2,$$

$$\nu_{\text{Treatment}} = G - 1 \tag{18-22}$$

$$SS_{\text{Error-Between}} = SS_{\text{Between-subject}} - SS_{\text{Treatment}},$$

$$\nu_{\text{Error-Between}} = N - G \tag{18-23}$$

$$SS_{\text{Within-subject}} = \sum_{g=1}^{G}\sum_{i=1}^{n_g}\sum_{t=1}^{T} \left(x_{git} - \bar{X}_{i\cdot}\right)^2,$$

$$\nu_{\text{Within-subject}} = N(T - 1) \tag{18-24}$$

$$SS_{\text{Time}} = \sum_{t=1}^{T} N(\bar{X}_{\cdot t} - \bar{X})^2, \ \nu_{\text{Time}} = T - 1 \tag{18-25}$$

$$SS_{\text{Treatment} \times \text{Time}} = \sum_{g=1}^{G}\sum_{t=1}^{T} n_g(\bar{X}_{gt} - \bar{X})^2,$$

$$\nu_{\text{Treatment} \times \text{Time}} = (G - 1)(T - 1) \tag{18-26}$$

$$SS_{\text{Error-within}} = SS_{\text{Within-subject}} - SS_{\text{Time}} - SS_{\text{Treatment} \times \text{Time}},$$

$$\nu_{\text{Error-within}} = \nu_{\text{Within-subject}} - \nu_{\text{Time}} - \nu_{\text{Treatment} \times \text{Time}} = (N - G)(T - 1) \tag{18-27}$$

The mean squares (MS) can be calculated as the SS divided by the corresponding ν from the above formulas. Further, we can obtain the F statistic for testing the main effects of treatment with the ratio of $MS_{\text{Treatment}}$ divided by $MS_{\text{Error-Between}}$. Meanwhile, the F statistic for testing the main effects of time is the ratio of MS_{Time} and $MS_{\text{Error-Within}}$, and the F statistic for testing the interactions between treatment and time effects is the ratio of $MS_{\text{Treatment} \times \text{Time}}$ and $MS_{\text{Error-Within}}$. The components and calculations are displayed in the following ANOVA table (Table 18.17).

Table 18.17 ANOVA for repeated measures data with a completely randomized design

Variation Source	Sum of squares	Degree of freedom	Mean square	F
Total	SS_{Total}	ν_{Total}		
Between-subject effects	$SS_{\text{Between-subject}}$	$\nu_{\text{Between-subject}}$		
Treatment	$SS_{\text{Treatment}}$	$\nu_{\text{Treatment}}$	$MS_{\text{Treatment}}$	$\frac{MS_{\text{Treatment}}}{MS_{\text{Error-Between}}}$
Error of between-subject	$SS_{\text{Error-Between}}$	$\nu_{\text{Error-Between}}$	$MS_{\text{Error-Between}}$	
Within-subject effects	$SS_{\text{Within-subject}}$	$\nu_{\text{Within-subject}}$		
Time	SS_{Time}	ν_{Time}	MS_{Time}	$\frac{MS_{\text{Time}}}{MS_{\text{Error-Within}}}$
Treatment × Time	$SS_{\text{Treatment}\times\text{Time}}$	$\nu_{\text{Treatment}\times\text{Time}}$	$MS_{\text{Treatment}\times\text{Time}}$	$\frac{MS_{\text{Treatment}\times\text{Time}}}{MS_{\text{Error-Within}}}$
Error of within-subject	$SS_{\text{Error-Within}}$	$\nu_{\text{Error-Within}}$	$MS_{\text{Error-Within}}$	

18.4.3. *The Calculation and analysis of Example 18.4*

Descriptive results of the data from Example 18.4 are listed in Table 18.18. The results of Box's M test for homogeneity of covariance matrix between groups and the Mauchly's test for sphericity of covariance matrix structure are displayed in Table 18.19. The difference of covariance matrix between groups was not significant ($P = 0.0530$), which met the prerequisite of ANOVA. However, the covariance matrix structure violated the assumption of sphericity ($P = 0.026$). Therefore, the degrees of freedom of F statistics for within-subject effects should be adjusted by an estimated ε, which was 0.599 based on the Greenhouse-Geisser method or 0.731 based on the Huynh-Feldt method.

The results of the ANOVA are displayed in Table 18.20. The interactions between treatment and time effects were statistically significant ($P = 0.016$), which means that the time trends of weight gains between the two groups were different (Figure 18.4). Therefore, although the general means were different between the two groups, if the means were different between the two groups at a specific time point, we need to test further. Likewise, the significant main effects of

Table 18.18 Descriptive statistics of the repeated measures data from Example 18.4 ($\bar{X} \pm SD$)

Treatment group	Repeated factor (Time)				General mean of group
	t_1	t_2	t_3	t_4	
Group 1	27.625 ± 6.739	32.875 ± 5.768	31.000 ± 3.338	30.000 ± 3.703	30.375 ± 5.203
Group 2	20.125 ± 4.612	25.750 ± 4.713	29.625 ± 3.777	33.875 ± 4.704	27.344 ± 6.670
General mean of time point	23.875 ± 6.791	29.313 ± 6.279	30.313 ± 3.516	31.938 ± 4.553	28.859 ± 6.128

Table 18.19 Results of homogeneity test and sphericity test for the covariance matrix of the data from Example 18.4

		Statistic			Adjustment coefficient, ε	
Test	Method	Name	Value	P-value	Greenhouse-Geisser	Huynh-Feldt
Homogeneity	Box's M test	F	0.903	0.530	—	—
Sphericity	Mauchly's test	χ^2	12.810	0.026	0.599	0.731

Table 18.20 The results of repeated measures ANOVA of data from Example 18.4

Variation source	SS	ν	Adjusted ν (G-G method)	MS	F	P
Total	2365.735	63				
Between-subject effects	478.485	15				
Treatment	147.016	1		147.016	6.209	0.026
Error of between-subject	331.469	14		23.676		
Within-subject effects	1887.250	48				
Time	586.172	3	1.798	326.093	8.616	0.002
Treatment × Time	348.672	3	1.798	193.969	5.125	0.016
Error of within-subject	952.406	42	25.166	37.845		

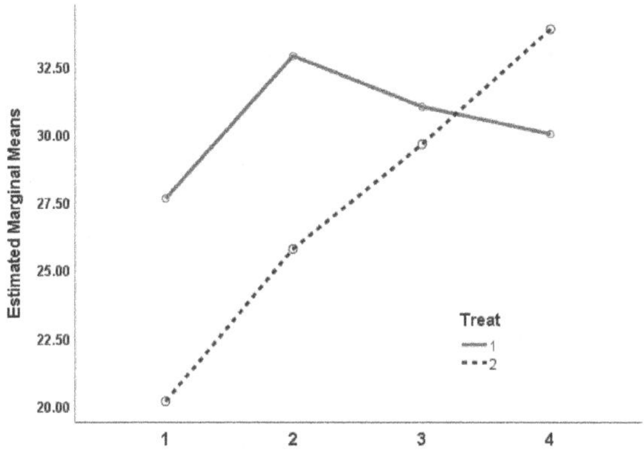

Figure 18.4 The trend over time of average weight gains (gram) of the two groups

time ($P = 0.002$) showed that the general means of the four periods were not all equal, but we need to further test group by group if the general means of the four periods are different.

18.4.4. *The multiple comparisons of time points or trend analysis*

Considering the non-zero interactions between treatment and time effects in Example 18.4, the multiple comparisons of time points were conducted group by group separately. The results of sphericity test of covariance structure and the results of repeated measures ANOVA are displayed in Table 18.21 and Table 18.22, respectively.

For Group 1, the assumption of sphericity cannot be rejected ($P = 0.388$). However, given the small sample size, the power of the test might be not high enough to reject the assumption of sphericity. Therefore, the degrees of freedom of F statistics in ANOVA were still adjusting. The effects of time were not significant ($P = 0.257$), so that no multiple comparisons were required for different time points.

For Group 2, differences in means between different time periods were significant ($P = 0.002$), so, multiple comparisons were conducted subsequently (Table 18.23). Multiple comparisons among time points were conducted using several methods such as

Table 18.21 Mauchly's sphericity test of covariance matrix separately for the two groups in Example 18.4

			Adjustment coefficient, ε	
Groups	χ^2	P	Greenhouse-Geisser method	Huynh-Feldt method
Group 1	5.286	0.388	0.621	0.838
Group 2	12.455	0.031	0.476	0.564

Table 18.22 Results of the repeated measures ANOVA separately for the two groups in Example 18.4

Groups	Variation source	SS	ν	Adjusted ν (G-G method)	MS	F	P
Group 1	Total	839.500	31				
	Between-subject	192.000	7		27.429		
	Within-subject	647.500	24				
	Time	114.750	3	1.863	61.582	1.508	0.257
	Error	532.750	21	13.044	40.844		
Group 2	Total	1379.219	31				
	Between-subject	139.469	7		19.924		
	Within-subject	1239.750	24				
	Time	820.094	3	1.428	574.431	13.679	0.002
	Error	419.656	21	9.994	41.992		

Table 18.23 Results of polynomial contrasts of repeated factor (time) for Group 2 in Example 18.4

Source	SS	ν	MS	F	P
Time					
Linear	814.506	1	814.506	18.372	0.004
Quadratic	3.781	1	3.781	0.376	0.559
Cubic	1.806	1	1.806	0.326	0.586
Error (Time)					
Linear	310.344	7	44.335		
Quadratic	70.469	7	10.067		
Cubic	38.844	7	5.549		

polynomial, Helmert, profile, and so on. The principle of polynomial method is to test the linear, quadratic, cubic, (and/or higher order) trends of the means with time. For Group 2 here, the highest order of time was cubic because there were four time points. The results of trend test for Group 2 are displayed in Table 18.23. As shown in the table, only the linear trend was significant ($P = 0.004$), suggesting that the weight gain increased linearly with time (the dotted line in Figure 18.4).

18.4.5. *Other methods for repeated measures data*

The dependent variable must be continuous and normally distributed in repeated measures ANOVA. Meanwhile, the repeated factor is discrete or categorical. Moreover, the time points or repeated number of observations must be uniform for all subjects. The format of the dataset for statistical software must be a wide style with each case representing a specific subject and each variable representing a specific level of the repeated factors. A case will be deleted in the process of ANOVA if there is a missing value at any level of the repeated factor, which may result in loss of information. Therefore, the method of repeated measures ANOVA is fairly restrictive in practice.

Data from repeated measures design with different observation time points/intervals, different numbers of observations, or with missing values are also usually considered as longitudinal data. The analytic methods for longitudinal data include generalized estimated equation (GEE), multilevel linear model, multilevel generalized linear model, and so on, which can be used to analyze flexible types of repeated measures data. Moreover, GEE and a multilevel generalized linear model can be used to analyze dependent variables of any member of the exponential distribution family. Chapter 28 will cover the multilevel model.

18.5. Report writing

The report of the results of ANOVA should usually include the following aspects: (1) The design type and the testing objectives; (2) The descriptive statistics; (3) The ANOVA method, F and P values; and (4) The method and results of multiple comparisons. The reporting format of ANOVA may differ depending on the design type. The reporting of the study results for the four examples in this chapter are illustrated in the following sections.

18.5.1. *Reporting results of Example 18.1 (Randomized Blocked Design)*

To compare the effect of five types of disinfectant (A, B, C, D, E) on bacteria inhibition, four species of bacteria were cultured by five dishes, each under the same condition. The dishes were then randomly assigned to treatment with one of the disinfectants. The diameter of inhibition zone was measured as an indicator of effect. The mean and standard deviation ($\bar{x} \pm s$, mm) of A, B, C, D, E disinfectant groups were 17.75 ± 6.08, 18.50 ± 6.76, 18.25 ± 4.99, 17.50 ± 8.35 and 13.00 ± 4.83 respectively. The results of two-way ANOVA showed that the difference among five types of disinfectant was statistically significant ($F = 3.95$, $P = 0.029$) at the significance level of 0.05. Meanwhile, the difference of mean diameters among four species of bacteria was also significant ($F = 34.37$, $P < 0.001$).

Then, post hoc multiple comparisons for 5 types of disinfectants were conducted with Student-Newman-Keuls test. The results showed that the difference between E and each of the other disinfectants was significant at the level of 0.05. However, no differences between any two types of the other disinfectants (A, B, C, D) were significant.

18.5.2. *Reporting results of Example 18.2 (Crossover Design)*

To explore the bioequivalence of two preparations of cyclosporine microemulsifying oral solutions, an experiment with a two-stage crossover design was conducted. Twenty volunteers ordered by weight were randomly divided into two equal groups. Participants in Group A were assigned to orally take the test preparation at stage I and take the reference preparation at stage II after a washout period of one week. Participants in Group B were assigned to take the two preparations in a reversed order. The area under the curve (AUC) of blood concentration vs. time was the measurement to be compared.

The mean and standard deviation ($\bar{x} \pm s$) of the test and reference preparations were 16.224 ± 2.120 and 16.223 ± 2.530 respectively; those of the two stages were 16.692 ± 1.742 and 15.756 ± 2.721 respectively; and those of the two groups were 15.743 ± 2.060 and 16.705 ± 2.484 respectively.

The results of ANOVA for crossover design indicated that the mean difference between the two preparations was not significant ($F = 0.000$, $P = 0.998$); nor was that between the two stages ($F = 4.293$, $P = 0.053$); and nor was that between the two orders ($F = 1.093$, $P = 0.310$).

18.5.3. *Reporting results of Example 18.3 (2 × 2 Factorial Design)*

To detect the main effect and interaction of two medications (A and B) on lowering serum cholesterol in hypercholesteremia patients, a 2×2 factorial design was used in an experiment. Twenty patients meeting the inclusion criterion were randomly divided into 4 treatment groups with 5 patients in each group. Subjects in Group 1 were given none of medications A and B as a control group; treatment of Group 2 was given A only and treatment of Group 3 was given B only; and Group 4 was given both A and B. The amount of decrease in serum cholesterol after a course of treatment was analyzed as the effect indicator.

The sample means and standard deviations ($\bar{x} \pm s$, mmol/L) of these 4 groups were 0.9438 ± 0.1987, 1.2009 ± 0.1271, 1.0452 ± 0.1343 and 2.0226 ± 0.1927, respectively.

The result of ANOVA for factorial designed data indicated that the interaction of A and B was statistically significant ($F = 23.42$, $P < 0.001$). The effect of A was stronger when it was used simultaneously with B than it was used solely (0.9744 vs. 0.2571), which showed that the interaction was synergistic. Meanwhile, the main effects of A and B were both statistically significant ($F_A = 68.77$, $P < 0.001$; $F_B = 38.46$, $P < 0.001$).

18.5.4. *Reporting results of Example 18.4 (Repeated Measures Design)*

Repeated measures ANOVA requires homogeneity and sphericity of the covariance matrix of measures at repeated factor levels. The reports should include the test results of homogeneity and sphericity first. The following are the reports of the results from Example 18.4.

In a nutritional experiment, 16 animals of the same species with similar age in months were randomly assigned to two equal-size groups and were fed by two different kinds of feedstuff. They were weighted every two weeks and the weight gains were recorded at four consecutive time points.

The sample means and standard deviations ($\bar{x} \pm s$, g)of the weight gains at the four time points in Group 1 were 27.625 ± 6.739, 32.875 ± 5.768, 31.000 ± 3.338 and 30.000 ± 3.703, respectively; and those in Group 2 were 20.125 ± 4.612, 25.750 ± 4.713, 29.625 ± 3.777 and 33.875 ± 4.704, respectively.

The result of Box's test showed that the assumption of the equality of covariance matrices should not be rejected ($F = 0.903$, $P = 0.530$). The result of Mauchly's test of sphericity showed that the assumption of the covariance matrix being spherical was violated ($\chi^2 = 12.810$, $P = 0.026$), so that the degrees of freedom of F statistic for within-subjects effect should be adjusted. The estimated adjustment factor of Greenhouse-Geisser Epsilon was 0.599.

The ANOVA results for repeated measurement showed that the interaction between treatment and time was significant ($F = 5.125$, $P = 0.016$); the main effect of the treatment was significant ($F = 6.209$, $P = 0.026$); and the main effect of time was also significant ($F = 8.616$, $P = 0.002$). ANOVA was then conducted separately for the two treatment groups. The results showed that the difference among the 4 time points in Group 1 was not significant ($F = 1.508$, $P = 0.257$), while that in Group 2 was significant ($F = 13.679$, $P = 0.002$). Comparison with polynomial transformation for different time points in Group 2 indicated that the weight gain linearly increased with time ($F = 18.372$, $P = 0.004$).

18.6. Case discrimination

Case 18.1 A researcher enrolled 13 patients with gallbladder cholesterol calculus and took their gallstones to study the effects of dissolution stone by methyl tert-butyl ether (MTBE). Three stones of similar shape and weight were selected from each patient. Each of the stones from the same subject was randomly allocated into one of three groups: MTBE supplemented by ultrasound, MTBE by perfusion, and MTBE in static state. The duration before complete dissolution is listed in Table 18.24. The author analyzed the data using t-test to compare means between any two groups. The questions are: (1) Is the data analysis method correct? (2) What problems does this data analysis method lead to?

Case 18.2 A doctor wanted to test how medications A and B affected patients with iron-deficiency anemia (IDA). He recruited 12 IDA patients and randomly allocated them to four groups. Three participants in Group 1 were given both A and B; Group 2 were only given A and Group 3 were only given B; and Group 4 were given neither A nor B. In order to avoid violating the requirements of medical ethics, all participants were on a special high-iron diet under the guidance of a doctor during the entire study period. After a month of treatment, the increase in red blood cells was recorded for each participant, and the data are shown in Table 18.25. The doctor analyzed the data using ANOVA, and the study results are displayed in Table 18.26.

Table 18.24 Time spent (minutes) of stone dissolution by three MTBE methods on 13 subjects

Treatment method	No. of subject													Mean	Standard deviation
	1	2	3	4	5	6	7	8	9	10	11	12	13		
Supplemented by ultrasound	40	30	25	32	22	13	8	12	8	10	14	10	20	18.77	10.37
By perfusion	43	36	30	35	35	16	15	30	13	18	16	15	25	25.77	10.75
In static state	644	690	645	390	420	700	690	570	670	690	660	712	676	624.46	105.15

Table 18.25 Increase of red blood cell ($\times 10^{12}$/L) of 12 IDA patients after one-month treatment

Group	Treatment	Increase of red blood cell ($\times 10^{12}$/L)			n_i	ΣX_i	ΣX_i^2	$\overline{X_i}$
Group 1	A + B + High iron diet	2.1	2.2	2	3	6.3	13.25	2.1
Group 2	A + High iron diet	1.3	1.2	1.1	3	3.6	4.34	1.2
Group 3	B + High iron diet	0.9	1.1	1	3	3.0	3.02	1.0
Group 4	High iron diet	0.8	0.9	0.7	3	2.4	1.94	0.8
Total					12	15.3	22.55	1.275

Table 18.26 The results of ANOVA for data in Table 18.25

Variance source	SS	ν	MS	F	P
Total	3.043	11			
Between groups	2.963	3	0.987	98.750	<0.001
Within groups	0.080	8	0.010		

Please answer:

(1) Was the right data analysis method used? If not, how can you improve the data analysis method?
(2) Please draw a statistical conclusion based on your analysis.

Case 18.3 To study the effect of an adjuvant agent for chemotherapy on improving white blood cell count, a clinical trial with a treatment period of two-week drug use and one-week withdrawal was conducted. Two hundred postoperative cancer patients were randomly allocated to two groups, and each received treatment in two phases. During the first phase of the trial, participants in Group 1 were treated with both chemotherapeutic drug and the adjuvant agent, while Group 2 participants were only given chemotherapeutic drug. After a washout period, all the subjects entered the second phase of the trial where the treatment regimen was interconverted. That means that Group 1 only used chemotherapeutic drug and

Table 18.27 Descriptive statistics and t-test for means of the logarithm of WBC count between two groups

Treatment	Phase I	Phase II
Chemotherapeutic drug and the adjuvant agent	8.4154 ± 0.1818	8.3403 ± 0.1804
Chemotherapeutic drug only	8.3756 ± 0.1814	8.3019 ± 0.1940
	$t = 1.5470$, $P = 0.1235$	$t = 1.4469$, $P = 0.1495$

Group 2 used both chemotherapeutic drug and the adjuvant agent during the second stage. The type and dose of the chemotherapeutic drug for all the subjects were kept the same from the beginning to the end of the trial.

The count of white blood cells was used to measure the curative effect, and each patient was examined at the end of the first and the second stage. The researcher used log transform for the count of WBC because the data were right-skewed. The researcher then calculated the mean and standard deviation for each group at each stage. He then compared the population means between two groups using t test for each stage. The results are displayed in Table 18.27.

He concluded that the adjuvant agent might not be effective in improving WBC because the P values of t-tests were greater than 0.05.

Questions:

Are there any problems with these analyses? How would you analyze the data?

Case 18.4 To test the effect of Drug A and Drug B on weight control, 80 female subjects with body mass index (BMI) over 25 kg/m^2 were randomly allocated to two groups. Participants were asked to take the given drug for 6 months. The BMI was the study outcome, and each subject was measured BMI three times: at the beginning of the study, at the end of the third month, and at the end of the sixth month.

Data from this experiment were analyzed using repeated measures ANOVA. The results are displayed in Table 18.28 and

Table 18.28 Descriptive statistics of BMI (kg/m^2) for the two groups at three time points

Drug	Baseline	The end of the third month	The end of the sixth month
A	27.96 ± 1.39	24.74 ± 1.43	24.72 ± 1.32
B	27.95 ± 1.15	25.53 ± 1.22	23.85 ± 1.53

Table 18.29 Results of repeated measures ANOVA for the data of Case 18.4

Source	*SS*	*df*	*MS*	*F*	*P*
Treatment	0.05	1	0.05	0.02	0.8985
Error of between-subject	257.23	78	3.30		
Time	588.94	2	294.47	274.21	0.0000
Treatment × Time	27.40	2	13.70	12.76	0.0000
Error of within-subject	167.53	156	1.07		
Total	1041.16	239	4.36		

Table 18.29. The P value of Mauchly's sphericity test was 0.795, so that the covariance matrix of measurement at time points was supposed to be spherical.

Question:

The P value for testing interaction between treatment and time was less than 0.0001, but the P value for the main effect of treatment was 0.8985 (Table 18.29). How do you interpret the results? Can you conclude that the effect difference between Drug A and Drug B is not statistically significant?

18.7. Computer experiments (Reference to electronic materials exp18.1 to exp18.4)

Experiment 18.1 To analyze the data of Example 18.1 with SPSS

To learn the software implementation and the interpretation of the results of ANOVA for randomized block design by SPSS.

Experiment 18.2 To analyze the data of Example 18.2 with SPSS

To learn the software implementation and the interpretation of the results of ANOVA for 2 × 2 factorial design by SPSS.

Experiment 18.3 To analyze the data of Example 18.3 with SPSS

To learn the software implementation and the interpretation of the results of ANOVA for 2-stage crossover design by SPSS.

Experiment 18.4 To analyze the data of Example 18.4 with SPSS

To learn the software implementation and the interpretation of the results of ANOVA for repeated measurements design by SPSS.

18.8. Frequently asked questions and summary

18.8.1. *Frequently asked questions*

1. **Q:** What will happen if the data of randomized block design are analyzed with one way ANOVA?

A: If the data of randomized block design are analyzed by one way ANOVA, the total variance will be decomposed into between-treatment and within-treatment variance, which means that the variance between blocks is mixed with variance of within treatments. This would lead to an overestimate of the variance of random error, so that the F value would become smaller, and the power would become lower for testing the treatment effect.

2. **Q:** What will happen if you analyze the data from a factorial designed experiment using one way ANOVA?

A: The subjects in a factorial designed experiment are usually randomly divided into several groups, similar to those from a completely randomized design. Therefore, the conclusion of whether the population means are equal in all groups can be drawn from the results of one way ANOVA. If the null hypothesis of equal population means is not rejected, we may conclude that the differences in population means between groups with any combination of factor levels are not statistically significant. This means that the main effect of any factor and all the interactions are not significant and further analysis is not necessary. Conversely, if the null hypothesis is rejected, we need to further analyze the causes for the difference in effects among groups. We could decompose the between-group variance into main effect of each factor and interactions generated by any factors and divide the MS of each part by MS of error to get its own F statistic and the corresponding P value. In short, analyzing the data from a factorial designed experiment by one way ANOVA would be incomplete. The results of one-way ANOVA are not useful for determining the source of the difference among groups.

3. Q: How to understand the concepts of main effect and interaction effect?

A: The main effect of a factor is the effect of the variable itself on the dependent variable averaged across the levels of any other factors. In other words, main effects are essentially the overall effect of a factor. Interaction refers to the joint influence of two or more factors on dependent variable. A statistical interaction occurs when the effect of one factor on the dependent variable *changes* depending on the level of another factor.

In an experiment with a factorial design, a non-zero main effect of a factor indicates that the population means of dependent variable at different levels of the factor are not equal. If factor A and factor B exhibit interaction, the effect of factor A changes at different levels of B, and vice versa. If interaction of A and B exists, while the main effect of A is zero, we cannot assert that A is ineffective, because the individual effect might be covered up by the interaction. Figure 18.5 illustrates such a situation where the interaction effect between factors A and B exists, but the main effect of factor A is nearly zero. Therefore, the test result for the main effect in ANOVA is meaningless when the interaction is statistically significant. In this case, the individual effect of A should be analyzed separately at a given level of B.

Additionally, if the experiment includes three or more factors, we should consider not only interactions between any two factors, but also more complex interactions. For example, the secondary interaction among three factors indicates that the interaction between

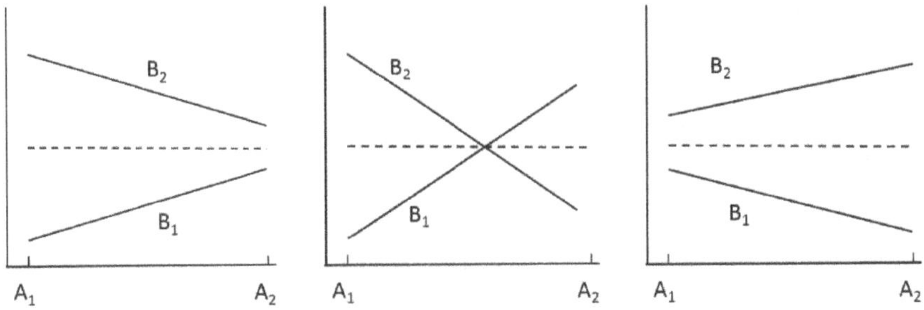

Figure 18.5 Several possible diagrams for the following situations: Interaction effect between factors A and B exists, but the main effect of factor A is nearly zero. The solid lines represent means of A1 and A2 at given levels of B (B1 or B2). The dotted line is the connecting line of gross population means of A1 and A2.

factors A and B changes depending on the level of factor C. In practice, higher order interactions are usually ignored due to their complexity and difficulty in interpretation.

18.8.2. *Summary*

1. This chapter mainly introduces the ANOVA method of data analysis for randomized block design, two-stage crossover design, 2×2 factorial design and repeated measurement design. The sum of squares (SS) of observations with randomized block design can be decomposed into SS of between treatment groups, SS of between blocks, and SS of residual. The SS of observations with two-stage crossover design is decomposed into SS of between treatment groups, SS of two stages, SS of individuals and SS of residuals. For 2×2 factorial design, the SS of observations is decomposed into SS of main effect of factor A, SS of main effect of factor B, SS of interaction and SS of residual. For repeated measurement data, the observations within an individual are not independent so that the method of ANOVA depends on the result of a sphericity test for the covariance matrix.
2. The prerequisites of ANOVA including independence, normality, and homoscedasticity of the observations should be determined before conducting the ANOVA. However, small sample size usually limits the power of hypothesis testing for these assumptions.

Therefore, in practice, we often speculate whether these assumptions are met by using scatter plots of residuals and we may use nonparametric methods instead when any assumptions are violated.

3. To explain the results from data with factorial design or repeated measures design, the significance of the test for interaction should be first focused. If the interaction is significant, we should explain the main effect cautiously and further analyze the main effect of a factor at a fixed level of the other factor. On the contrary, if the interaction is not significant, the SS of interaction may be combined with that of residuals in ANOVA to simplify the results. Diagrams are useful to illustrate the results and their interpretation.

Think and Practice

I. Best Choice

1. For data with the randomized block design, which of the following equations is correct? ( )
   A. $SS_{\text{Total}} = SS_{\text{Treatment}} + SS_{\text{error}}$ B. $SS_{\text{Total}} = SS_{\text{block}} + SS_{\text{error}}$ C. $SS_{\text{Total}} = SS_{\text{treatment}} + SS_{\text{block}} + SS_{\text{error}}$ D. $MS_{\text{Total}} = MS_{\text{treatment}} + MS_{\text{block}} + MS_{\text{error}}$ E. None of the above.
2. What kind of ANOVA can replace paired t-test? ( )
   A. ANOVA of completely randomized design B. ANOVA of randomized block design C. ANOVA of crossover design D. ANOVA of repeated measurement design E. None of the above
3. For the ANOVA of two-stage crossover design, which of the following equations is correct? ( )
   A. $SS_{\text{Total}} = SS_{\text{treatment}} + SS_{\text{stage}} + SS_{\text{error}}$ B. $SS_{\text{Total}} = SS_{\text{treatment}} + SS_{\text{order}} + SS_{\text{individual}} + SS_{\text{error}}$ C. $SS_{\text{Total}} = SS_{\text{treatment}} + SS_{\text{stage}} + SS_{\text{individual}} + SS_{\text{error}}$ D. $SS_{\text{Total}} = SS_{\text{treatment}} + SS_{\text{stage}} + SS_{\text{order}} + SS_{\text{error}}$ E. None of the above.
4. For the ANOVA of repeated measurement design, the total variance can be decomposed into ( ).
   A. between-subject variance and within-subject variance. B. between-treatment variance and variance of among levels

of repeated factor. C. individual variance and random error. D. variance of among levels of repeated factor and random error. E. None of the above.

II. Questions for Reflection

1. What are the differences between randomized block design and completely randomized design in design and data analysis?
2. For the data of Group 2 in Example 18.4, please try to analyze them using repeated measurement ANOVA by the "General Linear Model → Repeated Measures" and using two-way ANOVA by the "General Linear Model → Univariate" in SPSS software. Then, please compare the results from these two types of analyses to find the difference between the test for the main effect of time in repeated measures ANOVA and the test for time in two-way ANOVA. What can you learn from the comparison? Please contemplate the relationship between repeated measures ANOVA and two-way ANOVA for randomized block design.

III. Questions on Calculation

1. Every three of 36 experimental rats were matched as a block by similar weights, and 12 blocks resulted in total. The three rats in every block were randomly allocated to three treatment groups. The effect indicator of this experiment was the excretion of amino nitrogen in the urine. After the calculation, we got $SS_{\text{Total}} = 162$, $SS_{\text{block}} = 8$ and $SS_{\text{treatment}} = 110$. Please list the results in an ANOVA table for these data and draw a conclusion.
2. Every three of 18 patients with thrombocytopenia idiopathic were matched as a block by similar illness degree and age. There were six blocks in total. The three patients in a block were randomly allocated to be treated by Drug A, B, or C. Increment of blood platelet was recorded at the end of the experiment, and the data are shown in Table 18.30. Please determine whether there is difference in the treatment effects among the 3 treatments.

Table 18.30 Increment of blood platelet (10^{12}/l) in patients with thrombocytopenia idiopathic after treated

	Block					
Treatment	1	2	3	4	5	6
A	3.8	4.6	7.6	8.6	6.4	6.2
B	6.3	6.3	10.2	9.2	8.1	6.9
C	8.0	11.9	14.1	14.7	13	13.4

Table 18.31 Phagocytic index of 20 rats in an experiment of adjuvant

Benzene-free group		Benzene-injected group	
No adjuvant	Adjuvant	No adjuvant	Adjuvant
3.80	3.88	1.85	1.94
3.90	3.84	2.01	2.25
4.06	3.96	2.10	2.03
3.85	3.92	1.92	2.10
3.84	3.80	2.04	2.08

3. To study the effect of an adjuvant treatment, an animal experiment was conducted. Twenty rats were randomly divided into two groups with 10 each. The 10 rats in one group were subcutaneously injected benzene with a dose of 0.3ml/kg, three times per week until the count of white blood cells decreased 50% or so. Rats in the other group were not injected benzene as controls. The 10 animals in each group were further randomly divided into two groups and one group was given the adjuvant but the other group was not. The experiment results were shown in Table 18.31. Please do analysis.
4. A double-blind trial was conducted to explore the effect of a medication on alleviating pain for dysmenorrhea women. Thirty dysmenorrhea women were randomly divided into two groups.

Table 18.32 Scores of VAS for Pain by 30 dysmenorrhea women in a double-blind trial

Group 1			Group 2		
No. of Subject	1st period: Using medication	2nd period: Using placebo	No. of Subject	1st period: Using placebo	2nd period: Using medication
1	43	34	16	28	47
2	34	31	17	37	31
3	48	31	18	29	36
4	34	27	19	34	39
5	25	13	20	26	36
6	43	25	21	33	42
7	37	30	22	35	46
8	34	22	23	34	51
9	39	30	24	34	43
10	42	22	25	47	37
11	38	36	26	22	42
12	41	26	27	40	43
13	28	32	28	30	46
14	35	27	29	40	39
15	42	29	30	38	31

Subjects in Group 1 were given the medication when experiencing pain during the first menstrual period, but they were given a placebo during the second menstrual period. Subjects in Group 2 were given placebo during the first menstrual period but given the medication during the second period. The degree of pain of each subject was assessed using the Visual Analog Scale For Pain two times in her two menstrual periods. A higher score on the scale means a higher degree of pain. The data were shown in Table 18.32. Please analyze the data to determine if the medication is effective.

5. To evaluate the effects of a drug on the heart rate variability (HRV, millisecond), 20 patients with abnormal HRV following inclusion criteria were randomly divided into two groups (treatment and control). Every patient was measured HRV four

Table 18.33 HRV measurements (millisecond) at four time points for 20 patients with abnormal HRV

Treatment group					Control group				
No.	Before treatment	First week	Second week	Third week	No.	Before treatment	First week	Second week	Third week
1	45.3	52.4	61.0	70.4	11	36.1	41.8	48.3	63.0
2	40.3	48.7	54.9	66.4	12	42.0	46.8	53.8	67.4
3	41.0	48.8	54.8	68.8	13	43.7	50.5	53.2	69.2
4	38.0	44.9	52.7	63.0	14	41.4	46.2	54.3	64.7
5	42.7	50.8	56.7	70.2	15	41.5	50.0	53.6	65.7
6	39.1	45.1	55.3	64.9	16	45.0	52.4	57.5	70.6
7	43.1	52.3	56.5	69.1	17	42.2	47.8	53.2	70.3
8	39.3	46.2	56.9	67.8	18	42.5	45.4	55.8	68.7
9	41.9	48.0	57.3	65.4	19	37.0	42.7	48.1	61.9
10	37.8	44.7	54.1	65.0	20	35.5	40.8	45.9	59.5

times: before trial, at the end of the first, second and third week after starting the trial. The data were shown in Table 18.33. Please analyze the data and draw statistical conclusion.

Acknowledgements

The authors would like to express their deep gratitude to Professor Junling Wang and Doctor Edward Chiyaka, who worked at College of Pharmacy, University of Tennessee Health Science Center. Prof. Wang and Dr. Chiyaka revised and polished this chapter patiently and selflessly. The authors would also like to thanks Dr. Zhongshang Yuan, an associate professor working at Shandong University, who gave some valuable advice for this chapter.

References

[1] Yuanjie, J, Liangping, H, Dehe, C. Statistical analysis for quantitative data with crossover design and SAS solutions. *Pharm Care Res.* 2012;12(3):172–174. (in Chinese)

[2] Songlin, Y, Huiyun, X. *Methods for Analyzing Repeated Measures Data and SAS Programs.* [M] Beijing: Science Press; 2004:3. (in Chinese)
[3] Hongyun, L, Lei, C. *Longitudinal Data Analysis Methods and its Applications.* [M] Beijing, Educational Science Publishing House; 2005:5. (in Chinese)
[4] Bernard, R.*Fundamentals of Biostatistics.* 8th ed. Boston, MA:Brooks/Cole; 2015.

Liu Jing, Liu Yi

CHAPTER 19

MULTIPLE LINEAR REGRESSION

The interaction between factors is very common in the field of biomedical research. For example, height is not only affected by genetic factors, but also by nutritional status, physical exercise, living environment, etc.; blood pressure is related to not only age but also family history, diet, and labor intensity; the score of health-related Quality of Life (QoL) is influenced by physiological, psychological, social, environmental and many other factors. This chapter describes how multiple linear regression analysis can be used to quantitatively characterize the effects of multiple factors on the outcome variable such as height and blood pressure acting on health-related QoL score.

19.1. Overview

1. Multiple linear regression

Multiple linear regression is an important classical multi-factor analysis method, which is an extension of the simple linear regression and it applies regression equation to quantitatively describe linear dependency between a dependent variable Y and multiple independent variables. Multiple linear regression focuses on only one dependent variable; therefore, it is also called univariate linear regression. When multiple dependent variables are included in the model, we often name it as multivariate linear regression or multivariate linear model.

2. Variable selection and optimal model

Many independent variables may be involved in the process of establishing multiple linear regression, some of which may not be important. There may be a larger measurement error, also may be highly correlated with each other and influence the effect of the regression model, therefore we need to select valuable variables. The variable selection process must be very careful not to exclude the key independent variables, which significantly affect the outcome. Detailed selection methods will be introduced later.

3. Interaction effect

The concept of interaction effect has been mentioned in the previous chapter "analysis of variance in a factorial design." People also often consider whether there is an interaction effect in multiple linear regression analysis. We say there is an interaction effect between two independent variables if the linear relationship between an independent variable and the dependent variable changes along with another independent variable value. The interaction effect is also called an effect modification and the interacting variable is called an effect modifier.

19.2. Multiple linear regression model

19.2.1. *Setting the scene*

Example 19.1. In Chapter 9, in the study of the relationship between nitric oxide (NO) concentration (ppm) and traffic flow (per thousand car), temperature (°C), humidity (%), wind speed (m/s), etc., we only consider the effect of traffic flow on the NO concentration and established the simple linear regression equation to predict NO concentration with traffic flow only. It is known that the atmospheric concentration of NO could also be affected by the temperature, humidity, wind speed, and many other factors, therefore, to predict the concentration of NO more effectively, these predictive factors should also be included in the linear regression equation.

Namely, a simple linear regression equation that includes one independent variable is extended to a multiple linear regression equation including multiple independent variables. Now, we still use this example to illustrate the basic concept and principle of the multiple linear regression, see Chapter 9, Table 9.1 for the data.

According to the basic principles and steps of the simple correlation and regression analysis described earlier, the scatter plot between NO concentration and the number of passing cars in the unit time (per thousand), the temperature (°C), the humidity (%), the wind speed (m/s), are shown separately (Figure 19.1).

It can be seen from the scatter plot, the concentration of NO is positively correlated with traffic flow, and negatively correlated with wind speed, while there is no linear correlation with temperature and humidity. Simple linear correlation analysis shows that the correlation coefficient between the concentration of NO and traffic flow is

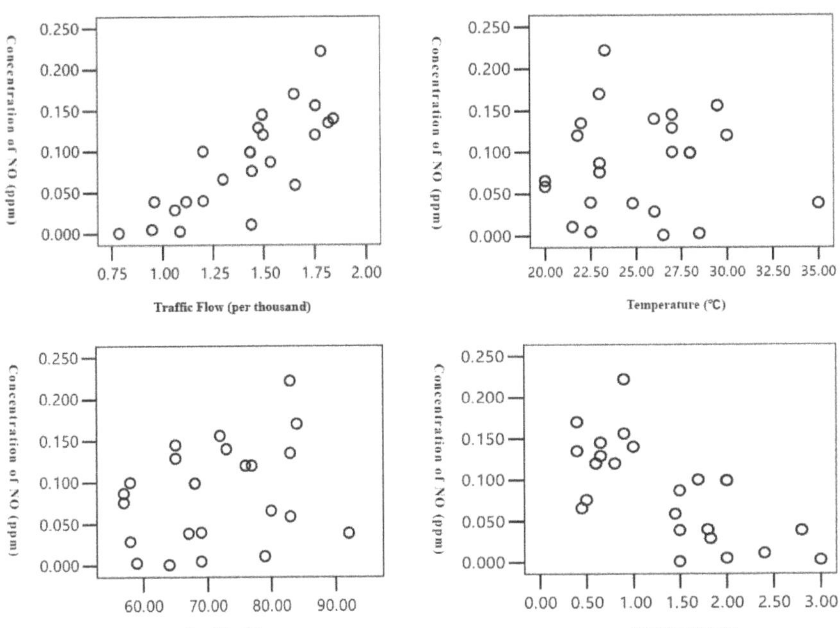

Figure 19.1 Scatter plot between NO concentration and traffic flow, temperature, humidity, and wind speed

0.808 and that between the concentration of NO and wind speed is −0.680, both the correlation coefficients have statistical significance. However, the correlation coefficients between the concentration of NO and temperature and humidity have no statistical significance, which means their overall correlation coefficients cannot be considered as non-zero. Through the above analysis, it can be preliminarily concluded that the concentration of NO is related to the traffic flow and wind speed.

Based on the research objectives and the collected data, the following questions are intended to be answered:

1. Did the number of cars passing in a unit time (per thousand), temperature (°C), humidity (%) and wind speed (m/s) affect the concentration of NO (ppm)?
2. How to quantitatively describe the effect of these factors on the concentration of NO?
3. Which factor had the greatest effect on the concentration of NO? Which factor had the least impact?
4. How to use these factors to predict the concentration of NO and how well does it work?

19.2.2. *Descriptive statistics*

1. Estimation of regression coefficients

Multiple linear regression model is an extension of simple linear regression model, the equation can be written as

$$\mu_{Y|x_1,x_2,\ldots,x_p} = \beta_0 + \beta_1 X_1 + \beta_2 X_2 + \cdots + \beta_P X_P \tag{19-1}$$

The regression equation of the sampling population can be written as

$$\hat{Y} = b_0 + b_1 X_1 + b_2 X_2 + \cdots + b_p X_p \tag{19-2}$$

Among which, $\hat{Y}$ is the estimation of the mean of dependent variable Y when the value of each independent variable is fixed. b_0 is called the constant term or Y-intercept, which is the estimation of a parameter β_0, which means the estimation of the mean of dependent variable Y while the value of each independent variable is zero. b_i is called the partial regression coefficient of variable X_i, which is the estimation of a parameter β_i, which means the dependent variable Y would change a b_i unit in average while the independent variable X_i change one unit and other variables in the equation keep unchanged.

Multiple linear regression analysis usually adopts least square (LS) method to estimate partial regression coefficients. The basic principle is searching for a set of suitable partial regression coefficients $(b_0, b_1, b_2, \ldots, b_p)$ to establish multiple linear regression equation and let the residual sum of squares between the observed values of the dependent variable Y_i and the estimate of the regression equation $\hat{Y}_i$ reach minimal value. The partial regression coefficients satisfying this condition are the estimated value obtained by the least square method.

Although the parameter estimation method of multiple linear regression analysis is the same as that of simple linear regression analysis; the computational cost becomes quite large due to the increase of the number of independent variables. Generally, statistical software is used to complete the parameter estimation.

According to the LS principle, with the help of statistical software, the fitted multiple linear regression equation of NO concentration by traffic flow (X_1), temperature (X_2), humidity (X_3), and wind speed (X_4) based on the sampling data is:

$$\hat{Y} = -0.142 + 0.116X_1 + 0.004X_2 - 6.55 \times 10^{-6}X_3 - 0.035X_4$$

2. Regression equation

If we want to establish a linear regression equation to predict NO concentration (Y) by only traffic flow (X_1) and wind speed (X_4), the equation can be written as:

$$\hat{Y} = b_0 + b_1X_1 + b_4X_4$$

Among which, b_4 means that the NO concentration will change b_4 ppm in average when the traffic flow is fixed and wind speed increases one unit (1m/s).

The partial regression coefficients cannot compare with each other directly. Since independent variables have their own units of measurement and different degrees of variation, it is impossible to directly compare the partial regression coefficients to reflect the contribution of each independent variable to the dependent variable. If the contribution of each independent variable to the dependent variable has to be compared, the original observed data should be standardized firstly, i.e.

$$X_i' = \frac{X_i - \bar{X}_i}{S_i} \tag{19-3}$$

Then the regression model is fitted with the standardized data, the obtained partial regression coefficients b_i' are named standardized partial regression coefficients. As the standardized partial regression coefficients b_i' have no measurement scale, they can be compared directly to reflect the contribution of each independent variable to the dependent variable Y. For example, if we want to compare the contribution of traffic flow and wind speed on the concentration of NO, the original data must be standardized first and then the standardized partial regression coefficients b_1' and b_4' can be obtained, next we compare the value of b_1' and b_4' directly to determine which factor influences the NO concentration more.

3. Questions to Answer

This multiple linear regression equation is estimated from a sampling data, and we need to answer three questions before using this equation for prediction or control:

(1) Does the regression equation make sense in general? Which means whether there is a linear relationship described by this regression equation in the population?
(2) How well does the regression equation work? What is the percentage of variation that these four independent variables can account for the dependent variable?
(3) Whether all four independent variables can affect the dependent variable Y? Which means whether the corresponding partial regression coefficients in the population $(\beta_1, \beta_2, \beta_3, \beta_4)$ estimated by the partial regression coefficients learned from the sampling data (b_1, b_2, b_3, b_4) equal to zero?

These three questions are all about inferring the overall characteristics from the sample information, so the next task is to make statistical inferences.

19.2.3. *Statistical inference*

1. Hypothesis test for regression equation

Analysis of variance (ANOVA) is usually used to test the significance of the regression equation. The null hypothesis is

$$H_0 : \beta_1 = \beta_2 = \beta_3 = \beta_4 = 0.$$

The basic ideas of ANOVA towards multiple linear regression are similar to that of simple linear regression stated in Chapter 9. The total sum of squares SS_{total} of dependent variable Y is divided into regression sum of squares $SS_{\text{regression}}$ and residual sum of squares SS_{residual}, and the degrees of freedom change a little accordingly, $\nu_{\text{total}} = n - 1$ (n is the sample size), $\nu_{\text{regression}} = p$ (p is the number of variables), and $\nu_{\text{residual}} = n - p - 1$. The ratio between each sum of squares and their degrees of freedom is denoted as MS, and the ratio between $MS_{\text{regression}}$ and MS_{residual} is denoted as F. It has been proved that F follows F distribution when the null hypothesis is true.

The results of the ANOVA are shown in Table 19.1. The P value in the table is smaller than 0.001, and we reject H_0 according to $\alpha = 0.05$, which means the regression equation composed of these four independent variables is statistically significant to explain the change of NO concentration.

The coefficient of determination, or the determination coefficient, can be calculated from the results in the ANOVA table to reflect the

Table 19.1 ANOVA test for the significance of the regression equation

Variation source	*df*	*SS*	*MS*	*F*	*P*
Regression	4	0.064	0.016	17.59	<0.001
Residual	19	0.017	0.001		
Total	23	0.081			

effect of the regression equation. The calculation formula of coefficient of determination R^2 is:

$$R^2 = \frac{SS_{\text{regression}}}{SS_{\text{total}}} \tag{19-4}$$

In this case, we can get the $R^2 = 0.79$, it means that the regression equation works well and 79% variations of NO concentration can be explained by those four variables.

In addition to R^2, adjusted $R^2(R^2_{ad})$ is often used in multiple linear regression analysis, the calculation formula for which is:

$$\begin{aligned} R^2_{ad} &= 1 - \frac{MS_{\text{residual}}}{MS_{\text{total}}} = 1 - \frac{SS_{\text{residual}}/(n-p-1)}{SS_{\text{total}}/(n-1)} \\ &= 1 - R^2\left(\frac{n-1}{n-p-1}\right) \end{aligned} \tag{19-5}$$

The R^2_{ad} in this case is 0.743.

It has been found that R^2 keeps growing even when we add more independent variables with a small contribution to the dependent variable in the equation, and this is the defect of R^2. While R^2_{ad} just overcomes the defect, the R^2_{ad} may decrease when we add more independent variables with a small contribution to the dependent variable in the equation, so it is often used in the variable selection of multiple linear regression analysis.

Taking square root of R^2 as the multiple correlation coefficient.

$$R = \sqrt{\frac{SS_{\text{regression}}}{SS_{\text{total}}}} \tag{19-6}$$

The multiple correlation coefficient means the degree of linear correlation between Y and $(X_1, X_2, X_3, \ldots, X_P)$ ranging from 0 to 1. It can be proved that the multiple correlation coefficient equals to the simple correlation coefficient between $Y$and $\hat{Y}$.

$$R = corr(Y, \hat{Y})$$

Similarly, the adjusted multiple correlation coefficient R_{ad} is obtained by taking the square root of R^2_{ad}.

2. Hypothesis testing for the regression coefficient

Due to the sampling error, even if the population partial regression coefficient is equal to zero, it is possible to obtain a sample partial regression coefficient as non-zero. Therefore, a hypothesis test of the partial regression coefficient is needed to infer whether the overall partial regression coefficient is zero. If the overall partial regression coefficient is zero, then the corresponding independent variable has no effect on the dependent variable.

The t test is used to test whether the overall partial regression coefficient is zero or not. The assumption of the test is:

$$H_0 : \beta_i = 0$$

$$H_1 : \beta_i \neq 0$$

$$\alpha = 0.05$$

The t test statistic is

$$t_{bi} = \frac{b_i}{S_{bi}} \tag{19-7}$$

Where, S_{bi} is the ith standard error of partial regression coefficient

The results of the four-partial regression coefficient hypothesis tests in Example 19.1 are shown in Table 19.2.

It can be seen from the Table 19.2 that the effects of traffic flow, temperature, and wind speed influence the concentration of NO, there is a statistically significant difference ($P < 0.05$), but there is no statistically significant difference on the effect of humidity ($P > 0.05$). In addition, it can be found that the traffic flow has the

Table 19.2 The results of t test of partial regression coefficient and standardized partial regression coefficient

Variable	*df*	b	Standard error	t	P	b'
Traffic flow X_1	1	0.116	0.027	4.23	0.0005	0.592
Temperature X_2	1	0.004	0.002	2.36	0.0289	0.273
Humidity X_3	1	-6.55×10^{-6}	0.001	−0.01	0.9925	−0.001
Wind speed X_4	1	−0.035	0.011	−3.21	0.005	−0.448

greatest influence on the concentration of NO, followed by the wind speed and the temperature successively, according to the value of the standardized partial regression coefficient.

19.2.4. *Selection of independent variables*

According to the above analysis of Example 19.1, not all the independent variables considered in advance have statistically significant effects on the dependent variable. The purpose of multiple linear regression analysis is to establish an optimal regression model, the independent variables contained in the model are statistically significant on the dependent variable. Therefore, in the process of multiple regression analysis, the independent variables need to be screened, the independent variables, which have no influence on the dependent variables should be removed from the model, and include the independent variables, which have statistically significant effect on the dependent variables in the model. Questions like, how to determine the criteria for an independent variable to be entered or removed, how to filter variables, and what are the commonly used strategies for variable screening will be discussed next.

1. Statistical criteria for independent variable screening

(1) The reduced residual sum of squares (SS_{residual}) or the increase in the determination coefficient (R^2) determines the variable selection. If there is a large reduction in residual sum of squares or increase in the determination coefficient after an independent variable is rolled into the model, it is indicated that the variable has great influence on Y, and can be included; on the contrary, if there is little influence on Y, the variable cannot be included. The disadvantage of this standard is that for each additional rolling of variable, residual sum of the squares will always decrease, and the determination coefficient will always increase, even if the statistically insignificant independent variable is added, so that it tends to select all the variables.

(2) The reduced residual mean square (MS_{residual}) or the increased standardized determination coefficient (R^2_{ad}). The equation of

residual mean square is:

$$MS_{\text{residual}} = \frac{SS_{\text{residual}}}{n-p-1} \tag{19-8}$$

According to the formula of the residual mean square, as the number of the independent variable increases, the residual sum of the squares in the numerator as well as the degree of freedom $(n-p-1)$ in the denominator reduces. If the added independent variable is not statistically significant, then the residual mean square in the numerator is not reduced greatly, and the degree of freedom in the denominator is reduced more, so the value of the residual mean square does not decrease. In order to reduce the residual mean square, the independent variable introduced into the model must have a greater influence on Y, so the residual mean square is reduced further. If an introduced independent variable has little effect on Y, the residual sum of squares SS_{residual} in the numerator is decreased less and the denominator $(n-p-1)$ is decreased more. As a result, the value of residual mean square MS_{residual} increases rather than decreasing, hence, such independent variable is not recommended to roll into the model.

The criterion of reduction for residual mean square MS_{residual} is equivalent to the increase of standardized determination coefficient R^2_{ad}. This criterion takes into account the number of independent variables in evaluating the fitting effect and is more reasonable than the previous one.

(3) The reduced of C_P statistic, C_P statistic is defined as:

$$C_P = \frac{SS_{\text{residual},p}}{MS_{\text{residual},T}} + 2(p+1) - n \tag{19-9}$$

In the formula, the $SS_{\text{residual},p}$ is denoted as the residual sum of squares when regression with p independent variables, and the $MS_{\text{residual},T}$ is denoted as the residual mean square when regression with all independent variables. This statistic was proposed by Mallows (citation). The complete meaning of this criterion is selecting smaller C_P and the model with the value of C_P closer to its number of unknown parameters. The criterion, which requires smaller C_P

statistics conforms to the principle of statistical modeling: On the one hand, there cannot be too many independent variables, so that the equations are easy to understand and explain, and the workload and research costs are reduced. On the other hand, the independent variables cannot be too few to ensure a certain accuracy of estimation and prediction. Therefore, the criterion for the smaller C_P statistics is relatively more respected.

In addition to the above criterions, there are other criteria, such as the largest U_P and Akaike information criterion (AIC), which are not introduced here. Readers can read related monographs.

2. Algorithms for variable selection

There are some common algorithms for selecting independent variables, including forward regression, backward regression, stepwise regression, and optimal subset regression. Most statistical software uses the value of the "partial regression sum of squares" as the basis for each step of the selection of variables. It represents the part of the regression sum of squares, which is increased or decreased after introducing or removing an independent variable based on the original regression equation. When the value reaches a certain level, the variable can be rolled into the model or eliminated out of the model. The specific threshold can be determined by the F statistic.

For example, to determine whether an independent variable can be rolled into the current equation, the following test can be performed

H_0: P variables are better
H_1: $P+1$ variables are better

The following formula is used as the test statistic generally

$$F = \frac{SS_{\text{residual}}(H_0) - SS_{\text{residual}}(H_1)}{SS_{\text{residual}}(H_1)/(n-p-2)} \tag{19-10}$$

Among them, the degree of freedom is $\nu_1 = 1$ in the numerator and the degree of freedom is $\nu_2 = n - p - 2$ in the denominator. $SS_{\text{residual}}(H_0)$ and $SS_{\text{residual}}(H_1)$ respectively represent the residual sum of squares in the model when P independent variables are rolled into and the residual sum of squares in the model when $P+1$ independent variables are rolled into. The difference between them is called the partial regression sum of squares of the $P+1$ variables. Given the α value, F_α can be found in the F distribution table, by one-sided threshold with degrees of freedom equal to 1 and $n-p-2$. If $F \geq F_\alpha$, then H_0 is rejected, the corresponding independent variable can be rolled into the model; otherwise, without H_0 being rejected, the corresponding independent variable cannot be rolled into the model.

(1) Forward method

The independent variables are rolled into the regression equation one by one. The first selected independent variable meets the requirement when the partial regression sum of squares is the largest one and H_0 is rejected after F test. A critical value $F_{\text{inclusion}}$ is specified, then the following selected independent variable that meets the requirement when the partial regression sum of squares is the largest one and H_0 is rejected after the F test. You will have to keep carrying out the same procedure for the rest of the independent variables until no H_0 can be rejected. The forward regression only considers whether variables outside the model can be rolled into the model.

(2) Backward method

The independent variables are removed from the equation one by one. First, a total regression is performed on all suitable variables, then the independent variable when its partial regression sum of squares is the least and the H_0 cannot be rejected after F test will be removed, until none of the variables can be removed further. The backward regression only considers whether there are variables in the model that should be rejected if they do not meet the requirements.

(3) Stepwise method

Combining the above two methods, after each step forward, it is necessary to be considered that an independent variable becomes not statistically significant and should be excluded. Two critical value $F_{\text{exclusion}}$ and ($F_{\text{inclusion}} > F_{\text{exclusion}}$) are specified in advance. When an independent variable has the largest partial regression sum of squares and its $F \geq F_{\text{inclusion}}$, the variable should be included in the equation. Similarly, when an independent variable has the smallest partial regression sum of squares and its $F \geq F_{\text{exclusion}}$, the variable should be excluded from the equation. Such inclusion and exclusion procedures are performed alternately until no variable can be included or excluded from the equation. Note that the adjusted critical value of $F_{\text{imclusion}}$ and $F_{\text{exclusion}}$ would change the result of regression. If there are more variables to be included, you can reduce the critical value $F_{\text{imclusion}}$. If there are fewer variables to be included, you can increase the critical value $F_{\text{exclusion}}$.

(4) Optimal subsets method

When there are p independent variables, all possible subsets of independent variables are used in regression equations, then the number of the equation is $(2^p - 1)$. According to a certain selection criterion of variables, one or several optimal regression subsets are selected by comparing the degree to which each subset meets the criterion, which is called "optimal subsets regression". It is also possible to specify the minimum (or maximum) number of variables appearing in the subset in advance, and then implement the selection of the "optimal" subset within the certain scope of all possible variables in different subsets. This method is only suitable in the condition if the number of independent variables is not too large.

For the same dataset, the independent variables selected by the above four methods respectively are not all the same and are not the "optimal subsets". When the number of independent variables is large, statistical methods are rough in screening variables. Therefore, it cannot be used as a final conclusion, nor replace the professional knowledge related to the problem. Before implementing regression, we must sort out the independent variables by professional knowledge, distinguish between direct and indirect factors, primary and secondary factors, clarify the relationship among them, and avoid analyzing all of them without distinguishing. Through the screening of the model and the interpretation of professional knowledge, we can find a model that satisfies both the statistical requirements and professional knowledge. This is the "optimal model" that the researchers hope for.

Table 19.3 Parameter estimation and statistics for two regression models

				Estimates of model				
R^2	R^2_{ad}	C_P	MS_{residual}	*Intercept*	X_1	X_2	X_3	X_4
0.787	0.755	3.00	.0008	−0.142	0.116	0.004	—	−0.035
0.787	0.743	5.00	.0009	−0.142	0.116	0.004	−6.6E-6	−0.035

The data of Example 19.1 was analyzed by stepwise method, and the model containing three independent variables was obtained. Comparing with the model containing all four independent variables (see Table 19.3 for details), according to the value of R^2, R^2_{ad}, C_P, and MS_{residual}, it can be considered that the model containing three independent variables is better than the model containing four independent variables, so the final regression equation can be written as:

$$\hat{Y} = -0.142 + 0.116X_1 + 0.004X_2 - 0.035X_4$$

Traffic flow, temperature and wind speed are better to predict the concentration of NO in the air.

19.3. The applications of multiple linear regression

19.3.1. *The application of multiple linear regression in biomedicine*

Multiple linear regression is widely used in biomedical researches, which can be summarized in the following aspects.

1. Establish a linear relationship between a dependent variable and multiple independent variables quantitatively. For example, establish a linear relationship between the size of the lung capacity and the variables, such as height, weight, age, and gender.
2. Screen risk factors. For example, screen the risk factors of hypertension.
3. Estimate variables that are difficult to measure by variables that are easier to measure. For example, by establishing a multiple

linear regression equation for infant body surface area with measurement of the height, weight, and age, while the body surface area can be estimated easily with the use of other variables.

4. Predict dependent variables by independent variables. For example, the concentration of NO in the air can be predicted by variables, such as wind speed, traffic flow, and temperature.
5. Control independent variables by the dependent variable. For example, in the condition of constant temperature and wind speed, by prescribing the upper limit to the concentration of NO in the air, the value of the traffic flow can be calculated.

19.3.2. *Preconditions and analysis of residuals*

The precondition for multiple linear regression analysis is the same as simple linear regression, which requires the data to satisfy linearity, independency, normal distribution and equal variance, abbreviated as LINE. Linearity refers to a linear tendency between the dependent variable Y and independent variables. Independency means that the individual observations are independent of each other. Normal distribution means that given the value of independent variables, the corresponding Y follows a normal distribution. Equal variance refers to a constant variance of Y for different values of X, denoted with σ^2.

How to check whether the data meet the four preconditions? A simple and practical method is the analysis of residuals. Residual is defined as $Y - \hat{Y}$. The examination of the residual plot is a direct and effective informal method. For example, the normal probability plot or histogram of residuals can be used to check normality. The scatter plot of residuals and the fitted value of the dependent variables can be used to check whether the model satisfies linearity and equal variance. If the plot tends to be a curve, the nonlinear functions or appropriate variable transformation should be considered in the model. If the scatter plot is in the shape of a trumpet, it suggests that the equal variances do not hold. If there exists a significant structure in the residual plot based on time points, the role of time variables or individual independence should be considered.

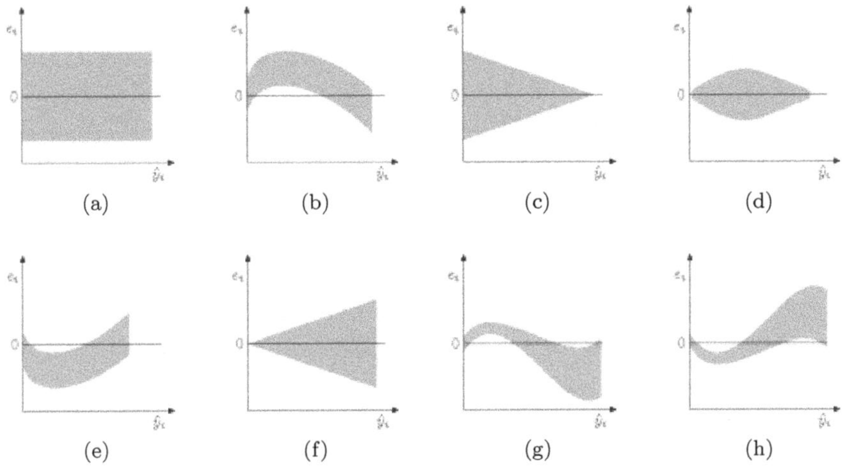

Figure 19.2 Scatter plots of residuals

Several scatter plots of residuals are shown in Figure 19.2. The ordinate represents the residual e and the abscissa represents the fitted value $\hat{Y}$ of the dependent variable.

If the points are randomly distributed in the zonal region centered on $e = 0$ and parallel to the horizontal axis, as shown in Figure 19.2(a), it can be considered to basically satisfy the assumptions of linearity and equal variance. The scatter plot in Figure 19.2(b) or (c) shows a curve trend indicating nonlinear data. Figure 19.2(d), (e) or (f) shows that the residuals change with the fitted values $\hat{Y}_i$ indicating unequal variances of data. Figure 19.2(g) or (h) shows that the residuals change with the fitted values $\hat{Y}_i$ and it has a curve shape, which indicates that the data satisfy neither linearity nor equal variances.

Regarding the verification of independence, in addition to drawing the residual plot, it can also be judged by calculating the Durbin-Watson statistic. The value of the statistic is generally between 0 and 4. If the residuals are independent of each other, the value is around 2. If the value is close to 0 or 4, it is suggested that independence is not satisfied. Durbin-Watson statistic can be calculated by many statistical software.

If the analysis of residuals shows that the data does not satisfy the assumptions of LINE, commonly handling methods are as follows:

1. If the data are nonlinear, consider modifying the model or using curve fitting.
2. If the data does not meet normality or equal variances, variable transformation is generally applied to satisfy the assumption of normality and variance homogeneity. The common transformation methods include logarithmic transformation, square root transformation, reciprocal transformation, etc., which are better used for independent variables.
3. If there is no variance homogeneity, the following methods can be used to estimate the partial regression coefficients such as the weighted least square method. The specific principles can be found in other monographs.

19.3.3. *Multi-collinearity*

In addition to the preconditions for linearity, independency, normality and equal variance, the relationship between independent variables should also be considered when performing multiple linear regression analysis. When random independent variables are highly correlated, it is said to be multi-collinearity between them. Collinearity brings a lot of trouble to regression estimation and inference. For example, it can make extremely instability for the estimation value of regression coefficient, which shows a large standard error causing that an important independent variable is not statistically significant to enter the equation. It can even lead to the opposite and unexplained professional significance, because of the large or small, or positive or negative regression coefficient of the sample.

Example 19.2. Feng Chen (1991) reported a case. There were 22 cases of fetal fertilization age Y (week) and fetal shape measurement variables: length X_1 cm, head circumference X_2 cm, weight $X_3\, g$. The regression equation for Y about X_1, X_2, X_3 was as:

$$\hat{Y} = 11.012 + 1.693X_1 - 2.159X_2 + 0.007X_3$$

Among them, the coefficient of the head circumference X_2 was less than zero, which seemed that larger the head circumference, smaller the age, which was contrary to common sense. The reason was the strong correlation between the three independent variables resulting in multiple collinearity. Calculation found that the correlation coefficient between head circumference and body length was 0.997, 0.947 of that between head circumference and body weight, and 0.944 between body length and body weight, all of which were statistically significant. In fact, in the above regression equation, X_1 and X_3 not only simply reflected their contribution to the regression, but also included the contribution of X_2 to the regression. The excessive contribution of X_1 and X_3 to the regression could only be neutralized by the negative coefficient of the X_2.

What should be done if there is a multiple collinearity among the independent variables? The easiest way is to delete the variable with the largest measurement errors, the most missing data and the least important or unsatisfactory variables in terms of profession. In addition, principal component regression methods can also be used (Chapter 24).

19.3.4. *Dummy variables*

The independent variables in multiple linear regression analysis can be continuous variables (such as age, blood pressure, etc.), and binary variables (such as gender), except the unordered categorical variables. Unordered categorical variables must be transformed into several binary variables before introducing into a regression model. If original variables have k possible categories, then $(k-1)$ binary variables can be used instead. This process is called "dummying" and the resulting $(k-1)$ binary variables are called "dummy variables".

19.3.5. *Interaction effects*

In multiple linear regression, the most straightforward way to estimate the interaction of two independent variables is to introduce a new independent variable, which is equal to the product of two independent variables that may have interaction effects. The interaction of two independent variables is called first-order interaction, and second-order interaction for three independent variables, and so on.

The following example shows how to determine whether there are interaction effects, how to introduce interaction effects in the model, and how to interpret the results.

Example 19.3. A study investigated 3,334 women with heart disease to learn about the relationship between serum high-density lipoprotein (HDL), cholesterol (mg/dl) and body mass index (BMI, kg/m^2). Considering diabetes (DIABETES) may be an influencing factor of HDL levels, a linear regression equation was established with independent variables of BMI and diabetes, and a dependent variable of HDL. The results are shown in Table 19.4.

The results in Table 19.4 show that both BMI and DIABETES are influencing factors of HDL, and the model assumes the trends of the mean level of HDL changing with BMI are the same between diabetic non-diabetic women, showing the same partial regression coefficient (−0.391).

Considering that the change regulation of the HDL mean level with BMI may be different in diabetic and non-diabetic groups, the regression lines of HDL with respect to BMI in the diabetic and non-diabetic groups are established, respectively (Figure 19.3).

The two lines are not parallel. The decline rate of HDL level in diabetic patients with increasing BMI is slower than that of the non-diabetic group, indicating that DIABETES affects the effect of

Table 19.4 Linear regression equations with independent variables of body mass index and diabetes

Variable	Coefficient	*SE*	*t*	*P*	95% *CI*	
BMI	−0.391	0.017	−22.531	0.000	−0.426	−0.357
DIABETES	−4.783	0.092	−52.207	0.000	−4.962	−4.603
CONSTANT	67.551	0.363	185.847	0.000	66.839	68.264

$F = 2441.323$, $P = 0.000$; $R^2 = 0.594$, $R^2_{adj} = 0.594$, $\sqrt{MSE} = 2.02$.

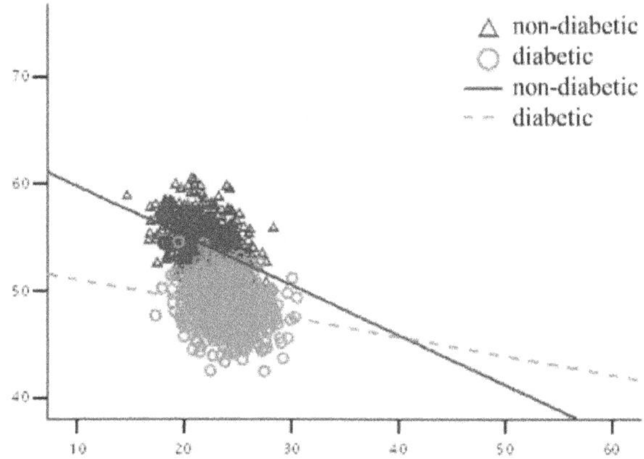

Figure 19.3 The linear regression plot of BMI and HDL

Table 19.5 The results of linear regression with interaction items, independent variables of BMI and diabetes

Variable	Coefficient	*SE*	*t*	*P*	95% CI	
DIABETES	−11.340	0.965	−11.755	0.000	−13.231	−9.448
BMI	−0.735	0.053	−13.822	0.000	−0.839	−0.631
DMBMI	0.278	0.041	6.828	0.000	0.198	0.358
CONSTANT	75.544	1.225	61.672	0.000	73.142	77.945

$F = 1665.379$, $p = 0.000$; $R^2 = 0.600$, $R^2_{adj} = 0.600$, $\sqrt{MSE} = 2.01$.

BMI on HDL. In other words, DIABETES and BMI may have an interactive effect on HDL.

A new independent variable (DMBMI) introduced in the multiple linear regression model is defined as the product of BMI and DIABETES, which describes the relationship between two independent variables and the reaction variables.

Since the two independent variables are already in the model, the product item can be interpreted as an interaction effect. The fitting results of the model are shown in Table 19.5. The partial regression coefficient of the interaction item indicates the difference in the rate of HDL changing with BMI between the diabetic group and the non-diabetic group.

The meaning of the partial regression coefficient can be explained more clearly by the regression equation below.

$$\hat{Y} = b_0 + b_1 DIABETES + b_2 BMI + b_3 DMBMI$$

$$\text{DIABETES} = \begin{cases} 1 & \text{diabetic} \\ 0 & \text{non-diabetic} \end{cases}$$

So, for non-diabetic women:

$$\hat{Y} = b_0 + b_2 BMI$$

where, b_2 reflects the effects of BMI in non-diabetic women.

As for women with diabetes, there are

$$\hat{Y} = b_0 + b_1 + (b_2 + b_3) BMI$$

where, $(b_2 + b_3)$ reflects the effects of BMI in women with diabetes. The partial regression coefficient b_3 characterizes the difference in the BMI between the diabetic group and the non-diabetic group. The variable "diabetes or not" affects the effect of BMI, in other words, the combination of "diabetes or not" and BMI has an interactive effect on HDL.

The above case introduces the introduction of interaction effects and the interpretation of the results. When considering multiple independent variables, the model will become huge and complex if the interaction effects are in all the independent variables. If it needs to introduce an interaction item to the model? Which interaction variables should be analyzed for independent variables? One of the important bases is professional background knowledge. Based on it, the interaction effects can be incorporated into the model for analysis if considering the possible interaction are not reflected, or in the condition that the residual analysis does not satisfy the conditions such as normality and linearity.

19.4. Results report

The results of the analysis of multiple linear regression models should include the following:

1. The purpose of multiple linear regression analysis: quantitatively characterize the linear relationship between a dependent variable and multiple independent variables, select factors that are statistically significant to the dependent variable, control confounding factors, predict, control, and so on.
2. Determining the independent and dependent variables for analysis.
3. Verifying that the data meets the prerequisites for multiple linear regression.
4. Methods for fitting linear models and methods for selecting independent variables.
5. Determining if there is collinearity between independent variables.
6. Whether the interaction between the independent variables and the dependent variable is considered in the analysis.
7. Whether there are abnormal values in the data.
8. The final model and the statistics reflecting the fitting effect of the model, such as the coefficient of determination, the adjusted coefficient of determination, the residual mean square, and so on.
9. Finally, a table is often used to summarize the results of the analysis.

The table includes the following main statistics: the estimated value of the partial regression coefficient, the standard deviation of the partial regression coefficient, the standard partial regression coefficient, the t value, the P value, and sometimes the 95% confidence interval of the partial regression coefficient. The goodness of fit and analysis of variance results are generally listed as remarks below the table.

The following paragraph is a brief summary of the results of the analysis of Example 19.1.

In order to describe the linear association between Nitric Oxide Y and a set of exploratory variables, including traffic flow X_1, temperature X_2, humidity X_3, and wind speed X_4, a multiple linear regression model was developed by a stepwise method. Table 19.6 showed the main statistics of the final model.

The results indicated that the dependent variable Y was affected by exploratory variables X_1, X_2, X_4. The exploratory variable X_1

Table 19.6 Parameter estimation of regression model

Variable	Unstandardized coefficients b	Standard error	Standardized coefficients	t	P
Intercept	−0.142	0.058	—	−2.452	0.024
Traffic flow X_1	0.116	0.025	0.808	4.699	0.000
Temperature X_2	0.004	0.002	0.273	2.430	0.025
Wind speed X_4	−0.035	0.010	−0.448	−3.316	0.003

$^*F = 24.687,\ p < 0.001, R^2 = 0.787.$

had the biggest effect on Y according to the values of standardized coefficients. R^2 suggested that the three independent variables could explain 78.7% of the variation of Y, and the final model fitted the data well.

19.5. Case analysis

Case 19.1 Prediction of hospital inpatients

Shi Lei (1991) published data on the number of outpatient visits X_1, bed utilization X_2, bed turnover X_3 and inpatients Y in his hospital from 1970 to 1989 (see Table 19.7), and established a linear regression equation predicting Y by X_1, X_2 and X_3 (Chinese Health Statistics, 1991, 8 (6)). The main results of multiple linear regression analysis are listed below (see Table 19.8 for details).

The author used a stepwise regression method to establish a multiple regression equation. The independent variables are the number of outpatients and the number of bed turnovers, and the dependent variable is the number of hospitalized patients. The results in Table 19.8 were obtained, and the regression effect was considered to be very good. However, the reader Xiao Ming made a residual analysis chart (Figure 19.4) and considered that the regression effect is not good. Please arbitrate, who is right and who is wrong?

Table 19.7 Statistical material of the second affiliated hospital of Chongqing medical University from 1970 to 1989

Year	Inpatients Y	Outpatients (ten thousand) X_1	Bed utilization (%) X_2	Bed turnover X_3
1970	6349	49.8	94.25	19.84
1971	6519	38.1	98.50	20.37
1972	5952	36.6	89.86	18.80
1973	5230	36.0	86.00	16.34
1974	5411	32.3	83.29	16.91
1975	5277	37.8	77.88	18.07
1976	3772	34.1	92.62	17.96
1977	3846	42.2	86.57	18.31
1978	3866	38.1	84.29	18.41
1979	5142	39.5	89.29	20.61
1980	7724	55.8	97.63	21.72
1981	8167	63.0	96.53	23.33
1982	8107	65.2	93.43	21.91
1983	7998	66.1	94.45	21.05
1984	7331	65.4	93.03	19.96
1985	6447	60.1	91.79	18.81
1986	4869	56.9	88.94	15.82
1987	5506	57.7	91.79	16.01
1988	5741	53.4	99.03	16.59
1989	5568	48.7	94.93	19.09

Table 19.8 Parameter estimation for multiple linear regression models

Variable	Unstandardized coefficients		Standardized coefficients	t	P
	b	Std. Error			
Intercept	−3219.628	1505.165		−2.139	0.047
X_1	59.834	15.780	0.512	3.792	0.001
X_3	327.553	85.725	0.515	3.821	0.001

$^*F = 24.39,\ P < 0.001\ R^2 = 0.861.$

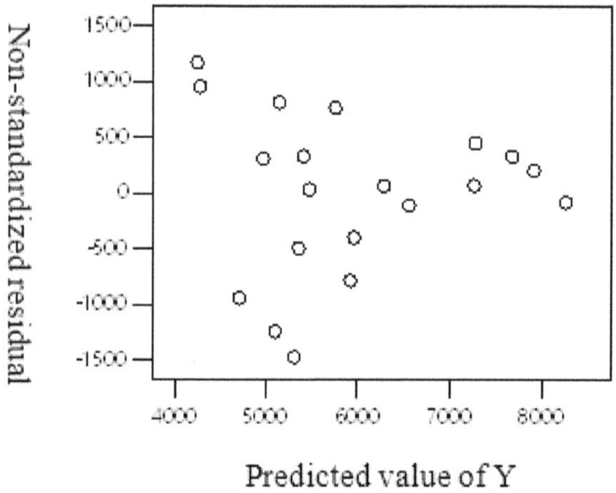

Figure 19.4 Residual analysis

19.6. Computer experiments (See Electronic resources exp19.1 to exp19.3)

Experiment 19.1 Using SPSS to achieve the calculation of multiple linear regression Learn to fit multiple linear regression models, write regression equations and test results.

Experiment 19.2 Using SPSS to implement the calculation of multiple linear regression with interaction effects Learn to fit multiple linear regression models with interaction terms, write regression equations and test results.

Experiment 19.3 Using SPSS to examine multi-collinearity Investigate the effects of multiple collinearity on regression and diagnose multiple collinearity.

19.7. Common questions and summary

19.7.1. *Frequently asked questions*

1. What should I do if the dependent variable is an ordered or categorical variable?

Multiple linear regression analysis requires that the dependent variable is continuous random variable such as blood pressure, height, and weight. However, in medical research, some dependent variables are often categorical variables. For example, the classification of cardiac function is an ordered categorical variable, although there is a difference between the levels, the difference between level 1 (unrestricted physical activity) and level 2 (lightly limited physical activity) is not the same as the difference between level 3 (physical activity is obviously limited) and level 4 (cannot engage in any physical activity and symptoms at rest), which means the numbers 1, 2, 3, and 4 here only represent different levels, and do not represent the actual values. In addition, unordered categorical variables are also common in medical research, such as treatment outcomes divided into healing and death. When the dependent variable is an ordered or unordered categorical variable, multiple linear regression cannot be used to perform multivariate analysis on the data. Other multivariate analysis methods such as logistic regression can be considered.

2. Is the screening of independent variables necessary?

In the previous section, the statistical criteria and selecting strategies for independent variables in multiple linear regression analysis were introduced. Is the screening of independent variables necessary in practical applications? Sometimes it is not necessary and sometimes it is necessary. Whether or not to select the variables depends on the theory, experience, and actual conditions of the materials. The final model must not only meet the requirements of statistics, but more importantly, it can be reasonably explained professionally.

3. How to judge whether there is multi-collinearity

A simple method is to calculate the correlation coefficient matrix for all independent variables. If the correlation coefficient between two independent variables exceeds 0.9, it will bring about the problem of collinearity; if the correlation coefficient is below 0.8, there is generally no problem. In addition, statisticians have proposed two statistics to help determine whether there are multiple collinearity problems, which are the variance inflation factor (VIF) and tolerance.

The following briefly introduces the principle and calculation method of VIF. Suppose there are p independent variables, and each independent variable is treated as a dependent variable and the remaining independent variables are subjected to multiple linear regression analysis. R_j^2 represents the coefficient of determination of a multiple linear regression equation when the j_{th} independent variable is treated as a dependent variable. For each multiple linear regression equation, the VIF is defined as:

$$VIF_j = \frac{1}{1 - R_j^2} \tag{19-11}$$

If the j_{th} independent variable is closely related to the remaining independent variables, then R_j^2 is close to 1, and VIF_j is larger. The results suggest that when the variance inflation factor is greater than 4, there may be a collinearity problem; if the variance inflation factor is greater than 10, the collinearity problem is serious.

Tolerance is the reciprocal of the variance inflation factor. If the tolerance is less than 0.25, there may be a collinearity problem; if the tolerance is less than 0.10, the collinearity problem is severe.

19.7.2. *Summary*

1. Multiple linear regression is an extension of simple linear regression to study the linear dependence of a dependent variable with multiple independent variables. Multiple linear regression is often used in medical research to screen for risk factors, control confounding factors, analyze interaction effects, predict and control, and so on.
2. The assumptions for multiple linear regression models are linear, independent, normal, and homogeneity of variance. Residual analysis is often used to examine whether the data meets these four prerequisites. If the prerequisites are not met, you can try to transform the variables, introduce interaction effects or change the model.
3. The least square method is often used to estimate model parameters in multiple linear regression analysis. The meaning of the partial regression coefficient in the model is the number of units in which the dependent variable changes on average when one independent variable changes by one unit while the value of the

other independent variables are fixed. Standardized partial regression coefficients are often used to compare the contribution of independent variables to the dependent variable. The coefficient of determination and the adjusted coefficient of determination are often used to evaluate the degree of fit of the model. Variance analysis is generally used for hypothesis testing of the entire regression model, and a t-test is often used for hypothesis testing of whether the overall partial regression coefficients are zero.

4. Methods for screening independent variables in multiple linear regression analysis include forward method, backward method, stepwise regression method, and optimal subset method. The indicators used to screen the independent variables are the residual sum of squares, the residual mean of squares, the coefficient of determination, the adjusted coefficient of determination, the C_p statistics, and so on.
5. When there is a strong correlation between the independent variables, multiple collinearity will occur, making the parameter estimation of multiple linear regression unstable or difficult to interpret.
6. General steps of multiple regression analysis: (1) single-factor model analysis; (2) stepwise screening of variables to establish a multi-factor model; (3) combining the results of single-factor and multi-factor models, when the two are contradictory, combined with professional knowledge to analyze the reasons. Also, pay attention to whether there is an interaction between variables.

Think and Practice

Best Choice

1. In the stepwise regression analysis, if the number of independent variables is increased, then ( ).
   A. The regression sum of squares and the residual sum of the squares are increased B. The regression sum of squares and the residual sum of the squares are decreased C. The total sum of squares and the regression sum of squares are increased D. The total sum of the squares is increased, and the residual sum of

the squares is decreased E. The total sum of squares and the regression sum of squares are decreased

2. Which of the following is wrong in the statistical criteria for independent variable screening? ( ).
   A. The reduction of the residual sum of squares SS_{residual} B. The increase of the coefficient of determination R^2 C. The reduction of the residual mean square MS_{residual} D. The increase of the adjust determination coefficient R^2_{ad} E. The increase of the C_p statistics
3. In the multiple linear regression analysis, the indicator that directly reflects the independent variable's interpretation of the percentage variation of the dependent variable is ( ).
   A. Complex correlation coefficient B. Simple correlation coefficient C. Coefficient of determination D. Partial regression coefficient E. Partial correlation coefficient
4. The collinearity in multiple linear regression analysis refers to ( ).
   A. Y has the same regression coefficient for each independent variable. B. Y has the same regression coefficient and intercept for each independent variable. C. Y has the same correlation coefficient with each independent variable. D. Y has a higher complex correlation with the independent variables. E. There is a high correlation between independent variables
5. In multiple linear regression analysis, if a constant K which is not zero is added to the value of an independent variable, there is ( ).
   A. The intercept and the partial regression coefficients are constant. B. The partial regression coefficient is K times the value of the original partial regression coefficient. C. The partial regression coefficient will change, but it is irregular. D. The intercept changes, but the values of all partial regression coefficients do not change. E. All partial regression coefficient values will not change

Questions for Reflection

1. What are the uses of multiple linear regression analysis?
2. Please explain the meaning of the least square method used for multiple linear regression parameter estimation?

Table 19.9 Contents of inorganic substances in bones

ID	Main side radius	Non-main side radius	Main side humerus	Non-main side humerus	Main side ulna	Non-main side ulna
1	1.103	1.052	2.139	2.238	0.873	0.872
2	0.842	0.859	1.873	1.741	0.590	0.744
3	0.925	0.873	1.887	1.809	0.767	0.713
4	0.857	0.744	1.739	1.547	0.706	0.674
5	0.795	0.809	1.734	1.715	0.549	0.654
6	0.787	0.779	1.509	1.474	0.782	0.571
...	...	...	...	...	...	...
25	0.915	0.936	1.971	1.869	0.869	0.868

Source: Practical Multivariate Statistical Analysis (Fourth Edition), Richard A. Johnson & Dean W. Wichern, translated by Lu Xuan, Tsinghua University Press. See the CD for details.

3. How to judge and analyze the interaction between independent variables?
4. What are the basic assumptions of a multiple linear regression model? How to judge if the data meets these assumptions? If the data does not meet the assumptions, what are the common treatment methods?

Question on Calculation

To determine whether older women doing exercising or increasing nutrition can slow down bone damage. At the beginning of the study, a researcher measured the inorganic content of bones by photon absorption. The measured values were recorded on the main and non-main sides of the three bones. The results are shown in Table 19.9. Multiple linear regression analysis was performed on the other bones using the two radius measurements as dependent variables, and appropriate regression models were proposed and fitted to analyze the residuals.

References

[1] Zhu, J, Chen, Z. Research on the multiple linear regression in non-invasive blood glucose measurement. *Biomed Mater Eng.* 2015; 26(Suppl 1): S447–S453.
[2] Dieguez-Santana, K, Pham-The, H, Villegas-Aguilar, PJ, *et al.* Prediction of acute toxicity of phenol derivatives using multiple linear regression

approach for Tetrahymena pyriformis contaminant identification in a median-size database. *Chemosphere.* 2016; 165: 434–441.
[3] Slinker, BK, Glantz, SA. Multiple linear regression: accounting for multiple simultaneous determinants of a continuous dependent variable. *Circulation.* 2008; 117(13): 1732–1737.

Yuantao Hao, Yanbo Zhang

CHAPTER 20

LOGISTIC REGRESSION

Multiple linear regression models are usually thought of as only being appropriate for continuous response variables that have a normal distribution with respect to the independent variables. Categorical variables are a common type of response variable in medical research, and examples include recurrence vs. non-recurrence, alive vs. dead, different tumor histological types (squamous carcinoma, adenocarcinoma, and large cell carcinoma), and therapeutic effects (cure, effective, improved, and ineffective). Because the relationships between these dependent and independent variables are nonlinear, when the range of dependent variables is not consistent with a linear combination of the independent variables, multiple linear regression is no longer suitable to analyze categorical dependent variables. In this chapter, logistic regression is introduced as an effective method to analyze the relationship between categorical dependent variables and corresponding independent variables. Logistic regression includes unconditional logistic regression for group data and conditional logistic regression for paired data. According to the type of dependent variable, logistic regression can be divided into binary logistic regression, multinomial logistic regression, and ordinal logistic regression. This chapter will introduce the above methods respectively.

20.1. Binary logistic regression

Example 20.1. Survival data of 50 patients with acute lymphoblastic leukemia (cohort study)

A physician collected survival data of 50 patients with acute lymphoblastic leukemia who had been treated for 1 year. The data are displayed in Table 20.1. X_1 is their leukocyte count at admission ($\times 10^9$/L). X_2 is lymph node infiltration (divided into three levels: 0, 1, 2). X_3 is whether the patient accepts consolidation therapy after remission (1: yes; 0: no), and Y is the observation result (1: death within 1 year; 0: survival for more than 1 year). He is wondering how to analyze these data. Please help him.

20.1.1. *Basic concepts of binary logistic regression model*

The dependent variable in Table 20.1 is binary. If its relationship with only one risk factor is considered, a chi-square test can be used. When its relationship with multiple influencing factors is considered, the Mantel–Haenszel stratification analysis method can be used to correct for multiple confounding factors in epidemiology subjects. However, this approach has some shortcomings. First, this method can control confounding factors but cannot describe their direction and effect size, and further, the interaction effects between the confounding factors cannot be considered. Second, it requires a large sample but can analyze only a small number of factors. With increasing numbers of factors, the layers thicken, and there are fewer samples in each cell. The frequency in some layers can even be 0, which makes analysis difficult, and the results can be unreliable. Third, the method focuses on the influence between factors and dependent variables while simultaneously adjusting for other factors. Logistic regression can be a good choice to analyze the influence of independent variables on the occurrence probability of dependent variables, because it can address the above problems faced by the Mantel–Haenszel method.

Previously, the theoretical model of multiple linear regression was $Y = \beta_0 + \beta_1 X_1 + \cdots + \beta_m X_m + e$.

Table 20.1 Survival data of 50 patients with acute lymphoblastic leukemia

No.	Leukocyte count X_1	Lymph node infiltration X_2	Consolidation treatment X_3	Result Y	No.	Leukocyte count X_1	Lymph node infiltration X_2	Consolidation treatment X_3	Result Y
1	2.5	0	0	1	26	4.7	0	0	1
2	1.2	2	0	1	27	6.0	0	0	1
3	173.0	2	0	1	28	128.0	2	1	1
4	3.5	0	0	1	29	3.5	0	1	1
5	119.0	2	0	1	30	35.0	0	0	1
6	39.7	0	0	1	31	62.2	0	0	0
7	10.0	2	0	1	32	2.0	0	0	0
8	62.4	0	0	1	33	10.8	0	1	0
9	502.2	2	0	1	34	8.5	0	1	0
10	2.4	0	0	1	35	21.6	0	1	0
11	4.0	0	0	1	36	2.0	2	1	0
12	34.7	0	0	1	37	2.0	0	1	0
13	14.4	0	1	1	38	2.0	0	1	0
14	28.4	2	0	1	39	3.4	2	1	0
15	2.0	2	0	1	40	4.3	0	1	0
16	0.9	0	1	1	41	5.1	0	1	0
17	40.0	2	0	1	42	244.8	2	1	0
18	30.6	2	0	1	43	2.4	0	0	0
19	6.6	0	0	1	44	4.0	0	1	0
20	5.8	0	1	1	45	1.7	0	1	0
21	21.4	2	1	1	46	5.1	0	1	0
22	6.1	0	1	1	47	1.1	0	1	0
23	2.8	0	0	1	48	32.0	0	1	0
24	2.7	2	1	1	49	12.8	0	1	0
25	2.5	0	0	1	50	1.4	0	1	0

In which the values of the independent variables are given, Y follows a normal distribution, and its value interval is $(-\infty, +\infty)$. The regression equation of the sample is $\hat{Y} = b_0 + b_1X_1 + \cdots + b_mX_m$.

However, if the dependent variable Y is a dichotomous variable with a value distribution of 0 or 1 (e.g., onset or not), the above model cannot handle the situation. For dichotomous variables, 1 represents a positive result (death, effectiveness, recurrence, etc.), which is generally researchers' primary concern, and 0 represents a negative result (survival, lack of effectiveness, no recurrence, etc.). The response of interest is binary, taking the value 1 with probability π and the value 0 with probability $1-\pi$. Researchers usually care about the relationship between probability π of $Y = 1$ and an independent variable. $\pi = P\{Y = 1|X_1, X_2, \ldots, X_m\}$, where the formula represents that under the effects of independent variables $X_1, X_2, \ldots, X_m$, the probability of Y is 1. In addition, $0 \leq \pi \leq 1$.

If a regression model is established directly between the influencing factors and the probability π of disease occurrence, the formula becomes $\pi = \beta_0 + \beta X$. Accordingly, the impossible situation that π is greater than 1 or less than 0 may occur. In epidemiology, the ratio of incidence probability π to the non-incidence probability $(1 - \pi)$ is usually called *odds*. The value range of *odds* is $(0, +\infty)$. If a variable has this value range, it cannot be used to establish a model directly using a linear combination of independent variables with value ranges $(-\infty, +\infty)$. To restrict probability π to the range of [0,1], we employ not probability π but the log-odds,

$$\text{logit}\pi = \ln\left(\frac{\pi}{1-\pi}\right). \tag{20-1}$$

This change converts the incidence probability π whose value interval is [0, 1] into logitπ, whose value interval is $(-\infty, +\infty)$. If we take $\log \text{it}\pi$ as the dependent variable, a logistic regression model can be established with several independent variables. The basic logistic function is given by

$$\text{logit}\pi = \beta_0 + \beta_1X_1 + \cdots + \beta_mX_m \tag{20-2}$$

or

$$\ln(odds) = \beta_0 + \beta_1X_1 + \cdots + \beta_mX_m$$

or

$$\ln\left(\frac{\pi}{1-\pi}\right) = \beta_0 + \beta_1 X_1 + \cdots + \beta_m X_m$$

Equation (20-2) is called a logistic regression model. The parameters $\beta_1, \beta_2, \ldots, \beta_m$ are named the partial regression coefficients of the logistic regression, and β_0 is a constant term.

To obtain the relationship between incidence probability and influencing factors, Formula (20-2) can be transferred as the following:

$$\pi = \frac{e^{\beta_0+\beta_1 X_1+\cdots+\beta_m X_m}}{1+e^{\beta_0+\beta_1 X_1+\cdots+\beta_m X_m}} \tag{20-3}$$

or

$$\pi = \frac{1}{1+e^{-(\beta_0+\beta_1 X_1+\cdots+\beta_m X_m)}} \tag{20-4}$$

Logistic regression has no special requirement for the type of independent variable: these can be numerical, categorical, or ordinal variables. Like multiple linear regression, logistic regression requires that the value of each observation be independent from each other.

20.1.2. *Parameter estimation of logistic regression and the epidemiological significance of parameters*

(1) Parameter estimation of logistic regression

To establish a logistic regression model, it is necessary to estimate the model's partial regression coefficients β_j according to the sample data. The dependent variable Y is a binary variable that has a binomial distribution. Estimation of the partial regression coefficient β_j is usually carried out by maximum likelihood estimation (MLE). Statistical software can be used to complete the calculation.

The main idea of MLE is to get "the most likely outcome of the current sample value." Thus, first, we calculate the theoretical probability of the current situation with the likelihood function. Second, we let it reach its maximum value so as to obtain the value of the unknown parameter. We take this value as the estimated value of the parameter and name it the "maximum likelihood estimation of the unknown parameter."

Based on these concepts, we construct the following likelihood function of the n currently observed cases according to the multiplication theorem of probability.

$$L = \prod_{i=1}^{n} P_i^{Y_i}(1 - P_i)^{1-Y_i} \quad i = 1, 2, \ldots, n \tag{20-5}$$

In the above formula, P_i is the probability of a positive result for the ith observation; Y_i: if the actual result is positive, $Y_i = 1$; otherwise, $Y_i = 0$. To simplify the calculation, the natural logarithm is taken of both sides of the likelihood function L to obtain the log likelihood function.

$$\ln L = \sum_{i=1}^{n} [Y_i \ln P_i + (1 - Y_i)\ln(1 - P_i)] \quad i = 1, 2, \ldots, n \tag{20-6}$$

When the logarithmic likelihood function reaches its maximum value, the corresponding parameter estimation $b_0, b_1, \ldots, b_m$ can be obtained by using the approximate calculation method of the MLE of the parameter $\beta_0, \beta_1, \ldots, \beta_m$. The following hypothesis test about logistic regression proceeds according to the logarithmic likelihood function and constructs the test statistics with the negative double value of the logarithmic likelihood function, $-2\ln L$. The formula of the regression equation of the sample is

$$\text{logit}P = b_0 + b_1X_1 + \cdots + b_mX_m$$

or

$$\ln(odds) = b_0 + b_1X_1 + \cdots + b_mX_m$$

or

$$\ln\left(\frac{P}{1-P}\right) = b_0 + b_1X_1 + \cdots + b_mX_m$$

In which P is the estimate of π. We used the SPSS software package to perform the statistical analysis in Example 20.1. The results are shown in Table 20.2.

(2) Meaning of parameters

In multiple linear regression, the constant term β_0 represents the average value of Y when all independent variables are 0. When all independent variables are 0, the logistic regression model is as follows:

$$\ln\left(\frac{\pi}{1-\pi}\right) = \beta_0, \quad \frac{\pi}{1-\pi} = e^{\beta_0}$$

In which β_0 is the logarithmic advantage of the occurrence rate for positive events when all independent variables are 0; e^{β_0} is the advantage of positive events.

In multiple linear regression, the partial regression coefficient β_j is statistically significant in that when other independent variables remain unchanged, there is an average change of Y for every unit of change of X_j. The logistic regression model is:

$$\ln(odds_0) = \beta_0 + \beta_1 X_1 + \cdots + \beta_j X_j + \cdots + \beta_m X_m$$

When 1 unit is added to X_j, the model becomes:

$$\ln(odds_1) = \beta_0 + \beta_1 X_1 + \cdots + \beta_j (X_j + 1) + \cdots + \beta_m X_m$$

When we subtract the latter from the former, the model changes to

$$\ln(odds_1) - \ln(odds_0) = \beta_j (X_j + 1) - \beta_j X_j = \beta_j$$
$$\ln(OR) = \beta_j, \quad OR_j = e^{\beta_j}$$

β_j represents the logarithmic dominance ratio of positive events before and after X_j changes by 1 unit under the condition that other independent variables are fixed and unchanged; e^{β_j} is the odds ratio (OR). If the probability of positive events is very small, the OR is approximately the relative risk, so β_j is the logarithmic relative risk of positive events after X_j changes by 1 unit vs. before the change; e^{β_j} is the relative risk.

When the dependent variable $Y = 1$ indicates "bad events" such as recurrence or death that are of concern to researchers, and the regression coefficient is $\beta_j > 0$, $OR > 1$, the increase of X_j may lead to an increase in the probability of events' occurrence. Here, X_j is a risk factor, whereas X_j is a protective factor. When $\beta_j = 0$, $OR = 1$, the independent variable has no effect on event occurrence.

Similar to multiple linear regression, the units of multiple independent variables can be different. However, we still need to compare the relative importance of each independent variable to the occurrence probability of an event. Logistic regression can be conducted after standardization of all independent variables. The results include the standardized partial regression coefficients of each independent variable and a comparison of their absolute values.

20.1.3. *Interval estimation of partial regression coefficient and dominance ratio*

When the sample size is large, the estimated value of the partial regression coefficient is b_j, calculated by the MLE method, and it approximately follows a normal distribution. The formula for the $(1-\alpha)$ confidence interval (CI) of β_j is $b_j \pm Z_{\alpha/2}SE(b_j)$:

Correspondingly, the $(1-\alpha)$ CI of OR_j is $e^{b_j \pm Z_{\alpha/2}SE(b_j)}$

After the hypothesis test ($\alpha = 0.05$), if the partial regression coefficient corresponding to an independent variable is not 0, the 95% CI of the OR value corresponding to the partial regression coefficient of this independent variable should not contain 1.

As in multiple linear regression, the estimated value of the parameter b_j is not 0, which does not mean that the population parameter β_j is not 0, nor does it mean that the population regression equation is true. After establishing the regression model and the partial regression coefficients in the model, a hypothesis test of the overall model and regression coefficients is needed.

20.1.4. *Hypothesis test of total model and regression coefficient*

(1) Hypothesis testing of the general model

H_0: The model including only the intercept terms,
H_1: The model including both intercepts and m independent variables.

The value of the logarithmic likelihood function ($\ln L$) can reflect the model's fitness. The model improves in tandem with an increase in value of the logarithmic likelihood function. In the $-2\ln L$ function, smaller values are better. The likelihood ratio test statistic value is as follows:

$$G = -2(\ln L_0 - \ln L_1) = -2\ln(L_0/L_1)$$

where, L_0 is the maximum likelihood corresponding to H_0, and L_1 is the maximum likelihood corresponding to H_1.

L_0 and L_1 are decimals, and $L_0 < L_1$. Both $\ln L_0$ and $\ln L_1$ are negative, and $\ln L_0 < \ln L_1$; thus, $-2\ln L_0 > -2\ln L_1$. This indicates that if a large sample size is used while H_0 is being established, G approximately follows the χ^2 distribution subject to m degrees of freedom. If the χ^2 value is much larger than the critical value of the χ^2 distribution of freedom m, or the P value is very small, then we reject H_0, and the logistic regression model with m independent variables can be considered to be established.

In general, the likelihood ratio test can be used to compare two models with different numbers of variables. Suppose m_0 is the number of variables in the model with fewer variables, and m_1 is the number of variables in the model with more variables, and $m_0 < m_1$.

H_0: The model with fewer variables is established,
H_1: The model with more variables is established.

When the sample size is large and H_0 is established, G approximately obeys the χ^2 distribution with $m_1 - m_0$ degrees of freedom. If the χ^2 value is much larger than the critical value of the χ^2 distribution with $m_1 - m_0$ degrees of freedom, or the P value is very small, then H_0 is rejected and the model with more variables is adopted. Otherwise, H_0 is not rejected and the model with fewer variables is adopted.

(2) Hypothesis test of regression coefficient

H_0: $\beta_j = 0 (j = 1, 2, \ldots, m)$,
H_1: $\beta_j \neq 0 (j = 1, 2, \ldots, m)$.

Construct the following test statistics for testing the hypothesis that the regression coefficient β_j equals 0:

$$Z = \frac{b_j - 0}{SE(b_j)}$$

$$\text{Wald } \chi^2 = \left[\frac{b_j}{SE(b_j)}\right]^2$$

where, b_j and $SE(b_j)$ are the estimated values of parameter β_j and its standard error. With a large sample and H_0 being true, Z obeys the standard normal distribution. Wald χ^2 obeys the χ^2 distribution with 1 degree of freedom. If the value of Wald χ^2 is much larger than the χ^2 critical value with 1 degree of freedom, we reject H_0, and β_j are not 0.

20.1.5. *Goodness of fit test*

Similar to linear regression, the goodness of fit test should be conducted according to the logistic regression equation. The goodness-of-fit test is used to check the consistency between the selected model and the actual data. The test can evaluate the consistency between the model's predicted value and the observed value.

The null hypothesis (H_0) assumes consistency between the frequency distributions of the actual observation and the model to predict the frequency distribution. The Hosmer–Lemeshow test can test the model's goodness of fit. Its essence is the Pearson χ^2 test, which compares the observed frequency and the model's predicted frequency. Such tests can be done by statistical software. If the test statistics do not exceed the critical value thresholds according to the corresponding degrees of freedom, and the critical value of the χ^2 distribution or the P value is large, then the model fitness is good. This shows that the model's prediction ability is strong and that it is suitable for prediction. In addition to the Hosmer–Lemeshow test, the Pearson and deviation tests are also commonly used goodness-of-fit test methods. These tests are based on the basic principle of the χ^2 test, and their results are generally similar to each other.

20.1.6. *Independent variables selection of logistic regression*

Variable selection methods in logistic regression are similar to those in multiple linear regression, including forward, backward, and stepwise methods. The test statistic is not the F statistic used by multiple regression, but instead, we adapt the likelihood ratio test. In practical application, if there are too many independent variables, univariate logistic regression can be used to incorporate the extra variables one by one; or, we can set the test level wider to obtain more candidate variables. For example, let $\alpha = 0.2$ be the initial selection of independent variables. The statistically significant independent variables can then be used to conduct multivariable logistic regression.

20.1.7. *Analysis of results presented in Example 20.1*

Solution: The results of the binary logistic regression model obtained with SPSS software are shown in Table 20.2.

The $-2\ln L$ statistic can be obtained by a hypothesis test after the overall model has been established. Values of $\chi^2 = 20.734$, $P < 0.001$ shows that at least one independent variable is statistically significant and the overall model has good fit. Table 20.2 shows the estimates of

Table 20.2 Results of binary unconditioned logistic regression analysis

						95% CI of OR	
Variable	b	$SE(b)$	Wald χ^2	P values	OR	Lower	Upper
Constant	1.697	0.659	6.635	0.010	5.455		
Leukocyte count X_1	−0.002	0.006	0.167	0.682	0.998	0.987	1.009
Lymph node infiltration X_2	0.792	0.487	2.643	0.104	2.208	0.850	5.738
Consolidation therapy X_3	−2.830	0.793	12.726	<0.001	0.059	0.012	0.279

the partial regression coefficient, *OR*, and its 95% CI. The results of the Wald χ^2 test show that the consolidation treatment of regression coefficients is statistically significant. Because the regression coefficient of consolidation treatment is negative, higher values of consolidation are associated with lower Y values. According to the reference level and *OR*, consolidation treatment is a protective factor. If other independent variables are fixed, the probability of death within 1 year among patients who undergo consolidation treatment is 0.059 times as high as that of patients who do not undergo consolidation treatment. The hypothesis test results for leukocyte count and lymph node infiltration are $P = 0.682$ and $P = 0.104$, respectively, and no significant influence of leukocyte count or impact of lymph node invasion degree on death has been found.

The results of the Hosmer–Lemeshow test show that $\chi^2 = 3.156$ and $P = 0.924$, indicating good fit.

The expression of the regression equation is:

$$\ln\left(\frac{P}{1-P}\right) = 1.697 - 0.002X_1 + 0.792X_2 - 2.830X_3$$

The probability prediction model of logistic regression can be established according to Table 20.2.

$$P = \frac{1}{1 + e^{-(1.697-0.002X_1+0.792X_2-2.830X_3)}}$$

20.1.8. *Binary logistic regression case: Case-control study*

Example 20.2. Risk factors of nasopharyngeal cancer
To find the risk factors of nasopharyngeal cancer, a case-control study was conducted on 105 new cases of nasopharyngeal cancer in the head and neck department of a tumor hospital and 130 healthy people. The information collected from the respondents is shown in Tables 20.3 and 20.4.

Solution: The stepwise method ($\alpha_{\text{in}} = 0.05$, $\alpha_{\text{out}} = 0.1$) is used for variable selection in Example 20.2. The results are shown in Table 20.5. The likelihood ratio test is used for the hypothesis test. The likelihood ratio value $\chi^2 = 77.413$, $P < 0.001$ indicates that

Table 20.3 Values of variables for 105 new cases of nasopharyngeal carcinoma and 130 healthy subjects

Variable	Explanation	Coding	Variable	Explanation	Coding
X_1	Gender	Female = 0; Male = 1	X_6	Smoke	No = 0; Yes = 1
X_2	Age	At the age of	X_7	Drink tea	No = 0; Yes = 1
X_3	Family history of nasopharyngeal cancer	No = 0; Yes = 1	X_8	Exercise for a long time	No = 0; Yes = 1
X_4	History of chronic rhinitis	No = 0; Yes = 1	X_9	Life stress	No = 0; Yes = 1
X_5	Occupational exposure to hazardous substances	No = 0; Yes = 1	Y	Group	Control = 0; Case = 1

Table 20.4 Original records of 105 new cases of nasopharyngeal carcinoma and 130 healthy subjects

No.	X_1	X_2	X_3	X_4	X_5	X_6	X_7	X_8	X_9	Y
1	0	68	0	0	0	0	0	0	1	0
2	0	22	0	0	1	0	1	1	1	0
...	...	...	...	...	...	...	...	...	...	...
234	0	33	1	0	0	0	0	0	0	1
235	1	44	0	1	1	1	1	1	0	1

at least one independent variable is significant and that the overall model has good fit. Table 20.5 shows the estimates of the partial regression coefficient, OR, and its 95% CI in the last model. The Wald χ^2 test results show that the four independent variables (family history of nasopharyngeal cancer, occupational exposure to harmful substances, smoking, and long-term exercise), are statistically significant. Based on the reference level and OR, family history of nasopharyngeal cancer, occupational exposure to harmful substances and smoking are risk factors for breast cancer, whereas long-term exercise is a protective factor for breast cancer. If other independent variables are fixed, the risk of nasopharyngeal cancer in patients with

Table 20.5 Results of binary classification unconditioned logistic regression analysis

						95% CI of *OR*	
Variable	b	$SE(b)$	Wald χ^2	P	OR	Lower	Upper
Constant	−0.855	0.246	12.108	0.001	0.425		
Family history of nasopharyngeal cancer X_3	2.202	0.451	23.879	<0.001	9.043	3.739	21.870
Occupational exposure to hazardous substances X_5	0.892	0.364	5.985	0.014	2.439	1.194	4.982
Smoke X_6	1.421	0.337	17.742	<0.001	4.143	2.138	8.027
Exercise for a long time X_8	−1.368	0.350	15.291	<0.001	0.255	0.128	0.505

a family history of nasopharyngeal cancer is 9.043 times higher than that in patients without a family history of nasopharyngeal cancer. In contrast, the risk of nasopharyngeal cancer in long-term exercisers is 0.255 times higher than that in non-long-term exercisers. Other risk factors have similar explanations.

A Hosmer–Lemeshow goodness of fit test on the model shows $\chi^2 = 0.921$ and $P = 0.988$, indicating that the model has good fit.

The expression for the regression equation is:

$$\ln\left(\frac{P}{1-P}\right) = -0.855 + 2.202X_3 + 0.892X_5 + 1.421X_6 - 1.386X_8$$

Because of the case-control nature of the study, the proportions of cases and controls are artificial. This does not represent the true case-control ratio in the natural population. The constant is not the logarithm of the population disease predominance estimation when the value of each independent variable is 0; therefore, the constant has no practical significance. The regression model cannot be directly used for prediction, as we need to know the true prevalence rate in the

Table 20.6 Effects of cell differentiation and Ki67 cell staining on three lung cancer histological types

		Histological types		
Cell differentiation	Ki67 cell staining	Squamous carcinoma $Y = 1$	Adenocarcinoma $Y = 2$	Large cell carcinoma $Y = 3$
I ($X_1 = 1$)	$+(X_2 = 1)$	10	17	26
	$-(X_2 = 0)$	5	12	50
II ($X_1 = 2$)	$+(X_2 = 1)$	21	17	26
	$-(X_2 = 0)$	16	12	26
III ($X_1 = 3$)	$+(X_2 = 1)$	15	15	16
	$-(X_2 = 0)$	12	12	20

population and correct for it as a constant. Please refer to related monographs for the specific formula.

Logistic regression not only applies to cohort study and case-control studies, but is also suitable for cross-sectional studies. However, because of space limitations, this text will not give further examples. The Thinking and Practice section gives an example of the latter type of problem, and readers can try to solve it by themselves.

20.2. Multinomial logistic regression model

Binary logistic regression can be extended to multinomial dependent variables, including categorical and ordinal variables.

20.2.1. *Multiple classification logistic regression*

Example 20.3. To study the relationship between lung cancer histological types (Y) and cell differentiation (X_1) and Ki67 cell staining (X_2), a set of data was collected (Table 20.6). Please analyze the data.

The Table 20.6 is a three-dimensional contingency table with a categorical variable as the outcome variable. The multinomial logistic regression model introduced in this section can be a good choice for quantitative analysis of the influence of various factors on the type of lung cancer tissue.

(1) Basic concept

In general, if the dependent variable has k categories, one of them is selected as a reference category, and $k-1$ logit models are fitted with respect to it.

Taking $k = 3$ as an example, if the third category is used as a reference category, two different logit models can be constructed.

$Y = 1$ vs. $Y = 3$:

$$\ln\left[\frac{\pi(Y=1)}{\pi(Y=3)}\right] = \beta_{10} + \beta_{11}X_1 + \beta_{12}X_2 + \cdots + \beta_{1m}X_m \qquad (20\text{-}7)$$

$Y = 2$ vs. $Y = 3$:

$$\ln\left[\frac{\pi(Y=2)}{\pi(Y=3)}\right] = \beta_{20} + \beta_{21}X_1 + \beta_{22}X_2 + \cdots + \beta_{2m}X_m \qquad (20\text{-}8)$$

The constant and partial regression coefficients in the above two equations are different. The meaning of the regression coefficients and the methods of parameter estimation and hypothesis testing are similar to those of binary logistic regression. However, unlike two-time binary logistic regression, the parameters of the above two regression equations are estimated using all of the data simultaneously.

(2) Analysis of results

Solution: Multinomial logistic regression analysis can be done using the multinomial logistic process in the SPSS software package. Taking large cell carcinoma as a reference, squamous cell carcinoma and adenocarcinoma are compared with it, and two generalized logit models are fitted. The likelihood ratio χ^2 value of the likelihood ratio test on the whole model is 22.227, $P < 0.001$, which indicates that at least one population regression coefficient among the independent variables is not 0 and that the model can be considered to be established. The goodness-of-fit test of the model shows that the Pearson χ^2 value is 7.358, $P = 0.289$, and the deviation test χ^2 value is 7.389, $P = 0.286$. These test results are consistent between the two methods, indicating that the model has good fit.

Table 20.7 Results of multinomial logistic regression analysis

Histological types		b	$SE(b)$	Wald χ^2	P	OR	95% CI of OR	
							Lower	Upper
Squamous carcinoma	Constant	−2.281	0.418	29.818	<0.001			
	Cell differentiation	0.628	0.180	12.192	<0.001	1.874	1.317	2.666
	Ki67 cell staining	0.649	0.283	5.257	0.022	1.914	1.099	3.335
Adenocarcinoma	Constant	−1.616	0.380	18.051	<0.001			
	Cell differentiation	0.345	0.173	3.995	0.046	1.413	1.007	1.982
	Ki67 cell staining	0.635	0.272	5.434	0.020	1.887	1.106	3.219

The first logit model compares squamous cell carcinoma with large cell carcinoma. According to the parameter estimation results, each time the cell differentiation increases by one level, the risk of having squamous cell carcinoma is elevated by 1.874 times that of large cell carcinoma, and patients with a high degree of cell differentiation are more susceptible to squamous cell carcinoma (Wald $\chi^2 = 12.192$, $P < 0.001$). Compared with Ki67 cell staining-negative patients, patients who are Ki67 cell staining-positive have 1.914 times the risk of large cell carcinoma, and Ki67 cell staining-positive patients are also more susceptible to squamous cell carcinoma (Wald $\chi^2 = 5.257$, $P = 0.022$). Model 1 is written as:

$$\ln\left[\frac{P(Y=1)}{P(Y=3)}\right] = -2.281 + 0.628X_1 + 0.649X_2 \tag{20-9}$$

The second logit model compares adenocarcinoma with large cell carcinoma. According to the parameter estimation results, each time the level of cell differentiation increases by one level, the risk of adenocarcinoma is elevated by 1.413 times that of large cell carcinoma, and patients with a high degree of cell differentiation are more susceptible to adenocarcinoma (Wald $\chi^2 = 3.995$, $P = 0.046$). Compared with Ki67 cell staining-negative patients, Ki67 cell staining-positive patients have 1.887 times higher risk of adenocarcinoma. Patients with positive Ki67 cell staining are more susceptible to adenocarcinoma (Wald $\chi^2 = 5.434$, $P = 0.020$).

Model 2 is written as:

$$\ln\left[\frac{P(Y=2)}{P(Y=3)}\right] = -1.616 + 0.345X_1 + 0.635X_2 \qquad (20\text{-}10)$$

With the above two regression equations, we can predict the probability that each individual belongs to each of the three categories: according to Equations (20-9) and (20-10), we can obtain:

$$\frac{P(Y=1)}{P(Y=3)} = e^{-2.281+0.628X_1+0.649X_2}$$

$$\frac{P(Y=2)}{P(Y=3)} = e^{-1.616+0.345X_1+0.635X_2}$$

$$P(Y=1) = \frac{e^{-2.281+0.628X_1+0.649X_2}}{1+e^{-2.281+0.628X_1+0.649X_2}+e^{-1.616+0.345X_1+0.635X_2}}$$

$$P(Y=2) = \frac{e^{-1.616+0.345X_1+0.635X_2}}{1+e^{-2.281+0.628X_1+0.649X_2}+e^{-1.616+0.345X_1+0.635X_2}}$$

$$P(Y=3) = \frac{1}{1+e^{-2.281+0.628X_1+0.649X_2}+e^{-1.616+0.345X_1+0.635X_2}}$$

20.2.2. *Ordinal variable logistic regression*

Example 20.4. A researcher wants to study the effect of gender (X_1) and treatment (X_2) on the treatment efficacy (Y) of a disease. The results are shown in Table 20.8. How can we analyze this data?

Table 20.8 Impact of gender and treatment on a certain disease

		Efficacy		
Gender	Treatment	Invalid ($Y = 1$)	Valid ($Y = 2$)	Cure ($Y = 3$)
Woman	New therapy ($X_2 = 1$)	6	5	16
$X_1 = 1$	Traditional therapy ($X_2 = 0$)	19	7	6
Man	New therapy ($X_2 = 1$)	7	2	5
$X_1 = 0$	Traditional therapy ($X_2 = 0$)	10	0	1

The above table is a three-dimensional contingency table with an ordinal variable as the result variable. To quantitatively analyze the impact of each influencing factor on the curative effect, the ordinal variables logistic regression introduced in this section can be a good choice.

(1) Basic concept

In practical applications, we often encounter dependent variables that are ordinal variables. For example, with the values for curative effect including "cure," "markedly effective," "improved," and "ineffective," a cumulative logit model based on cumulative probability can be fitted. When the variable Y is assigned, the level about which the researchers care most should be given the maximum value; if Y has k levels, $k-1$ cumulative logit models can be fitted according to $k-1$ dividing points.

Taking $k = 3$ as an example, the values of Y are 1, 2, and 3, while the occurrence probabilities of the three levels are π_1, π_2, and π_3, respectively, and $\pi_1 + \pi_2 + \pi_3 = 1$. These values can be fit to a pair of two-category logit models:

(1) Category 1 vs. 2 and 3,

$$\log\left[\frac{\pi_1}{\pi_2 + \pi_3}\right] = \beta_{10} + \beta_1 X_1 + \cdots + \beta_m X_m \tag{20-11}$$

(2) Categories 1 and 2 vs. 3,

$$\log\left[\frac{\pi_1 + \pi_2}{\pi_3}\right] = \beta_{20} + \beta_1 X_1 + \cdots + \beta_m X_m \tag{20-12}$$

The second model is equal to combining $Y = 1$ and $Y = 2$ together and comparing them with $Y = 3$ to form a binary variable model. Therefore, the ordinal variable logistic regression model is also called the cumulative logit model, and its parameter estimation can be conducted using the ordinal process of the SPSS software package.

The above cumulative logit model assumes that each of the independent variables has the same influence on the ratio of the cumulative probability in each cumulative model, which means the partial regression coefficients of the each of logit models are the same. However, the difference between the independent variables is reflected in the constant. According to the fitted cumulative logit model, the curves created by the cumulative probability of the response variable and the independent variable are parallel, but the intercepts are different. Therefore, the cumulative logistic regression model needs to be tested for parallelism, which is used to determine whether the regression coefficients of each independent variable are different in $k - 1$ different models. The SPSS software package uses the likelihood ratio test as its parallelism test. Any result of $P > 0.1$ indicates that the parallelism assumption is satisfied. Otherwise, the parallelism assumption is not satisfied. If the data do not satisfy the parallelism assumption, then the data are not suitable for cumulative logit regression. This may indicate that different categories of Y are essentially different. Thus, the abovementioned multinomial logistic regression model should be used.

The cumulative logit regression model's methods of parameter estimation and hypothesis testing are also similar to those of binary logistic regression. The regression equation is usually fitted using MLE.

(2) Analysis of results

Solution: The following results from SPSS take the lowest level of X as the reference. The likelihood ratio χ^2 value of the model's parallelism test is 1.469, and the P value is 0.480, which satisfies the parallelism assumption, and thus, cumulative logit regression can be used. The likelihood ratio test on the whole model shows that the likelihood ratio χ^2 value is 19.887, $P < 0.001$, indicating that the population partial regression coefficient of at least one independent variable is not 0, and that the model can be considered to be is established. Goodness of fit tests show that the Pearson χ^2 value is 1.910, $P = 0.752$, and the deviation value is 2.712, $P = 0.607$. Both methods show that the model has good fit (Table 20.9).

Using the ordinal process in SPSS to perform ordinal logistic regression analysis, the two cumulative logit models can be fitted whose two constant values are 1.813 and 2.667, respectively.

Table 20.9 Results of multi-classification ordinal logistic regression analysis

Variable	b	$SE(b)$	Wald χ^2	P	OR	95% CI for OR	
						Lower	Upper
Constant 1 (efficacy = 1)	1.813	0.557	10.607	0.001		0.722	2.904
Constant 2 (efficacy = 2)	2.667	0.600	19.780	<0.001		1.492	3.843
Gender	1.319	0.529	6.210	0.013	3.740	0.282	2.356
Treatment	1.797	0.473	14.449	<0.001	6.032	0.871	2.724

The regression coefficients of the two models are the same. The independent variables including gender and treatment are statistically significant ($P < 0.05$). For gender, $OR = e^{1.319} = 3.798$ with male gender as the reference level, meaning that women have a higher level of efficacy. For therapy, $OR = e^{1.797} = 6.032$, reflecting that with traditional therapy as a reference level, new therapy has improved effects. According to Equations (20-11) and (20-12), we obtain the following two regression equations:

$$\log\left[\frac{P(Y=1)}{1-P(Y=1)}\right] = 1.813 + 1.319X_1 + 1.797X_2$$

$$\log\left[\frac{P(Y=1)+P(Y=2)}{P(Y=3)}\right] = 2.667 + 1.319X_1 + 1.797X_2$$

Based on this, we can further predict the probability that individuals belong to three categories:

$$P(Y=1) = \frac{e^{1.813+1.319X_1+1.797X_2}}{1+e^{1.813+1.319X_1+1.797X_2}}$$

$$P(Y=1)+P(Y=2) = \frac{e^{2.667+1.319X_1+1.797X_2}}{1+e^{2.667+1.319X_1+1.797X_2}}$$

Thus,

$$P(Y=2) = \frac{e^{2.667+1.319X_1+1.797X_2}}{1+e^{2.667+1.319X_1+1.797X_2}} - \frac{e^{1.813+1.319X_1+1.797X_2}}{1+e^{1.813+1.319X_1+1.797X_2}}$$

and

$$P(Y = 3) = 1 - \frac{e^{2.667+1.319X_1+1.797X_2}}{1 + e^{2.667+1.319X_1+1.797X_2}}$$

20.3. Conditional logistic regression

Example 20.5. (1:1 matched case-control study) To study the risk factors of breast cancer in women, researchers randomly sampled 350 patients who were diagnosed with breast cancer from 1996 to 1997 in a city. A healthy control group was chosen according to the following two rules. First, the case and control should be the same gender. Second, the age difference between case and control should not be more than 2.5 years. The list of factors is shown in Tables 20.10 and 20.11. Please select the appropriate methods to analyze the risk factors of breast cancer in women.

20.3.1. *Conditional logistic regression*

Cases and controls are often matched according to confounders (such as gender and age) so as to control for some important confounders and improve efficiency. The most common is 1:1 matching, in which

Table 20.10 Values of factors for breast cancer in women

Variable	Coding	Variable	Coding
Education (X_1)	College degree and below = 0; College degree or above = 1	Family history of malignancy (X_5)	No = 0; Yes = 1
Body mass index (X_2)	Not more than 27 = 0; More than 27 = 1	Menarche age (X_6)	Not less than 14 years old = 0; Less than 14 years old = 1
Recently spiritual pressure (X_3)	No = 0; Yes = 1	Breast-feeding histories (X_7)	Yes = 0; No = 1
History of breast benign diseases (X_4)	No = 0; Yes = 1	Group (Y)	Control = 0; Case = 1

Table 20.11 Data of 350 pairs of women breast cancer cases and controls

	Case ($Y = 1$)							Control ($Y = 0$)						
No.	X_1	X_2	X_3	X_4	X_5	X_6	X_7	X_1	X_2	X_3	X_4	X_5	X_6	X_7
1	0	0	0	0	0	1	0	0	0	0	0	0	0	1
2	0	1	0	0	1	0	1	0	0	0	0	0	0	1
...	...	...			...	...	...	...	...			...	...	...
349	1	0	1	0	0	0	1	0	0	0	0	0	1	1
350	0	0	1	1	1	1	1	1	0	0	0	0	1	1

each matched group contains one case and one control. The case in each paired group is comparable with the control in the same pair, and there is no guarantee of comparability with the controls in other pairs. Therefore, it is necessary to establish the logistic regression model according to the exposure and incidence status of the subjects in each pair. These will provide additional pairing numbers to add to the data format for conditional logistic regression.

In each pair, the case is indicated by A and the control is indicated by B. $Y = 1$ refers to having the disease, with $Y = 0$ otherwise. The probability of only one within the pair having the disease is

$$P(\text{either } Y_A = 1 \text{ or } Y_B = 1) = P(Y_A = 1)P(Y_B = 0) + P(Y_A = 0)P(Y_B = 1) \tag{20-13}$$

When only one within the pair has the disease, the probability of A suffering from the disease is:

$$P(Y_A = 1 | Y_A = 1, Y_B = 0 \text{ or } Y_A = 0, Y_B = 1) = \frac{P(Y_A = 1)P(Y_B = 0)}{P(Y_A = 1)P(Y_B = 0) + P(Y_A = 0)P(Y_B = 1)} \tag{20-14}$$

Let

$$P(Y_A = 1) = \frac{e^{(\beta_0 + \beta_1 X_1^A + \beta_2 X_2^A + \cdots + \beta_m X_m^A)}}{1 + e^{(\beta_0 + \beta_1 X_1^A + \beta_2 X_2^A + \cdots + \beta_m X_m^A)}} \tag{20-15a}$$

$$P(Y_B = 1) = \frac{e^{(\beta_0+\beta_1 X_1^B+\beta_2 X_2^B+\cdots+\beta_m X_m^B)}}{1+e^{(\beta_0+\beta_1 X_1^B+\beta_2 X_2^B+\cdots+\beta_m X_m^B)}} \qquad \text{(20-15b)}$$

$$P(Y_A = 0) = \frac{1}{1+e^{(\beta_0+\beta_1 X_1^A+\beta_2 X_2^A+\cdots+\beta_m X_m^A)}} \qquad \text{(20-15c)}$$

$$P(Y_B = 0) = \frac{1}{1+e^{(\beta_0+\beta_1 X_1^B+\beta_2 X_2^B+\cdots+\beta_m X_m^B)}} \qquad \text{(20-15d)}$$

We can substitute the above four equations into Equation (20-16) and simplify it as

$$P(\text{either } Y_A = 1 | Y_A = 1, Y_B = 0 \text{ or } Y_A = 0, Y_B = 1)$$
$$= \frac{e^{(\beta_0+\beta_1 X_1^A+\beta_2 X_2^A+\cdots+\beta_m X_m^A)}}{e^{(\beta_0+\beta_1 X_1^A+\beta_2 X_2^A+\cdots+\beta_m X_m^A)} + e^{(\beta_0+\beta_1 X_1^B+\beta_2 X_2^B+\cdots+\beta_m X_m^B)}} \qquad \text{(20-16)}$$

or

$$P(Y_A = 1 | \text{ either } Y_A = 1, Y_B = 0 \text{ or } Y_A = 0, Y_B = 1)$$
$$= \frac{1}{1+e^{[\beta_1(X_1^A-X_1^B)+\beta_2(X_2^A-X_2^B)+\cdots+\beta_m(X_m^A-X_m^B)]}} \qquad \text{(20-17)}$$

The left side of Equation (20-17) is a conditional possibility that refers to the probability of the case having the disease under the condition that anyone within the pair has the disease. Thus, any model built according to this equation is called a conditional logistic regression model. To avoid confusion, the logistic regression model in the previous section is called the unconditional logistic regression model.

The conditional logistic regression model uses the maximal likelihood to estimate the parameters, as in the unconditional logistic regression model. Further, the two models have the same hypothesis test of partial regression coefficients and goodness-of-fit tests.

Here, the estimates of coefficients $b_1, b_2, \ldots, b_m$ (and accordingly $e^{b_1}, e^{b_2}, \ldots, e^{b_m}$) have the same meaning as before and can still be used to describe variable risk. However, Equations (20-16) and (20-17) show that the constant in each regression cannot be estimated, as they can be reduced in the index of the denominator on the right side of the equation. Thus, the conditional logistic regression model can be used only to analyze risk factors, not for prediction.

20.3.2. *Results*

All the categorical variables are set to the lowest level (level 0) as their baseline. After the stepwise regression (in which $\alpha_{\text{in}} = 0.05$ and $\alpha_{\text{out}} = 0.1$), variables X_1, X_2, X_3, X_4, and X_5 finally enter the equation. The value of the likelihood ratio χ^2 is 74.828, and $P < 0.001$, which means at least one partial regression coefficient is not 0 and that the model can be considered to be successfully established.

Table 20.12 shows that all five variables' partial regression coefficients have statistical significance. Considering the baseline setting of each variable and their *OR* values, the results of Wald χ^2 tests suggest that education, body mass index, recent spiritual pressure, history of benign breast diseases, and family history of malignancy have a relatively close association with the occurrence of breast cancer. Taking history of benign breast diseases as an example, its *OR* is 6.686, suggesting that this factor might increase the risk of breast

Table 20.12 Results of conditional logistic analysis for screening the risk factors

						OR 95% CI	
Variable	b	$SE(b)$	Wald χ^2	P value	*OR*	Lower	Upper
Education (X_1)	0.611	0.243	6.297	0.012	1.841	1.143	2.966
Body mass index (X_2)	1.097	0.477	5.283	0.022	2.997	1.175	7.639
Recently spiritual pressure (X_3)	1.369	0.263	27.084	<0.001	3.931	2.348	6.583
History of breast benign diseases (X_4)	1.900	0.533	12.725	<0.001	6.686	2.354	18.993
Family history of malignancy (X_5)	0.607	0.259	5.498	0.019	1.835	1.105	3.047

cancer to 6.686 times the baseline value. Other variables can also be explained as above.

20.4. Format of result report

The appropriate reporting format of logistic regression results should include sufficient information to address the following:

(1) Aim of the analysis
(2) Basic statistical description of independent variables
(3) Methods of variable selection
(4) A statistical table which reporting the regression coefficient, standard error (SE), *P* value, *OR* estimates values, and their 95% CI.

For example, the result of Example 20.7 can be reported as below:

To investigate the risk factors of nasopharyngeal carcinoma, a case-control study was conducted including 105 cases and 130 controls. For data analysis, unconditional logistic regression analysis was applied, and the variables was selected by stepwise procedure.

The results of logistic regression analysis are shown in Table 20.5. The results showed that family history of nasopharyngeal carcinoma, occupational exposure to hazardous substance, smoking, exercise was significantly associated with the outcome ($P < 0.05$). The *OR*s with 95% CI were 9.043(3.739–21.870), 2.439(1.194–4.982), 4.143(2.138–8.027), and 0.255(0.128–0.505), respectively.

20.5. Other examples

Example 20.6. A new anti-influenza granule acute was developed to treat children with acute upper respiratory tract infection. In the phase three clinical trial of that new medication, a total of 428 cases were included from 5 general hospitals of the experimental center. The dependent variable is the curative effect (1: drug is effective for the disease and 0 stands for ineffective). The main independent variable is whether take the new Granules ($X_1 = 1$ means have the new anti-influenza granule acute, $X_1 = 0$ means have the control medication). Other factor that might influence the curative effects

Table 20.13 The number of cases treated in 5 sub-centers and the treatment outcomes

Sub-centers No.	Trial group		Control group	
	Effective	Ineffective	Effective	Ineffective
1	35	27	10	10
2	47	18	15	7
3	63	21	18	
4	26	22	9	6
5	46	17	14	8

is center variable, which suggests the clinical trial center that cases is originally from (X_2). After allocation, there were 322 cases in the trial group and 106 cases in the control group. The number of cases treated and the treatment outcomes of 5 clinical trial centers are shown in Table 20.13.

Before putting the medication into market, the interaction effects between the center variable and the drugs should be fully investigated. The center variable, X_2, is a nominal variable with 5 levels, so it was coded as four dummy variables D_1, D_2, D_3, D_4 and center 1 was taken as the reference. The interaction term between the center and the drug is also taken as a variable in logistic regression function while doing analysis by SPSS. The final results of the stepwise logistic regression are shown in Table 20.14. As is shown in Table 20.14, the medication variable and the interaction variable have been removed which proved the interaction effect was not exist.

Question: Whether the model building, variable selecting methods and the explanation of the interaction terms are appropriate?

Example 20.7. To investigate the risk factors of depression in adult patients (older than 18 years old), 294 samples were randomly selected from the adults in the city. Among them, 50 are patients with depression, and 244 are controls without depression. Three possible risk factors were included, which include gender X_1 (0 is male and 1 is female), age X_2 (age/10), and health condition X_3 (1 represents very good, 2 represents good, 3 represents fine, 4 represents bad).

Table 20.14 The final results of the stepwise logistic regression in SPSS software

Variables	b	$SE(b)$	Wald χ^2	Df	P	OR
D	—	—	11.688	4	0.020	—
D_1	0.713	0.325	4.818	1	0.028	2.039
D_2	0.798	0.308	6.700	1	0.010	2.220
D_3	0.027	0.337	0.007	1	0.935	1.028
D_4	0.680	0.325	4.362	1	0.037	1.973
Constant	0.196	0.222	0.778	1	0.378	1.216

Table 20.15 The risk factor analysis on adult depression problems

Variables	b	$SE(b)$	Wald χ^2	P	OR	Standard b
Constant	0.4057	0.1255	10.450	<0.001	1.5004	—
X_1	2.0683	0.4475	21.362	<0.001	7.9114	1.0457
X_2	−1.3890	0.3264	18.109	<0.001	0.2493	−1.7200
X_3	1.3791	0.2736	25.407	<0.001	3.9713	1.4634

The results of the logistic regression formulation with three factors are displayed in Table 20.15.

Questions: (1) According to Table 20.15, some researchers draw the following conclusions. Firstly, gender, age, and health condition were related to the adult depression. Secondly, female, younger, and bad health condition were the risk factors of adult depression. Thirdly, the *OR*s showed that gender had the largest effect on the depression, followed by health condition, and age had the smallest effect. Are these conclusions right? Why?

(2) Other researchers believed that with an increase of every 10 years in age, the risk of the depression will possibly decrease 25%, and with a decrease of 20 years old, the risk of developing depression would possibly decrease 50% each. Is this conclusion right? Please explain.

20.6. Computer exercises

(For more details, please see electronic resources from exp20-1 to exp20-4)

Experiment 20.1 Variable selection by using binary logistic regression

With binary logistic procedure in SPSS software, the binary logistic regression can be used to select the risk factors and predict the outcome.

Experiment 20.2 Multinomial logistic regression by using SPSS

With the multinomial logistic procedure, disordered multi-classification logistic regression can be used to select the risk factors and predict the outcome.

Experiment 20.3 Ordinal multi-classification logistic regression

With Ordinal Regression procedure in SPSS software, the Ordinal multi-classification logistic regression can be used to select the risk factors and predict the outcome.

Experiment 20.4 Conditional logistic regression by using Cox regression

With Cox regression procedure in SPSS software, the conditional logistic regression can be used to select the risk factors.

20.7. Frequently asked questions and summary

20.7.1. *Frequently asked questions*

1. If the code of dependent variable was changed, for example, the code of dependent variable of 20.2 was changed, and 1 was set as the control group,0 was the case group. What the logistic regression results will change?

Currently code 1 in binominal variable Y stands for case group while 0 represents control group. when switch the code for two groups, that is, 1 represents control group label and 0 represents case group label, the absolute value of regression coefficient in two functions will not change, however, the sign will change. In general, the outcome value of concern should be set a higher score. In most cases, 1 would be coded as case group.

2. At least, how many samples is required when applying logistic regression model?

When using a logistic regression model, several or even dozens of candidate independent variables need to be introduced into the logistic regression model. To make sure there are enough samples for each level of each variable, and to ensure the stability of the parameter estimations in each model and to avoid the over fitting problems, in common cases, it is believed that the number of samples should be at least 10–20 times larger than the number of independent variables independent variables where the outcome is rare happened. What's more, there should be at least 30–50 samples on each side of case and control groups. Please see section 15 for more details about sample size calculation.

3. Which logistic regression model should we use to make prediction?

There are mainly two purposed of Logistic regression. The first one is to analyze the risk factors and to give the corresponding *OR* for each independent variable. The other one is to predict the probability of occurrence for each sample. For study with cohort or cross-sectional design, the predict possibility can be calculated directly by using unconditional logistic regression function. For study with nested case-control design, the Unconditional logistic regression can also be used to establish the model for group case-control data, but the constant term needs to be corrected before it can be used for probability prediction. For the matched case-control data, conditional logistic regression can be used. However, since the constant cannot be estimated, it cannot be used for probability prediction, and it can only be used for risk factor analysis.

4. If the purpose of establishing a logistic regression model is to predict clinical diagnosis or prognosis, from which aspects can the prediction effect of the model be verified?

The model prediction effect evaluation includes three aspects. The first one is discrimination, which means the model's ability of discriminating the high- and low-risk people. ROC analysis is often applied to calculate the area under curve (AUC). AUC over 0.7 represents the high discrimination of the model. Please read section 14 for more details. The second one is calibration, which stands for the goodness of the model's fitness. Hosmer–Lemeshow test is adopted to compare the actual and predicted number of calibrations, and the larger P value is, the better their calibration is. Calibration curve also can be used. It is a scatter graph of the actual and predicted incidence rates, and the scatter should be close to a 45-degree line. The third is clinical relevance, which means the model's usage in disease prevention or the development of clinical intervention measures or screening strategies. In addition, from the dataset perspective, the validation of the prediction effect of the model includes internal and external validation. The internal validation divides the original data into the modeling sample and the validation sample, or adopts the method of cross-validation. The external validation collects a new data for validation.

20.7.2. *Summary*

1. The dependent variable of logistic regression is the classification variable. According to the types of dependent variables, logistic regression can be divided into binary logistic regression, multinomial logistic regression, and ordered multi-classification logistic regression. Independent variables can be quantitative, ordinal or, nominal variables. For quantitative variables, it is usually more efficient to introduce the variables without any transformation. Besides, these variables can also be transformed into hierarchical variables or disordered classification variables when necessary. The ordinal independent variables can be firstly analyzed in the form of dummy variables. If the dominant ratio between adjacent grades is approximately constant, the variables can be assigned with specific values, and then those variables can be introduced into the equation as the discrete quantitative variables. For multinomial independent variables, the equation must be introduced in

the form of dummy variables, and the dummy variables of a single independent variable should be in/out equation at the same time in the variable selection. According to different types of study design, logistic regression can be divided into non-conditional logistic regression and conditional logistic regression. Such regression has been widely used in cohort studies, case-control studies and cross-sectional studies.

2. Like the multiple linear regression, after the logistic regression equation is obtained, it is necessary to carry out hypothesis test for the regression equation, including the hypothesis test for each partial regression coefficient and the hypothesis test for the regression equation. Wald test and likelihood ratio test are commonly used. If the equation is established, goodness of fit test should be carried out to evaluate the degree of fitting between the equation and data.
3. The results report of logistic regression should include: Statistical description of independent and dependent variables; selecting method of independent variables; partial regression coefficients, which are reported in a statistic form, standard error, value of test statistic, *OR*s with its confidence interval and evaluation of equation goodness of fit.

Think and Practice

I. Best Choice

1. The dependent variables of Logistic regression can be ( ).
   A. binomial variables B. ordinal variables C. multinomial variables D. continuous quantitative variables E. A, B, and C are all right
2. In order to explore the influence of risk factors (including treatment, tumor infiltration degree and histological types, etc.) on the survival time in patients with lung cancer, the patients were followed up and observed. The patients were divided into two categories, including the patients' survival time not more than

2 years and more than 2 years. The most suitable statistical analysis method for this sample is ( ).
A. analysis of variance B. linear regression analysis C. multiple linear regression analysis D. logistic regression analysis E. survival analysis

3. The independent variables can be applied to logistic regression are ( ).
A. binomial variables B. ordinal variables C. multinomial variables D. continuous quantitative variables E. All above

4. In Logistic regression, if change the code of the independent variables "hypertension history" from 0,1 to 0,2 with the other variables unchanged, the partial regression coefficient of the "hypertension history" will turn to ( ).
A. the partial regression coefficient remains unchanged. B. partial regression coefficient is half of the original. C. partial regression coefficient is twice of the original. D. partial regression coefficient is $e^{1/2}$ of the original. E. partial regression coefficient is e^2 of the original.

5. The relationship between Logistic regression coefficients and OR is ( ).
A. $\beta > 0$ is equal to $OR > 1$ B. $\beta > 0$ is equal to $OR < 1$ C. $\beta = 0$ is equal to $OR = 1$ D. $\beta < 0$ is equal to $OR < 1$ E. A, C, and D are right.

6. If the independent variable in Logistic regression is a multinomial variable, firstly it should be coded as dummy variables, then together with other independent variables, variable selection procedure can be conducted, which of the following method should be adopted ( ).
A. Software automatic screening of the forward process B. Software automatic screening of the backward process C. Software automatic screening of the stepwise process D. Several dummy variables should be considered as a factor, and should in/out regression equation as a whole E. A, B, and C are right.

7. The regression coefficients in logistic regression $\beta_j (j = 1, 2, \dots, m)$ can be interpreted as follows: the change $\ln(odds)$ that caused by

the change of one unit of the jth risk factor X_j when the values of other risk factors are certain. Which is the correct description of the relationship between β_j and OR_j ( )?
A. If the risk factor X_j is a binary variable, when $X_j = 1, 0$, $\beta_j = \ln OR$. B. If the risk factor X_j is a level variable, when $X_j = k_1, k_0$, $\beta_j = \frac{1}{k_1 - k_0} \ln OR$ C. If the risk factor X_j is continuous variable, β_j is the increasing/decreasing value of $\ln OR$ caused by the change of one unit of X_j. D. If the risk factor X_j is a level variable, when $X_j = k_1, k_0$, $\beta_j = \frac{1}{k_1} \ln OR$ E. A, B, and C are right.

II. Open Questions

1. In order to study the risk factors of smoking among teenagers, researchers selected students from one of the graded-one classes in urban and suburban area, respectively by using cluster sampling. For data analysis a logistic regression method was applied to screen the risk factors. Is it appropriate to use logistic regression method in this case? Please explain why.?
2. The categorical independent variables are often assigned to different values. For example, if the values of long-term exercise and smoking were assigned to the independent variables in Example 20.7, how the logistic regression result would change?
3. What is the effect of using unconditioned logistic regression in the analysis of paired case-control studies?

III. Questions on Calculation

1. To investigate the risk factors of the emergency surgery of patients with acute myocardial infarction (AMI), two hundred patients were included with detailed medical records in the past 5 years (only 3 factors were listed in Table 20.16 for sake of simplification). For the outcome, $P = 0$ means successful rescue surgery, and $P = 1$ means failed and death; While for risk factors, $X_1 = 1$ indicates that shock had occurred before the surgery, and $X_1 = 0$ indicates that shock had not occurred before the surgery; $X_2 = 1$ means heart failure occurred before surgery, and $X_2 = 0$ means no heart failure

Table 20.16 Data of risk factors for AMI patients

$P = 0$ (successful in rescue)				$P = 1$ (failure to rescue and death)			
X_1	X_2	X_3	N	X_1	X_2	X_3	N
0	0	0	35	0	0	0	4
0	0	1	34	0	0	1	10
0	1	0	17	0	1	0	4
0	1	1	19	0	1	1	15
1	0	0	17	1	0	0	6
1	0	1	6	1	0	1	9
1	1	0	6	1	1	0	6
1	1	1	6	1	1	1	6

occurred before surgery; $X_3 = 1$ indicates that the patient has AMI symptoms for more than 12 hours before surgery, $X_3 = 0$ indicates that the patient has AMI symptoms for less than 12 hours before surgery questions:

(1) Which factors might affect the success of AMI surgery?
(2) How to predict the outcome (success or failure) of AMI patients?

Yanhong Luo, Yuan Wang

CHAPTER 21

SURVIVAL ANALYSIS

In logistic regression we are interested in how risk factors are associated with the presence or absence of an event. Sometimes, however, we are interested in how a risk factor or treatment affects the time to an event. Time-to-event data is analyzed in a number of applied fields such as laboratory studies of animals and clinical and epidemiological studies in humans. Survival analysis is a collection of statistical methods used to describe, explain, or predict the occurrence and timing of events. Often the event of interest is death, hence the name "survival analysis." It has now become one of the most important fields in statistics.

21.1. Basic concepts of survival analysis

Example 21.1: Prognosis in patients with bladder tumors

A urologist selected 30 patients with surgically treated bladder tumors at a hospital between 2006 and 2010 and recorded the times from surgery to death. The study factors and explanations are shown in Table 21.1. The follow-up end-point was December 30, 2010. Patient outcomes including follow-up data were obtained from medical records (Table 21.2).

The survival data consists of three parts; research factors (age, grade, size, and relapse), survival time, and event of interest.

Table 21.1 Variable coding of survival data in patients with bladder tumors

Variable	Explanation	Coding
age	Age	years
grade	Tumor grade	1 (level I); 2 (level II); 3 (level III)
size	Tumor size (cm)	0 (<3.0); 1 (≥3.0)
relapse	Whether relapsed or not	0 (no); 1 (yes)
start	Surgery date	month/day/year
end	Termination date	month/day/year
time	Survival time	months
status	Outcome	0 (censored); 1 (death)

Such datasets are known as "triple" data, and the following aspects thereof can be analyzed:

1. Estimation: To estimate the survival rate, survival curve, and median survival time in a group of individuals, such as patients with bladder tumors <3.0 cm in size.
2. Comparison: To compare the survival curves of two or more groups, such as patients with tumors ≥3.0 cm in size vs. patients with tumors <3.0 cm in size, to investigate relationships between prognosis and tumor size.
3. Identifying potential risk/prognostic factors: To assess relationships between predictors and time-to-event, for example, "Do age, tumor grade, tumor size, and/or relapse influence survival time in patients with bladder tumors?"

21.1.1. *Survival time and censoring*

Survival time or time-to-event refers to the duration from a clear and well-defined starting point to the occurrence of the outcome of interest. The starting point may be the date of the first diagnosis, admission to a hospital, or the initiation of a therapy. In clinical trials the appropriate starting point is the time of randomization. The event can be the development of a disease, response to a treatment, relapse, or death. Therefore survival time can be the time from exposure to cancer incidence in an epidemiological cohort study, the time from randomization to recurrence in a cancer clinical trial, the time from remission of leukemia to relapse, or the time from diagnosis of cancer to death due to the cancer. Overall survival (OS) and progression-free survival (PFS), which are common measures of survival time in clinical trials, are widely used in composite events. OS generally refers to the period from the date of group randomization to death for any reason. PFS generally refers to the time from group randomization to a pre-identified determinant of disease progression such as distant tumor metastasis, secondary primary tumor, or death. In engineering research the end-point event is usually referred to as a failure, and the survival time is also known as the failure time.

1. Complete data

During a follow-up period researchers may observe a given end-point event in some subjects, and these exact survival time data are called complete data. Among the first six patients in Table 21.2, patients with IDs 2, 5, and 6 all died from bladder tumors, thus their survival time data were complete.

2. Censored data

Censoring occurs when we are unable to collect a complete set of data for a subject and have incomplete information about the time-to-event. Three common situations where an individual's survival time is right-censored are the following:

(1) The end-point event had not occurred by the end of the study, such as in patient ID 1 in Table 21.2.
(2) Lost to follow-up for non-study-related reasons such as failure to continue treatment, refusal to visit the required facility, or relocation such as in patient ID 3 in Table 21.2.
(3) Death from causes other than the event of interest (in cause-specific survival analyses). For example, patient ID 4 in Table 21.2 died from coronary heart disease.

Right censoring is the most common form of censoring in medical studies, of which we know that the true survival time of a patient is commonly greater than a given value, often marked with a "+"

Table 21.2 Survival data in patients with bladder tumors ($n = 30$)

ID (1)	age (2)	grade (3)	size (4)	relapse (5)	start (6)	end (7)	time (8)	status (9)	PI (10)	S(t) (11)
1	62	1	0	0	02/20/2006	12/30/2010	59	0	1.680	0.256
2	64	1	0	0	03/05/2006	08/12/2010	54	1	1.680	0.256
3	52	2	0	1	04/09/2006	12/03/2009	44	0	4.339	0.018
4	60	1	0	0	06/06/2006	10/27/2010	53	0	1.680	0.512
5	59	2	1	0	07/20/2006	06/21/2008	23	1	4.438	0.662
6	59	1	1	1	08/19/2006	09/10/2009	37	1	3.737	0.249
7	63	1	1	0	09/16/2006	10/20/2010	50	1	2.758	0.139
8	62	1	0	0	09/20/2006	09/18/2009	36	1	1.680	0.859
9	50	1	1	0	09/26/2006	03/22/2009	30	1	2.758	0.760
10	26	1	1	1	11/04/2006	05/25/2010	43	1	3.737	0.110
11	43	2	1	0	01/10/2007	11/08/2009	34	1	4.438	0.131
12	62	1	0	0	02/16/2007	11/10/2010	45	1	1.680	0.646
13	67	1	0	0	03/09/2007	08/18/2010	42	1	1.680	0.785
14	70	2	0	0	03/28/2007	07/20/2010	40	1	3.360	0.328
15	56	1	0	1	04/03/2007	11/10/2009	32	1	2.659	0.747
16	85	2	0	1	04/15/2007	11/20/2008	19	1	4.339	0.801
17	65	1	0	1	08/06/2007	09/28/2009	26	1	2.659	0.894
18	54	3	1	1	11/10/2007	12/09/2008	13	1	7.097	0.155
19	62	2	0	0	02/19/2008	07/20/2010	29	1	3.360	0.659
20	52	3	0	0	03/14/2008	07/02/2010	28	1	5.040	0.163
21	63	2	1	0	06/10/2008	09/01/2010	27	1	4.438	0.446
22	50	3	1	1	06/15/2008	04/14/2009	10	1	7.097	0.517
23	83	2	1	1	09/03/2008	09/20/2010	25	1	5.417	0.246
24	61	3	1	0	10/10/2008	06/13/2010	20	1	6.118	0.181
25	57	3	1	1	01/16/2008	12/20/2009	11	1	7.097	0.396
26	63	2	0	1	02/17/2009	04/20/2010	14	1	4.339	0.845
27	72	3	1	1	05/10/2009	05/12/2010	12	1	7.097	0.276
28	56	3	1	1	09/15/2009	06/17/2010	9	1	7.097	0.638
29	73	3	1	1	12/19/2009	07/26/2010	7	1	7.097	0.759
30	54	3	1	1	03/10/2010	09/20/2010	6	1	7.097	0.879

PI:prognostic index; S(t): survival function. See Section 21.4.

on the upper right of the time. Censoring that is random and non-informative is usually required in order to avoid bias in a survival analysis. That is, if subjects had been followed beyond the censored time-point they would have had the same probability of survival as those not censored at that time-point.

Survival time may be expressed in hours, days, weeks, months, or years from the beginning of follow-up until an event occurs. Most survival analysis methods are based on survival time sorting, underpinning a need for accuracy. Because survival time data are usually not normally distributed or the distribution is unknown, this chapter only introduces non-parametric and semi-parametric methods of survival analysis.

21.1.2. *Probability of survival and probability of death*

The interval-specific probability of survival is the conditional probability that someone who is alive and under observation at the start of an interval will survive to the end of that interval. Annual probability of survival is the probability that the number of people who are alive at the beginning of a year will survive to the end of that year.

$$p = \frac{\text{Number of alive in the interval}}{\text{Number at risk at the start of this interval}} \tag{21-1}$$

The interval-specific probability of death is the conditional probability that someone who is alive and under observation at the start of an interval will be dead by the end of that interval. Annual probability of death is the probability that the number of people at risk of death at the beginning of a year will be dead by the end of that year.

$$q = \frac{\text{Number of death in the interval}}{\text{Number at risk at the start of this interval}} \tag{21-2}$$

If the interval is the same, then $p = 1 - q$.

21.1.3. *Survival function and hazard function*

Let the survival time (random variable) be denoted by t. The survival function is defined as the probability that an individual survives longer than t. The survival function summarizes survival data by providing survival probabilities at different time-points. $S(t)$ ranges between 0 and 1. In the absence of censoring, an estimate of $S(t)$ could be obtained by simply calculating the proportion of individuals still alive at selected values of t:

$$\hat{S}(t) = P(T > t) = \frac{\text{Number of patients surviving longer than } t}{\text{Total number of patients in the study}} \tag{21-3}$$

Conversely, in the presence of censoring the survival function can be estimated as the product of conditional probabilities of survival:

$$S(t) = P(T > t) = p_1 \cdot p_2 \cdots p_t = S(t_{t-1}) \cdot p_t \tag{21-4}$$

Where $p_i(i = 1, 2, \ldots, t)$ is the interval-specific probability of survival, so the survival function is also known as the cumulative survival function.

The hazard function describes the risk of death during an interval of time after t, conditional on the subject having survived to time t, and is also called the conditional probability of failure.

$$h(t) = \lim_{\Delta t \to 0} \frac{P(t \leq T < t + \Delta t \,|T \geq t)}{\Delta t} \tag{21-5}$$

The hazard function is also known as the instantaneous failure rate, force of mortality, and age-specific failure rate. Note that $h(t)$ is a rate rather than a probability, and the range is 0 to $+\infty$.

All survival functions are monotone, non-increasing functions. In contrast to the survival function, the hazard function summarizes survival data by focusing on failures. The hazard function may be increasing, decreasing, remaining constant, or exhibiting a bathtub-shaped course, or it may possess some other characteristics. Considering that the hazard function is usually more informative with regard to the underlying mechanism of failure than the survival function, the survival analysis model is usually given in the form of $h(t)$ (see Section 21.4 for further details).

21.2. Estimation of survival functions

Nonparametric methods for the estimation of survival functions include the life-table method (also known as the actuarial method) and the product-limit (PL) method. Both estimates are generated on the same basis, that is, the cumulative survival function $S(t)$ at the end of a specified interval is then given by the product of the interval-specific survival proportions for all intervals up to and including the specified interval. The only difference is that the PL estimates are based on individual survival times, whereas in the life-table method survival times are grouped into intervals. The PL estimate can be considered a specific variant of the life-table estimate, where each interval contains only one observation.

21.2.1. *Life-table method*

In some situations it is not possible to know or to record the exact time when an event occurs. Sometimes the only available information is that the event occurred during a certain period of time, for example, the death or censoring of certain individuals at follow-up occurs between two visits at a cancer registry, or similarly imprecise data derived from other large surveillance systems. One approach is to divide the entire period of observation into a series of time intervals then estimate the conditional (interval-specific) survival proportion for each interval. This is one of the oldest and most widely used methods for non-parametric analysis and presentation of right-censored data.

Example 21.2. A total of 374 patients with malignant tumors were collated and followed up at intervals of 1 year. The information needed to estimate the cumulative survival rate is shown in columns 1–5 in Table 21.3.

1. Calculate the effective number of people at risk (the number of people at risk just before the beginning of the interval). In the presence of censoring it is assumed that censoring occurs uniformly throughout the interval. Therefore, people who are lost to follow-up or withdraw during the interval are deemed to have been exposed to a risk of death for one half of the interval, that is, $n_i = n_i' - c_i/2$ (see column 6 in Table 21.3).
2. Calculate the conditional proportion dying (q_i) and conditional proportion surviving (p_i) in each interval (see columns 7 and 8 in Table 21.3).

$$q_i = \frac{d_i}{n_i} \quad p_i = 1 - q_i \tag{21-6}$$

3. Calculate the survival rate (see column 9 in Table 21.3). The 1-year survival rate in patients with malignant tumors was 75.94%, the 2-year survival rate was 55.62%, and so on.

Table 21.3 Life-table estimation of survival rate

ID i (1)	Years since diagnosis $t_i \sim$ (2)	Number of death d_i (3)	Number of censored c_i (4)	Number at risk n'_i (5)	Effective number at risk n_i (6)	Conditional proportion dying q_i (7)	Conditional proportion surviving p_i (8)	Cumulative proportion surviving $\hat{S}(t_i)$ (9)	Standard error of survival rate $SE[\hat{S}(t_i)]$ (10)
1	0∼	90	0	374	374.0	$90/374.0 = 0.2406$	0.7594	0.7594	0.0221
2	1∼	76	0	284	284.0	$76/284.0 = 0.2676$	0.7324	$0.7594 \times 0.7324 = 0.5562$	0.0257
3	2∼	51	0	208	208.0	$51/208.0 = 0.2452$	0.7548	$0.5562 \times 0.7548 = 0.4198$	0.0255
4	3∼	25	12	157	151.0	$25/151.0 = 0.1656$	0.8344	$0.4198 \times 0.8344 = 0.3503$	0.0248
5	4∼	20	5	120	117.5	$20/117.5 = 0.1702$	0.8298	$0.3503 \times 0.8298 = 0.2907$	0.0239
6	5∼	7	9	95	90.5	$7/90.5 = 0.0773$	0.9227	$0.2907 \times 0.9227 = 0.2682$	0.0235
7	6∼	4	9	79	74.5	$4/74.5 = 0.0537$	0.9463	$0.2682 \times 0.9463 = 0.2538$	0.0233
8	7∼	1	3	66	64.5	$1/64.5 = 0.0155$	0.9845	$0.2538 \times 0.9845 = 0.2499$	0.0233
9	8∼	3	5	62	59.5	$3/59.5 = 0.0504$	0.9496	$0.2499 \times 0.9496 = 0.2373$	0.0232
10	9∼10	2	5	54	51.5	$2/51.5 = 0.0388$	0.9612	$0.2373 \times 0.9612 = 0.2281$	0.0232

Note: Forty-seven patients have survival times of more than 10 years.

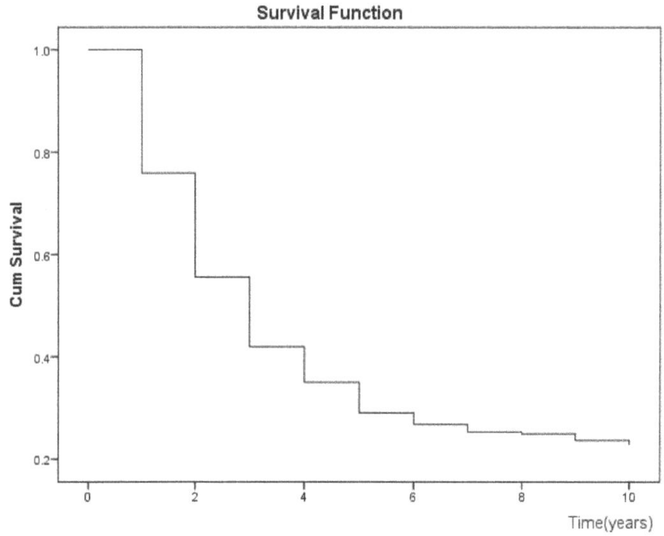

Figure 21.1 Survival curve in patients with malignant tumors

The survival curve is the plot of $S(t)$(vertical axis) against t(horizontal axis). If the vertical axis is $h(t)$, it is known as the hazard curve. The survival and hazard curves of the patients with malignant tumors in Example 21.2 are shown in Figures 21.1 and 21.2, respectively. It can be seen that the risk of death is higher 1 year after diagnosis, gradually decreases 2 years later, and slightly increases after 8 years.

21.2.2. *PL method*

Example 21.3. Consider the data in Table 21.2. The survival times (months) of 14 patients with bladder tumors <3.0 cm in size and 16 patients with bladder tumors $\geq$3.0 cm in size are listed below. Estimate the survival functions of the two groups.

Tumors <3.0 cm in size: 14, 19, 26, 28, 29, 32, 36, 40, 42, 44^+, 45, 53^+, 54, 59^+

Tumors $\geq$3.0 cm in size: 6, 7, 9, 10, 11, 12, 13, 20, 23, 25, 27, 30, 34, 37, 43, 50

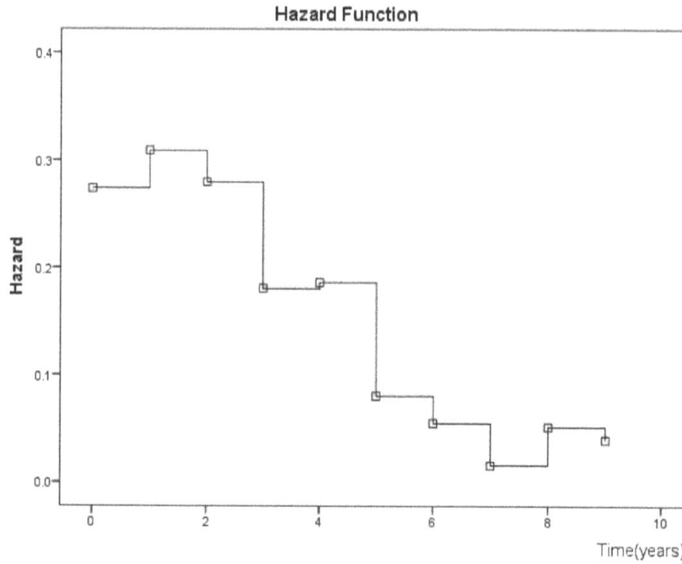

Figure 21.2 Hazard curve in patients with malignant tumors

Taking the group with tumors <3.0 cm in size as an example, 14 patients with survival data ($n = 14$) is a small sample and contains censored times. The survival rate can be estimated by the PL method. In that method, the cumulative survival rate is a "product" of the conditional probability of survival and the estimates are limited to the time interval in which the observations fall. This standard non-parametric technique for estimating the survival function was proposed by Kaplan and Meier (1958), and is called the Kaplan–Meier estimator.

1. Rank the survival times (t_i) in ascending order. If a censored observation has the same value as an uncensored observation, the latter should appear first, as shown in column 2 in Table 21.4.
2. List the number of deaths d_i and the number of censored entries c_i in the interval (t_i, t_{i+1}), as shown in columns 3 and 4 in Table 21.4.
3. Calculate the number of people at risk n_i. The number of deaths and the number of censored before t_i should be subtracted (i.e., $n_i = n_{i-1} - d_{i-1} - c_{i-1}$). See column 5 in Table 21.4.

Table 21.4 The PL estimator in patients with bladder tumors <3.0 cm in size

ID i (1)	Time (month) $t_i \sim$ (2)	Number of events d_i (3)	Number of censored c_i (4)	Number at risk n_i (5)	Conditional proportion dying q_i (6)	Conditional proportion surviving p_i (7)	Cumulative proportion surviving $\hat{S}(t_i)$ (8)	Standard error of survival rate $SE[\hat{S}(t_i)]$ (9)
1	14	1	0	14	$1/14 = 0.0714$	0.9286	0.9286	0.0688
2	19	1	0	13	$1/13 = 0.0769$	0.9231	$0.9286 \times 0.9231 = 0.8572$	0.0935
3	26	1	0	12	$1/12 = 0.0833$	0.9167	$0.8572 \times 0.9167 = 0.7858$	0.1097
4	28	1	0	11	$1/11 = 0.0909$	0.9091	$0.7858 \times 0.9091 = 0.7144$	0.1207
5	29	1	0	10	$1/10 = 0.1000$	0.9000	$0.7144 \times 0.9000 = 0.6429$	0.1281
6	32	1	0	9	$1/9 = 0.1111$	0.8889	$0.6429 \times 0.8889 = 0.5715$	0.1323
7	36	1	0	8	$1/8 = 0.1250$	0.8750	$0.5715 \times 0.8750 = 0.5001$	0.1336
8	40	1	0	7	$1/7 = 0.1429$	0.8571	$0.5001 \times 0.8571 = 0.4286$	0.1323
9	42	1	0	6	$1/6 = 0.1667$	0.8333	$0.4286 \times 0.8333 = 0.3571$	0.1281
10	44^+	0	1	5	$0/5 = 0.0000$	1.0000	$0.3571 \times 1.0000 = 0.3571$	0.1281
11	45	1	0	4	$1/4 = 0.2500$	0.7500	$0.3571 \times 0.7500 = 0.2678$	0.1233
12	53^+	0	1	3	$0/3 = 0.0000$	1.0000	$0.2678 \times 1.0000 = 0.2678$	0.1233
13	54	1	0	2	$1/2 = 0.5000$	0.5000	$0.2678 \times 0.5000 = 0.1339$	0.1130
14	59^+	0	1	1	$0/1 = 0.0000$	1.0000	$0.1339 \times 1.0000 = 0.1339$	0.1130

4. Calculate the conditional probability of death q_i and the probability of survival p_i (see columns 6 and 7 in Table 21.4).
5. Calculate the survival rate $\hat{S}(t_i)$ (see column 8 in Table 21.4). The 14-month survival rate of patients with bladder tumors <3.0 cm in size is 92.86%, and the 19-month survival rate is 85.72%, and so on. Note that the PL estimator does not change at censoring times. Drops only occur at event times. Of course, censored subjects are excluded from the future number at risk, and do not count as failures either.

The survival curve yielded by the PL method is a step function. The survival curves for patients with tumors <3.0 cm in size and those with tumors $\geq$3.0 cm in size (calculation table omitted) are shown in Figure 21.3. A flat survival curve indicates a higher survival rate or a longer survival time, as shown in Figure 21.3 in the group

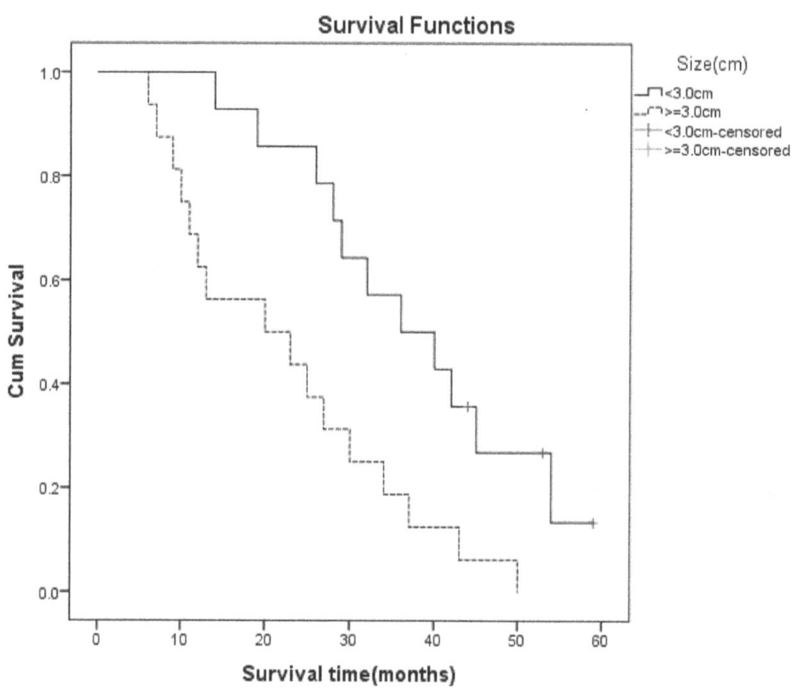

Figure 21.3 Survival curves in patients with tumors <3.0 cm in size and tumors $\geq$3.0 cm in size

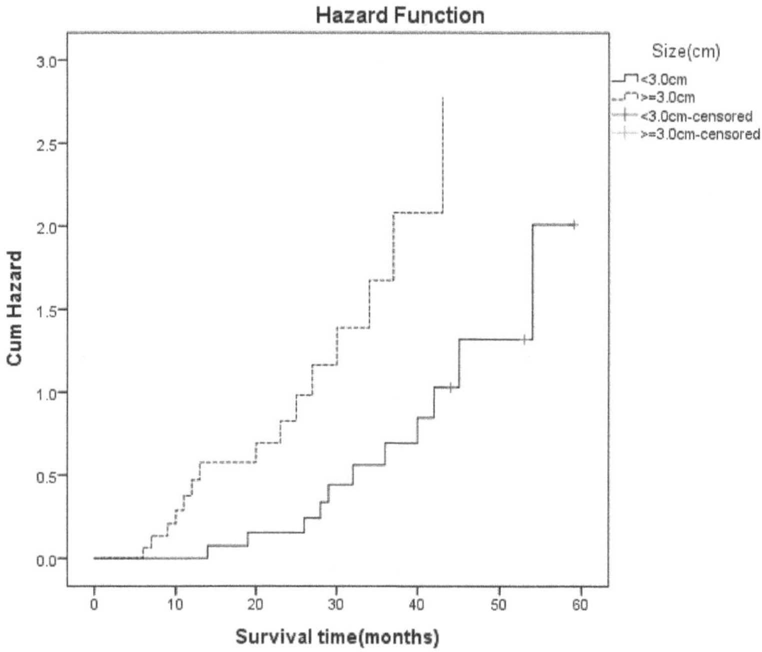

Figure 21.4 Hazard curves in patients with tumors <3.0 cm in size and tumors ≥ 3.0 cm in size

with tumors <3.0 cm in size. A steep survival curve indicates a lower survival rate or a shorter survival time, as shown in Figure 21.3 in the group with tumors ≥ 3.0 cm in size. The hazard curves of the two groups are shown in Figure 21.4. The longer the time, the higher the risk of death in both groups, and the risk of death is greater in the group with tumors ≥ 3.0 cm in size.

The most commonly used summary statistic in survival analysis is median survival time. The longer the median survival time the better the prognosis, and vice versa. A simple estimate of the median can be derived from survival curves estimated via the PL method as the time t at which $\hat{S}(t_i)$ is 0.5. The estimated median survival times from Figure 21.3 are approximately 36 months in patients with tumors <3.0 cm in size and 20 months in patients with tumors ≥ 3.0 cm in size. A more accurate estimate can be obtained using linear interpolation.

21.2.3. *Interval estimation of survival rate*

The survival rate $\hat{S}(t_i)$ calculated from the sample data is a point estimate based on which a confidence interval (CI) can be estimated. The standard error of the PL estimator is estimated via Greenwood's formula:

$$SE[\hat{S}(t_i)] = \hat{S}(t_i)\sqrt{\sum_{t_j \le t_i} \frac{d_j}{n_j(n_j - d_j)}} \tag{21-7}$$

We can easily construct $(1-\alpha)\cdot 100\%$ point-wise CIs for the survival function at a fixed time from the asymptotic normality of the estimator:

$$\hat{S}(t_i) \pm Z_{\alpha/2} \cdot SE[\hat{S}(t_i)] \tag{21-8}$$

where $Z_{\alpha/2}$ is the upper critical value of the standard normal distribution corresponding to the two-sided area α, when $\alpha = 0.05$, $Z_{0.05/2} = 1.96$.

Standard error of $\hat{S}(t_4)$ in Table 21.4 is

$$\begin{aligned} SE[\hat{S}(t_4)] &= 0.7144 \times \sqrt{\frac{1}{14 \times 13} + \frac{1}{13 \times 12} + \frac{1}{12 \times 11} + \frac{1}{11 \times 10}} \\ &= 0.1207 \end{aligned}$$

The 95% CI of the survival rate is $0.7144 \pm 1.96 \times 0.1207 = (0.4778-0.9509)$.

21.3. Comparison of survival curves

In many studies the primary objective is to compare survival in different groups of patients. These groups may be defined based on sex, tumor stage at the time of diagnosis, and histological type, among other parameters. In clinical trials groups will often be defined based on the treatment/s administered. Cumulative survival probabilities are calculated separately for each group and the two survival curves are plotted on the same graph for comparison (Figure 21.3). Traditional statistical methods such as the chi-square test discussed in Chapter 7 are not appropriate for comparing proportions of survivors. The most common methods used are the log-rank test and the Breslow test, which take the whole follow-up period into account and do not require any assumptions about the distribution of the survival function.

21.3.1. *Log-rank test*

Example 21.4. Following Example 21.3, compare the survival curves of patients with bladder tumors <3.0 cm in size and tumors ≥3.0 cm in size.

Let $S_1(t)$ and $S_2(t)$ be the respective survival functions of the two groups. The null hypothesis is:

H_0: $S_1(t) = S_2(t)$, for all $t > 0$

The alternative hypothesis is:

H_1: $S_1(t) \neq S_2(t)$, for some $t > 0$
$\alpha = 0.05$

The log-rank test is based on the difference between the observed number of events and the expected number of events in each group in cases where there is no difference between the two groups:

$$\chi^2 = \frac{\left[\sum (d_{gi} - T_{gi})\right]^2}{\sum V_{gi}} \tag{21-9}$$

$$V_{gi} = \frac{n_{gi}(n_i - n_{gi})(n_i - d_i)d_i}{n_i^2(n_i - 1)} \tag{21-10}$$

where d_{gi} is the number of observed events at each event time in each group, T_{gi} is the number of expected events at each event time in each group, and V_{gi} is the estimate of variance of the observed number in each group. The test statistic follows a chi-square distribution with (number of groups − 1) degrees of freedom.

Using the survival data in Example 21.4 we would like to statistically test the differences between the survival distributions in the two groups.

1. Rank all the event times (t_i) in ascending order, as shown in column 2 in Table 21.5.

Table 21.5 A log-rank test comparing survival curves of patients with tumors <3.0 cm in size and patients with tumors ≥3.0 cm in size

ID	Time (months)	Tumor size <3.0 cm				Tumor size ≥ 3.0 cm				Total	
i	t_i	n_{1i}	d_{1i}	T_{1i}	V_{1i}	n_{2i}	d_{2i}	T_{2i}	V_{2i}	n_i	d_i
(1)	(2)	(3)	(4)	(5)	(6)	(7)	(8)	(9)	(10)	(11)	(12)
1	6	14	0	0.4667	0.2489	16	1	0.5333	0.2489	30	1
2	7	14	0	0.4827	0.2497	15	1	0.5172	0.2497	29	1
3	9	14	0	0.5000	0.2500	14	1	0.5000	0.2500	28	1
...											
Total		—	11	17.5416	5.8064	—	16	9.4584	5.8064	—	27

2. List the number of people at risk n_{gi} (see columns 3 and 7 in Table 21.5) and the number of deaths observed d_{gi} (see columns 4 and 8 in Table 21.5) at time t_i in each group. The total number at risk n_i and deaths d_i are shown in columns 11 and 12 in Table 21.5.
3. Calculate the number of deaths expected T_{gi} at time t_i in each group. The estimated expected number of deaths at an event time is obtained via the same formula as that used to calculate the expected numbers in Chapter 7.

$$T_{gi} = \frac{n_{gi}d_i}{n_i} \tag{21-11}$$

   A single 2×2 contingency table like Table 21.6 is created for each event time t_i. Using the first event time as an example, the expected number of deaths in patients with tumors <3.0 cm in size is $14 \times 1/30 = 0.4667$, and that in patients with tumors ≥3.0 cm in size is $16 \times 1/30 = 0.5333$. The respective numbers of deaths at time t_i in each group are shown in columns 5 and 9.
4. Calculate the total numbers of observed and expected deaths in each group. In the group with tumors <3.0 cm in size the observed deaths $A_1 = 11$ and the expected deaths $T_1 = 17.5416$. In the group with tumors ≥3.0 cm in size the corresponding values are $A_2 = 16$ and $T_2 = 9.4584$. $A_1 + A_2 = T_1 + T_2 = 27$, which can be

Table 21.6 Calculation table of expected deaths

Group	Dead	Alive	At risk
Tumor <3.0 cm	0	14	14
Tumor ≥3.0 cm	1	15	16
Total	1	29	30

used to check the calculation. Respective estimations of variance V_{gi} are shown in columns 6 and 10, and $V_1 = V_2 = 5.8064$.

5. Calculate the chi-square statistic using Formula (21-9).

$$\chi^2 = \frac{(11 - 17.5416)^2}{5.8064} = \frac{(16 - 9.4584)^2}{5.8064} = 7.369$$

$$df = 1$$

Because $P < 0.01$ we reject the null hypothesis and conclude that survival time in patients with tumors <3.0 cm in size differed significantly from that in patients with tumors ≥3.0 cm in size.

21.3.2. *Breslow test*

The Breslow test is also known as the Wilcoxon test and has been referred to as a weighted log-rank test. The formula to calculate the chi-square statistic is as follows:

$$\chi^2 = \frac{\left[\sum w_i(d_{gi} - T_{gi})\right]^2}{\sum w_i^2 V_{gi}} \tag{21-12}$$

where w_i is a positive weight and $w_i = n_i$. The Breslow test gives more weight to deaths at earlier time-points and is consequently more sensitive to differences early in the follow-up period, when the number at risk is larger. This kind of weight is appropriate when short-term survival is of more interest. The log-rank test is a specific case in which all w_i are equal to 1 irrespective of the number at risk at the time of the failure, and thus is more sensitive to differences in the right tails than the Breslow test.

Using the Breslow test in Example 21.4, $\chi^2 = 7.631, P < 0.01$, thus the conclusion is the same as that derived using the log-rank test.

21.3.3. *Practical notes*

1. The log-rank test and the Breslow test can be readily applied to more than two groups. If the time interval is small enough to cause deaths in each interval $d_{gi} \leq 1$, the test of the null hypothesis depends only on the order of the occurrence of death rather than the time at which death occurs. Therefore, the log-rank statistic is a rank-based test statistic, hence the name "log-rank" test.
2. The ratio of the number of deaths observed (A) to that expected (T) assuming the null hypothesis is called the relative death ratio, and the relative risk (RR) is the ratio of relative deaths in two groups.

$$RR = \frac{A_1/T_1}{A_2/T_2} \tag{21-13}$$

   This quantity expresses how much larger the failure rate is in one group compared to another. Because it is < 1 in this case it indicates that group 1 has the more favorable survival rate. Using the data shown in Table 21.5 in patients with tumor sizes <3.0 cm and ≥3.0 cm:

$$RR = \frac{A_1/T_1}{A_2/T_2} = \frac{11/17.5416}{16/9.4584} = 0.37$$

   We can conclude that patients with tumors <3.0 cm in size have 0.37 times the risk of death as patients with tumors of ≥3.0 cm in size. Correspondingly, the patients with tumors ≥3.0 cm in size would have 2.69 times death risk as patients with tumor <3.0 cm ($RR = 1/0.37 = 2.69$).
3. The log-rank test is a univariate method of analysis. When comparing survival curves in relation to a particular prognostic factor, it is important to establish whether the groups are similar with regard to other prognostic factors. If they are not, we need to

use Cox's proportional hazards regression modeling to adjust for other potentially confounding factors.

21.4. Cox's proportional hazards regression model

Chapters 19 and 20 introduce the use of multiple linear regression and logistic regression to analyze influencing factors. Often survival times are not normally distributed and they may include censoring, which linear regression is no longer appropriate. Logistic regression can predict the presence or absence of events, but not the time-to-events, and the outcome remains the same regardless of whether an event occurs earlier or later. Moreover, logistic regression cannot incorporate the incomplete information resulting from censored observations.

Currently Cox's proportional hazards regression modeling — "Cox regression" for short — is the most commonly used multivariate analysis for survival data. Cox regression examines relationships between survival and one or more explanatory variables irrespective of the distribution of survival time.

21.4.1. *Cox regression*

1. Model structure

The general Cox regression model takes the form:

$$h(t) = h_0(t)\exp(\beta_1 X_1 + \beta_2 X_2 + \cdots + \beta_m X_m) \tag{21-14}$$

where $X_1, X_2, \ldots, X_m$ represent predictors or independent variables, for example, age, sex, clinical indicators, and biomarkers at the time of entry into the study; $h(t)$ is the hazard rate at time t for a set of m fixed predictors; $h_0(t)$ is the baseline hazard function and can be regarded as the hazard function for an individual whose predictors all have values of 0; and $\beta_1, \beta_2, \ldots, \beta_m$ are regression coefficients corresponding to the independent variables. Cox regression modeling effectively partitions the contributions of time and predictors to the hazard function into two multiplicative components:

(1) The baseline hazard function specifies how the hazard function changes as a function of time when there is no predictor effect.
(2) The exponential term involves a simple linear combination of the predictors through their respective coefficients, and does not depend on time. The coefficients characterize the relative effects of different predictors on the hazard.

Cox regression is considered a semi-parametric multiplicative form of modeling because the baseline hazard function can take any form and the predictors enter the model via a linear combination. Notice that there is no constant term (intercept) in the linear combination; the constant is absorbed in the baseline hazard.

2. Proportional hazards assumption

Cox modeling can generate an estimate of hazard for a particular individual relative to baseline hazard at a particular point in time. It is easy to see that based on Equation (21-14), if we look at two individuals with different values of the predictors, then the hazard ratio (HR),or risk ratio is:

$$\begin{aligned} HR = \frac{h_a(t)}{h_b(t)} &= \frac{h_0(t)\exp(\beta_1 X_{a1} + \beta_2 X_{a2} + \cdots + \beta_m X_{am})}{h_0(t)\exp(\beta_1 X_{b1} + \beta_2 X_{b2} + \cdots + \beta_m X_{bm})} \\ &= \exp[\beta_1(X_{a1} - X_{b1}) + \beta_2(X_{a2} - X_{b2}) + \cdots + \beta_m(X_{am} - X_{bm})] \end{aligned} \tag{21-15}$$

which is constant, independent of time, in that the model assumes that the ratio of the hazard functions for any two individuals remains constant over a follow-up period. This is known as the proportional hazard (PH) assumption. Using the Equation (21-15) logarithm, we obtain:

$$\begin{aligned} \ln HR &= \ln h_a(t) - \ln h_b(t) \\ &= \beta_1(X_{a1} - X_{b1}) + \beta_2(X_{a2} - X_{b2}) + \cdots + \beta_m(X_{am} - X_{bm}) \end{aligned} \tag{21-16}$$

If we graph the log hazards for any two individuals, the PH property implies that the hazard functions should be strictly parallel.

3. Interpretation of parameters

In the multiplicative model, if all the predictors are fixed at time zero the hazard rates of two individuals with different predictor values are proportional. So, $\beta_j (j = 1, 2, \ldots, m)$ is the natural logarithm of the HR for a one-unit increase in the variable X_j when the other variables remain fixed.

$$\ln HR_j = \beta_j \quad HR_j = \exp(\beta_j) \tag{21-17}$$

A positive parameter estimate indicates that the hazard increases with increasing values of the predictor and $HR_j > 1$; whereas a negative estimate indicates that the hazard decreases with increasing values of the predictor and $HR_j < 1$.

4. Parameter estimation and hypothesis testing

The likelihood function for the Cox model of Equation (21-14) can be factored into two parts, where one part depends on both $h_0(t)$ and the coefficients and the other part depends on the coefficients alone. What partial likelihood does, in effect, is to discard the first part and treat the second part — the partial likelihood function — as though it was an ordinary likelihood function. By finding values of coefficients that maximize the partial likelihood, estimates of coefficients can be obtained. The main advantage of the Cox model is that we can estimate the coefficients, without having to estimate $h_0(t)$. Another interesting property of partial likelihood estimates is that they only depend on the ranks of the event times, not their numerical values. This implies that any monotonic transformation of the event times will leave the coefficient estimates unchanged. For example, we could add a constant to the event time, multiply the event time by a constant, or take the logarithm, all without producing any change in the coefficients.

The estimate of 95% CI of β_j can be obtained as follows:

$$\beta_j : b_j \pm Z_{0.05/2} S_{b_j} \tag{21-18}$$

where $S_{b_1}, S_{b_2}, \ldots, S_{b_m}$ are the standard errors of the regression coefficients.

A 95% CI for the HR can be obtained by using the CI for coefficients:

$$HR : \exp(b_j \pm Z_{0.05/2} S_{b_j}) \qquad (21\text{-}19)$$

The hypothesis-testing procedures are similar to those used in logistic regression. One is the likelihood ratio test, which is frequently used for the removal of insignificant variables, the introduction of new variables, or comparisons between models with different predictors. Another is the Wald test, which is used for either the removal of insignificant variables or the introduction of new variables. Both statistics utilize the chi-square method for hypothesis testing, and the degree of freedom is the number of parameters tested in the model.

21.4.2. *Examples*

The forward, backward, and stepwise selection procedures discussed in the context of linear regression and logistic regression are applicable in Cox regression. Moreover, significance level α may range from 0.10 to 0.15 (in studies with less variables or exploratory studies), or from 0.01 to 0.05 (in studies with more variables or confirmatory studies). Multivariate Cox regression analysis can be used to examine the influence of one or more factors on survival time when other factors are controlled. Specific applications include the identification of predictive prognostic factors, multivariate survival prediction, and comparisons between groups after adjustment for confounding factors.

1. Identification of predictive prognostic factors

Example 21.5. Using the data in Table 21.2 we wish to identify from the four predictors a subset of variables that affect the hazard the most significantly, and consequently, the length of survival. We fit the Cox model to the data, $\alpha_{\text{entry}} = 0.05, \alpha_{\text{removal}} = 0.10$, variable selection = forward. The results are shown in Table 21.7.

Table 21.7 shows that tumor grade, tumor size, and relapse are significant independent prognostic predictors in bladder tumor patients. The positive regression coefficients (as opposed to negative values) indicate that these factors are positively associated with

Table 21.7 Results of multivariate Cox regression analysis of 30 bladder tumor patients

Variable	Regression coefficient	Standard error	Wald chi-square	P value	Hazard ratio	HR 95% CI	Standardized estimate
grade	1.680	0.382	19.385	<0.001	5.37	(2.54, 11.34)	1.419
size	1.078	0.460	5.493	0.019	2.94	(1.19, 7.24)	0.546
relapse	0.979	0.460	4.525	0.033	2.66	(1.08, 6.56)	0.498

death, rather than negatively (or "inversely") associated with it. The analysis suggests that if the tumor grade increases by one the risk of dying increases 4.37 times, after adjusting for tumor size and relapse. Patients with tumors ≥3.0 cm in size would have 2.94 times the risk of death as patients with tumors <3.0 cm in size. The estimated risk of dying in patients with relapse is 1.66 times higher than that for patients without relapse.

The influence of these three factors can be ranked by standardized regression coefficients:

$$b'_j = b_j \cdot S_j \quad j = 1, 2, \ldots, m \tag{21-20}$$

where S_j is the standard variation of X_j. As indicated by the values in the last column in Table 21.7, tumor grade contributes most to the risk of death.

2. Multivariate survival prediction

The hazard function in patients with bladder tumors is as follows:

$$h(t) = h_0(t)\exp(1.680 \times \text{grade} + 1.078 \times \text{size} + 0.979 \times \text{relapse})$$

The greater the value of the exponent, the higher the hazard rate, and the worse the prognosis, and this linear combination is known as the prognostic index (PI). The PI in Example 21.5 is:

$$1.680 \times \text{grade} + 1.078 \times \text{size} + 0.979 \times \text{relapse}$$

In patient ID 1, grade = 1, size = 0, and relapse = 0, thus:

$$\text{PI} = 1.680 \times 1 + 1.078 \times 0 + 0.979 \times 0 = 1.680$$

In patient ID 3, grade = 2, size = 0, and relapse = 1, thus:

$$\text{PI} = 1.680 \times 2 + 1.078 \times 0 + 0.979 \times 1 = 4.339$$

The PIs of the 30 bladder tumor patients are shown in column 10 in Table 21.2, above. To facilitate the formulation of individual treatments and guide patient treatment plans in an effort to improve survival, it is helpful to divide patients into several risk groups (2–5 groups) based on PI percentiles, such as low, intermediate, and high-risk groups.

It may be possible to estimate the probability of survival of a newly assessed individual using a given set of predictors at time t and Cox regression modeling:

$$\hat{S}(t) = [\hat{S}_0(t)]^{\exp(\sum b_j X_j)} \tag{21-21}$$

where $\hat{S}_0(t)$ is a baseline survival function estimator.

$$\hat{S}_0(t) = \exp[-\hat{H}_0(t)] \tag{21-22}$$

The Breslow's estimator of the baseline cumulative hazard function is

$$\hat{H}_0(t) = \sum_{t_{(i)} \leq t} \frac{d_i}{\sum\limits_{i \in R_i} \exp(\sum b_j X_j)} \tag{21-23}$$

where $t_{(i)}$ denotes the distinct i-th death times, d_i is the number of deaths at time t_i, and R_i is the risk set at time t_i. Estimates of survival probabilities in the 30 patients in Example 21.5 are shown in column 11 of Table 21.2. Patient ID 1 has a tumor grade of I, a tumor <3.0 cm in size, and is without relapse, and their estimated 59-month survival probability is 25.6%. Patient ID 3 has a tumor grade of II, a tumor <3.0 cm in size, and has undergone relapse, and their estimated 44-month survival probability is 1.8%.

3. Comparisons between groups after adjusting for confounding factors

Often one is interested in comparing times-to-event in two or more groups. If the groups are similar in all respects other than the parameter being investigated, the non-parametric methods discussed in Section 21.3 may be used directly. With reference to the data in Table 21.2, if the purpose of the analysis is to investigate survival in relation to tumor size, log-rank testing is applicable assuming that other potentially influential factors with regard to survival such as age, tumor grade, and relapse are homogeneous between the groups. In cases where such parameters are not homogenous, it is often desirable to adjust for the influences of potentially confounding factors. First tumor size is entered, followed by variable selection procedures for the other three variables age, tumor grade, and relapse, then a Cox regression model is generated.

21.4.3. *Checking the PH assumption*

The validity of Cox regression analysis relies heavily on the PH assumption, and its appropriateness should always be assessed. Various methods have been proposed for this purpose. In the case of categorical predictors, Kaplan–Meier survival curves can facilitate quick and easy estimation of proportional hazards. When there is crossing between survival curves, the PH assumption is not met. We prefer the $\ln[-\ln \hat{S}(t)]$ plot. If the PH assumption holds, $\ln[-\ln \hat{S}(t)]$ vs. time should be approximately parallel. Using the tumor sizes listed in Table 21.2 as an example dataset, a graph of $\ln[-\ln \hat{S}(t)]$ vs. time with approximately parallel curves is shown in Figure 21.5. We do not have enough evidence to say that the PH assumption is not met with respect to tumor size.

21.5. Reporting results

General principles for reporting statistical results in survival analysis:

1. General description: Include the purpose of the analysis, the dates or events that constituted the beginning and the end of the time-period analyzed, the circumstances under which data were censored, sample sizes, the numbers of all types of events analyzed, the amount of censored data, and the follow-up duration (range and mean).
2. Estimation of survival rate: Specify the statistical methods used to estimate the survival rate. Consider presenting the complete set of results, either as graphs (e.g., Kaplan–Meier plots) or tables, or a combination of both. Provide the estimated survival probability at appropriate follow-up times (with CIs), and the number of participants at risk of death at each time-point, in every individual

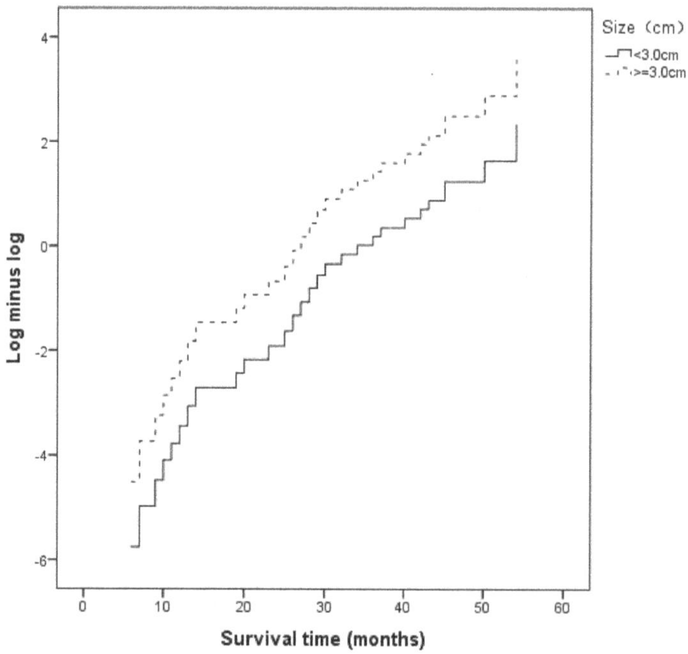

Figure 21.5 $\ln[-\ln\hat{S}(t)]$ vs. time for tumor size

group. Report median survival times (with CIs), because these are often useful with regard to comparing results obtained in a current investigation with those obtained in previous studies.

3. Survival curve comparisons: Specify the statistical methods used to compare two or more survival curves. When comparing survival curves in conjunction with references to hypothesis testing, report the test statistic and corresponding P values of comparisons.
4. Analysis of influencing factors: Describe the regression model used to assess associations between potential predictors and survival or time-to-event. Report selection method, significance levels, and measure/s of risk (e.g., HRs) considered for each explanatory variable, with corresponding CIs and P values. Confirm that the assumption of PH in the Cox model is met.

By way of examples, reporting of survival rate estimations, survival curve comparisons, and Cox regression analysis of potentially predictive factors in patients with bladder tumors in Table 21.2 is shown below.

Kaplan–Meier estimates in groups with tumors <3.0 cm in size and ≥3.0 cm in size are shown in Figure 21.3. The respective median survival times in the two groups were 36 months and 20 months. There were more deaths over time in the group with tumors ≥3.0 cm in size than in the group with tumors <3.0 cm in size (log-rank test chi-square = 7.369, $P = 0.007$). In multivariate Cox proportional hazards regression analysis tumor grade (HR = 5.37; 95% CI: 2.54–11.34, $P < 0.001$), tumor size (HR = 2.94; 95% CI: 1.19–7.24, $P = 0.019$), and relapse (HR = 2.66; 95% CI: 1.08–6.56, $P = 0.033$) are significant predictors of death (Table 21.7).

21.6. Case study

Case 21.1: A physician collected survival data pertaining to 30 postoperative lung cancer patients, but subsequently lost contact with one of those patients due to incorrect telephone number and postal address details. He considered utilizing the following methods in the data analysis:

(1) Remove the patient from the analysis dataset.
(2) Retain the patient in the analysis dataset, but leave the last follow-up time missing and analyze automatically through SPSS.
(3) Record the last follow-up time as the scheduled date an attempt was made to contact the patient in accordance with the study protocol (e.g., "01 September 2016").

In addition to this problem pertaining to a patient who was lost to follow-up, the physician also noticed that there was another problem with the dataset that the median survival time was calculated as 10 months, but the raw data indicated that a patient recorded as having a survival time of "10 months" in fact lived until the end of the follow-up period.

Questions

(1) Is it appropriate to classify this case as "lost to follow-up"? Why? What is the right way to code it?

(2) If another patient died of cerebral infarction, how to code this patient?
(3) Are the physician's findings inconsistent with the definition of median survival time? Why?

Case 21.2: To evaluate the effects of two treatments, 12 patients were treated by Physician A (group 1) and 13 patients were treated by physician B (group 2). Kidney function was assessed in all patients, and scored as 0 for normal, or 1 for abnormal. In the "status" column 0 indicates censoring and 1 indicates death. Time is measured by days after treatment. The data are shown in Table 21.8.

Physician A summarized Table 21.9 based on the event of death. Fisher's exact test yielded $P = 0.097$ (i.e., >0.05), indicating that there was no statistically significant difference in efficacy between the two treatments.

Physician B used multiple linear regression considering time-to-event only, and adjusted for kidney function. Table 21.10 shows his results, which are consistent with those generated by physician A.

Table 21.8 Survival in two groups of patients with kidney disease undergoing treatment by two different physicians ($N = 25$)

ID	group	kidney	time	status	ID	group	kidney	time	status
1	1	1	8	1	13	2	0	180	1
2	1	0	852	0	14	2	0	632	1
3	1	1	52	1	15	2	0	2240	0
4	1	0	220	1	16	2	0	195	1
5	1	1	63	1	17	2	0	76	1
6	1	0	8	1	18	2	0	70	1
7	1	0	1976	0	19	2	1	13	1
8	1	0	1296	0	20	2	1	23	1
9	1	0	1460	0	21	2	0	1296	1
10	1	1	63	1	22	2	0	210	1
11	1	0	1328	0	23	2	0	700	1
12	1	0	365	0	24	2	1	18	1
					25	2	0	1990	0

Table 21.9 Comparison of efficacy between two treatments

Group	Mortality	Survival	Total	Mortality (%)
1	6	6	12	50.0
2	11	2	13	84.6
Total	17	8	25	68.0

Table 21.10 Multiple linear regression analysis of 25 patients

Variable	b	$SE(b)$	t	P
constant	914.817	211.229	4.331	<0.001
group	−137.271	261.838	−0.524	0.605
kidney	−821.701	291.346	−2.820	0.010

Questions

(1) Did physicians A and B use appropriate statistical analysis methods? Why or why not?
(2) Conduct an appropriate analysis based on the data and the research purposes.

21.7. Computer experiment

Refer to electronic resources exp 21-1 to exp 21-3. Survival analysis methods and SPSS procedures are shown in Table 21.11.

Experiment 21.1: Using the life-table method to estimate survival rates

Learn how to use the life-tables procedure in SPSS to estimate survival rate, plot survival curves, and hazard curves.

Table 21.11 Survival analysis methods and SPSS procedures

Research purposes	Univariate analysis and SPSS procedure	Multivariate analysis and SPSS procedure
Estimating survival functions	Kaplan–Meier method (Kaplan–Meier procedure) Life table method (Life tables procedure)	Proportional hazards model (Cox regression)
Comparing survival curves	Log-rank test (Kaplan–Meier procedure)	Proportional hazards model (Cox regression)
Analyzing influencing factors	Log-rank test (Kaplan–Meier procedure)	Proportional hazards model (Cox regression)

Experiment 21.2: Using the Kaplan–Meier method to estimate survival rates and compare survival curves

Learn how to use the Kaplan–Meier procedure in SPSS to calculate survival rate and its CI, and estimate the median survival time. Use the log-rank test and the Breslow test to compare survival curves and obtain relevant statistics and P values. Plot the survival curves and hazard curves.

Experiment 21.3: Cox regression

Learn how to use the Cox regression procedure in SPSS to select independent predictors and fit the Cox regression model. Explain the HR and 95% CI of each variable.

21.8. Frequently asked questions and summary

21.8.1. *Frequently asked questions*

1. When estimating the CI of survival rate, it may fall outside the interval (0 to 1). How is this dealt with?

The CI of survival rate may fall outside the interval of 0 to 1 because of a skewed distribution when the survival rate is close to 0 or close to 1. This can be remedied by using transformations such as

$\ln[-\ln \hat{S}(t)]$.

$$\hat{\upsilon}(t) = \ln[-\ln \hat{S}(t)]$$

$$SE[\hat{\upsilon}(t)] = \frac{SE[\hat{S}(t)]}{\left|\ln \hat{S}(t)\right| \cdot \hat{S}(t)}$$

The 95% CI of $\hat{S}(t)$ is

$$\hat{S}(t)^{\exp\{\pm 1.96 SE[\hat{\upsilon}(t)]\}}$$

2. We have considered the log-rank test to compare survival functions over a range of time-points. How do we compare K survival curves at a predetermined fixed point in time, such as 2 years post-diagnosis or 3 years post-diagnosis?

Suppose we are interested in comparing the survival rates of two different groups at a fixed point in time. Using the Kaplan–Meier estimates of the survival rates in Table 21.4 and the estimated variances of these survival rates from Equation (21-7), we obtain the Z-test statistic, which is the square root of the chi-square quadratic form with one degree of freedom:

$$Z = \frac{\hat{S}_1(t) - \hat{S}_2(t)}{\sqrt{SE^2[\hat{S}_1(t)] + SE^2[\hat{S}_2(t)]}}$$

which, when H_0 is true, has a standard normal distribution for large samples. In Example 21.3 the estimated respective 2-year survival rates in the groups with tumors <3.0 cm in size and tumors ≥ 3.0 cm in size are $\hat{S}_1(2) = 0.8571$ and $\hat{S}_2(2) = 0.4375$, and the corresponding standard error estimates are $SE[\hat{S}_1(2)] = 0.0935$ and $SE[\hat{S}_2(2)] = 0.1240$.

$$Z = \frac{0.8571 - 0.4375}{\sqrt{0.0935^2 + 0.1240^2}} = 2.70$$

Patients with tumors <3.0 cm in size were significantly more likely to survive for 2 years than patients with tumors ≥ 3.0 cm in size ($P < 0.01$).

3. What are the differences among the three multivariate analysis methods, multiple linear regression, logistic regression, and Cox regression? (Table 21.12)

Table 21.12 Differences among multiple regression, logistic regression, and Cox regression

	Multiple linear regression	Logistic regression	Cox regression
Dependent variable and its distribution	Continuous variable Normal distribution	Categorical variable Binomial distribution	Binary variable and survival time No requirement
Independent variables	Continuous variable or categorical variable	Continuous variable or categorical variable	Continuous variable or categorical variable
Censoring permitted	No	No	Yes
Model	$\mu_Y = \beta_0 + \Sigma\beta_j X_j$	$\text{logit}(\pi) = \beta_0 + \sum \beta_j X_j$	$h(t) = h_0(t)\exp(\sum \beta_j X_j)$
Variables selection	Forward, backward, and stepwise	Forward, backward, and stepwise	Forward, backward, and stepwise
Parameter estimation	Least square method	Maximum likelihood method	Maximum partial likelihood method
Parameter test	F-test and t-test	Likelihood-ratio test and Wald test	Likelihood-ratio test and Wald test
Parameter explanation	Increment of the mean of Y caused by each unit increase of X_j	Log of OR caused by each unit increase of X_j	Log of HR caused by each unit increase of X_j
Application	Analysis of influencing factors, comparisons adjusting for confounders, and prediction (estimating Y)	Analysis of influencing factors, comparisons adjusting for confounders, and prediction (estimating π)	Analysis of influencing factors, comparisons adjusting for confounders, and prediction (estimating $S(t)$)

4. What is the sample size requirement in Cox regression?

It requires a large sample size. A common rule of thumb is that at least 10 events are required per variable. Refer Chapter 15 for more information about sample size estimation.

21.8.2. *Summary*

1. Survival analysis is concerned with analyzing the occurrence and timing of events (time-to-event data). A typical feature of survival data is that we usually have incomplete information about survival times due to censoring. The event of interest includes death from a certain cause, development of a disease, response to treatment, and recurrence of a disease, among other things. Survival analysis is used to estimate or compare survival curves, and explore related factors.
2. Non-parametric methods used to estimate survival rates include the life-table method and the PL method. In the life-table method survival times are grouped into intervals, whereas the PL estimate is based on individual survival times. Both estimates are based on the product of the interval-specific survival proportions.
3. The log-rank test and the Breslow test are non-parametric methods used to compare two or more survival curves. The log-rank test may be more sensitive to long-term differences than the Breslow test, whereas the Breslow test is more sensitive to differences early in the follow-up period.
4. The Cox proportional hazards regression model is a semi-parametric multiplicative model. It is used for the analysis of influencing factors, survival predictions, and survival comparisons, and it can incorporate adjustment for confounding factors.

Think and Practice

I. Best Choice

1. Which of the following can be analyzed using survival analysis? ( )
   A. The length of time between a group of people being exposed to a risk factor and the occurrence of a specific disease. B. The

Table 21.13 Follow-up data from remission to relapse

ID	Date of remission	Date of finishing observation	Outcome	Survival time (days)
1	2000.04.01	2000.09 06	Relapse	158
2	2001.11.05	2002.02.05	Death	91
3	2000.07.15	2000.12.10	Relapse	147
4	2001.05.20	2001.08.25	Lost to follow-up	96
5	2002.09.03	2002.12.31	Remission	119

length of time that women with breast hyperplasia remain symptom-free after treatment. C. The length of time from surgery to death in patients with lung cancer. D. The length of time from treatment to remission in patients with acute leukemia. E. All of the above.

2. Table 21.13 contains follow-up data derived from patients with acute leukemia, from remission after drug treatment to their first relapse.
   Which of the above survival times are censored? ( )
   A. ID 1 and ID 3 B. ID 1 and ID 2 C. ID 2, ID 4, and ID 5 D. ID 2, ID 3, and ID 4 E. ID 1, ID 2, and ID 3
3. Which statement below is correct with regard to the log-rank test? ( )
   A. The log-rank test compares the survival curves of different groups. B. The log-rank test compares survival rates at a fixed point in time. C. The log-rank test is a parametric method used to compare survival curves. D. In the log-rank test the observed deaths in all groups should be equal to the expected deaths. E. In the log-rank test the degree of freedom is 1.
4. Comparing the log-rank test with the Breslow test: ( )
   A. The log-rank test is more sensitive to short-term differences between groups. B. The log-rank test is more sensitive to long-term differences between groups. C. The Breslow test is more sensitive to long-term differences between groups. D. Both tests are equally sensitive to long-term differences between groups.

E. Both tests are equally sensitive to short-term differences between groups.

5. In Cox regression modeling it is required that the HR of two individuals: ( )

   A. Increases with time B. Decreases with time C. Increases with time at the beginning and then decreases D. Does not change with time E. Changes depending on specific situations

II. Questions for Reflection

1. State the applications and related statistical methods used in survival analysis.
2. How are censored data used when estimating survival rates in the life-table method and the PL method?
3. Both Cox regression and logistic regression can be used to analyze prognoses in clinical research. What are the differences between them?
4. What is the meaning of "HR" in Cox regression, and how would you explain HR?

III. Questions on Calculations

1. Consider 100 patients with esophageal cancer. The respective numbers of deaths in the 1st, 2nd, and 3rd years after surgery are 10, 20, and 30. Assume no censoring, and calculate the conditional survival probability for each year and the survival function.
2. A total of 42 patients with acute leukemia who experienced complete or partial remission were included in a clinical trial. Each patient was randomized to receive either 6-mercaptopurine (6-MP) or a placebo, then followed up until their leukemia returned (relapsed) or until the end of the study. Estimate the survival functions in the two groups, and test the significance of the difference between the survival functions in the two groups (Table 21.14).

Table 21.14 Remission duration (in months) in children with acute leukemia taking 6-MP or a placebo

Placebo group:	1	1	2	2	3	4	4	5	5	8	8	8	8	11	11	12	12	15	17	22	23
6-MP group:	6	6	6	6^+	7	9^+	10	10^+	11^+	13	16	17^+	19^+	20^+	22	23	25^+	32^+	32^+	34^+	35^+

Table 21.15 Survival in 949 patients with ovarian cancer

Years after diagnosis	Deaths	Censored
0∼	731	18
5∼	52	16
10∼	14	75
15∼	10	33

3. Survival data derived from a cohort of 949 patients with ovarian cancer are shown in Table 21.15. Estimate the survival function.
4. Using the data given in Example 21.5, recode "tumor grade" as a categorical variable with three categories (i.e., two dummy variables) and perform Cox regression analysis as in Example 21.5. Interpret the results and compare your results with those shown in Table 21.7.
5. Check the PH assumption in the Cox regression model for the other two variables grade and relapse in Example 21.5.

Hongmei Yu, Yan Guo

CHAPTER 22

DISCRIMINANT ANALYSIS AND CLASSIFICATION TREE

In the medical field, doctors discriminate the types of diseases suffered by patients according to their symptoms, signs, and results of laboratory examinations. Disease diagnosis is a classification problem. For example, the differences between diabetic and healthy people can be found by their symptoms, signs, and laboratory examinations. If the differences are expressed as a classification rule, new patients with suspected diabetes can be diagnosed by this rule. Computer Expert diagnostic system is this way.

According to the number of categories of the outcome, there are two kinds of classification problems, binary classification and multi-classification. Because multiple collections are often crowded together and there are overlapping phenomena, the discriminant effect of multi-classification is usually not as good as that of two-classification. Therefore, it is suggested that the multi-classification problem be transformed into several binary classification problems. This chapter introduces the discriminant analysis and classification tree method for binary classification problems.

22.1. Basic principles of discriminant analysis

Discriminant analysis is a supervised classification method used to determine the category of an individual. It learns rules from a set of "training samples" and then classifies the individuals according to some observed indicators.

Example 22.1. A doctor collected data of 25 patients with coronary heart disease and 25 normal persons (Table 22.1). The doctor intended to use this data to determine whether a person has coronary heart disease or not.

There are five variables in the data. X_1 = Age, X_2 = Systolic Pressure, X_3 = Cholesterol, X_4 = Three Acyl glycerol, X_5 = Blood Sugar. According to the measured data (training sample), the discriminant function can be established by discriminant analysis.

$$Y = 0.290X_1 + 0.765X_2 + 0.360X_3 - 0.128X_4 + 0.446X_5 \quad (22\text{-}1)$$

Then the values of 5 variables of a new individual are substituted into the formula to calculate the Y value. If $Y > 0$, the person is classified as a coronary heart disease patient, otherwise, a normal person.

Fisher's discriminant method and Bayes' discriminant method are mostly popular. Here is a brief introduction to the basic concept of these two methods.

22.2. Introduction to two discriminant methods

22.2.1. *Fisher's discriminant method*

There are two categories, $g = 1$ and $g = 2$.

The basic principle of the binary Fisher's discriminant method is to project two groups of p-dimensional data to a certain direction, so that the same group of points can be as close as possible along this direction, while different groups of points can be separated as far as possible, so as to achieve the purpose of classification. The steps are as follows.

1. According to the criterion of "maximum ratio of inter-group variance to intra-group variance," p eigenvalues and corresponding eigenvectors are extracted from the training sample with known classification, so the discriminant coefficients $b_i (i = 1, 2, 3, \ldots, p)$ and linear discriminant functions

$$Y = b_1X_1 + b_2X_2 + \cdots + b_pX_p \quad (22\text{-}2)$$

are obtained.

2. Cut-off point and classification rules are determined.

Table 22.1 Data of 25 patients with coronary heart disease and 25 normal persons

First category (coronary heart disease): $g = 1$								Second category (normal): $g = 2$							
	Variables								Variables						
No	X_1	X_2	X_3	X_4	X_5	Value of DF	Category	No	X_1	X_2	X_3	X_4	X_5	Value of DF	Category
1	61	23	5.1	1.0	5.2	1.1719	1	1	63	13	4.0	0.5	4.6	−1.9212	0
2	66	17	6.1	2.3	5.6	0.1296	1	2	55	17	5.1	1.4	5.6	−0.4748	0
3	64	25	5.3	0.6	5.7	2.1286	1	3	64	14	5.6	1.1	6.1	−0.5042	0
4	73	19	4.8	1.5	5.9	0.6099	1	4	59	16	4.6	0.6	6.0	−0.5060	0
5	59	19	7.6	2.8	6.1	1.1236	1	5	40	16	3.3	0.8	5.6	−1.8351	0
6	66	19	5.8	1.6	5.1	0.4447	1	6	59	20	6.0	2.0	4.7	0.3264	1
7	55	19	4.7	0.5	5.3	−0.0864	0	7	56	13	3.5	1.1	4.7	−2.4103	0
8	47	16	4.3	1.6	4.8	−1.6611	0	8	53	18	5.4	0.5	4.8	−0.3286	0
9	83	23	4.1	1.5	4.7	1.2114	1	9	57	13	4.7	0.6	5.4	−1.5397	0
10	81	17	4.9	1.1	5.1	0.1483	1	10	45	15	4.8	0.8	4.4	−1.8078	0
11	73	24	5.8	1.7	5.0	1.9014	1	11	60	16	4.0	1.1	5.3	−1.0730	0
12	76	23	5.1	1.8	5.5	1.6456	1	12	60	20	4.3	1.0	4.9	−0.0677	0
13	66	24	5.8	0.9	5.4	1.9662	1	13	70	18	5.0	3.9	6.5	0.1662	1
14	67	22	2.8	0.6	5.3	0.3051	1	14	59	16	4.9	1.6	4.8	−1.0307	0
15	70	22	5.7	1.0	5.3	1.4870	1	15	72	16	4.8	1.7	4.9	−0.6230	0
16	70	13	6.7	0.9	5.8	−0.2132	0	16	58	20	4.0	1.0	4.0	−0.6083	0
17	75	23	6.1	1.9	5.0	1.7952	1	17	58	17	3.2	0.9	4.2	−1.6006	0
18	71	16	4.7	1.1	9.3	1.1472	1	18	41	16	5.6	3.9	6.2	−1.1757	0
19	75	17	4.5	0.8	8.7	1.2686	1	19	47	12	4.8	0.8	5.0	−2.2757	0
20	66	23	5.0	0.9	4.9	1.1938	1	20	62	19	3.5	0.6	4.7	−0.5885	0
21	61	21	4.6	2.3	5.4	0.3191	1	21	69	20	5.5	1.1	5.2	0.8046	1
22	72	23	4.2	1.1	4.9	1.0384	1	22	45	13	3.4	0.9	6.0	−2.2613	0
23	63	19	5.1	0.9	5.6	0.3849	1	23	61	17	4.2	0.8	5.2	−0.6929	0
24	73	20	5.5	1.4	9.5	2.9818	1	24	53	13	4.8	0.6	5.2	−1.7098	0
25	58	20	3.4	1.7	5.3	−0.4505	0	25	80	23	4.3	0.8	5.8	1.7464	1

3. For each new individual, the values of $X_1, X_2, \ldots, X_p$ are substituted into the discriminant function, and the calculated Y value is compared with the cut-off point to determine which category the new individual belongs to, either $g = 1$ or $g = 2$.

22.2.2. *Bayes' discriminant method*

The basic principle of the binary Bayes' discriminant method is to generate 2 classification functions related to the probabilities for any individual belonging to 2 categories respectively according to the criterion of "minimum misjudgment loss"; and to determine the affiliation of any new individual according to the values of 2 classification functions.

The classification function of Bayes' discriminant method is as follows

$$\begin{aligned} Y_1 &= C_{10} + C_{11}X_1 + C_{12}X_2 + \cdots + C_{1p}X_p, \\ Y_2 &= C_{20} + C_{21}X_1 + C_{22}X_2 + \cdots + C_{2p}X_p. \end{aligned} \tag{22-3}$$

where the values of $C_{j0}, C_{j1}, C_{j2}, \ldots, C_{jp}$ $(j = 1, 2)$ can be calculated based on training sample.

Then for any individual, the corresponding values of $X_1, X_2, \ldots,$ X_p are substituted into the classification functions to calculate the values of Y_1 and Y_2. If $Y_1 > Y_2$, the individual is classified as category $g = 1$; if $Y_1 < Y_2$, the individual is classified as category $g = 2$; and if $Y_1 = Y_2$, the judgment can be made randomly.

For any individual in the population, without knowing any specific characteristics, if the probability of belonging to category j is $q_j, j = 1, 2$, then q_j is called a prior probability of an individual belonging to category j. When the prior probability is considered, the classification function can be defined as

$$\begin{aligned} Y_1 &= C_{10} + C_{11}X_1 + C_{12}X_2 + \cdots + C_{1p}X_p + \ln(q_1) \\ Y_2 &= C_{20} + C_{21}X_1 + C_{22}X_2 + \cdots + C_{2p}X_p + \ln(q_2) \end{aligned} \tag{22-4}$$

If the observed values of $X_1, X_2, \ldots, X_p$ are known as $x_1, x_2, \ldots, x_p$, the $P(j \mid x_1, x_2, \ldots, x_p)$ is called a posterior probability. The formulas for posterior probabilities are

$$
\begin{aligned}
P(g = 1 \mid x_1, x_2, \ldots, x_p) &= \frac{\exp(Y_1)}{\sum_{j=1}^{2} \exp(Y_j)}, \\
P(g = 2 \mid x_1, x_2, \ldots, x_p) &= \frac{\exp(Y_2)}{\sum_{j=1}^{2} \exp(Y_j)}
\end{aligned}
\qquad (22\text{-}5)
$$

For an individual, if the observation values of $X_1, X_2, \ldots, X_p$ are known, the posterior probability can be used to judge whether the individual belongs to category 1 or 2.

22.3. Dichotomy classification tree

Classification tree is a non-linear discriminant method. Classification tree grows a tree recursively by using splitting rules based on predictor variables. Compared with the classical linear models, this method can produce intuitive and easy-to-explain tree structure without making constrained parametric assumptions. As an alternative to linear models, classification trees have been useful in the medical field for disease diagnosis and prognostic prediction.

According to tree structures, we will introduce the dichotomy classification tree and the trichotomous classification tree, respectively.

22.3.1. *Classification and regression trees*

Classification and regression tree (CART) algorithm is developed by Breiman and others in 1984. This method originates from the expert system, which can help doctors to diagnose whether a patient has certain disease or not. Usually, the doctor can diagnose the disease according to the patient's medical history and clinical manifestations. If the diagnosis is not confirmed, further examinations will be carried out until a certain diagnosis is made. The process of analysis of CART is very similar to clinical diagnostic thinking of doctors. The CART consists of classification trees for categorical dependent variable and regression trees for continuous dependent variable.

The CART method constructs the tree model recursively from top to bottom. Its structure is similar to an inverted tree, consisting of trunk and many branches. There are many nodules in the tree, which are usually represented by circular or rectangular frames, called tree nodes. A circular frame is used to represent a non-terminal node (or internal node), and a rectangular frame is used to represent a terminal node. In different cases, the number of layers of trees could be different. Generally, a tree has only one root node, which can also be regarded as an internal node. Each internal node is split into two sub-nodes according to certain splitting rules, which are called left sub-node and right sub-node respectively. Figure 22.1 is a diagram of a tree structure.

The process of constructing a classification tree is more complex. There are three sets of problems to be solved for constructing a classification tree in CART as follows.

1. What are the nodes? Which nodes are the internal or terminal nodes in a tree? What is the root node, the father node, and the son node? These are the basic elements of a tree model.

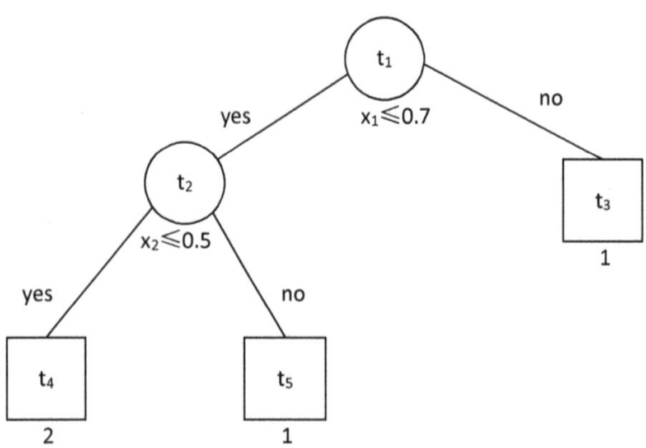

Figure 22.1 Diagram of a tree structure

2. How to split the father nodes into the son nodes, that is, how to use training data to make a tree grow from the root node gradually?
3. When does a node become a terminal node, that is, how to use termination conditions to stop a tree growing? How to make trees of moderate size by pruning algorithm?

22.3.2. *Tree growing*

1. Two basic concepts

(1) Impurity function

The impurity function of a node is a function used to evaluate the consistency of the individuals contained in the node. There are three kinds of impurity functions frequently used.

① Gini impurity function: $I(t) = \sum_{i \neq j} p(i \mid t)p(j \mid t)$
② Misclassification error impurity function: $I(t) = 1 - \max_i p(w_i \mid t)$
③ Mutual entropy or discreteness impurity function: $I(t) = -\sum_{i \neq j} p(i \mid t) \log(p(j \mid t))$

(2) The recursive splitting rule

This is a process from one subset to two subsets. CART defines a split rule S_p for selecting best variables and thresholds to maximize decreasing of impurity function.

$$\Delta I(s_p, t) = I(t) - [I(t_L)p_L + I(t_R)p_R]$$

That is to make the whole tree the purest.

2. The process of tree growth

First, at the root node, the impurity function value before splitting is calculated. Then, the algorithm searches through the predictor variables one by one. For each variable, the algorithm finds the optimal split; compares all optimal splits and selects the variable and threshold with the best split. In other words, the algorithm searches for the best variable and threshold to maximize decreasing of impurity function. Finally, the algorithm applies the variable and corresponding threshold of the best split for the root node, and the root node is divided into two son nodes. Any son node that meets any of the termination conditions will be recognized as the terminal node, and the split will be stopped; otherwise, the son node will be splitted continuously.

For any node, including root node, the split termination conditions are as follows:

(1) Small node: The number of individuals at the node is smaller than a number set in advance.
(2) Pure node: All the individuals in the node are subject to the same category.
(3) Empty node: There are no individuals in the node.

If the splitting stops, the process of tree growth is completed.

22.3.3. *Tree pruning*

If the algorithm described in the previous section leads to too many splits, the misclassification rate calculated from the training sample will falsely appear lower; however, too less splits might result in a misclassification rate that is truly higher than that of the optimal-sized tree. The motivation for pruning the tree is to achieve an optimal size and an unbiased estimate of the misclassification rate.

First, the largest tree is generated, which is denoted as $T_{\max}$. Then, starting from $T_{\max}$, the sub-branches with terminal nodes are pruned off continually until the tree has only the root node. A sequence of sub-trees $T_{\max}, T_1, T_2, \ldots, T_k$ with decreasing number of nodes is generated, and the final sub-tree will be selected among them.

22.3.4. *Tree evaluation*

How do we select the "optimal tree" from the sub-trees? The CART uses the test sample and cross-validation to evaluate each sub-tree.

The establishment of classification tree model often requires a large sample size, but in practice, due to various reasons, the sample size is relatively insufficient, which requires to reuse the sample data. Cross-validation is a method to make full use of the training sample. Generally, the whole training sample is randomly divided into 10 sub-samples of the same size, so that the attributes of each sub-sample are similar. Nine sub-samples are used to generate a saturated tree, and a sequence of sub-trees $(T_{\max}, T_1, T_2, \ldots, T_k)$ are obtained by tree pruning, then the "misclassification cost" of each sub-tree is calculated with the remaining sub-sample. Those steps are repeated 10 times and the sub-tree with the minimum or near minimum "misclassification cost" is selected as the "optimal sub-tree." In addition, the "misclassification cost" can be measured by weighted sum of the probabilities of two kinds of misclassification with the losses caused by two kinds of misclassification as the weighted coefficients. If the losses caused by the two kinds of misclassification are equal, the "misclassification cost" can be measured by the sum of the probabilities of two kinds of misclassification.

From the introduction above, we can see that the basic idea of CART method is very simple. Starting from the root node, CART chooses the optimal branch of the optimal variable at each sub-node to build a large tree. Then prune the tree to get a sequence of sub-trees and select the best sub-tree with the least cost of misclassification. Finally, the tree can be used to classify and predict the new samples.

22.4. Trichotomous classification tree

For the dichotomous classification tree algorithm, each node is always divided into two parts referring to two distinct categories, with the result that the individuals located around the cutoff point cannot be all correctly classified, and thus some of them inevitably suffer from misclassification. To solve such a problem, we proposed an alternative approach, named logistic regression-based trichotomous classification tree (LRTCT) (Zhu YK, Fang JQ. *Medical Decision Makin*, 2016; 36(8): 973–989).

22.4.1. *Diagrams of dichotomous and trichotomous classification trees*

Next, we would illustrate the difference between dichotomy and trichotomy by a simple example with only two predictor variables. On the left of Figure 22.2, we have a training sample in the two-dimensional feature space of $X1$ and $X2$, with Δ and $+$ representing two types of individuals respectively. The dichotomous classification tree divides the two-dimensional space into upper and lower parts at $X2 = 5$; accordingly, the root node is divided into two son nodes according to weather $X2$ is less than 5. In the second step, the lower part is divided into two parts at $X1 = 3.5$, with one mainly including $+$ and another mainly including Δ; the upper part is divided into two parts at $X1 = 6.5$, with one mainly including $+$ and another mainly including Δ. Correspondingly, on the right of Figure 22.2, the two son nodes are divided into two parts respectively, forming four terminal nodes finally denoted as $+$ or Δ. As a result, a rule has been set up: Any individual who falls into the root node with $+$ will be classified as $+$, and who falls into the root node with Δ will be classified as Δ. In this way, from the left image, if the tree is applied to the training sample, two Δ will be misclassified as $+$ and one $+$ will be misclassified as Δ.

The two-dimensional sample points on the left of Figure 22.3 and that on the left of Figure 22.2 are the same. Firstly, on the left of Figure 22.3, at $X1 = 2$ and $X1 = 6$ the trichotomous classification tree divides the two-dimensional space into 3 parts, left, middle,

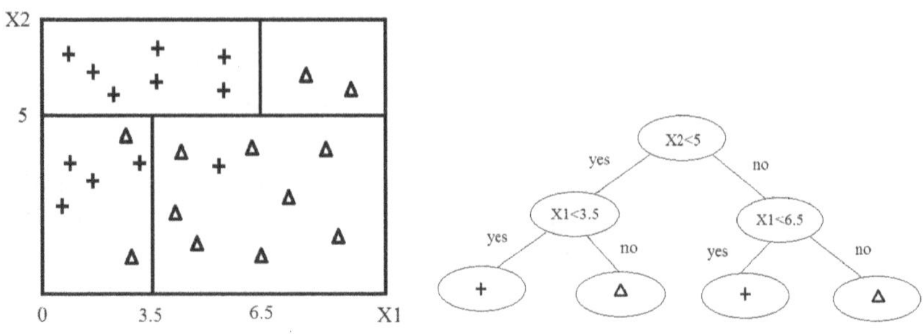

Figure 22.2 Diagram of space partition and tree structure of dichotomous classification trees

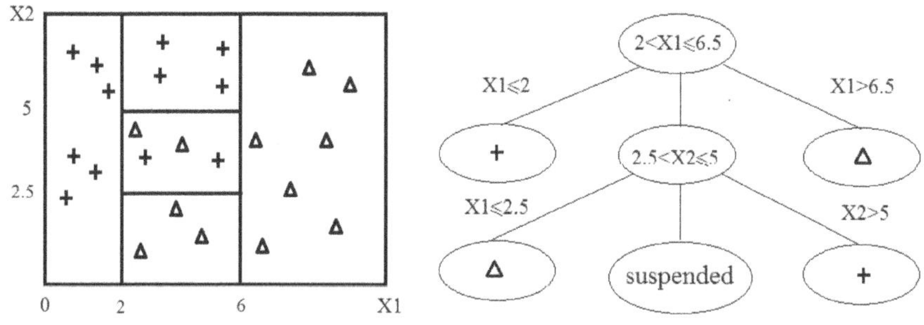

Figure 22.3 Diagram of space partition and tree structure of trichotomous classification trees

and right. Accordingly, on the right of Figure 22.3, the root node is divided into three son nodes, left, middle and right, according to whether $X1$ is outside the interval $(2, 6.5)$; the left and right nodes are "pure," marked with $+$ and Δ, respectively; the middle node is "non-pure" to be processed in the next step. Next, back to the left of Figure 22.3, the interval $(2, 6.5)$ is divided into 3 parts; the upper and lower parts are "pure," and the middle is "non-pure." Accordingly, on the right of Figure 22.3, the left and right son nodes are marked with Δ and $+$, respectively, while the middle node is "suspended."

22.4.2. *The LRTCT algorithm*

1. Tree growth

Similar to other classification trees, tree growth in LRTCT is a recursive process of splitting the training sample. The core algorithm of it is to establish the splitting rule and the stopping rule.

(1) The recursive splitting rule

The splitting rule involves two issues: first, how to select an optimal variable from all predictor variables for splitting; and second, how to find the optimal thresholds (cut-off points) from the possible values of the splitting variable. A single predictor variable is selected as the splitting variable for the root node, but from the second layer on, besides a single predictor variable, the linear combination of predictors could also be the candidate of splitting variable.

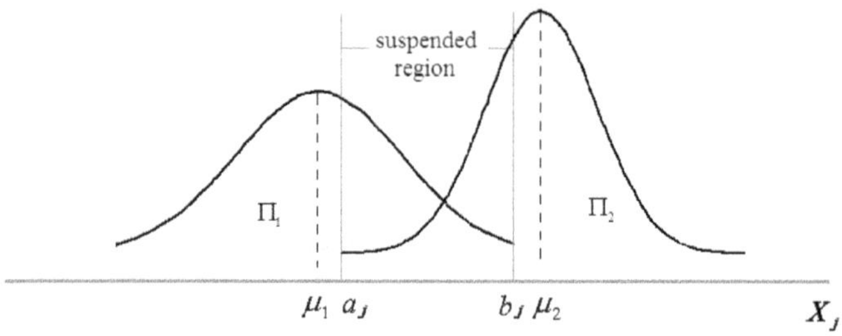

Figure 22.4 Diagram of trichotomy based on the optimal splitting variable

The root node is denoted by $t^{(0)}$. For each variable X_j ($j = 1, 2, \ldots, p$), as shown in Figure 22.4, there will be an overlapping portion of the setting of X_j in two categories with the threshold values denoted by

$$a_j = \max(\min_{X_j \in T_1^{(0)}} X_j, \min_{X_j \in T_2^{(0)}} X_j), \tag{22-6}$$

$$b_j = \min(\max_{X_j \in T_1^{(0)}} X_j, \max_{X_j \in T_2^{(0)}} X_j). \tag{22-7}$$

where $T^{(0)} = \cup_{i=1}^{2} T_i^{(0)}$ is the training sample for $t^{(0)}$; $i = 1, 2$ indicates the two categories. The $T^{(0)}$ could be divided into three subsets based on three intervals of X_j, $(-\infty, a_j)$, $[a_j, b_j]$, and $(b_j, +\infty)$.

Let p_{Lj}, p_{Rj} denote the proportions of the individuals in the population $T^{(0)}$ that meet $\{X_j < a_j \,|T^{(0)}\}$ and $\{X_j > b_j \,|T^{(0)}\}$ respectively, define the discrimination power (DP) of X_j, by

$$DP(X_j) = p_{Lj} + p_{Rj}. \tag{22-8}$$

Then, a search is made through all $X_j (j = 1, 2, \ldots, p)$ to find the optimal splitting variable X_{j_*}, which has the greatest discrimination power, that is,

$$DP(X_{j_*}) = \max_{j=1,2,\ldots,p} DP(X_j). \tag{22-9}$$

The optimal splitting variable is denoted as $X^{(1)}$, and the corresponding splitting threshold values are denoted as $a^{(1)}$ and $b^{(1)}$.

The node $t^{(0)}$ is divided into the left son node $t_L^{(0)} = \{X^{(1)} < a^{(1)} \,|\, t^{(0)}\}$, the right son node $t_R^{(0)} = \{X^{(1)} > b^{(1)} \,|\, t^{(0)}\}$ and the middle son node $t_M^{(0)} = \{a^{(1)} \le X^{(1)} \le b^{(1)} \,|\, t^{(0)}\}$. In $t_L^{(0)}$ and $t_R^{(0)}$, the heterogeneity in category is as low as possible to achieve the highest "purity"; the $t_L^{(0)}$ and $t_R^{(0)}$ will serve for assertive discrimination, the overlapping portion $t_M^{(0)}$ is suspended. If $t_M^{(0)}$ does not meet the given stopping rule of recursive splitting, then it is denoted by $t^{(1)}$, and being splitted in the next step.

For $t^{(1)}$, with each of $X_j(j = 1, \ldots, p,\ X_j \neq X^{(1)})$ incorporating with $X^{(1)}$ as candidate independent variables to conduct $p - 1$ times of stepwise logistic regression, getting $p - 1$ combination variables denoted by $\log it\ P_j(j = 1, 2, \ldots, p,\ X_j \neq X^{(1)})$; Taking these $p - 1$ combination variables and all $X_j(j = 1, \ldots, p)$ to be candidate splitting variables, the one with the greatest discrimination power is selected as the optimal splitting variable denoted by $X^{(2)}$, and the corresponding splitting threshold values are denoted as $a^{(2)}$ and $b^{(2)}$. The node $t^{(1)}$ is divided into the left son node $t_L^{(1)} = \{X^{(2)} < a^{(2)} \left| t^{(1)} \right.\}$, the right son node $t_R^{(1)} = \{X^{(2)} > b^{(2)} \left| t^{(1)} \right.\}$ and the middle son node $t_M^{(1)} = \{a^{(2)} \le X^{(2)} \le b^{(2)} \left| t^{(1)} \right.\}$. The $t_L^{(1)}$ and $t_R^{(1)}$ will serve for assertive discrimination, and $t_M^{(1)}$ is suspended. If $t_M^{(1)}$ does not meet the stopping rule for recursive splitting, then it is denoted by $t^{(2)}$ and being splitted in the next step through a similar recursive partitioning process. In general, for any son node $t^{(k)}$, $k \ge 1$, not only the single predictor variables, but also all possible linear combinations of used variables and each of the unused predictor variables (generated by logistic regression) are considered, among which the one with the greatest discrimination power is used for partition until the stopping rule for splitting is met.

(2) The stopping rule of recursive splitting

In order to prevent over fitting, for any middle son node $t_M^{(k)}$, $k \ge 0$, if any one of the following conditions is met, then the recursive splitting should stop.

① The layer of the tree is less than an constant, which is set in advance as the maximum depth.
② The proportion of the individuals in the middle son node $t_M^{(k)}$ is less or equal a constant proportion, which is set in advance.

③ The proportions of the individuals in the left and right son nodes after splitting of $t_M^{(k)}$, are less or equal a constant proportion, which is set in advance.

2. Discriminant of the final layer

With the above stopping rule of recursive splitting the LRTCT algorithm allows to retain a portion of individuals being "suspended" at the last layer, for whom there are two possible choices: One is to further collect information of other variables and continue the "trichotomous classification," which conforms to the principles of clinical ethics; Second is to regard it as a termination node, if necessary, using all variables to make a binary logistic regression for clinical reference. The advantage of LRTCT is that we can find a subset of individuals, who are difficult to be classified with the existing predictor variables and must be "suspended." We prefer the former choice to avoid leading to more misclassification, while the latter should not be used as a conclusion, which is "for reference only." Although we do not encourage people to make assertive classifications for the individuals in the final layer, if one insists on doing so, we would suggest using logistic regression model considering prior probability.

According to Chapter 20 of this book, the general equation for binary logistic regression without considering prior probabilities is

$$\text{logit } P = \beta_0 + \sum_j^m \beta_j X_j \tag{22-10}$$

$$\text{or } P = \frac{1}{1 + \exp[-(\beta_0 + \sum_j^m \beta_j X_j)]} \tag{22-11}$$

If the proportions of the individuals of the two categories are different, it is necessary to consider the influence of prior probability in logistic regression model. Let q is the prior probability of $Y = 1$, the logistic regression equation considering the prior probability is

$$\text{logit } P' = \beta_0' + \sum_j^m \beta_j X_j \tag{22-12}$$

$$\text{or } P' = \frac{1}{1 + \exp[-(\beta_0' + \sum_j^m \beta_j X_j)]} \tag{22-13}$$

where P' is the adjusted prediction probability, and

$$\beta_0' = \beta_0 + \ln \frac{q}{1-q}$$

It can be proved that if $q = 0.5$, then $P' = P$. When the value of P is small or large, the P' is more reasonable.

In summary, the steps of applying logistic regression considering prior probability to discriminate the individuals in the final layer are as follows:

(1) With regardless of prior probability, the logistic regression model

$$P = \frac{1}{1 + \exp[-(\beta_0 + \beta_1 X_1 + \cdots + \beta_m X_m)]}$$

is applied to the sample data in the final layer to get the estimates of $\hat{\beta}_0, \hat{\beta}_1, \ldots, \hat{\beta}_m$;

(2) Given the values of $X_j (j = 1, \ldots, m)$, the value of P and adjusted prediction probability
P' of the individual are calculated by

$$P' = \frac{qP}{qP + (1-q)(1-P)}$$

(3) If $P' > 0.5$, the individual is classified as category $Y = 1$, otherwise $Y = 0$.

In practical problems, the prior probability q is often unknown, and can be estimated by the proportion of individuals with $Y = 1$ in the final layer.

22.5. Validation of classification

The classification model must be validated. Validation is to classify individuals one by one with the established classification rules and find out sensitivity (TPR), specificity (TNR), total misclassification rate, and ROC curve. Validation includes retrospective validation and prospective validation. Retrospective validation, also known as internal validation, is to use the original training samples for validation. Prospective validation, also known as external validation, is to use the testing samples that have not participated in the establishment of discriminant models for validation. The sensitivity (TPR), specificity (TNR), and total misclassification rate can be well estimated by prospective validation. Prospective validation is necessary in application. Only when the prospective validation has a better discriminant effect, that is, a higher correct rate, we can think that a discriminant model has a stronger discriminant ability and can be used in application. Therefore, training sample is used to establish discriminant rules, and testing sample is used to carry out prospective validation. Testing sample also needs reliable data with correct classification, and enough sample size. In the application, the collected sample can be randomly divided into two groups, one group as training sample and one group as testing sample.

In addition to prospective validation based on testing sample, we can also approximately reach the goal of prospective validation based on the training sample by leave-one-out (LOO) approach. The method is as follows: suppose there are n individuals in the training sample. Leaving the first individual out, we use linear discriminant or classification tree to establish a discriminant rule based on the remaining $n-1$ individuals and evaluate the first individual by using the rule; then putting the first individual back, and leaving the second individual out, use linear discriminant or classification tree to establish a discriminant rule based on the remaining $n-1$ individuals and evaluate the second individual by using the rule ... Repeating such a leaving-one-out process for n individuals in turn, we can evaluate the discriminant rule for n times so as to get the estimation of sensitivity (TPR), specificity (TNR), and total misclassification rate. The LOO approach is also called Jackknife. It is often extended as follows: divide the training sample into k groups; leave one group out in turn for evaluation; establish discriminant rule based on remaining $k-1$ groups; summarize the evaluation data for k groups. This is the general approach of cross-validation, which can be used as a supplement to the prospective validation.

22.6. Report writing

A report for classification analysis mainly contains:

1. Basic statistical description of data sets.

2. Classification method.
3. Validation method.
4. Summary tables and figures for results of validation.

Take Example 22.2 for instance, results of a classification tree model are reported as follows.

Example 22.2. The Wisconsin breast cancer dataset was collected by Dr. William H. Wolberg, the University of Wisconsin Hospitals, Madison. It consisted of 683 complete observations on 9 predictor variables (denoted by $X_1, \ldots, X_9$) with integer values ranging between 1 and 10, and a binary response variable. In all of the observations, 444 were benign cases and 239 were malignant cases.

The tree structure diagrams of CART and LRTCT for the WBCD were plotted in Figure 22.5. The data sets were randomly divided into 10 groups for cross validation. The results were summarized in Table 22.2.

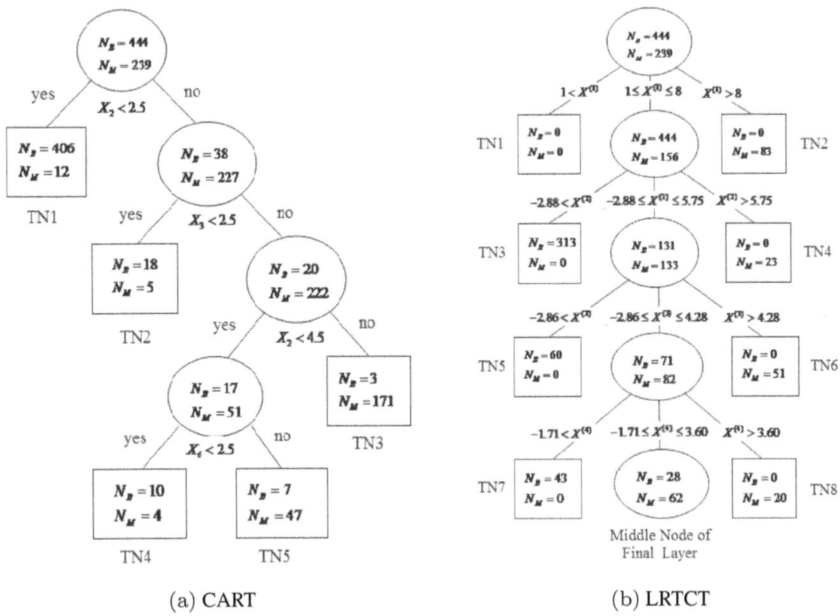

(a) CART (b) LRTCT

Figure 22.5 Tree structure diagrams of CART and LRTCT

Table 22.2 The classification results of CART and LRTCT

		Proportion of Sub-population	TPR	TNR
LRTCT	$t_{ALL} - t_{FLM}$	87.49	0.9727	0.9896
	t_{FLM}	12.51	0.7484	0.8446
	t_{ALL}	100	0.9236	0.9772
CART	—	100	0.9368	0.9534

Note: t_{ALL} represented all the terminal nodes; t_{FLM} represented the middle node of the final layer; and $t_{ALL} - t_{FLM}$ represented all the terminal nodes except the middle node of the final layer.

Table 22.3 Classification results of Fisher's linear discriminant analysis and CART

Method	TPR	TNR
Fisher's	0.762	0.868
CART	0.524	0.974

For classification results of all terminal nodes except the middle node of the final layer, the LRTCT consistently performed superior to the CART did. For classification results of all terminal nodes as a whole, LRTCT also consistently performed superior to CART did.

22.7. Case discrimination

Experiment 22.1: A study was conducted to diagnose a certain disease using the data of known outcomes as training sample. Fisher's linear discriminant analysis and CART classification tree method were constructed respectively and the training sample was substituted for retrospective validation. The results were shown in Table 22.3. Please evaluate the classification results of the two methods.

22.8. Computer experiments

Experiment 22.1: Using SPSS to fit a discriminant analysis model for Example 22.1.

To learn the operational process of fitting a discriminant analysis model by using SPSS.

Experiment 22.2: Using SPSS to fit a CART tree model for Example 22.2.

To learn the operational process of fitting a CART model by using SPSS.

Experiment 22.3: Using the software R to fit a LRTCT model for Example 22.2 tree model for Example 22.2.

To learn the operational process of fitting a LRTCT model by using R package"TriCTree."

22.9. Frequently asked questions and summary

22.9.1. *Frequently asked questions*

1. How to validate the effect of classification method?

Generally, retrospective validation and prospective validation are necessary to validate the effect of classification. Some studies inappropriately omitted prospective validation because lack of cases. Any retrospective validation even with a satisfied outcome does not mean that the classification method is really good since the results of retrospective validation are often over optimistic.

2. Compared with traditional linear discriminant analysis and dichotomy classification tree, what are the advantages of LRTCT in medical diagnosis?

Commonly used linear discriminant analysis requires that the predictor variables approximately follow a multivariate normal distribution in each group. However, it can hardly be met in practice so that the results of linear discriminant analysis sometimes are not satisfied.

For binary classification problems, both linear discriminant analysis and existing dichotomy classification trees adopt the rule of "black or white." Compared with them, the method of LRTCT believes that there is a "gray region" between black and white, and keeps cautious to the gray region.

In order to minimize the harm of a possible incorrect diagnosis, the LRTCT seeks zero-error discriminant for the training sample in the left and right terminal nodes of each layer. In addition, LRTCT tries to save the number of predictor variables according to the principle of "discriminate as you can." In each run of the LRTCT algorithm, the ambiguous individuals in the middle node are postponed temporarily so as to be classified in next run. With introducing new predictor variables, the middle nodes are splitted recursively, until the termination conditions are satisfied. At the end of the tree growth process, the individuals in the middle node of the final layer could be regarded as a subset of individuals, who are difficult to be classified with the existing predictor variables. It is immoral to give them an arbitrary diagnosis. However, by logistic regression with consideration of prior probability, if necessary, LRTCT can inform these individuals with the risk and probability of disease and suggest them to add new examinations before making final diagnosis.

22.9.2. *Summary*

The core idea of linear discriminant analysis is to establish a discriminant function based on the training sample; then for application, the values of predictor variables of individuals are substituted into the discriminant function, and they can be classified according to the value of the discriminant function.

Compared with the classical linear model, classification tree is a non-linear discriminant method. Classification tree can produce intuitive and easy-to-explain tree structure without making constrained parametric assumptions. As an alternative to classical statistical methods, classification trees have been useful in the medical field for disease diagnosis and prognostic prediction.

Given a set of information, there must be a part of individuals easy to be diagnosed and another part difficult to be diagnosed.

In order to avoid the disadvantage of "one-size-fits-all," the trichotomous classification tree would try best to differentiate the 2 parts. In diagnostic study, we pay attention to "easy to be diagnosed" individuals and make a distinction between "positive" and "negative." In other applications, we pay attention to those "difficult to be diagnosed" individuals and make further exploration. After decades of development, classification technology has been widely valued and applied in telecommunications, banking, insurance, retail, medical, and other industries. LRTCT algorithm is also expected to be applied in the above areas in the future.

Think and Practice

1. UCI database is a database for algorithmic testing provided by the University of California Irvine. There are 322 datasets for classification problems. Please download some datasets from http://archive.ics.uci.edu/ml/datasetshtml, analyze them with different classification methods, compare and evaluate the classification results of different classification methods.
2. As dichotomous linear discriminant analysis, Fisher's discriminant and Bayes' discriminant are equivalent in terms of discriminant effect. Please verify this rule through the data and statistical software of Example 22.1, and think: What is the difference between Fisher's discriminant and Bayes' discriminant?

Yanke Zhu, Jiqian Fang

CHAPTER 23

CLUSTER ANALYSIS

Cluster analysis is a multivariate statistical method, which aims to classify objects, such as samples and variables, into different groups based on the idea of "birds of a feather flock together." Through cluster analysis, the objects in the same cluster are highly similar, whereas objects in different clusters are dissimilar.

At present, cluster analysis has become a common multivariate statistical method in the fields of biology, sociology, education, and so on. It has also been widely used in the medical domain.

23.1. The basic idea of cluster analysis

23.1.1. *Examples*

Example 23.1 In order to investigate the psychological status of the elderly over 60 years old in a certain region, psychological assessment was carried out on 20 elderly people. This research applied a self-rating scale, which included 10 psychological clinical symptoms such as somatization (X1), obsessive-compulsive symptoms (X2), interpersonal sensitivity (X3), depression (X4), anxiety (X5), hostility (X6), phobia (X7), paranoia (X8), psychosis (X9), sleep and diet (X10). The data of each symptom score was shown in Table 23.1. Please discuss how many groups of the psychological status for these 20 elderly people can be classified based on their 10 psychological symptoms scores; and explore how many clusters of the psychological symptoms can be grouped.

Table 23.1 Psychological evaluation data for 20 elderly people

ID	X1	X2	X3	X4	X5	X6	X7	X8	X9	X10
1	22	20	17	15	16	19	20	20	22	22
2	8	12	11	10	14	17	10	14	11	15
3	7	7	8	7	5	10	8	7	5	5
4	10	15	5	10	14	12	11	9	11	9
5	11	17	19	11	21	20	29	12	21	22
6	10	12	12	10	11	12	8	10	3	6
7	22	23	16	20	20	20	19	24	13	13
8	18	10	11	16	12	16	16	12	14	14
9	6	6	7	9	9	7	5	6	5	8
10	11	11	12	15	15	20	13	16	18	14
11	16	22	18	16	20	11	17	20	18	21
12	11	8	7	14	12	10	11	5	15	12
13	17	13	22	17	18	15	9	15	15	14
14	23	30	25	10	13	27	23	16	14	22
15	11	18	22	9	15	13	18	16	12	18
16	8	11	14	13	9	11	11	12	15	11
17	11	15	20	15	11	21	21	12	12	21
18	12	8	13	17	18	14	14	16	16	15
19	7	5	10	4	4	7	7	8	6	3
20	17	18	8	13	13	13	18	18	10	13

Example 23.2 In order to study the severity of the brain aging, researchers tested eight aspects of 100 normal people of different ages. The eight variables were: age (X1), picture memory (X2), digital width memory (X3), graphic sequential memory (X4), digits number of mental arithmetic (X5), time of mental arithmetic (X6), stepping distance (X7), pace (X8). The data of each variable was shown in Table 23.2. Please discuss how many groups of the 100 normal people can be classified.

23.1.2. *The basic idea of cluster analysis*

In practice, the problems are often complex, however, categorizing similar objects in a cluster will make them simple to deal with. For example, biologists classify organism into different kingdoms, phyla,

Table 23.2 Assessment data of brain-related variables for 100 normal people

ID	X1	X2	X3	X4	X5	X6	X7	X8
1	62	13	7	7	18	4	49	5
2	60	14	7	2	4	5	36	6
3	42	16	9	8	3	5	12	3
4	62	13	7	7	6	5	44	3
5	59	10	7	14	5	5	19	7
6	65	6	7	2	10	1	16	10
7	44	14	9	14	3	4	43	4
8	20	17	9	14	4	5	45	4
9	20	17	9	9	3	4	45	4
10	58	17	5	4	6	3	27	8
11	64	9	5	14	6	3	34	7
12	69	2	8	5	7	4	28	4
...	...	...	...	...	...	...	...	...
94	19	17	9	14	3	3	39	4
95	53	16	8	6	2	3	40	4
96	26	14	9	14	3	2	39	4
97	41	17	9	2	10	4	39	4
98	65	16	7	7	7	3	36	5
99	60	6	9	6	4	5	28	6
100	61	13	6	5	14	1	39	5

classes, orders, families, genera, species based on the biological characteristics; sociologists classify human beings into workers, peasants, soldiers and intellectuals based on different occupations; education departments classify schools into different categories according to their infrastructure, teaching, scientific research level, teaching management and learning culture. The purpose of cluster analysis is using digital information to achieve "classification."

Cluster analysis is an exploratory statistical analysis method. According to the purpose of clustering, it can be divided into two different categories: sample-clustering and variable-clustering. Sample-clustering, known as Q-type clustering, refers to the method of classifying n subjects into clusters. It classifies subjects with similar characteristics into one cluster based on the characteristics of the related observations. The purpose of the sample-clustering is to find out the commonalities among subjects. For example, we can use Q-type clustering method to divide the subjects into several clusters with different intelligence levels. Variable-clustering, known as R-type clustering, classifies the variables with similar characteristics into one cluster according to the similarity of m variables. The purpose of the variable-clustering is to reduce the dimension of variables and select representative variables. For example, we can use R-type clustering method to classify the 11 test variables and to select representative variables for the Wechsler Children's Intelligence Scale in a psychological research. In Example 23.1, Q-type clustering can be used to classify 20 elderly people based on the 10 psychological symptom scores; R-type clustering can be used to classify the 10 psychological symptoms.

23.1.3. *Procedure of cluster analysis*

Three steps involved in clustering regardless of Q-type clustering or R-type clustering are:

1. Standardization of the raw data. For the raw data, different measurement units always interfere the calculation and comparison in the process of cluster analysis. Therefore, the raw data needs to be standardized to eliminate the influence of the data dimension on numerical size.
2. Clustering statistics selection. The key of clustering is selecting the clustering statistics. Clustering statistics are used to indicate the degree of similarity among samples or variables. Distance is the most commonly statistic used in Q-type clustering, and similarity degree is the most common statistic used in R-type clustering.
3. Clustering methods selection. Selecting clustering methods are the most important step in cluster analysis. According to the clustering statistics, appropriate clustering methods are selected to classify samples or variables with similar characteristics into one group. This chapter will focus on two common but important clustering methods in sample-clustering and variable-clustering: System clustering and K-means clustering.

23.2. Sample-clustering

23.2.1. *Sample clustering statistics*

In sample-clustering, there are n samples, p variables are measured for each sample. According to the data of each variable of every sample, we can get n points representing the n samples in the p-dimensional space.

The raw data matrix is:

$$\mathbf{X} = \begin{bmatrix} \mathbf{X}_1^T \\ \mathbf{X}_2^T \\ \vdots \\ \mathbf{X}_n^T \end{bmatrix} = \begin{bmatrix} x_{11} & x_{12} & \cdots & x_{1p} \\ x_{21} & x_{22} & \cdots & x_{2p} \\ \vdots & \vdots & & \vdots \\ x_{n1} & x_{n2} & \cdots & x_{np} \end{bmatrix}$$

where x_{ij} $(i = 1, 2, \ldots, n;\ j = 1, 2, \ldots, p)$ is the value of the jth variable of subject i. $\mathbf{X}_i^T$ denotes the ith row of the matrix.

The raw data is transformed by standardization. The transformation formula is: $x_{ij}^* = \frac{x_{ij} - \bar{x}_j}{s_j}$, x_{ij}^* denotes the standardized data; $\bar{x}_j = \frac{1}{n}\sum_{i=1}^{n} x_{ij}$ denotes the mean of the jth variable; $s_j = \sqrt{\frac{1}{n-1}\sum_{i=1}^{n}(x_{ij} - \bar{x}_j)^2}$ denotes the standard deviation of the jth variable. Therefore, the normalized matrix can be expressed as follows:

$$\mathbf{X}^* = \begin{bmatrix} \dfrac{x_{11} - \bar{x}_1}{s_1} & \dfrac{x_{12} - \bar{x}_2}{s_2} & \cdots & \dfrac{x_{1p} - \bar{x}_p}{s_p} \\ \dfrac{x_{21} - \bar{x}_1}{s_1} & \dfrac{x_{22} - \bar{x}_2}{s_2} & \cdots & \dfrac{x_{2p} - \bar{x}_p}{s_p} \\ \vdots & \vdots & & \vdots \\ \dfrac{x_{n1} - \bar{x}_1}{s_1} & \dfrac{x_{n2} - \bar{x}_2}{s_2} & \cdots & \dfrac{x_{np} - \bar{x}_p}{s_p} \end{bmatrix}$$

For convenience, we still use the symbols of the raw matrix to represent the standardized transformation matrix. The similarity degree between any two samples can be measured by the distance between two points in the p-dimensional space. Let d_{ij} denote the distance between $\mathbf{X}_i$ and $\mathbf{X}_j$.

23.2.1.1. *Distances between samples*

A variety of measurements have been proposed for calculating distance. The commonly used measurements for distance are:

(1) Euclidean distance: Euclidean distance can be used to measure the degree of similarity between two samples based on the continuous data. The formula is:

$$d_{ij} = \sqrt{(x_{i1} - x_{j1})^2 + (x_{i2} - x_{j2})^2 + \cdots + (x_{ip} - x_{jp})^2} = \sqrt{\sum_{k=1}^{p} (x_{ik} - x_{jk})^2} \quad (23\text{-}1)$$

(2) Manhattan distance: Manhattan distance d_{ij} is calculated by the sum of absolute values of the differences between two variables in each dimension. The formula is:

$$d_{ij} = |x_{i1} - x_{j1}| + |x_{i2} - x_{j2}| + \cdots |x_{ip} - x_{jp}| = \sum_{k=1}^{p} |x_{ik} - x_{jk}| \quad (23\text{-}2)$$

(3) Minkowski distance: The formula of Minkowski distance is:

$$d_{ij} = \sqrt[q]{|x_{i1} - x_{j1}|^q + |x_{i2} - x_{j2}|^q + \cdots |x_{ip} - x_{jp}|^q} = \sqrt[q]{\sum_{k=1}^{p} |x_{ik} - x_{jk}|^q} \quad (23\text{-}3)$$

The definition of Minkowski distance is intuitive and the calculation is simple. From equation (23-3), we can see that Minkowski distance is identical to Manhattan distance when $q = 1$, and is identical to Euclidean distance when $q = 2$.

(4) Mahalanobis distance: $\sum$ denotes the covariance matrix between two variables.

$$\sum = \begin{pmatrix} \sigma_1^2 & \sigma_{12}^2 & \cdots & \sigma_{1p}^2 \\ \sigma_{21}^2 & \sigma_2^2 & \cdots & \sigma_{2p}^2 \\ \cdots & \cdots & \cdots & \cdots \\ \sigma_{p1}^2 & \sigma_{p2}^2 & \cdots & \sigma_p^2 \end{pmatrix}$$

The formula of Mahalanobis distance is:

$$d_{ij} = (\mathbf{X}_i - \mathbf{X}_j)^T \boldsymbol{\Sigma}^{-1} (\mathbf{X}_i - \mathbf{X}_j) \qquad (23\text{-}4)$$

Mahalanobis distance is known as generalized Euclidean distance. It considers not only the differences between the variables but also the covariances. If $\sum = I$ (unit matrix), the Mahalanobis distance is identical to the square of the Euclidean distance.

23.2.1.2. *Distances between clusters*

Distance between clusters is a statistic to measure the similarity of clusters. When there is more than one sample in each cluster, many methods can calculate the distance between clusters. Different measurements for distances will lead to different clusters. We will introduce five commonly calculation methods used for distances. Let G_1, G_2 denote two different clusters, each cluster contains n_1, n_2 samples, respectively; D_{12} denote the distance between G_1, G_2.

(1) Nearest neighbor: There are $n_1 n_2$ distances, $d_{ij}, i = 1, 2, \ldots, n_1$, $j = 1, 2, \ldots, n_2$, between n_1 samples in G_1 and n_2 samples in G_2, and the distance between G_1 and G_2 can be defined as: $D_{12} = \underset{i \in G_1, j \in G_2}{Min}(d_{ij})$.
(2) Furthest neighbor: The distance between two clusters can be defined as: $D_{12} = \underset{i \in G_1, j \in G_2}{Max}(d_{ij})$.
(3) Average linkage: It is known as between-groups linkage. The distance between G_1 and G_2 is defined as: $D_{12} = \frac{\sum_{i=1}^{n_1} \sum_{j=1}^{n_2} d_{ij}^2}{n_1 n_2}$. Average linkage can entirely reflect the individual information of every sample, and is one of the best methods for calculating the distance between clusters in cluster analysis.

(4) Centroid clustering: Let $\bar{\mathbf{X}}^{(1)} = (\bar{x}_1^{(1)}, \bar{x}_2^{(1)}, \ldots, \bar{x}_p^{(1)})$ and $\bar{\mathbf{X}}^{(2)} = (\bar{x}_1^{(2)}, \bar{x}_2^{(2)}, \ldots, \bar{x}_p^{(2)})$ denote the mean vectors (center of gravity) of G_1, G_2 respectively. The components are the mean values of every variable in the clusters. In brief, use the distance between centroids to represent the distance between clusters in clustering samples.
(5) Wald's method: This method is based on the condition that the distance measurement between samples are Euclidean distances. It is only used for sample-clustering. The statistical idea of this method comes from analysis of variance, that is, the correct classification should satisfy that the sum of squares of deviation between samples within one cluster is relatively small, and the sum of squares of deviation between clusters is relatively large.

The sum of squares of deviations is the sum of squared Euclidean distances of each sample in cluster to the center of gravity. The sum of squares of deviation method is superior to the centroid clustering in many cases due to the better classification effect and the wider application, while the method is sensitive to outliers.

In the following, we will introduce two commonly used and important clustering methods: Hierarchical clustering and K-means clustering.

23.2.2. *Hierarchical clustering*

Hierarchical clustering analysis is known as pedigree clustering. It is mainly used for variable-clustering and sample-clustering. Hierarchical clustering is the most commonly used clustering methods in practical work. The advantage of hierarchical clustering analysis is the methods of the similarity measurements and results representing are abundant when samples (or variables) are clustered. However, the limitation is that once sample (or variable) is assigned to a specific group, the classification results will not change. Moreover, the hierarchical clustering method needs to calculate the similarity coefficient repeatedly. When the sample sizes or the variable numbers are too large, the computing speed is obviously slow. Furthermore, it is vulnerable to the outliers. This section will mainly introduce sample-clustering.

23.2.2.1. *Basic ideas of hierarchical clustering*

Hierarchical clustering is based on the distances between selected samples and clusters. Firstly, each aimed subject is treated as one cluster, that is, each cluster only contains one sample; after that, calculate the distance between clusters, and merge two closest clusters into a new cluster; then calculate the distance between the new cluster and the other clusters, and merge the two closest clusters... and repeat it step by step. Each merge will reduce one cluster. Gradually, all the samples are merged into one cluster.

The whole clustering process can be plotted as a hierarchical diagram or a dendrogram. And the samples can be classified based on the characteristics of the dendrogram.

In the process of clustering calculation, different calculation methods for distances between clusters will lead to different clustering results. How to choose a better result can be judged by the professional knowledge in practice.

23.2.2.2. *Specific procedure of hierarchical clustering*

(1) Each sample is treated as a cluster, that is, each cluster only contains one sample; calculate the distance between clusters, and form a distance matrix. The distance matrix is a symmetric matrix.
(2) Merge two closest clusters into a new cluster, and then calculate the distance between the new cluster and the other clusters to form a new distance matrix.
(3) According to the second step, merge the two clusters with the smallest distance, until all samples are merged into one cluster.
(4) Plot the hierarchical diagram and analyze it. Combining with the professional knowledge, make appropriate classification based on the specific problems and clustering results.

23.2.2.3. *Implementation of hierarchical clustering*

In Example 23.1 it has two purposes: one is to classify 20 elderly people according to 10 psychological symptoms scores; the other is to group the 10 psychological symptoms by variables. We use the Q-type clustering and R-type clustering to answer this two questions respectively. SPSS software will perform the Q-type clustering in this section.

Firstly, standardize the raw data of 10 mental symptom scores for 20 elderly people to eliminate the influence of dimension. Based on the standardized data, the psychological status of 20 elderly people is classified, that is, 20 elderly people are clustered by hierarchical clustering. Secondly, each elderly person is regarded as a cluster. Choose the Euclidean distance to calculate the distance between samples, and select the between-groups linkage to calculate the distance between clusters (the default method in SPSS). The output dendrogram is shown in Figure 23.1.

Twenty elderly people can be classified into three groups based on the dendrogram and professional analysis. The results are:

The first group includes four elderly people, numbered 3, 6, 9, 19; the second group includes 12 elderly people, numbered 2, 4, 5, 8, 10, 12, 13, 15, 16, 17, 18, 20; the third group includes four elderly people, numbered 1, 7, 11, 14.

According to the scale scores, the elderly people who are in the first group have the lower psychological scores, and the psychological status is poorer; the psychological scores of the third group are higher, and the psychological status is better.

23.2.3. *K-Means clustering*

In hierarchical clustering, with the increase of clustering sample sizes, the calculation amount will increase rapidly and the clustering results will be very complicated and difficult to analyze. In addition, once the samples are classified in hierarchical clustering, they will not change. To overcome these shortcomings in hierarchical clustering, the dynamic clustering method is proposed. K-means clustering is one of the most commonly used clustering methods in dynamic

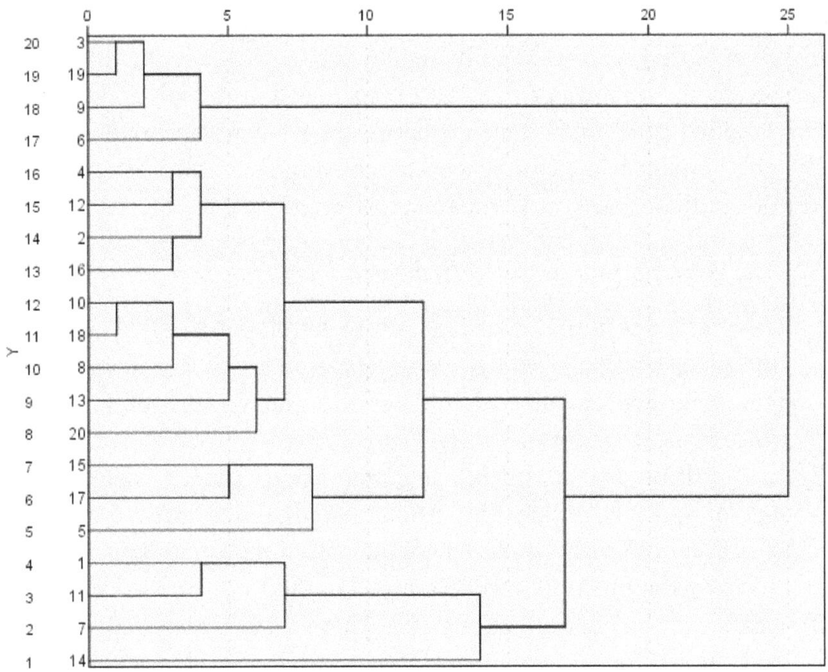

Figure 23.1 Hierarchical clustering results for 20 elderly people

clustering. It was proposed by James MacQueen in 1967. After more than 50 years of development, K-means has been considered to be the most classical distance-based clustering algorithm, and also an important branch of data mining.

23.2.3.1. *The basic idea of K-means clustering*

The idea of K-means clustering is inspired by the iteration idea in computational mathematics. It begins with rough classification and modifies it based on some principle until the classification is reasonable. The basic idea of K-means clustering is specifying the number of clusters and assuming k clusters to be classified firstly, then select k subjects from the raw data as the initial agglomeration points based on some principles. Except the initial agglomeration points, all the subjects are classified one by one based on the distance between them. Each subject is classified into the nearest cluster to the initial agglomeration point. The new agglomeration points are updated in the mean of this cluster. Finally, repeat the steps above for the second classification adjustment, ..., and continue it until all the subjects are classified and no further adjustments need to be made. Generally, the classification can reach the convergence state after several iteration adjustments in K-means clustering.

23.2.3.2. *Specific procedure of K-means clustering*

(1) Designate the number of clusters to be classified as k, and randomly select k subjects as agglomeration points to form k clusters. The centers of each cluster are the vectors of k subject observations, denoted by $X_1, X_2, \ldots, X_k$.
(2) In addition to k initial agglomeration points, select subject Y, and calculate the Euclidean distance between Y and $X_1, X_2, \ldots, X_k$. Y is classified into the nearest cluster. Repeat this process until all subjects are classified into k clusters.
(3) Calculate the cluster centers of k clusters got by the second step, and obtain the new agglomeration points of k clusters, denoted by $X_1^*, X_2^*, \ldots, X_k^*$.
(4) Compare the new agglomeration points of k clusters with the previous one. If the cluster center changes, turn to step 2 or step 5.
(5) When the agglomeration point does not change, the iteration stops and the clustering results are output.

From the steps above, we can see that the principle of K-means clustering is very simple. One of its distinct features is the iterative process. We have to check whether the classification of each subject is correct or not repeatedly. If not correct, we need to adjust it. When all the subjects are adjusted, the center is modified, and then the next iteration process proceeds. If all subjects have been correctly classified in one iteration, there will be no adjustment, the clustering center will not change, and the algorithm will be successfully completed. It should be noted that the number of clusters should be known in advance in the K-means clustering method, that is, the number of clusters k needs to be specified by researchers based on their professional knowledge. However, it is difficult to determine the number of classifications in advance in practical analysis sometimes. In this case, researchers can repeatedly try to classify the data into different clusters according to the specific problems, then choose a reasonable classification based on the actual situation.

23.2.3.3. *Implementation of K-means clustering*

The aim of Example 23.2 is to classify 100 normal people based on the eight related variables. SPSS software will perform the K-means clustering in this section. In order to eliminate the influence of dimension, the raw data is standardized before classification. In this case, we specify the number of clusters k = 4, and the clustering process is iterated 12 times. The center of gravity of the four clusters after K-means clustering is shown in Table 23.3. The number of samples in each cluster is shown in Table 23.4.

Table 23.3 K-means clustering centers

	Cluster			
	1	2	3	4
X1(age)	62	65	58	38
X2(picture memory)	13	8	13	17
X3(digital width memory)	7	6	8	8
X4(graphic sequential memory)	4	8	6	11
X5(digits number of mental arithmetic)	15	7	5	4
X6(time of mental arithmetic)	2	2	4	4
X7(stepping distance)	45	28	33	42
X8(pace)	5	8	5	4

Table 23.4 The number of subjects in each cluster

	Classification	Number of people
Cluster	1	6
	2	11
	3	44
	4	39

23.3. Variable-clustering

23.3.1. *Variable-clustering statistics*

Distances are commonly-used clustering statistics in sample-clustering. In variable-clustering, similarity is a statistic to depict the relationship between variables, and it is a quantity to characterize the similarity between variables.

23.3.1.1. *Similarity between variables*

There are many methods for calculating similarity, such as Pearson correlation, cosine, contingency coefficient, etc. The greater the absolute value, the closer the relationship between the variables and the higher the similarity.

(1) Pearson correlation:

$$r_{st} = \frac{\sum_{k=1}^{n} (x_{ks} - \bar{x}_s)(x_{kt} - \bar{x}_t)}{\sqrt{\left[\sum_{k=1}^{n} (x_{ks} - \bar{x}_s)^2\right]\left[\sum_{k=1}^{n} (x_{kt} - \bar{x}_t)^2\right]}}$$

(2) Cosine:

$$r_{st} = \cos\theta_q = \frac{\sum_{k=1}^{n} x_{ks}x_{kt}}{\sqrt{\left[\sum_{k=1}^{n} x_{ks}^2\right]\left[\sum_{k=1}^{n} x_{kt}^2\right]}}$$

(3) Contingency coefficient:

$$r_{st} = \sqrt{\frac{\chi^2}{\chi^2 + n}}$$

where r_{st} denotes the similarity coefficient between the sth variable and the tth variable; n is sample size. x_{ks} denotes the value of the sth variable in the tth sample of continuous variables. $\bar{x}_s$ is the mean of the sth variable; and χ^2 is the Pearson χ^2 value of the $R \times C$ contingency table formed by the frequency of the two categorical variables.

23.3.1.2. *Similarity between clusters*

Similarity between clusters is a statistic used to measure the similarity between one cluster (a group of variables) and another cluster (a group of variables). When there is more than one variable in each cluster, many methods can calculate the similarity between clusters. Different measurements for similarity will lead to different clusters. Let R_{12} denote the similarity between G_1 and G_2. Two commonly used calculation methods for similarity between clusters are as follows:

(1) Nearest neighbor: If we have p_1 variables in G_1 and p_2 variables in a G_2, there will be p_1p_2 similarity coefficients. Hence the similarity between two clusters can be defined as: $R_{12} = \underset{s\in G_1, t\in G_2}{Max}(r_{st})$
(2) Furthest neighbor: similarity between two clusters can be defined as: $R_{12} = \underset{s\in G_1, t\in G_2}{Min}(r_{st})$

In the following, we will use the hierarchical clustering method introduced in section 23.2 to cluster variables. The processes of clustering variables are similar to the sample-clustering when clustering variables with hierarchical clustering method. We only need to change the clustering subject (each sample) of sample-clustering into variables and change the clustering statistics of sample-clustering into variable-clustering statistics. The other steps are consistent with the sample-clustering.

23.3.2. *Hierarchical clustering method for variable-clustering*

The second aim of the Example 23.1 is to cluster 10 psychological symptoms of 20 elderly. SPSS software will perform the R-type clustering in this section.

Standardize the raw scores data of 10 psychological symptom of the 20 elderly people. Based on the standardized data, 10 psychological symptoms are clustered by variables. Each variable is treated as a cluster, select the cosine to calculate the similarity, and choose

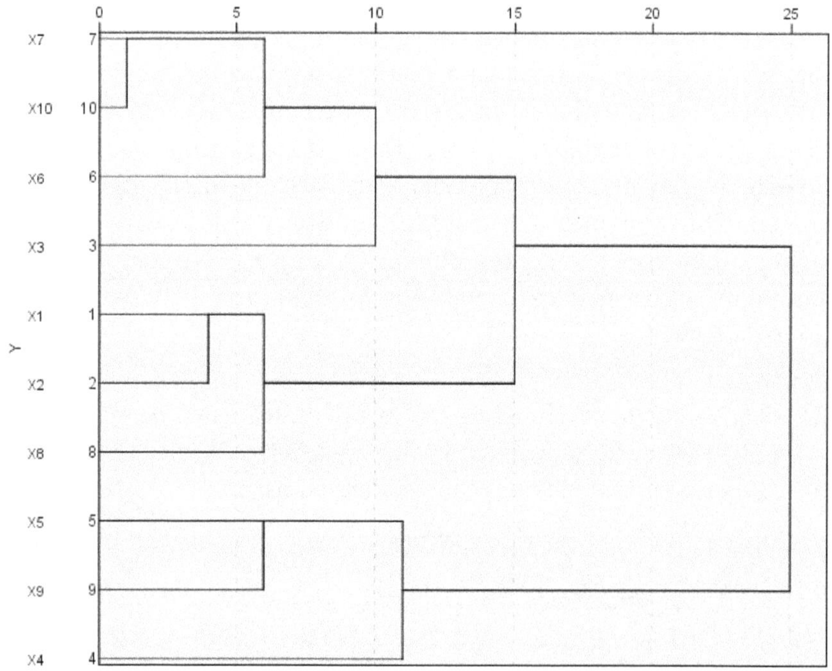

Figure 23.2 Hierarchical clustering results for 10 psychological symptoms

furthest neighbor to calculate the similarity between clusters. The output dendrogram is shown in Figure 23.2.

Ten psychological symptoms can be classified into three clusters based on the dendrogram and professional analysis. The results are: the first cluster includes interpersonal sensitivity (X3), hostility (X6), phobia (X7), sleep and diet (X10); the second cluster includes somatization (X1), obsessive-compulsive symptoms (X2), paranoia (X8); the third cluster includes depression (X4), anxiety (X5), psychiatric (X9).

23.4. Result writing

Results of the cluster analysis are as follows:

1. The purpose of clustering.
2. Types of clustering.

3. The clustering statistics selection.
4. The clustering methods selection.
5. Explanation of the dendrogram and clustering results.

The following are the English results report in Example 23.1.

We would classify 20 elderly people based on the psychological scores. It belongs to sample-clustering. Euclidean distance is selected as the cluster statistic. Hierarchical clustering analysis is used to achieve this clustering.

From the results of Figure 23.1 and professional analysis for the Example 23.1, 20 elderly people are classified into three groups. No. 3, 6, 9, 19 are clustered into the first group; No. 2, 4, 5, 8, 10, 12, 13, 15, 16, 17, 18, 20 are clustered into the second group; No. 1, 7, 11, 14 are clustered into the third group.

According to the scale scores, the elderly who are in the first group have the lower psychological scores, and the psychological status is poorer; the psychological scores of the third group are higher, and the psychological status is better.

23.5. Case discrimination

Case 23.1 In order to compare the distribution of TCM syndromes in different stages of diabetic retinopathy, 750 patients with diabetes were selected, including 250 patients in DR subclinical stage, nonproliferative stage and proliferative stage respectively. The researchers inquired 106 TCM syndromes of all patients in detail, and divided them into four groups according to no, light, medium and heavy symptoms. In this case, please discuss methods used to compare the distribution of TCM syndromes in different stages of diabetic retinopathy.

23.6. Computer experiments (See Electronic Resources exp 23.1 to exp 23.3)

Experiment 23.1 Using SPSS software to implement sample-clustering in Example 23.1

Please use hierarchical clustering method to classify the 20 elderly people based on the 10 psychological symptoms scores.

Experiment 23.2 Using SPSS software to implement sample-clustering in Example 23.2

Please use K-means clustering method to classify the 100 normal subjects based on the values of eight variables.

Experiment 23.3 Using SPSS software to implement variable-clustering in Example 23.1

Please use hierarchical clustering method to classify 10 psychological symptoms based on the 10 psychological symptoms scores for the 20 elderly people.

23.7. Frequently asked questions and summary

23.7.1. *Frequently asked questions*

1. The differences between discriminant analysis and cluster analysis?

Discriminant analysis is a supervised learning method, which requires some prior information. It divides the given objects into several types (or groups). Observations of various types of known subjects have been obtained. It establishes discriminants according to certain criteria, and then classifies the unknown subjects using discriminant analysis. Cluster analysis is an unsupervised learning method. There is no prior information for the type of a given subject to be classified. It is necessary to determine the classification by cluster analysis.

2. How to prove the results of clustering are meaningful?

Cluster analysis is an unsupervised learning method. There is no specific standard to prove whether the clustering results are right or wrong. There are three general methods for judging: 1) Verifying and interpreting the clustering results by the realistic logic. The experts should agree with this clustering result; 2) Setting some evaluation criteria in advance, such as the compactness within the cluster and the alienation between the clusters; 3) Illustrating the differences between different clusters through visualization. Therefore, a good clustering result should be consistent with common sense recognition, and the general direction of it can be recognized by experts in related fields either.

3. The differences between hierarchical clustering and K-means clustering in cluster analysis?

Hierarchical clustering is a method to classify similar samples or variables into a cluster. It is mainly used for variable-clustering and small sample-clustering. It is characterized by the fact that once the sample (or variable) is assigned to a particular group, the classification results will not change. While K-means is a dynamic clustering method. The number of clusters needs to be specified before K-means clustering. One of its distinct features is the iterative process. We have to check whether the classification of each subject is correct or not repeatedly, if not correct, we need to adjust it. When all the subjects are adjusted, the center is modified. The next iteration will proceed until all subjects are not needed to be adjusted.

Hierarchical clustering needs to calculate similarity coefficients repeatedly. When the sample sizes and variables are too large, the computing speed is obviously slow. While the K-means clustering algorithm is fast and simple, this is suitable for fast clustering of high-dimensional data.

23.7.2. *Summary*

1. Cluster analysis is often used for exploratory data analysis, and it should be interpreted closely with the professional knowledge. Meanwhile, we can try many clustering methods to get better classification results.
2. The raw data should be preprocessed before clustering analysis, such as deleting the invalid and missing data. Standardization the raw data is also needed in order to eliminate the influence of dimension on clustering results.
3. In clustering analysis, whether sample-clustering or variable-clustering, three steps involved are as follows: (1) Standardize

the raw data; (2) Select the clustering statistics; (3) Select the clustering methods.

4. Reasonable results of sample classification should have larger differences between clusters and smaller differences within intra-cluster. After classification, variance analysis or multivariate analysis of variance can be used to test whether the differences between clusters are statistical significance.
5. In addition to the introduced sample-clustering and variable-clustering in this chapter, there are also two-way clustering methods considering both sample and variable observations. This chapter will not introduce, and you can refer to other books or online enquiries for self-learning.
6. For clustering methods, this chapter only introduces hierarchical clustering and K-means clustering. Others such as fuzzy clustering, neural network clustering, and some special clustering analysis methods in data mining are not introduced in this chapter. Readers can learn from other books.

Think and Practice

I. Questions for reflection

1. Please describe the basic idea of hierarchical clustering and its clustering process in brief.
2. Please describe the basic idea of K-means clustering and its clustering process in brief.

References

[1] Kaitai, F. *Practical Multivariate Statistical Analysis*. Shanghai, China: East China Normal University Press; 1989.
[2] Feng, C. *Medical Multivariate Statistical Analysis Method*. Beijing: China Statistics Press; 2000.
[3] Jiqian, F. *Statistical Methods for Biomedical Research*. Beijing: Higher Education Press; 2007.

Xiaonan Wang, Yanxia Luo

CHAPTER 24

PRINCIPAL COMPONENT ANALYSIS AND FACTOR ANALYSIS

In the medical research, the researchers usually analyzed the problems systematically from multi-dimensionality, so they may measure several observed variables to reflect different aspects of the subject. However, the importance varies among variables and the information provided by the observed variables may be correlated. Researchers try to summarize these variables using fewer uncorrelated underlying variables. The latter is done to reflect most of the information provided by the original variables and reduce the dimensionality of a data set. Cluster analysis of variable in the previous chapter plays an important role of dimensionality reduction, while no new variables generate during the procedure of cluster analysis. Both principal component analysis (PCA) and factor analysis (FA) explored in this chapter may generate new variables in the process of dimensionality reduction, which can be applied for further analysis.

24.1. Principal component analysis

24.1.1. *Definition of PCA*

PCA was originally invented in 1901 by Karl Pearson and then advanced by Harold Hotelling. It is a multivariate statistical technique that applies a linear transformation to extract a few comprehensive variables by reducing the number of variables based on the correlation among multiple quantitative variables. Specifically, it is a method to recombine the large number of original multiple variables into a small number of new uncorrelated comprehensive variables. Meanwhile, the extracted comprehensive variables can reflect the maximum possible information of the original variable. Although the number of comprehensive variables is equal to the number of original variables after linear transformation, we only extract the first k comprehensive variables, which can present most of the information contained in the original data to obtain dimensionality reduction. These uncorrelated comprehensive variables are linear combinations of the original variables, called principal components. This procedure could reduce the dimensionality of data and eliminate the correlation between the original variables for further statistical analysis.

24.1.2. *The basic theory of PCA*

The original p variables are linearly combined into the new comprehensive variables to find the first linear combination C_1 that has maximum variance $Var(C_1)$. C_1 is also called the first principal component. If $Var(C_1)$ is not sufficient to represent the information of the original p variables, the second linear combination C_2 irrelevant to C_1 needs to be identified so that $Cov(C_1, C_2) = 0$ and $Var(C_2)$ reaches maximum and the C_2 is called the second principal component. By analogy, we can find linear combinations called the third principal component C_3 and the fourth principal component C_4 respectively, which is irrelevant to the other principal components. The latter principal component is uncorrelated with the previous, and their variances are decreasing successively.

24.1.3. *The computational procedure and application examples of PCA*

The computational procedure of PCA includes estimation of principal component, determination of the number of principal components, explanation of practical significance of principal components, and calculation of principal component score.

Suppose we have a set of p original variables $X_1, X_2, \ldots, X_p$, with means $\bar{X}_1, \bar{X}_2, \ldots, \bar{X}_p$ and standard deviations $S_1, S_2, \ldots, S_p$, respectively. We should standardize all original variables from the equation $x_i = \frac{X_i - \overline{X}_i}{S_i}, i = 1, 2, \ldots, p$

1) Estimate principal component

Denote the first principal component by C_1, which is the linear combination of $x_1, x_2, \ldots, x_p$.

$$C_1 = a_{11}x_1 + a_{12}x_2 + \cdots + a_{1p}x_p \tag{24-1}$$

C_1 should have the maximum variance than any other linear combinations and also put the constraints $a_{11}^2 + a_{12}^2 + \cdots + a_{1p}^2 = 1$.

Similarly, we can also search for the second principal component C_2. It should be another linear combination of $x_1, x_2, \ldots, x_p$.

$$C_2 = a_{21}x_1 + a_{22}x_2 + \cdots + a_{2p}x_p \tag{24-2}$$

$Var(C_2)$ is maximized among all possible combinations on the premise that C_2 is irrelevant to C_1 and $a_{21}^2 + a_{22}^2 + \cdots + a_{2p}^2 = 1$.

According to this principle, $k(k \leq p)$ principal components $C_1, C_2, \ldots, C_k$ are extracted, which have the following properties:

① Principal components $(C_1, C_2, \ldots, C_k)$ are uncorrelated with each other. Namely for any pairs i and j, the correlation coefficient between C_i and C_j is zero, $Cov(C_i, C_j) = 0$.
② The variance of the principal components decreases in sequence, which means $Var(C_1) \geq Var(C_2) \geq \cdots \geq Var(C_k) \geq 0$.
③ The sum square of the coefficients of each principal component is equal to 1 that is $a_{i1}^2 + a_{i2}^2 + \cdots + a_{ip}^2 = 1$ $(i = 1, 2, \ldots, k)$.

2) Determine the number of principal components

There are two criteria for principal components extraction. One is dependent on the cumulative variations explained by these components and the other is specified in advance by the researcher. The variance of the principal component is also called eigenvalue $Var(C_i) = \lambda_i$, for example the ith eigenvalue is denoted as λ_i. In applications, we can roughly decide the percentage of variations we want to retain and thus to decide how many principal components are kept. ① Keep the principal component that the corresponding eigenvalue is above 1 and drop the rest principal components that the corresponding eigenvalue is less than 1. This is a general rule to worth considering. ② Keep the principal component when the percentage of cumulative variance reaches 80%. ③ Keep the principal component based on the scree plot. If retaining a principal component adds only slightly to the cumulative variation, this principal component should be dropped. In some cases, we may decide the number of principal components in advance directly. For example, we can decide the number of principal components according to the dimensionality of the scale while evaluating structure validity of the scale. Therefore, the number of principal components dependents on the type of problem. It is also worth to point out that the number of the principal components should be less than the number of original variables in order to reduce the dimensionality.

3) Explain the practical significance of the principal component

Let C_i represent the ith principal component and x_j represent the jth random variable, the correlation coefficient between them is:

$$Corr(C_i, x_j) = a_{ij}\sqrt{Var(C_i)} = a_{ij}\sqrt{\lambda_i} \tag{24-3}$$

The correlation coefficient reflects the strength and direction. With the help of the latter, we can interpret the professional significance of principal components.

4) Calculate the principal component score

Principal components are also used as the intermediate step for further analysis. In the process, principal component scores play a role of intermediate step. The ith principal component score can be calculated from $C_i = a_{i1}x_1 + a_{i2}x_2 + \cdots + a_{ip}x_p$.

[**Example 24.1**] The researcher selected 2,250 adults over 35 years old in one region randomly and conducted physical examination and laboratory biochemical tests to explore the influencing factors of blood pressure. A total of 2,235 valid questionnaires were obtained,

Table 24.1 Biochemical test results of 2,235 adults in one region

ID	BMI (X_1)	WG (X_2)	TG (X_3)	CHO (X_4)	HDL-C (X_5)	Glu (X_6)	SBP (Y_1)	DBP (Y_2)
1	21.38	69.00	177.80	160.10	35.90	71.00	124.00	68.67
2	18.05	76.00	85.20	171.30	55.10	94.65	102.67	76.00
3	17.64	68.40	110.00	171.10	49.20	75.69	110.00	75.33
...	...	...	...	...	...	...	...	...
2233	27.40	88.00	67.90	162.70	42.80	94.15	155.33	90.00
2234	27.41	74.00	187.10	156.10	41.40	94.53	112.00	72.00
2235	34.42	77.20	73.80	183.90	57.30	75.39	108.67	72.67

Table 24.2 Total variance explained

Component	Eigenvalues λ	% of Variance	Cumulative %
1	2.291	38.178	38.178
2	1.261	21.012	59.190
3	0.991	16.513	75.703
4	0.815	13.584	89.287
5	0.404	6.732	96.018
6	0.239	3.982	100.000

and the data were shown in Table 24.1. Multiple linear regression was fitted with body mass index (BMI), waist circumference (TG), triglyceride (TG), total cholesterol (CHO), high-density lipoprotein cholesterol (HDL-C), and blood glucose (Glu) as predictors. Dependent variables were systolic blood pressure (SBP) and diastolic blood pressure (DBP) (See data24-1.sav). The collinearity diagnosis results identified collinearity between BMI, WC, TG, CHO, HDL-C and Glu. Please reduce the data dimensionality by PCA.

In this example, PCA was conducted with statistical package for the social sciences (SPSS). We can observe the detailed step from the proceeding section in computer experiments. Table 24.2 listed the eigenvalues, variance explained and cumulative variance explained.

Two principal components were kept according to the criteria of $\lambda \geq 1$, accounting for 59.190% total variation. In the terms of the criteria that cumulative variance reaches 80%, four principal

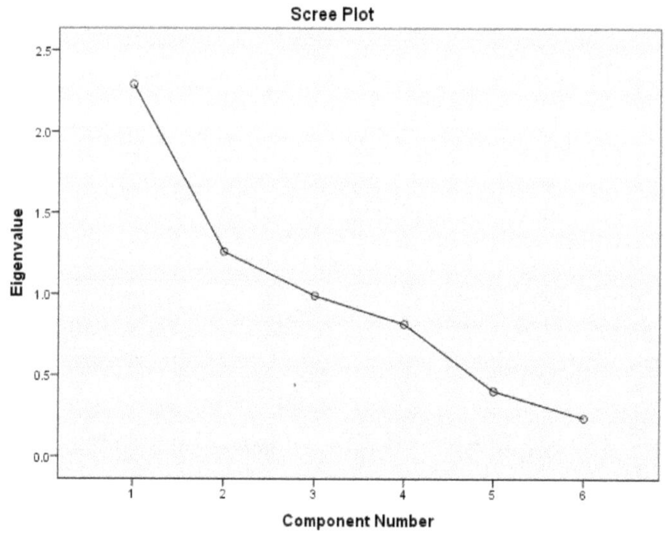

Figure 24.1 Scree plot

components were extracted. Considering that the eigenvalue of the third principal component is 0.991, close to 1, and the cumulative variance increase slightly if retaining the fourth principal component (Figure 24.1) from the scree plot, we kept the top three principal components, which accounted for 75.703% total variation in this example. The component matrix was shown in Table 24.3, from which we can list three principal component formulations.

$$C_1 = 0.816x_1 + 0.854x_2 + 0.665x_3 + 0.335x_4 - 0.490x_5 + 0.317x_6$$

$$C_2 = -0.040x_1 - 0.009x_2 + 0.013x_3 + 0.820x_4 + 0.699x_5 + 0.313x_6$$

$$C_3 = 0.401x_1 + 0.330x_2 - 0.367x_3 + 0.029x_4 + 0.313x_5 - 0.698x_6$$

In the above process, we use the principal component analysis to reduce the six original variables into three independent principal components on the premise of keeping sufficient information of the original variables, and the three principal components accounted for 75.703% variation. Furthermore, three principal components as predictors may be included in the multiple linear regression model, with systolic and diastolic blood pressures as dependent variables,

Table 24.3 Component matrix

Standardized variable	PC1 (C_1)	PC2 (C_2)	PC3 (C_3)
x_1	**0.816**	−0.040	0.401
x_2	**0.854**	−0.009	0.330
x_3	**0.665**	0.013	−0.367
x_4	0.335	**0.820**	0.029
x_5	−0.490	**0.699**	0.313
x_6	0.317	0.313	**−0.698**

respectively. Using the principal components as independent variables in the regression analysis will avoid problems of collinearity and reduce the number of original variables. PCA can also be performed in logistic regression analysis and cox regression analysis to avoid collinearity.

24.2. Factor Analysis

PCA and FA are two commonly used methods for dimensionality reduction. Different from PCA, FA aims to identify the underlying common factors supported by measurable original variables with minimum loss of information and makes the common factors to be easily interpreted. While evaluating the structural validity of a scale, we can apply FA if we want to summarize the less latent properties from original variables that could not be measured directly. Briefly, FA is a statistical method to find the common "latent variables" from many "explicit variables." FA includes exploratory factor analysis (EFA) and confirmatory factor analysis (CFA), both of which are based on the correlation matrix of the observed variables. EFA is abbreviated as FA, which assumes that researchers have no clear idea about the internal structure of variables and the underlying common factors and the results depend entirely on the known data. For example, the SCL-90 symptom self-rating scale, one of the most widely used mental health test scales in the world, includes 90 items in 10 domains: somatization, compulsive symptoms, interpersonal sensitivity, depression, anxiety, hostility, terror, paranoia, psychosis and others. Suppose we know nothing about the structure and latent common factors of the scale in advance, EFA could be performed to find common factors and then explore the relationship between the items and the common factors. Suppose we have known clearly that the scale is composed of 10 independent domains in advance, CFA could be performed to confirm whether the structure of the scale is the case.

24.2.1. *The basic theory of exploratory factor analysis*

The basic theory of EFA is to extract a less independent and abstract comprehensive variables (also called common factors) from multiple measurable variables, and each comprehensive variable could be represented in a linear combination of common factors.

Suppose we have a set of p random original variables $X_1, X_2, \ldots, X_p$ and $x_1, x_2, \ldots, x_p$ is the standardized variables, then p principal components $C_1, C_2, \ldots, C_p$ could be obtained.

$$\begin{aligned} C_1 &= a_{11}x_1 + a_{12}x_2 + \cdots + a_{1p}x_p \\ C_2 &= a_{21}x_1 + a_{22}x_2 \cdots + a_{2p}x_p \\ &\cdots \\ C_p &= a_{p1}x_1 + a_{p2}x_2 + \cdots + a_{pp}x_p \end{aligned} \tag{24-4}$$

So, we can compute

$$\begin{aligned} x_1 &= a_{11}C_1 + a_{21}C_2 + \cdots + a_{k1}C_k + \cdots + a_{p1}C_p \\ x_2 &= a_{12}C_1 + a_{22}C_2 + \cdots + a_{k2}C_k + \cdots + a_{p2}C_p \\ &\cdots \\ x_p &= a_{1p}C_1 + a_{2p}C_2 + \cdots + a_{kp}C_k + \cdots + a_{pp}C_p \end{aligned} \tag{24-5}$$

Suppose k is the number of common factors. The top k common factors are kept in the above equation, and the "error" terms are recorded as $\delta_1, \delta_2, \ldots, \delta_p$. Apply them into formula 24-5 and we can obtain:

$$
\begin{aligned}
x_1 &= a_{11}C_1 + a_{21}C_2 + \cdots + a_{k1}C_k + \delta_1 \\
x_2 &= a_{12}C_1 + a_{22}C_2 + \cdots + a_{k2}C_k + \delta_2 \\
&\cdots \\
x_p &= a_{1p}C_1 + a_{2p}C_2 + \cdots + a_{kp}C_k + \delta_p
\end{aligned} \tag{24-6}
$$

If we let $F_j = \frac{C_j}{\sqrt{Var(C_j)}}$ and $C_J = \sqrt{Var(C_j)}F_j$, then replace them in equation (24-6):

$$
\begin{aligned}
x_1 &= l_{11}F_1 + l_{12}F_2 + \cdots + l_{1k}F_k + \delta_1 \\
x_2 &= l_{21}F_1 + l_{22}F_2 + \cdots + l_{2k}F_k + \delta_2 \\
&\cdots \\
x_p &= l_{p1}F_1 + l_{p2}F_2 + \cdots + l_{pk}F_k + \delta_p
\end{aligned}
$$

Where $l_{ij} = a_{ij}\sqrt{Var(C_j)}$ is actually the correlation coefficient between x_i and C_j, which is called "factor loading," indicating the degree of influence for the latent factor F_j to x_i. The larger the absolute value of l_{ij}, the closer relationship between x_i and F_j. F_j is the common factor with mean 0 and standard deviation 1, appearing in the expression of every measurable variable. δ_i is the personality factor, reflecting the total influence of other potential factors besides k common factors on x_i.

Model assumptions of EFA are as follows:

① x_i $(i = 1, 2, \ldots, p)$ are random variables.
② $\delta_i(i = 1, 2, \ldots, p)$ are random normal distribution variables, which satisfy mean is 0 and variance is constant.
③ $\delta_i(i = 1, 2, \ldots, p)$ are independent.
④ F_j $(j = 1, 2, \ldots, k)$ are random independent variables, which satisfy mean is 0 and variance is 1.
⑤ δ_i and F_j are mutually independent.

24.2.2. *The computational procedure and application examples of exploratory factor analysis*

The computational procedure of PCA may be summarized as the standardization of original variables, construction of correlation matrices, determination of the number of common factors and extraction of common factors, factor rotation, interpretation to factor structure and calculation of factor score.

1) Standardization of the original variables

If there are p original variables represented as $X_1, X_2, \ldots, X_p$, the mean and standard deviation of original variables are calculated as $\bar{X}_1, \bar{X}_2, \ldots, \bar{X}_p$ and $S_1, S_2, \ldots, S_p$, respectively. The normalized original variables denote as$x_1, x_2, \ldots, x_p$ could be obtained from the equation

$$x_i = \frac{X_i - \overline{X}_i}{S_i}, i = 1, 2, \ldots, p$$

2) Construction of the correlation matrix

KMO test (Kaiser-Meyer-Olkin test) and Bartlett's spherical test are commonly used method to infer whether the data are applicable for FA via testing the correlation matrix. The former is a relative index of correlation and partial correlation, which is used to test whether the partial correlation between variables is small enough. KMO could be obtained from the equation

$$KMO = \frac{\sum\sum_{i \neq j} r_{ij}^2}{\sum\sum_{i \neq j} r_{ij}^2 + \sum\sum_{i \neq j} a_{ij}^2} \tag{24-7}$$

Where r_{ij} is the correlation coefficient and a_{ij} is the partial correlation coefficient between two random variables, which is the correlation coefficient after controlling the influence of other variables. The value of KMO is from 0 and 1. It means the higher intricate correlation between variables when KMO value is closer to 1 and the data is applicable for FA. According to the opinion of Kaiser, FA performs better when KMO$>$ 0.9. Or else we cannot apply FA when KMO $<$ 0.5.

Bartlett's sphericity test is applied to determine whether the correlation matrix is an identity matrix, the null hypothesis of which is "the correlation matrix is an identity matrix," and the alternative hypothesis is "the correlation matrix is not an identity matrix." It can be inferred the test statistic obeys with χ^2 distribution when the null hypothesis is valid. A P value less than 0.05 indicates that the correlation matrix is not the identity matrix and the data is applicable for factor analysis. Otherwise, the correlation matrix is the identity matrix, which indicates FA should not be performed.

3) Determination the number of common factors and extraction of common factors

There are several methods to extract common factors, and the most commonly used is the principal component method, which was introduced in the previous section of this chapter. The other methods include iterative principal components, unweighted least squares, generalized least squares, the maximum likelihood method and so on.

The criteria for determining the number of common factors are the same with determining the number of principal components. Depend on the eigenvalue, the proportion of cumulative eigenvalues in the total variance and professional interpretation, which can be read for reference in 24.1.3.

4) Factor rotation

Via factor analysis, we not only aim to find out the common factors, but also to interpret the professional meaning of them. However, the practical significance is usually ambiguous and difficult to interpret whether the common factors are extracted by the principal component method or other methods. Faced with such problems, factor rotation could be applied. The essence of factor rotation is to make the factor load "polarized" to 0 and 1, resulting in as big difference as possible such that, different new common factors could be closely related to different subsets of variables. The number of new and old common factors remains unchanged after factor rotation.

The commonly used factor rotation methods are varimax rotation and oblique rotation. Varimax rotation means that the maximum dispersion of the loads of each variable on every common factor, which could maintain the characteristics of non-correlation between the new common factors. Oblique rotation does not deliberately ensure that there is no correlation between the new public factors, but more emphasis on increasing the factor load "polarized" to make the significance of the new public factors clearer.

The eigenvalue, contribution rate and cumulative contribution rate of Example 24.1 are shown in Table 24.2, and the unrotated factor loads matrix between common factors and the variables are shown in Table 24.3. The factor loads matrix after varimax rotation are shown in the Table 24.4.

Compared with the unrotated factor loads in Table 24.3, the factor loads after varimax rotation "polarized" to 0 and 1. The practical meaning of each principal component should be explained after determining the number of principal components. Generally, the magnitude of factor load is taken as the basis. The bigger of the absolute value is, the greater contribution of variables to the common factors. When the absolute value of factor load ≥ 0.5, we may consider that the variable has a great influence on the common factor. According to this criterion,x_1 (body mass index) and x_2 (waist circumference) have the biggest load on F_1 and the factor load of them are both bigger than 0.5. Therefore, it can be considered that body mass index and

Table 24.4 Factor loads matrix after varimax rotation

Standardized variable	Common factor 1(F_1)	Common factor 2(F_2)	Common factor 3(F_3)
x_1	**0.909**	0.037	−0.014
x_2	**0.908**	0.123	−0.006
x_3	0.407	**0.625**	−0.145
x_4	0.275	0.355	**0.764**
x_5	−0.307	−0.306	**0.799**
x_6	−0.069	**0.820**	0.092

waist circumference are mainly controlled by F_1. Combining with the professional knowledge, these two variables represent the degree of obesity. Thus, the first common factor can be considered as "obesity factor." x_3 (triglycerides) and x_6 (blood glucose) have the largest load on F_2, and the factor load of them are both bigger than 0.5, which suggest triglycerides and blood glucose are mainly controlled by F_2. Combining with the professional knowledge, increased triglyceride level or increased blood glucose level is the diagnostic criteria of metabolic syndrome, hence the second common factor can be regarded as "metabolic syndrome factor." x_4 (total cholesterol) and x_5 (high-density lipoprotein cholesterol) have the largest load on F_3, and the factor load of them are both bigger than 0.5. We concluded that the total cholesterol and high-density lipoprotein cholesterol are mainly controlled by F_3. The third common factor could be regarded as "cholesterol factor".

In the principal component analysis, triglycerides, body mass index and waist circumference belong to the same principal component, which is not easy to explain professionally. However, this problem was reasonably solved after varimax rotation via factor analysis. For the purpose of practical applications, we can achieve factor rotation to get clear interpretations.

We could obtain the following function from the component matrix after varimax rotation:

$$x_1 = 0.909F_1 + 0.037F_2 - 0.014F_3$$

$$x_2 = 0.908F_1 + 0.123F_2 - 0.006F_3$$

$$x_3 = 0.407F_1 + 0.625F_2 - 0.145F_3$$

$$x_4 = 0.275F_1 + 0.355F_2 + 0.764F_3$$

$$x_5 = -0.307F_1 - 0.306F_2 + 0.799F_3$$

$$x_6 = -0.069F_1 + 0.820F_2 + 0.092F_3$$

Factor component score coefficient matrix of Example 24.1 is shown in Table 24.5:

Table 24.5 Factor component score coefficient matrix after varimax rotation

Standardized variable	Common factor 1(F_1)	Common factor 2(F_2)	Common factor 3(F_3)
x_1	0.508	−0.181	0.039
x_2	0.487	−0.106	0.042
x_3	0.077	0.451	−0.112
x_4	0.116	0.220	0.619
x_5	−0.058	−0.217	0.634
x_6	−0.226	0.723	0.046

Then we can conclude:

$$F_1 = 0.508x_1 + 0.487x_2 + 0.077x_3 + 0.116x_4 - 0.058x_5 - 0.226x_6$$
$$F_2 = -0.181x_1 - 0.106x_2 + 0.451x_3 + 0.220x_4 - 0.217x_5 + 0.723x_6$$
$$F_3 = 0.039x_1 + 0.042x_2 - 0.112x_3 + 0.619x_4 + 0.634x_5 + 0.046x_6$$

The above model is the same as the distribution of factor composition matrix after rotation.

24.2.3. *Confirmatory factor analysis*

Previously introduced methods are EFA because we have no prior knowledge of the factor structure of the original variables and also donot know the number of factors. The answer is only available after the analysis. Different from EFA is confirmatory factor analysis (CFA), which was developed on the basis of EFA and presented in 1969 by K.G.Joreskog, a statistician at the University of Apassala in Sweden. When researchers have prior knowledge on the intrinsic structure between the measurable variables and the potential factors, namely, which measurable variables may be affected by which potential factors, only aim to determine the load size of the measurable variables on the potential factors and verify the goodness-of-fit between the structure and the actual data, the CFA may be achieved. Details of CFA are presented in Chapter 27.

24.3. Result report

Result report of FA should include: ① The applicable conditions of FA. ② The method, number and cumulative contribution rate of extracting common factors. ③ The factor load matrix after rotation. Using Example 24.1, we may report:

Kaiser-Meyer-Olkin Measure of Sampling Adequacy is 0.572 and p value in Bartlett's Test of Sphericity is less than 0.001, which indicates the model assumption of FA is satisfied. Based on PCA, 3 common factors (components)are extracted and the cumulative variance is 75.703%. Table 24.2 lists the initial eigenvalues and total variance explained and Table 24.4 shows the factor loads matrix after varimax rotation.

24.4. Case discrimination

[**Case 24.1**] The following table lists the examination results of 70 patients with brain trauma admitted to hospital. $X_1, X_2, X_3, X_4, X_5, X_6$ represent the blood loss from CT (ml), severity of illness ($1 = $ light, $2 = $ medium, $3 = $ heavy), systolic blood pressure (mmHg), diastolic blood pressure (mmHg), ALT (U/L) and AST (U/L).

(1) The author conducted PCA on the original variable $X_1, X_2, X_3, X_4, X_5, X_6$ and extracted three principal components according to the principle of eigenvalue ≥ 1, the cumulative contribution proportion is 87.049%. Do you consider the analysis reasonable? Please give your reason.
(2) Furthermore, the author listed the equation of factor component score as follow according to the result of factor component matrix. What is your opinion on this?

$$F_1 = 0.635x_1 + 0.605x_2 + 0.709x_3 + 0.572x_4 + 0.466x_5 + 0.644x_6$$

$$F_2 = -0.178x_1 - 0.092x_2 - 0.483x_3 - 0.555x_4 + 0.811x_5 + 0.699x_6$$

$$F_3 = -0.592x_1 - 0.656x_2 + 0.383x_3 + 0.506x_4 + 0.232x_5 + 0.160x_6$$

Table 24.6 Examination results of 70 patients with brain trauma admitted to hospital

ID	X1	X2	X3	X4	X5	X6	ID	X1	X2	X3	X4	X5	X6
1	0	1	99	63	20	19	36	10	3	96	59	90	44
2	0	1	101	53	11	21	37	10	1	102	67	186	115
3	0	1	102	67	23	33	38	10	2	110	82	12	8
4	10	2	103	65	24	30	39	10	1	111	66	39	50
5	0	1	103	62	10	30	40	10	2	114	73	32	28
6	0	1	103	62	20	21	41	10	2	119	78	36	29
7	0	1	106	75	21	33	42	10	2	125	82	42	21
8	10	2	107	64	21	41	43	10	2	128	83	15	23
9	10	2	109	68	85	47	44	10	2	139	77	29	32
10	0	1	109	68	9	10	45	10	1	139	72	29	32
11	0	1	110	74	12	15	46	10	1	140	85	59	66
12	0	1	110	80	20	18	47	10	2	148	82	49	58
13	0	1	112	81	20	37	48	10	2	211	107	15	72
14	0	1	112	64	19	23	49	13	1	137	87	16	19
15	8	2	118	78	16	25	50	15	1	116	65	27	36
16	0	1	119	75	40	38	51	15	2	129	91	26	19
17	0	1	120	81	11	18	52	20	2	103	65	24	30
18	0	1	121	85	105	98	53	20	1	108	73	18	23
19	0	1	122	62	28	32	54	20	2	117	57	29	73
20	0	1	126	81	53	31	55	25	1	113	71	8	14
21	0	1	130	88	21	22	56	30	2	136	71	329	174
22	0	1	131	85	26	26	57	30	2	140	82	29	20
23	20	2	134	77	17	64	58	50	2	161	74	10	18
24	0	1	137	84	24	32	59	60	3	160	70	23	58
25	0	1	137	92	62	21	60	60	2	173	117	12	32
26	0	1	138	93	92	86	61	70	2	123	81	3	12
27	0	1	142	100	14	29	62	70	2	143	87	203	174
28	0	1	165	102	32	27	63	70	2	162	84	10	12
29	0	1	168	105	22	17	64	80	2	141	71	23	36
30	3	1	118	68	23	35	65	100	2	95	61	17	17
31	3	3	130	89	29	52	66	100	3	127	85	81	95
32	5	2	124	81	10	26	67	100	2	137	87	16	19
33	5	2	172	116	23	30	68	100	3	140	88	9	18
34	8	2	108	75	25	25	69	100	3	162	81	20	108
35	10	2	87	47	10	12	70	120	2	137	109	20	32

Table 24.6 (*Continued*)
Total variance explained

	Initial eigenvalues		
Component	Total	% of Variance	Cumulative %
1	2.231	37.184	37.184
2	1.729	28.817	66.002
3	1.263	21.047	87.049
4	0.411	6.843	93.892
5	0.247	4.123	98.016
6	0.119	1.984	100.000

Extraction method: PCA.

Component Matrix[a]

	Component		
	1	2	3
the blood loss from *CT*	0.635	−0.178	−0.592
severity of illness	0.605	−0.092	−0.656
systolic blood pressure	0.709	−0.483	0.383
diastolic blood pressure	0.572	−0.555	0.506
ALT	0.466	0.811	0.232
AST	0.644	0.699	0.160

24.5. Computer experiments (See electronic resources exp24-1)

[Experiment 24.1] Using SPSS software to implement FA in Example 24.1.

24.6. Frequently asked questions and summary

24.6.1. *Frequently asked questions*

1. The main applications of PCA.

   ① Synthesizing the original variables. PCA aims to represent the main information of the original variables using a small number of principal components. Methodologically speaking, it uses few uncorrelated new variables to reflect most of the information provided by the original correlated variables and can avoid the collinearity, which lays a foundation for further statistical analysis.

② Exploring the impact of multiple original variables on individual characteristics. As an exploratory analysis technique, the structure of loading matrix may be implemented to explore the relationship between each principal component and multiple original variables, and clarify the impact of the original variables of each principal component further, followed by extracting the principal component.

③ Making comprehensive evaluation of the sample. The proportion of variance of the principal component of total variance could be calculated. In the further analysis, we could construct a comprehensive evaluation function to evaluate the sample comprehensively using the proportion as the weight.

④ Predicting the properties of new sample and classifying the sample.

2. The main applications and points for attention about FA.
   Applications: [①] Reflecting most information of the original observed samples comprehensively. [②] Understanding the underlying nature of observed samples. [③] Evaluating structural validity of the scale.
   Points for attention: [①] The sample size of FA should not be too small, at least five times as much as the number of variables. The sample size at least 10 times as the number of variables may perform better in conducting FA. [②] The requirement of FA for variables should meet the multivariate normal distribution. [③] Higher correlation between variables may perform better. It is not suitable to conduct FA when KMO is less than 0.5. [④] The common factors should have a clear practical significance.
3. Cluster analysis, PCA and FA all play the role of dimensionality reduction on original variables. What are the differences between them?

Cluster analysis is a multivariate statistical method to classify the samples or variables based on the idea of "birds of the same feathers flock together." Variables cluster plays a role of dimensionality reduction. But cluster analysis is essentially a classification method, and the main result is presented in the form of dendrogram, without generating new variables. Different from cluster analysis, new variables will be generated while performing PCA and FA. The new generated variables can be applied for further analysis, such as solving the collinearity problem in multiple regression analysis by replacing the original variables with new variables.

24.6.2. *Summary*

Both PCA and FA are the procedures that synthesize multiple correlated variables into few uncorrelated variables on the premise of losing less information. FA is related to PCA, but the two are not identical. The connections may be summarized as: ① Extracting common factors and principal components share a similar mathematical process, and PCA can be considered as a more basic version of FA. ② FA is an extension of PCA from the interpretation of results.

The difference may be summarized as the emphasis of analysis. PCA focuses on synthesizing information of the original variables, which is the linear combination of principal components and original variables, and its mathematical model is $C_i = a_{i1}x_1 + a_{i2}x_2 + \cdots + a_{ip}x_p$. FA focuses on explaining the dominance of the common factors to the original variables where the original variables are the linear combination of common factors and error factors. The mathematical model is $x_i = a_{1i}C_1 + a_{2i}C_2 + \cdots + a_{ki}C_k + \delta_i$.

FA includes EFA and CFA, both of which are based on the correlation matrix among observed variables. EFA is abbreviated as FA. It assumes that researchers have no prior knowledge about the internal structure of variables and the latent common factors, and its analysis results dependent on the known data completely. When the researchers have a clear understanding on the inner structure between measurable variables and latent factors, the CFA can be performed to verify goodness-of fit between the structure and the actual data.

Think and Practice

1. Best Choice

1. Choose one correct answer from the following statements about PCA. ( )
   A. It aims to find several principal components to represent the original variables.
   B. The extracted principal components are highly correlated.
   C. The extracted principal components are uncorrelated with each other.
   D. If the correlation matrix is identity matrix, the data is not suitable for PCA.
   E. Each principal component is a linear combination of the original variables.
2. If the original variables need to be standardized during the PCA, the common standardization method is ( )
   A. to transform the original variables between 0 and 1.
   B. to transform the original variables between -1 and 1.
   C. logarithmic transformation.
   D. standardized normal transformation.
   E. centralized transformation, named $X - \overline{X}$.
3. Which statement is correct about the interpretations of factor loading? ( )
   A. It is actually the correlation coefficient between x_i and C_j.
   B. The larger the value, the closer relationship between x_i and F_j.
   C. The range of its value is from 0 to 1.
   D. Its value must be more than 0.
   E. The sum of factor loadings' squares of each variable x_i on a principal component C_j is equal to 1.
4. Which statement is incorrect about the personality factor δ_i in factor analysis? ( )
   A. It is a random variable with normal distribution.
   B. It is the factor that only affects one observed variable.

Table 24.7 The development data of health services of 18 cities in Henan Province in 2004

Regions	The number of health institutions	The number of beds in health institutions	The number of health technicians	The number of doctors	The number of registered nurses	The number of beds in health institutions per thousand people	The number of doctors per thousand people	The number of registered nurses per thousand people
Zhengzhou	1648	29422	35666	14350	12009	4.52	2.21	1.85
Kaifeng	446	12183	14594	5640	4355	2.57	1.19	0.92
Luoyang	947	18209	21745	8340	6243	2.85	1.31	0.98
Pingdingshan	526	12925	15676	5835	4430	2.64	1.19	0.90
Anyang	1631	11701	15082	6434	3888	2.20	1.21	0.73
Hebi	328	4295	5246	1989	1485	3.00	1.39	1.04
Xinxiang	770	15412	20921	7709	5742	2.80	1.40	1.04
Jiaozuo	862	9860	14477	5433	3741	2.90	1.60	1.10
Puyang	596	8088	9935	3810	2763	2.27	1.07	0.78
Xuchang	357	8258	11530	4670	2554	1.84	1.04	0.57
Luohe	323	4918	7435	2819	1801	1.95	1.12	0.72
Sanmenxia	610	6304	8059	3218	2070	2.85	1.45	0.93
Nanyang	1004	17421	26314	9096	6357	1.63	0.85	0.59
Shangqiu	813	13408	20759	7096	4875	1.65	0.87	0.60
Xinyang	1330	9796	14673	6187	3296	1.25	0.79	0.42
Zhoukou	1016	13176	22155	8945	4618	1.24	0.84	0.43
Zhumadian	536	11891	17925	6845	4032	1.43	0.82	0.49
Jiyuan	78	1779	2039	951	480	2.71	1.45	0.73

Table 24.8 Exam scores of 30 students

Mathematics	Physics	Chemistry	Chinese	History	English
84	67	94	52	61	60
77	99	81	80	89	76
84	93	70	75	94	80
75	61	67	66	66	70
83	72	78	65	80	82
90	71	67	71	85	83
68	70	70	72	71	77
80	81	90	62	73	76
97	96	89	79	77	85
78	81	80	69	83	76
88	83	85	90	77	84
91	89	76	63	85	79
69	70	71	67	78	70
80	85	78	60	74	67
69	87	66	89	80	85
93	99	95	74	78	76
87	82	84	58	60	62
70	55	64	72	75	80
66	87	60	78	85	89
81	87	76	65	76	69
65	63	81	82	77	73
70	64	56	71	76	82
69	51	50	100	89	94
63	48	60	85	90	82
68	81	70	78	80	81
92	83	90	87	87	88
90	81	75	94	90	87
86	79	73	65	62	58
95	96	99	80	86	79
82	83	69	87	85	91

C. It indicates that the total influence of latent factors on x_i except k common factors.

D. δ_i and F_j are mutually independent.

E. δ_i is independent to each other.

2. Think and practice

1. Please introduce the concept and basic theory of PCA briefly.

2. Why are the principal components arranged according to the eigenvalues?
3. What is the effect of factor rotation analysis after preliminary factor analysis? Will the number of common factors change before and after factor rotation?
4. How to apply EFA and CFA in practical work correctly?

3. Calculations

1. The following table includes the development data of health services of 18 cities in Henan Province in 2004. Please try to analyze the factor structure by performing factor analysis (FA).
2. The following table shows the exam scores of Mathematics, Physics, Chemistry, History, English and Chinese of 30 senior high school students. Please select several comprehensive variables to represent the academic performance of these students by PCA.

References

[1] Song, W, Faming, P. *SPSS Statistical Analysis* [M]. Beijing: Tsinghua University Publishing House; 2014.
[2] Yanbo, Z. *Latent Variable Analysis* [M]. Beijing: Higher Education Publishing House; 2009.
[3] Jiafang, Z. *Medical Multivariate Statistical Methods* [M]. Wuhan: Huazhong University of Science and Technology Press; 2002.
[4] Nan, H. *SPSS for Windows Statistical Product and Service Solution Tutorial* [M]. Beijing: Tsinghua University Publishing House, Northern Jiaotong University Press; 2003.

Yongli Yang, Xuezhong Shi

Part IV

Selected Topics of Advanced Statistics

CHAPTER 25

META ANALYSIS

The best possible synthesis of available information is essential for medical researchers, health policy-makers, clinicians and other decision-makers. During the past 30 years, meta-analysis, a statistical procedure for systematically combining and analyzing the results of multiple scientific studies, has been applied with increasing frequency to health-related contexts, especially in the fields of clinical trials.

25.1. Introduction

25.1.1. *Definition*

The origins of pooling the results may be traced to statistician Pearson in 1904, who was the first researcher to report the use of formal techniques to combine data from different samples. Famous statistician Fisher (1932) presented a method for "combining the p-values" that were generated from statistically independent tests of the same hypotheses in the 1930s. The first article, which quantitatively synthesized the previous research in medicine, entitled "the powerful placebo" and written by Beecher, was published in 1955.

The term "meta-analysis" was coined by Glass in 1976, he wrote that "meta-analysis... refers to the statistical analysis of a large collection of analyses results from individual studies for the purpose of integrating the findings." Although Glass was involved in social science research, the term "meta-analysis" has been adopted within other disciplines and has proved particularly popular in clinical research. The rapid and vast increase in the number of meta-analyses being conducted during the past two decades is mainly due to the greater emphasis on evidence-based medicine (EBM) and the fast-growing need for high quality and reliable evidences to improve clinical decision-making and patient caring. A systematic review of the relevant external evidence provides a framework for the integration of the research, and meta-analysis offers a quantitative summary of the results. Nowadays, meta-analysis is not limited to a statistical approach, and defined as a systematic approach to identifying, appraising, synthesizing, and (if appropriate) combining the results of relevant studies to arrive at conclusions about the body of research.

25.1.2. *Objectives of meta-analysis*

Meta-analyses are conducted to assess the strength of evidence present on a disease and treatment. One aim is to determine whether an effect exists; another aim is to determine whether the effect is positive or negative and, ideally, to obtain a single summary estimate of the effect. The results of a meta-analysis can improve precision of estimates of effect, answer questions not posed by the individual studies, settle controversies arising from apparently conflicting studies, and generate new hypotheses. In particular, the examination of heterogeneity is vital to the development of new hypotheses.

(1) To increase statistical power

Meta-analysis effectively provides a gain in statistical power for average estimates. In clinical trials, a single study often cannot detect or exclude with certainty a modest, albeit clinically relevant, difference in the effects of two treatments. If data from more than one study are available and can be combined, the "sample size" and, thus, power increase, and relatively small effects can be detected or excluded with confidence.

It is important to be familiar with the type of data (e.g. dichotomous, continuous) that result from measurement of an outcome in an individual study, and to choose suitable effect measures for comparing intervention groups.

Most meta-analysis methods are variations on a weighted average of the effect estimates from the different studies.

Studies with no events contribute no information about the risk ratio or odds ratio. For rare events, the Peto method has been observed to be less biased and more powerful than other methods.

Variation across studies (heterogeneity) must be considered, although most Cochrane Reviews do not have enough studies to allow for the reliable investigation of its causes. Random effects meta-analyses allow for heterogeneity by assuming that underlying effects follow a normal distribution, but they must be interpreted carefully. Prediction intervals from random effects meta-analyses are a useful device for presenting the extent of between-study variation.

Many judgments are required in the process of preparing a meta-analysis. Sensitivity analyses should be used to examine whether overall findings are robust to potentially influential decisions.

(2) To improve estimate of effect size.

Meta-analysis has historically been useful in summarizing prior research based on randomized trials when individual studies are too small to yield a valid conclusion. Results from studies may disagree as to the magnitude of effects or, of more concern, as to the direction of effects. By integrating the actual evidence, meta-analysis allows a more objective appraisal, which can help to resolve uncertainties when the original studies, classic reviews, and editorial comments disagree. As an effective tool for quantitative synthesis, meta-analysis may resolve issues relating to inconsistent or conflicting results from studies, provide the pooled estimate of effect size with a more precise confidence interval, and draw an explicit conclusion.

(3) To assess the disagreement and generalizability of study results.

Studies for same topic may use different eligibility criteria for participants, different definitions of disease, different methods of measuring or defining exposure, or different variations of treatment. It means there is heterogeneity between studies. When heterogeneity is large enough to be detected by a statistical test, it is important to explore its source. Meta-analysis also systematically assesses the biases and confounding in primary studies. On the other hand, meta-analysis can contribute to considerations about the generalizability of study results. The findings of a particular study may be valid only for a specific population of patients with the same characteristics as those investigated in the trial. In particular, the examination of heterogeneity is vital to the development of new hypotheses.

(4) To answer new questions those were not previously posed in the individual studies.

Meta-analysis includes the epidemiological exploration and evaluation of results, new ideas (hypotheses) that were not posed in the individual studies can thus be developed and tested for further research and further original studies. Moreover, the results of the subgroup meta-analysis can evaluate safety in a subgroup of patients, or a rare adverse event in all patients.

25.2. The main stages involved in a meta-analysis

Meta-analysis should be viewed as an observational study of the evidence. The steps involved are similar to any other research undertaking: formulation of the problem to be addressed, collection and analysis of the data, and reporting of the results.

25.2.1. *Formulating the problem*

As with any research, a meta-analysis begins with a well-formulated question and design. Meta-analysis can, in general, be motivated by a number of factors. It can be conducted in an effect to resolve conflicting evidence, to answer the questions where the answer is uncertain or to explain variations in practice.

A well-formulated question is essential for determining the structure of a meta-analysis. For framing an answerable question in a meta-analysis, use the PICO framework.

PICO is an acronym for "Participant-Intervention-Comparison-Outcome." These components of the question, with the additional specification of types of study that will be included, form the basis of the pre-specified eligibility criteria for the review. Participant here refers to individuals or population of interest to us. Intervention needs to be as broadly or as narrowly defined keeping only the interventions of our interest. Note that meta-analyses are not necessarily restricted only to randomized controlled trials, these are now increasingly applied to observational study designs as well for example cohort and case control studies; in these situations, we refer to the specific exposure variables of our interest. Meta-analyses are also conducted for diagnostic and screening studies. Likewise, the comparison group is important as well. The comparison group can be "no intervention," or "placebo," or "usual treatment." The outcomes that we are interested in can be narrowly or broadly defined based on the objective of the meta-analysis.

Once the problem is defined, developing a detail study protocol is essential. A protocol is the blueprint for conduct of the meta-analysis. The protocol should clearly state the objectives, the background, the hypotheses to be tested, the subgroups of interest, and the proposed methods and criteria for identifying and selecting relevant studies and extracting and analyzing information. The statement of objectives should be concise and specific.

25.2.2. *Searching the relevant information*

It is important to identify all studies which could potentially contribute to the meta-analysis. In order to minimize problems associated with selection bias, a comprehensive, unbiased information search is essential, and a highly sensitive search strategy should be undertaken, that is, find as many studies as possible, although it may result in relatively low precision. In addition to conducting a search of the popular online biomedical databases, such as PubMed, EMBASE, Web of Science, Scopus and CENTRAL (Cochrane Central Register of Controlled Trials),we should attempt to obtain relevant information from subject-specific databases (e.g., CINAHL for nursing), dissertations and theses databases, grey literature (e.g., abstracts of conference), clinical trials registers, expert informants and pharmaceutical industry, especially those unpublished and ongoing studies.

25.2.3. *Selecting the studies eligible for inclusion*

Studies are chosen for meta-analysis on the basis of inclusion and exclusion criteria. Generally, highly restrictive eligibility criteria tend to give meta-analysis greater validity. But the criteria may be so restrictive and require so much homogeneity as to limit the eligible studies to only one or two studies, which is conflicting with one of the goals of meta-analysis as a method to increase statistical power. However, less restrictive criteria may lead to the accusation that the meta-analysis "mixes apples and organs."

The process of determining whether studies are eligible for inclusion should be systematic and rigorous. To ensure reproducibility and minimize bias in selecting studies, the key components about eligibility for a meta-analysis, including study population, study design, interventions or exposures, outcomes, and presence of a particular condition such as the severity of disease, dose or intensity of interventions, need to be addressed.

In practice, the citations or abstracts in databases are browsed in search process, and those obviously unrelated to the topic are eliminated. The full-text of the remaining articles is then collected. These articles are read quickly, and those clearly irrelevant ones are excluded. The remaining publications are then systematically reviewed to determine whether they are eligible for the meta-analysis based on predetermined criteria for eligibility. The reference lists of the articles that contain useful information are searched for more references, then the new publications retrieved, and the process is repeated again and again, until all potential on the topic are identified.

25.2.4. *Abstracting the data*

The process of abstraction of information from eligible studies should be reliable, valid, and free of bias. Standardized data collecting forms should be designed carefully to target the objectives of the review. The key components of a data collecting form generally include study characteristic with methods, participants, interventions, outcome measures and results.

To avoid the selection bias, assessment of eligibility of studies, and extraction of data from study reports, should be done by at least two people, independently, and experts should be consulted for disagreement. Furthermore, the abstractors should be blinded to the information of the author, the journal, and the funding sources to be identified. It is believed that these factors possibly influence the judgment of the abstractor.

25.2.5. *Assessing the risk of bias in included studies*

The validity of a study is the extent to which its design and conduct are likely to prevent systematic errors, or bias. Generally, in clinical trials, biases can be broadly categorized as selection bias, performance bias, detection bias, attrition bias, reporting bias and other biases that do not fit into these categories.

Numerous tools are developed for assessing the methodological quality of clinical trials. A widely used tool introduced by the Cochrane Collaboration for assessing risk of bias is a "risk of bias" table, which addresses the seven specific domains, i.e., sequence generation (selection bias), allocation sequence concealment (selection bias), blinding of participants and personnel (performance bias), blinding of outcome assessment (detection bias), incomplete outcome data (attrition bias), selective outcome reporting (reporting bias) and other potential sources of bias. The tool assigns a judgment for each entry involves assessing the risk of bias as "low risk," as "high risk," or as "unclear risk," with the last category indicating either lack of information or uncertainty over the potential for bias.

25.2.6. *Analyzing data and presenting results*

The process of quantitative combining the data is the key step for meta-analysis. The main procedures involved in the statistical analysis are: defining the outcome; heterogeneity test for the effect size; model choice (fixed-effect model or random effects model); pooled estimate of effect size (point estimate and confidence interval estimate); hypothesis test for overall effect size and graphic display of the results.

25.2.7. *Interpreting results and drawing conclusions*

Meta-analysis is essentially viewed as an observational study. The results of meta-analysis should be interpreted with caution in discussion.

Variation across studies (heterogeneity) must be considered. Investigating and explaining the source of heterogeneity are critically important component of meta-analysis, when there is "statistically significant" heterogeneity across studies.

Sensitivity analysis should be conducted to examine whether overall findings are robust to potentially influential decisions. For example, if the eligibility of some studies in the meta-analysis is dubious because they do not contain full details, sensitivity analysis may involve undertaking the meta-analysis twice: first, including all studies and second, only including those that are definitely known to be eligible.

Subgroup analysis is necessary when treatment effect varies according to patient-level covariance or trial-level characteristics. Ideally, if individual patient data in each eligible study can be obtained, a standardized subgroup analysis can be performed.

Bias may seriously influence the validity and reliability of results, which occurs at multiple steps in the process of meta-analysis, and more attention needs to be paid to detect and assess of the bias.

Finally, when reporting the conclusion, we should summarize the key finding, interpret the results in light of the total of available evidence, and suggest a future research agenda.

25.3. Statistical methods for meta-analysis

The primary studies included in meta-analysis may report several different end points. It is very important to select pooled statistic that is comparable across all studies. First, we should identify the data type for the outcome measurements. Here, we just consider outcome data to be of two most frequent types: one is measures based on dichotomous (or binary) data, where each individual outcome is one of only two possible categorical responses; another is measures based on continuous data, where each individual outcome is a measurement of a numerical quantity.

For dichotomous data, summary measure may generally be thought of as odds ratio (OR), risk ratio (RR, also called the relative risk), or risk differences (RD, also called the absolute risk reduction). OR is the ratio of the odds for the treated group to the odds for the control group, RR is the ratio of two probabilities, and RD is the difference between two probabilities. RD is easy to interpret, which reflects both the underlying risk without treatment and the risk reduction associated with treatment. Taking the reciprocal of the RD gives the "number needed to treat" (NNT), i.e., the number of patients needed to be treated to prevent one event, which is very useful in making a decision in clinical practice.

For continuous data, mean difference (also called weighted mean difference, WMD), can be used as a summary statistic when outcome measurements in all studies are made on the same scale, which measures the absolute difference between the mean value in two groups in a study. When there is no direct measure common to all studies, it is necessary to standardize the results of the studies to a uniform scale before they can be combined, and standardized mean difference (SMD), is used as a scale-free summary statistic, which is calculated as the difference of means divided by the variability of the measures.

There are at least two sources of variation to consider before combining summary statistics across studies. One is the inner- or within-study variation, which is derived from sampling error. In general, the sampling error may be relatively small for studies with large sample sizes, which means high degrees of precision and large weight would be given. The other is the inter- or between study variation.

Meta-analyses use either a fixed-effect or a random effects statistical model. A fixed-effect (FE) meta-analysis assumes all studies are estimating the same (fixed) treatment effect. In other words, there is no between study heterogeneity in the true treatment effect. The implication of this model is that the observed treatment effect estimates vary only because of chance differences created from sampling patients. By contrast, a random effects meta-analysis model assumes the observed estimates of treatment effect can vary across studies because of real differences in the treatment effect in each study as well as sampling variability (chance). Such heterogeneity in treatment effects may be caused by differences in study populations, interventions received, follow-up length, and other factors. Study weights are more balanced under the random-effects model than under the fixed-effect model. Large studies are assigned less relative weight and small studies are assigned more relative weight as compared with the fixed-effect model.

Most existing methods for meta-analysis yield a weighted average of the results of the individual studies, and what differs is the manner in which these weights are allocated and also the manner in which the uncertainty is computed around the point estimate thus generated. Here we introduce several classical statistical methods of meta-analysis.

25.3.1. *Statistical methods for dichotomous data*

Suppose there are K studies for binary discrete measurements included in the meta-analysis, whose data are in the form of 2×2 tables (see Table 25.1). We denote a_i, b_i, c_i, and d_i as the number of observations in each of the cells defined by the treatment and outcome table, with m_{1i} subjects in the treatment group and m_{2i} in the control group. OR, RR and RD are the three potential study summary statistics. OR and RR are typically analyzed on a logarithmic scale with normal distribution approximation, and the confidence intervals for OR and RR are also computed on the logarithmic

Table 25.1 Data for 2×2 table with a binary outcome

	Treated group (Exposed)	Control group (Not exposed)	Total
Success (Case)	a_i	b_i	n_{1i}
Failure (Control)	c_i	d_i	n_{2i}
Total	m_{1i}	m_{2i}	T_i

scale, and then transformed back to the original scale. RD defined for boundary values (proportions of 0 or 1), and is approximately normally distributed for the modest sample sizes.

(1) Fixed-effect model

A. Generic inverse-variance method

One of the most frequently used approaches in meta-analysis is commonly referred to as the generic inverse-variance method (I-V method), which can be applied to both dichotomous and continuous data. In the inverse variance method, the weight given to each study is chosen to be the inverse of the variance of the effect estimate (i.e. 1 over the square of its standard error). Thus, larger studies, which have smaller standard errors, are given more weight than smaller studies, which have larger standard errors. This choice of weights minimizes the imprecision (uncertainty) of the pooled effect estimate. For fixed-effect model, inverse-variance method allows meta-analysis with odds ratio, risk ratio, or risk difference risk as the measure of effect.

Example 25.1. Meta-analysis for effect of nitric oxide on mortality in acute lung injury

Acute lung injury (ALI) and acute respiratory distress syndrome (ARDS) are life-threatening diseases, which are characterized by severe hypoxemia, hypercapnia, and diffuse infiltration in the chest X-ray. Nitric oxide (NO) is a selective pulmonary vasodilator and has anti-inflammatory properties; the possibility of using inhaled NO generated considerable interest. Based on limited data on efficacy, clinicians rapidly adopted this therapy. However, whether inhaled NO can improve the final outcome of ALI/ARDS patients or whether it can reduce the mortality of ALI/ARDS patients, has been controversial in clinical practice, and the results reported in the literature are also inconsistent. Adhikari NK *et al.* published a meta-analysis at BMJ in 2007 that included nine RCT studies to quantitatively assess the effect of inhaled NO on mortality in patients with established ALI or ARDS. Table 25.2 presents data from the nine RCT.

Table 25.2 Data from nine RCTs investigating the effect of inhaled NO for ALI/ARDS

	NO group		Control group		
Studies	Death a_i	Case n_{1i}	Death c_i	Case n_{2i}	Risk ratio (RR_i)
1 Dellinger 1998	35	120	17	57	0.978
2 Michael 1998	11	20	9	20	.222
3 Troncy 1998	9	15	8	15	1.125
4 Lundin 1999	41	93	35	87	1.096
5 Payen 1999	48	98	46	105	1.118
6 Mehta 2001	4	8	2	6	1.500
7 Gerlach 2003	3	20	4	20	0.750
8 Park 2003	4	11	2	6	1.091
9 Taylor 2004	44	192	39	193	1.134

Source: Adhikari NK, Burns KE, Friedrich JO, *et al.* Effect of nitric oxide on oxygenation and mortality in acute lung injury: systematic review and meta-analysis. BMJ, 2007, 334 (7597):779–786.

Inverse-variance method is used to estimate a summary risk ratio and its 95% confidence interval for these data as follows:

① Calculate the risk ratio (RR_i) for each included study

$$RR_i = \frac{a_i}{n_{1i}} / \frac{c_i}{n_{2i}} = \frac{a_i n_{2i}}{c_i n_{1i}} \tag{25-1}$$

② Let $y_i = ln(RR_i)$, calculate the variance s_i^2 of y_i, and the weight w_i of y_i. The results are shown in Table 25.3

$$s_i^2 = \frac{1}{a_i} - \frac{1}{n_{1i}} + \frac{1}{c_i} - \frac{1}{n_{2i}} \tag{25-2}$$

$$w_i = 1/s_i^2 \tag{25-3}$$

③ Heterogeneity test

Q statistic is calculated for the test of heterogeneity. Assuming the meta-analysis includes k studies, then

$$Q = \sum w_i(y_i - \overline{y})^2 = \sum w_i y_i^2 - \frac{(\sum w_i y_i)^2}{\sum w_i} \tag{25-4}$$

Q is approximately distributed as a χ^2 distribution on $k-1$ degrees of freedom. This test assumes the null hypothesis that all the studies are homogeneous, or that each study is measuring an identical effect, and a P-value is given to test this hypothesis, i.e., it assesses whether observed differences in results are compatible with chance alone. A low P-value (or a large χ^2 statistic relative to its degree of freedom) provides evidence of heterogeneity of intervention effects (variation in effect estimates beyond chance).

However, the statistical power of the Q test is low in the (common) situation of a meta-analysis when studies have small sample size or are few in number, implying that a nonsignificant result must not be taken as evidence of no heterogeneity. That is why using a cut-off significance level of 0.10, rather than the conventional 0.05, has become a customary practice in meta-analysis.

A useful statistic for quantifying inconsistency is

$$I^2 = \frac{Q-(K-1)}{Q} \times 100\% \tag{25-5}$$

I^2 index describes the percentage of total variation across studies that are due to heterogeneity rather than chance. For example, an I^2 value of 10% indicates that only 10% of the total variability is due to true heterogeneity, and 90% is due to sampling error of the included individual studies. Negative values of $I^2$are put equal to zero so that I^2 lies between 0% and 100%. A value of 0% indicates no observed heterogeneity, and there is no absolute rule for what is considered an acceptable degree of heterogeneity. It has been suggested that $I^2 < 30\%$ could be considered "mild" heterogeneity, and I^2 between 30% and 50% to be "moderate" heterogeneity, and greater than 50% to be "severe" heterogeneity.

For Example 25.1, Q statistic is calculated using equation (25-4) and data presented in Table 25.3.

$$Q = \sum w_i(y_i - \overline{y})^2 = \sum w_i y_i^2 - \frac{(\sum w_i y_i)^2}{\sum w_i} = 2.317 - \frac{14.393^2}{144.731}$$
$$= 0.886$$

Table 25.3 Calculations used in the meta-analysis of inhaled NO for ALI/ARDS

Studies	y_i	s_i^2	w_i	w_iy_i	$w_iy_i^2$
1	−0.022	0.062	16.255	−0.363	0.008
2	0.201	0.102	9.802	1.967	0.395
3	0.118	0.103	9.730	1.146	0.135
4	0.092	0.031	32.558	2.980	0.273
5	0.112	0.023	43.774	4.883	0.545
6	0.405	0.458	2.182	0.885	0.359
7	−0.288	0.483	2.069	−0.595	0.171
8	0.087	0.492	2.031	0.177	0.015
9	0.126	0.038	26.331	3.313	0.417
Total			144.731	14.393	2.317

In this case, $df = 8, \chi^2_{(0.1,8)} = 13.36 > 0.886, P > 0.1$. At a critical value of 0.10, the null hypothesis that all studies are estimating the same underlying treatment effect is not rejected, it can be concluded that the studies are homogeneous. The value of another statistic, I^2 is 0%, suggesting no observed heterogeneity as well.

Thus, the test for heterogeneity of the effect of inhaled NO for ALI/ARDS between the included nine studies shows no statistical evidence for differences, and it would seem valid to combine the studies using a fixed-effect model.

④ Calculate the summary risk ratio. In this case, we use fixed-effect model to combine the risk ratio.

$$RR_{\text{I-V}} = \exp\left[\frac{\sum w_i \ln(RR_i)}{\sum w_i}\right] \tag{25-6}$$

Using equation (25-6) and data presented in Table 25.3, the combined risk ratio is given by

$$\begin{aligned} RR_{\text{I-V}} &= \exp\left[\frac{\sum w_i \ln(RR_i)}{\sum w_i}\right] = \exp\left[\frac{\sum w_i y_i}{\sum w_i}\right] \\ &= \exp\left[\frac{14.393}{144.731}\right] = \exp(0.0994) = 1.104 \end{aligned}$$

⑤ Calculate the 95% confidence interval for the summary risk ratio

$$\exp\left[\ln(RR_{\mathrm{I-V}}) \pm \frac{1.96}{\sqrt{\sum w_i}}\right] \tag{25-7}$$

In this case, the 95% confidence interval for the summary risk ratio is

$$\exp\left[\ln(RR_{\mathrm{I-V}}) \pm \frac{1.96}{\sqrt{\sum w_i}}\right] = \exp\left[0.0994 \pm \frac{1.96}{12.03}\right] = (0.938, 1.30)$$

⑥ Report the overall effect and graphical representation of the results

In Example 25.1, the combined risk ratio is 1.104, indicating that inhaled NO may increase the risk of death by 10.4%; the 95% confidence interval is 0.938 to 1.30, including 1, and thus the results is statistically non-significant. In general, the meta-analysis suggests that inhaled nitric oxide does not improve survival, and may even cause harm for patient with ALI/ARDS.

A forest plot is developed for use as a means of graphically representing the results of a meta-analysis, which is an essential tool to summarize information on individual studies, give a visual suggestion of the amount of study heterogeneity, and show the estimated common effect, all in one figure.

Figure 25.1 shows the forest plot of the meta-analysis from Example 25.1 created using RevMan 5. The nine included trials are identified by their principal author and date of publication on the left side. The number of events (deaths) and the total number of participants are shown for each treatment arm. The effect measure in Example 25.1 is risk ratio (RR), where values lower than 1.0 indicate that inhaled NO has lower risk of mortality than the control, and vice versa for values greater than 1.0. For each included trial, the estimated RR with a 95% confidence interval is shown both in numerical and graphical form in the forest plot. Each included study represented by a horizontal line. The point estimate of RR of the results of each study is represented as a square in the center of the line, and the size of the square is proportional to the weight of the trial, which indicates its relative impact on the calculations of the pooled effect. The width of the line shows the confidence intervals of the

Study or Subgroup	Nitric oxide Events	Nitric oxide Total	Control Events	Control Total	Weight	Risk Ratio IV, Fixed, 95% CI
Dellinger 1998	35	120	17	57	11.2%	0.98 [0.60, 1.59]
Gerlach 2003	3	20	4	20	1.4%	0.75 [0.19, 2.93]
Lundin 1999	41	93	35	87	22.5%	1.10 [0.78, 1.55]
Mehta 2001	4	8	2	6	1.5%	1.50 [0.40, 5.65]
Michael 1998	11	20	9	20	6.8%	1.22 [0.65, 2.29]
Park 2003	4	11	2	6	1.4%	1.09 [0.28, 4.32]
Payen 1999	48	98	46	105	30.2%	1.12 [0.83, 1.50]
Taylor 2004	44	192	39	193	18.2%	1.13 [0.77, 1.66]
Troncy 1998	9	15	8	15	6.7%	1.13 [0.60, 2.11]
Total (95% CI)		**577**		**509**	**100.0%**	**1.10 [0.94, 1.30]**
Total events	199		162			

Heterogeneity: Chi² = 0.89, df = 8 (P = 1.00); I² = 0%

Test for overall effect: Z = 1.20 (P = 0.23)

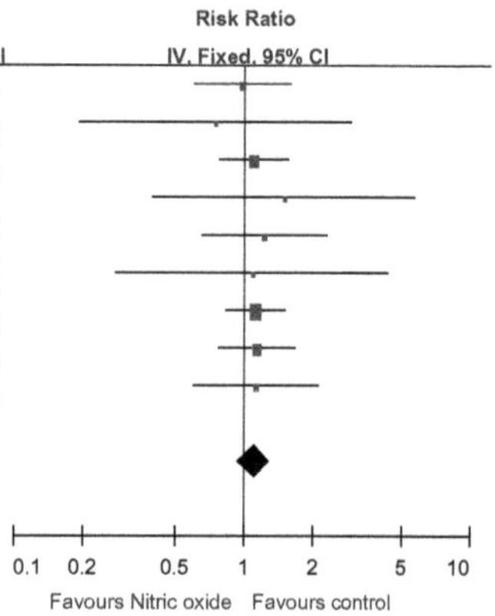

Figure 25.1 Forest plot for meta-analysis of inhaled NO for ALI/ARDS

effect estimate of individual studies. The diamond below the studies represents the overall effect, and its width shows the confidence intervals for the overall effect estimate.

In the forest plot, the solid vertical line in the center of the graph is called the "line of no effect," i.e., for studies that effect measure is ratio (e.g., risk ratio, odds ratio), the line of no effect is at 1; for studies that effect measure is difference (e.g., mean difference, risk difference), the line of no effect is at zero. When a horizontal line representing a study passes through the vertical "line of no effect," which indicates that the two treatments are not statistically different at the 95% confidence level. However, if horizontal line doesn't cross the vertical, it demonstrates a statistically significant effect. This same concept is also true for the overall effect at the bottom. In Figure 25.1, the total overall estimate of the risk ratio is presented in the row labeled "Total" and is equal to 1.10 (95% confidence interval is 0.94 to 1.30). It is represented graphically by the diamond; the center of the diamond equals the total overall estimated relative risk and the ends of the diamond indicate the limits of the 95% confidence interval. The meta-analysis therefore showed an overall 10% increase in the risk of mortality for inhaled NO relative to control treatment. Because the 95% confidence interval for the total overall estimate include 1.0, the increase in the risk of mortality is non-significant at the 5% level of significance. The P value for the test of significance of the total overall estimate was 0.23, as shown in the text "Test for overall effect: z = 1.20, P = 0.23," corroborating the inference from the 95% confidence interval. The value for z is the test statistic resulting from the statistical test used to derive the P value.

The forest plot also provides the information on statistical test for heterogeneity. As shown in Figure 25.1, I^2 statistic is equal to 0%, the test P value (quoted in brackets) is "1.00," which would indicate no heterogeneity between the included studies. The overall effect P value (quoted in brackets) is 0.23, and also shows no significant difference in mortality between inhaled NO group and control group for ALI/ARDS patients.

In Example 25.1, the effect measure is risk ratio. Generic inverse-variance method also can be used when the effect measure is odds ratio (OR) or risk difference (RD). The basic principles underlying the inverse-variance method is that the weight given to each study is chosen to be the inverse of the variance of the effect estimate. A fixed-effect meta-analysis using the inverse-variance method calculates a weighted average as

$$\theta_{I-V} = \frac{\sum (w_i y_i)}{\sum w_i} \tag{25-8}$$

Here, θ_{I-V} is the point estimate for the combined effect, which may be an $lnRR_{\text{combined}}$, $lnOR_{\text{combined}}$ or RD_{combined}, and y_i is the effect of the i_{th} inclusion study, which can be $lnRR_i$, $lnOR_i$ or RD_i. The calculation of the weight w_i is different, and the variance and weight of $lnRR_i$ are as shown in equations (25-2) and (25-3).

The weight of $lnOR_i$ is

$$w_i = 1/Var(lnOR_i) = 1 \Big/ \left(\frac{1}{a_i} + \frac{1}{b_i} + \frac{1}{c_i} + \frac{1}{d_i}\right) \tag{25-9}$$

The weight of RD is

$$w_i = 1/Var\,(RD) = 1 \Big/ \left(\frac{a_i b_i}{n_{1i}^3} + \frac{c_i d_i}{n_{2i}^3}\right) \tag{25-10}$$

The 95% confidence interval for the combined effect is

$$\theta_{I-V} \pm \frac{1.96}{\sqrt{\sum w_i}} \tag{25-11}$$

Note the statistical test for heterogeneity use the formula (25-4) and (25-5) to calculate the Q statistic, and I^2 statistic when adopting the inverse-variance method.

B. Mantel-Haenszel method

The Mantel-Haenszel method is a widely used approach for pooling data across strata. Since each study included in meta-analysis could be regarded as a stratum, Mantel-Haenszel method is appropriate for analyzing data for a meta-analysis. The method is based on the assumption of fixed-effect model, and the pooled measure is expressed as a combination of stratum-specific measures. Mantel-Haenszel method has been shown to have better statistical properties when there are a few events, and can be used when the measure of effect is odds ratio, risk ratio, and risk different, typical odds ratio.

Example 25.2. Meta-analysis of antibiotics versus placebo for common cold.

It is always controversial whether patients with upper respiratory tract infections in the common cold should be treated with antibiotics. To systematically assess the effectiveness of antibiotics in the treatment of the common cold, Arroll *et al.* collected the results from five RCTs comparing the antibiotics and placebo for common cold and conducted a meta-analysis. The outcome considered here is cure or general improvement in the first seven days after presenting symptoms. Table 25.4 gives basic information from the five trials included in the meta-analysis. The measure of effect is the odds ratio (OR), and the effect is combined by the Mantel-Haenszel method. Steps are as follows:

① Calculate the odds ratio (OR_i) and weight (w_i) for each included study. The results are shown in Table 25.4.

$$OR_i = \frac{a_i d_i}{b_i c_i} \tag{25-12}$$

$$w_i = \frac{b_i c_i}{T_i} \tag{25-13}$$

Here, $T_i = a_i + b_i + c_i + d_i$, as it is shown in Table 25.1.

Table 25.4 Data from five trials investigating the effectiveness of antibiotics versus placebo for the common cold

	antibiotics group		placebo group					
Studies	No. effective (a_i)	No. ineffective (b_i)	No. effective (c_i)	No. ineffective (d_i)	odds ratio (OR_i)	y_i	w_i	w'_i
1	67	87	69	86	0.96	−0.041	19.427	19.03
2	49	97	48	94	0.99	−0.011	16.167	16.08
3	166	8	83	4	1.00	0.00	2.544	2.54
4	9	4	10	6	1.35	0.300	1.379	1.59
5	117	12	56	3	0.52	−0.649	3.575	2.26
Total							43.092	41.5

Source: Sutton AJ, Abrams KR, Jones DR, *et al.* Methods for meta-analysis in medical research.

② Heterogeneity test

Let $y_i = lnOR_i$, calculate the Q statistic and I^2 statistic using equation (25-4), (25-5) and data presented in Table 25.4.

$$Q = \sum w'_i(y_i - \overline{y})^2 = \sum w'_i y_i^2 - \frac{(\sum w'_i y_i)^2}{\sum w'_i}$$

$$= 1.13 - \frac{(-1.914)^2}{41.5} = 1.042$$

Here, the weight, w'_i, is given by the inverse variance method, which is calculated by equation (25-9), and is not same as w_i calculated by equation (25-13).

In this example, $df = 4$, $\chi^2_{(0.1,4)} = 7.78 > 1.042, P > 0.1$, and $I^2 = 0$, thus, based on the Q statistic and I^2 statistic, it can be considered that five studies are homogenous.

③ Calculate the summary odds ratio. Here, fixed-effect model is adopted to pool the odds ratio.

$$OR_{M-H} = \frac{\sum w_i OR_i}{\sum w_i} = \frac{\sum (a_i d_i / T_i)}{\sum (b_i c_i / T_i)} \qquad (25\text{-}14)$$

Using equation (25-14), and data presented in Table 25.4, the combined odds ratio is given by

$$OR_{M-H} = \frac{\sum w_i OR_i}{\sum w_i} = \frac{\sum (a_i d_i / T_i)}{\sum (b_i c_i / T_i)} = \frac{40.914}{43.092} = 0.95$$

④ Calculate the 95% confidence interval for the summary odds ratio
First calculate the variance ($Var(lnOR_{M-H})$) of $lnOR_{M-H}$

$$Var(lnOR_{M-H}) = \frac{\sum F}{2(\sum R)^2} + \frac{\sum G}{2\sum R \sum S} + \frac{\sum H}{2(\sum S)^2}$$

Where $F = \frac{a_i d_i (a_i + d_i)}{T_i^2}$, $G = \frac{a_i d_i (b_i + c_i) + b_i c_i (a_i + d_i)}{T_i^2}$, $H = \frac{b_i c_i (b_i + c_i)}{T_i^2}$, $R = \frac{a_i d_i}{T_i}$, $S = \frac{b_i c_i}{T_i}$
The 95% confidence interval for combined $lnOR_{M-H}$ is

$$lnOR_{M-H} \pm 1.96\sqrt{Var(lnOR_{M-H})}$$

Thus the 95% confidence interval for summary odds ratio is given by

$$\exp\left[lnOR_{M-H} \pm 1.96\sqrt{Var\left(lnOR_{M-H}\right)}\right] \qquad (25\text{-}15)$$

In this example, F, G, H, R and S are calculated using the data presented in Table 25.4, and the $Var(lnOR_{M-H})$ is given by

$$Var\left(\ln OR_{M-H}\right) = \frac{\sum F}{2(\sum R)^2} + \frac{\sum G}{2\sum R \sum S} + \frac{\sum H}{2(\sum S)^2}$$
$$= 0.0063 + 0.012 + 0.0056 = 0.024$$

Using equation (25-15), the 95% confidence interval for summary odds ratio is

$$\exp\left(lnOR_{M-H} \pm 1.96\sqrt{Var\left(lnOR_{M-H}\right)}\right)$$
$$= \exp\left(ln0.95 \pm 1.96\sqrt{0.024}\right) = (0.70, 1.29)$$

⑤ Report the overall effect and graphical representation of the results

The combined odds ratio is 0.95, very close to 1, indicating that patient's recovery is very comparable in the antibiotic and placebo groups. The 95% confidence interval is 0.70 to 1.29, and around this estimate is reasonably wide, indicating considerable uncertainty in the pooled result. The conclusion that there is no evidence to suggest that antibiotics are effective at treating the common cold appears reasonable.

Forest plot for the meta-analysis in this case is omitted.

(2) Random effects model

The random effects model used in meta-analysis was described by DerSimonian and Laird in 1986, which was referred to as the D-L method. To undertake a random effects meta-analysis, the standard errors of the study-specific estimates are adjusted to incorporate a measure of the extent of variation, or heterogeneity, among the intervention effects observed in different studies. Therefore, studies are weighted with the inverse of their variance and the heterogeneity parameter.

Adjusted weight w_i^* for each of the studies is calculated as

$$w_i^* = \frac{1}{\tau^2 + (1/w_i)} \tag{25-16}$$

$$\tau^2 = \frac{(Q - (k-1))\sum w_i}{(\sum w_i)^2 - \sum w_i^2} \tag{25-17}$$

Where τ^2 is the between study variation, and Q is the heterogeneity test statistic defined in equation (25-4). Thus the random effects study weighting is given by the reciprocal of the sum of the between and within study variances, confirming that the random effect model reduces to the fixed-effect model when the between study variance τ^2 is estimated as 0.

In a heterogeneous set of studies, a random-effects meta-analysis will award relatively more weight to smaller studies than such studies would receive in a fixed-effect meta-analysis. This is because small studies are more informative for learning about the distribution of effects across studies than for learning about an assumed common intervention effect.

Note that a random-effects model does not "take account" of the heterogeneity, in the sense that it is no longer an issue. It is always preferable to explore possible causes of heterogeneity.

Example 25.3. Meta-analysis of main bleeding risks in patients with atrial fibrillation using a new oral anticoagulant versus warfarin

In recent years, several new oral anticoagulants (NOAC) have been developed. Ruff CT *et al.* performed a meta-analysis to compare the efficacy and safety of new oral anticoagulants with warfarin in patients with atrial fibrillation (AR) from four multi-center randomized controlled trials (RE-LY, ROCKET AF, ARISTOTLE, and ENGAGE AF-TIMI 48). Table 25.5 shows data about major bleeding in patients with atrial fibrillation who were treated with a new oral anticoagulant or warfarin in four included trials. The effect measure is the risk ratio (RR). The process of meta-analysis is as follows:

① Calculate the risk ratio (RR_i) for each included study.
② Let $y_i = ln(RR_i)$, calculate the variance s_i^2 of y_i, the weight w_i of y_i, also $w_i y_i$, $w_i y_i^2$, and the results are presented in Table 25.5.

Table 25.5 Data from four RCTs comparing major bleeding in patients with AR using NOAC or warfarin

	NOAC	Warfarin					
Studies	Events/Total	Events/Total	RR	y_i	w_i	w_i^*	$w_i^* y_i$
1	375/6076	397/6022	0.936	−0.066	205.977	37.237	−2.455
2	395/7111	386/7125	1.025	0.025	206.554	37.256	0.932
3	327/9088	462/9052	0.705	−0.350	199.916	37.034	−12.946
4	444/7012	557/7012	0.797	−0.227	265.791	38.816	−8.801
Total					878.238	150.344	−23.271

1: RE-LY; 2:ROCKETAF, 3:ARISTOTLE, 4:ENGAGEAF-TIMI 48. AR=atrial fibrillation. NOAC=new oral anticoagulant. RR=risk ratio.
Source: RuffCT, Giugliano RP, Braunwald E, *et al.* Comparison of the efficacy and safety of new oral anticoagulants with warfarin in patients with atrial fibrillation: a meta-analysis of randomised trials. Lancet, 2014, 383:955–962.

③ Heterogeneity test
Calculate the Q statistic and I^2 statistic using equation (25-4), (25-5) and data presented in Table 25.5.

$$Q = \sum w_i(y_i - \overline{y})^2 = \sum w_i y_i^2 - \frac{(\sum w_i y_i)^2}{\sum w_i}$$

$$= 39.12 - \frac{(-138.566)^2}{878.238} = 17.257$$

$$I^2 = \frac{Q-(K-1)}{Q} \times 100\% = 82.6\%$$

In this example, $df = 3$, $\chi^2_{(0.1,3)} = 6.25 < 17.257$, $P < 0.1$, and $I^2 = 82.6\%$, based on the Q statistic and I^2 statistic, it appears to be considerable heterogeneity between the trials. Hence, explorations of heterogeneity are essential, and it is clearly of interest to determine the causes of heterogeneity among results of those four RCTs. If we still wish to combine the results, it would appear that a random effects model would be more appropriate in conducting meta-analysis.

④ Calculate the between study variationτ^2
Using equation (25-17) and data presented in Table 25.5, τ^2 is given by

$$\tau^2 = \frac{(Q-(k-1))\sum w_i}{(\sum w_i)^2 - \sum w_i^2} = \frac{(17.257-(4-1))\times 878.238}{878.238^2 - 195702.227} = 0.022$$

⑤ Calculate the adjusted weight w_i^* by D-L method using equation (25-16). The results are shown in Table 25.5.

⑥ Calculate the combined risk ratio by D-L method

$$RR_{D-L} = \exp\left[\frac{\sum w_i^* \ln(RR_i)}{\sum w_i^*}\right] \qquad (25\text{-}18)$$

Entering the values from Table 25.5 into equation (25-18) gives the combined risk ratio

$$RR_{D-L} = \exp\left[\frac{\sum w_i^* \ln(RR_i)}{\sum w_i^*}\right] = \exp\left[\frac{\sum w_i^* y_i}{\sum w_i^*}\right]$$

$$= \exp\left[\frac{-23.271}{150.344}\right] = \exp(-0.155) = 0.857$$

⑦ Calculate the 95% confidence interval for the combined risk ratio

$$\exp\left[\ln(RR_{D-L}) \pm \frac{1.96}{\sqrt{\sum w_i^*}}\right] \tag{25-19}$$

In this case, the 95% confidence interval is calculated using equation (25-19)

$$\exp\left[\ln(RR_{D-L}) \pm \frac{1.96}{\sqrt{\sum w_i^*}}\right] = \exp\left[-0.155 \pm \frac{1.96}{12.261}\right]$$
$$= (0.73, 1.00)$$

⑧ Report the overall effect and graphical representation of the results

The combined risk ratio is 0.857, and the 95% confidence interval is 0.73 to 1.00, indicating that new oral anticoagulant is associated with a 14% non-significant reduction in major bleeding compared to warfarin.

Figure 25.2 shows the forest plot of the results of this meta-analysis, giving the summary information on each trial, visual suggestion of the heterogeneity test, and the estimate of the overall effect.

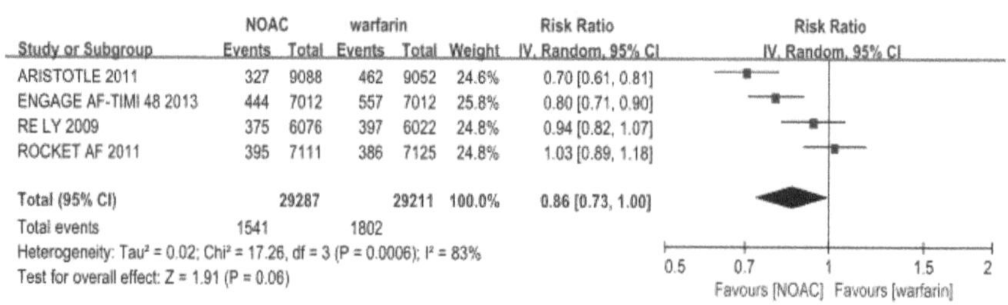

Figure 25.2 Forest plot for meta-analysis of major bleeding of NOAC vs. warfarin for atrial fibrillation

25.3.2. *Statistical methods for continuous data*

1. Fixed-effect model

Suppose n_{1i} and n_{2i} are the sample sizes, and x_{1i} and x_{2i} are the means, in the treatment and control group, respectively. Let $y_i = \overline{x}_{1i} - \overline{x}_{2i}$, with standard error, s_i, calculated as

$$s_i^2 = s_{p_i}^2\left(\frac{1}{n_{1i}} + \frac{1}{n_{2i}}\right), \quad s_{p_i}^2 = \frac{(n_{1i}-1)s_{1i}^2 + (n_{2i}-1)s_{2i}^2}{N_i - 2}$$

Where $N_i = n_{1i} + n_{2i}$, s_{1i}^2 and s_{2i}^2 are the treatment and control group variance, respectively, and $s_{p_i}^2$ is the estimate of the variance of the pooled sample, of the ith study.

(1) Outcomes defined on their original metric (mean difference), y_i is to be the measure of treatment effect, then the pooled estimate of the treatment effect is given by

$$y_{\text{combined}} = \frac{\sum w_i y_i}{\sum w_i}, w_i = \frac{1}{s_i^2} \tag{25-20}$$

The 95% confidence interval for the pooled effect is

$$y_{\text{combined}} \pm \frac{1.96}{\sqrt{\sum w_i}} \tag{25-21}$$

(2) Outcomes defined using standardized mean differences, the effect size of an experiment, d, is defined as

$$d_i = \frac{\overline{x}_{1i} - \overline{x}_{2i}}{s_{p_i}} \tag{25-22}$$

The variance of d_i, s_i^2, is difficult to compute exactly. However, if the underlying data can be assumed to be normal, the variance of d_i, can be estimated as

$$s_i^2 = \frac{N_i}{n_{1i}n_{2i}} + \frac{d_i^2}{2(N_i - 2)} \tag{25-23}$$

Thus, the point estimate of the combined effect size is given by

$$d_{\text{combined}} = \frac{\sum w_i d_i}{\sum w_i} w_i = \frac{1}{s_i^2} \tag{25-24}$$

The 95% confidence interval for the combined effect size is given by

$$d_{\text{combined}} \pm \frac{1.96}{\sqrt{w_i}} \tag{25-25}$$

Hegdes stated that the estimate d_i has small sample bias, and a correction equation has been derived

$$g_i = d_i \left(1 - \frac{3}{4N - 9}\right) \tag{25-26}$$

The variance of g_i, s_i^2, can be estimated as

$$s_i^2 = \frac{N_i}{n_{1i} n_{2i}} + \frac{g_i^2}{2(N_i - 3.94)} \tag{25-27}$$

In practice, if the sample sizes, n_{1i} and n_{2i}, are both large, the difference between d_i and g_i is almost negligible.

Example 25.4. Meta-analysis of antidepressant efficacy of agomelatine

Agomelatine is a novel antidepressant approved in February 2009 for use in the European Union. It is thought to act through a combination of antagonist activity at $5HT_{2C}$ receptors and agonist activity at melatonergic MT_1/MT_2 receptors. As such, for its unique pharmacology, agomelatine is not only used to treat major depressive disorder but also significantly improves sleep quality. Taylor D *et al.* conducted a meta-analysis of the effectiveness of agomelatine in antidepressant therapy. Table 25.6 shows data from five published RCTs, which comparing the effects of agomelatine and placebo in the treatment of depression. The main outcome was the change in mean scores on a depression rating scale at the end of treatment, using established depression rating scales such as the Hamilton rating scale for depression (HAM-D)7 or the Montgomery-Åsberg depression rating scale (MADRS). The summary measure of treatment effect is the standardized mean difference (SMD).

Table 25.6 Data from five published RCTs for the antidepressant efficacy of agomelatine versus placebo

Studies	Agomelatine group Cases (n_{1i})	Depression scale ($\overline{x}_{1i}$)	Standard deviation (s_{1i})	Cases (n_{2i})	Depression scale ([$\overline{x}_{2i}$)	Standard deviation (s_{2i})
1 Kennedy 2006	106	14.1	7.7	105	16.5	7.4
2 Loo 2002	135	12.8	8.2	136	15.3	8.9
3 Olie 2007	116	13.9	7.7	119	17	7.9
4 Stahl 2010	319	15.5	8.1	163	17.1	7.9
5 Zajecka 2010	317	15	7.8	167	16.6	8.4

Source: Taylor D, Sparshatt A, Varma S, *et al.* Antidepressant efficacy of agomelatine: meta-analysis of published and unpublished studies, BMJ. 2014, 348:g1888.

Table 25.7 Meta-analysis of the efficacy of published agomelatine versus placebo antidepressant treatment

Studies	d_i	s_i^2	w_i	$w_i d_i$	$w_i d_i^2$
1 Kennedy 2006	−0.318	0.019	52.737	−16.552	5.260
2 Loo 2002	−0.292	0.015	67.739	−19.580	5.719
3 Olie 2007	−0.397	0.017	58.721	−22.884	9.093
4 Stahl 2010	−0.199	0.009	107.870	−21.391	4.261
5 Zajecka 2010	−0.200	0.009	109.370	−21.745	4.343
Total			396.438	−102.153	28.676

① Calculate the difference d_i of the standardized mean of each included study: $d_i = \frac{\overline{x}_{1i}-\overline{x}_{2i}}{s_{p_i}}$, and the variance s_i^2 of d_i, the weight w_i and $w_i d_i, w_i d_i^2$. The results are listed in Table 25.7.

② Heterogeneity test

Calculate the Q statistic and I^2statistic using equation (25-4), (25-5) and data from Table 25.7.

$$Q = \sum w_i d_i^2 - \frac{(\sum w_i d_i)^2}{\sum w_i} = 28.676 - \frac{(-102.153)^2}{396.438} = 2.122$$

In this example, df=4, $\chi^2_{(0.1,4)} = 7.78 > 2.122, P > 0.1$, and I^2 =0, the results of heterogeneity test indicate that included studies are considered to be homogenous.

③ Calculate the pooled SMD and the 95% confidence interval for combined SMD using equation (25-24), (25-25).

$$d_{\text{combined}} = \frac{\sum w_i d_i}{\sum w_i} = \frac{-102.153}{396.438} = -0.26$$

$$d_{\text{combined}} \pm \frac{1.96}{\sqrt{\sum w_i}} = -0.26 \pm \frac{1.96}{19.911} = (-0.359,\ -0.161)$$

From the meta-analysis of the five RCTs, the point estimate of SMD is -0.26, i.e., on average, agomelatine reduced the scale score of patients with depression by 0.26 times the standard deviation compared with placebo. The 95% confidence interval for combined SMD is (−0.359, −0.161), excluding 0, indicating a statistically significant difference from 0. Compared with placebo, agomelatine reduced the scale score of patients with depression by 0.161 to 0.359 times of the standard deviation.

④ Report the overall effect and graphical representation of the results

Figure 25.3 is the forest plot showing the efficacy of published agomlelatine versus placebo in antidepressant treatment. The left side is the basic data for each included study, the estimated point, 95% *CI* of the SMD, combined SMD, heterogeneity test, and Z-test results for combined SMD.

25.3.3. *Random-effects model*

The meta-analysis of the random effects model of continuous variables can also be combined by the DerSimonian-Laird method whose

	Agomelatine			Placebo				Std. Mean Difference
Study or Subgroup	Mean	SD	Total	Mean	SD	Total	Weight	IV, Fixed, 95% CI
Kennedy 2006	14.1	7.7	106	16.5	7.4	105	13.3%	-0.32 [-0.59, -0.05]
Loo 2002	12.8	8.2	135	15.3	8.9	136	17.1%	-0.29 [-0.53, -0.05]
Olie 2007	13.9	7.7	116	17	7.9	119	14.7%	-0.40 [-0.65, -0.14]
Stahl 2010	15.5	8.1	319	17.1	7.9	163	27.3%	-0.20 [-0.39, -0.01]
Zajecka 2010	15	7.8	317	16.6	8.4	167	27.7%	-0.20 [-0.39, -0.01]
Total (95% CI)			993			690	100.0%	-0.26 [-0.36, -0.16]

Heterogeneity: Chi² = 2.10, df = 4 (P = 0.72); I² = 0%
Test for overall effect: Z = 5.14 (P < 0.00001)

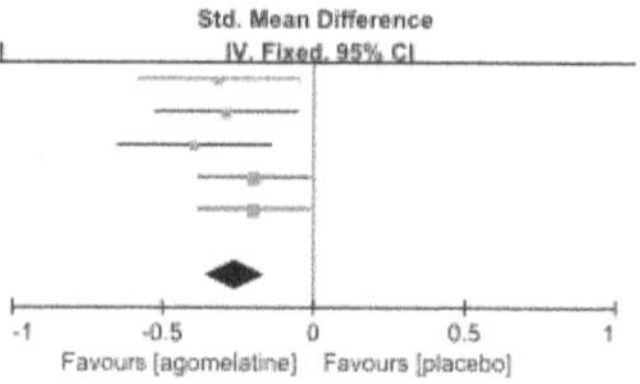

Figure 25.3 Forest plot presenting the results of the meta-analysis for the efficacy of published agomlelatine versus placebo in antidepressant treatment

principle is the same as the random effects model of the binary categorical variables, i.e., the adjusted weight w_i^* for each of the studies and the between study variation τ^2 should be calculated first, using equation (25-16) and (25-17), then the combined effect size is obtained by formula (25-20) or (25-24) using the corrected weight w_i^*.

25.4. Publication bias

Meta-analysis can be considered as an observational study of the evidence. In each step of meta-analysis, bias may be introduced intentionally or unintentionally, consciously or unconsciously. Biases often cause conflicting results of meta-analysis and threaten its internal validity and reliability.

Publication bias is usually used to refer to the greater likelihood of research with statistically significant results to be submitted and published compared with non-significant and null results. More generally, publication bias is the systematic error in a statistical inference by conditioning on the achievement of publication status. If a meta-analyst is restricted only to the published studies, then there is a risk that it will lead to biased conclusions because there may be many nonsignificant studies, which are often unpublished and hence are ignored, and it is quite possible that their combined effect, significant and nonsignificant studies together, may change the overall conclusion. Publication bias thus results from ignoring unavailable nonsignificant studies, and this is the familiar file-drawer problem.

Publication bias can originate from three sources: the authors, research sponsors, peer reviewers and editors of journals. First, the authors may be less likely write up and submit to journals when the results were considered to be negative or nonsignificant. Sometimes investigators may have resulted from multiple studies that could be publishable, and they usually focused on "wonderful results" and had no time for "negative results." Second, the editors and reviews of the journal may favor publication of positive results. Finally, the sponsor of the study may play an important role in generating publication bias, especially if it is a pharmaceutical company funded study. Many cases have been described in which the publication of studies with negative results has been suppressed by pharmaceutical companies. In addition, the publication of non-industry-sponsored studies may also be suppressed or delayed for various reasons.

Various methods have been introduced to detect and correct publication bias, but none of the available methods are entirely satisfactory for dealing with this problem. In practice, a funnel plot is frequently used to estimate the risk of publication bias in meta-analyses. The basic idea is that if the point estimates from individual studies are plotted against the inverse of the variances, or other surrogate for sample size, the points visualized together should produce a funnel shape, so they are scattered around the true value of the point estimate with the scattering narrowing as the standard errors decrease. That is, in such a plot, the effect size of studies is plotted against study sample size. If there is no publication bias, the plot would resemble an inverted funnel with a wide dispersion of results among studies of small size and a narrower range of study results for large studies. If the plot shows an asymmetrical and skewed shape, publication bias may present. This usually takes the form of a gap in the wide part of the funnel, which indicates the absence of small studies showing no benefit or harm. Figure 25.4 demonstrates two funnel plots based on simulated data. The left plot displays the simulated summaries for all the studies, which means absence of publication bias. The right plot displays the simulated summaries for studies that are statistically significant at the 0.05 level, which suggests the presence of publication bias.

The interpretation of the funnel plot is essentially subjective; many statistical methods have been developed to test funnel-plot asymmetry, including Begg's test and Egger's test. However, all available statistical tests have limitations, especially when the number of studies included is small and heterogeneity is large. It is always very important to recognize that publication bias is only one of many possible explanations for an asymmetric funnel plot in meta-analysis.

Locating unpublished studies and unpublished outcomes of published studies for inclusion may help to avoid publication bias, providing a better estimate of effectiveness or association. Clinical trial registration is a process by which details about the design and

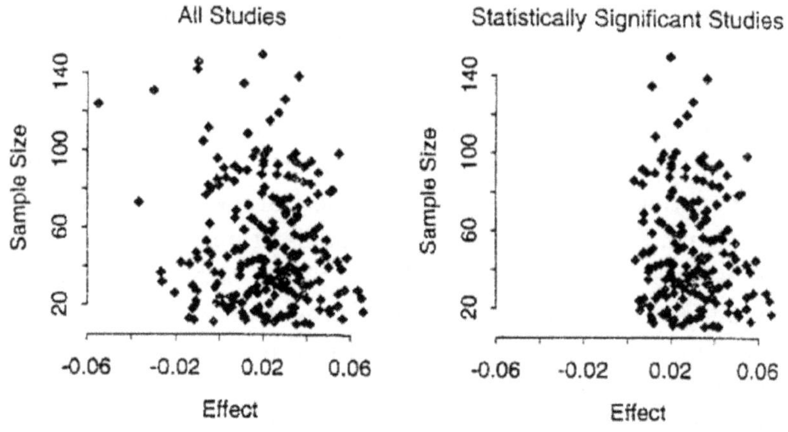

Figure 25.4 Two funnel plots based on simulated data. The left plot displays absence of publication, and the right displays the presence of publication bias
Source: Normand ST. (1999) Stat Med, 18:339.

conduct of a clinical trial are published (in an agreed format) in a publicly available resource, which typically is a website registry, ideal before study recruitment begins. Registration of clinical trials is required in some countries and is increasingly being standardized. The International committee of medical journal editors (ICMJE) advocated for registration of all clinical trials. Therefore, from 1st July 2005 onwards ICMJE consider only those clinical trials for publication, which have been registered before the start of patient recruitment. The WHO International Clinical Trials Registry Platform also advocated the registration of all clinical trials performed either on patients or healthy volunteers. It is also recommended that the complete trial details supplied during registration should be disclosed at public domain for the sake of transparency. Therefore, for obtaining reliable and accurate data for various health care interventions (drugs, diagnostics or therapeutic), registration of clinical trials is of paramount importance and makes the research more transparent, and reducing publication bias and selective reporting.

For example, Taylor D *et al.* systematically reviewed efficacy of agomelatine in people with depression in Example 25.4, it was necessary to consider whether there were unpublished trials. Therefore, in addition to undertaking a full electronic search of the databases, such as Medline, Embase, Cochrane Central Register of Controlled Trials, etc., they also searched trials registries for additional studies. They applied to the European Medicines Agency (EMA) for details of all studies submitted in support of regulatory approval of agomelatine. They also contacted the European manufacturer of agomelatine, Servier, and requested details of published and unpublished studies. Finally, they found four studies in the EMA, and there were full details of five further studies provided by the manufacturer, Servier. Twelve studies were included in the meta-analysis for comparing the antidepressant efficacy of agomelatine *vs.* placebo, and seven were unpublished from regulatory authorities EMA and from the manufacturer Servier. Heterogeneity in effect sizes was substantial with $I^2 = 66\%$ ($P < 0.001$). The random-effects model was adapted. Figure 25.5 is the forest plot of the meta-analysis containing published and unpublished studies, the results showed there was a significant difference favoring agomelatine (SMD 0.24, 95% confidence interval 0.12 to 0.35). This result is more conservative than the result obtained from five published studies (SMD 0.26, 95% confidence interval 0.16 to 0.36, Figure 25.2).

Figure 25.6 shows the funnel plots of standardized mean differences by publication status. Visual inspection of funnel plots showed no obvious evidence of funnel plot asymmetry for comparisons with placebo. The plots did, however, show evidence of publication bias: unpublished studies were more likely to show positive results. Overall, visual inspection of the forest plot and funnel plot shows that unpublished studies tend to have less favorable results for agomelatine.

Recently, the term "dissemination bias" was introduced to describe all forms of biases in the research-dissemination process, including outcome-reporting bias (selective reporting of some outcomes but not others), time-lag bias (rapid or delayed publication of research findings), multiple (duplication) publication bias (multiple or singular publication of research findings), language bias (publication of research findings in a particular language), citation bias (positive trials involving a medical intervention receive more citations

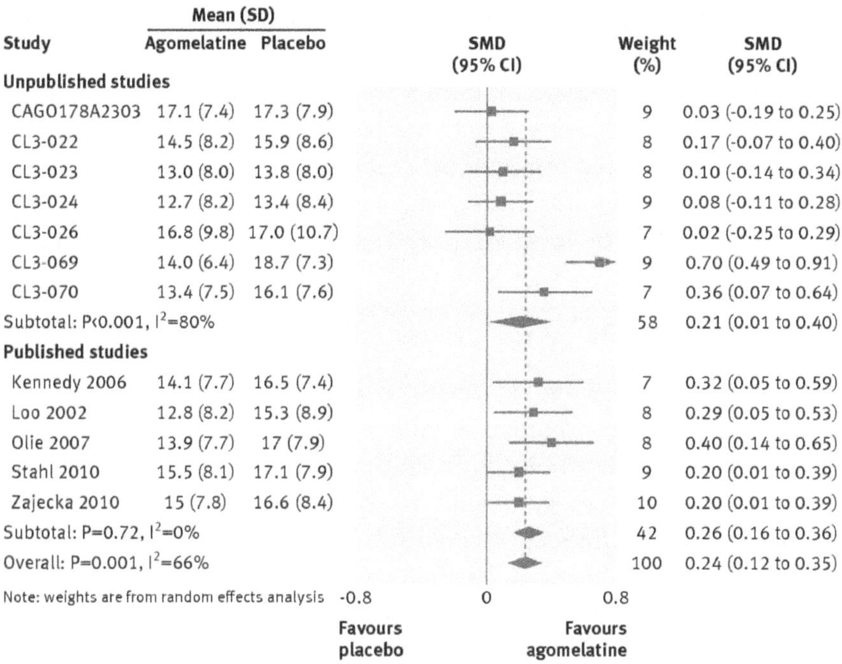

Figure 25.5 Forest plot for standardized mean differences (SMD) for agomelatine *vs* placebo in studies on antidepressant efficacy of agomelatine

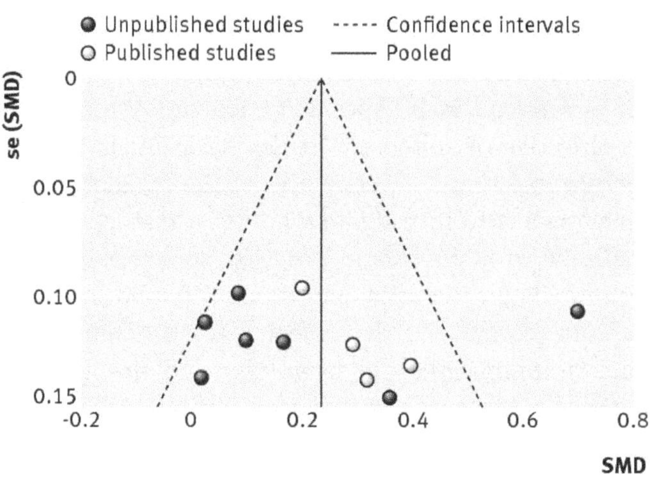

Figure 25.6 Funnel plot of standardized mean differences (SMD) for agomelatine *vs* placebo in studies on antidepressant efficacy

than neutral or negative trials of similar quality), location bias (publication of research findings in journals with different ease of access or levels of indexing in standard databases), gray-literature bias (studies might be not published and only available in PhD theses, conference proceedings, personal communications, and other forms of "gray" literature), and media-attention bias (studies that show up in the news are more likely to be included in analyses than those that do not).

25.5. Other methods for meta-analysis

The most frequently used methods of meta-analysis for dichotomous variable data and continuous variable data are outlined above. These effect estimates are combined across studies using a weighted average, with inverse variances as weights. In recent years, new approaches of meta-analysis for different types of data have been rapidly introduced. The following is a brief overview of the principles underlying the meta-analysis of diagnostic test accuracy and network meta-analysis.

25.5.1. *Meta-analysis of diagnostic test accuracy*

Meta-analysis of diagnostic test accuracy (DTA) studies, differs from the usual meta-analysis of therapeutic/interventional studies in that, it is required to simultaneously analyze a pair of two outcome measures such as sensitivity and specificity, instead of a single outcome. The main objective of systematic review of DTA, is to obtain more valid, generalizable summary estimates of the diagnostic accuracy of a test, which means to investigate whether a test is sufficiently sensitive or specific to fit its role in practice, to compare the accuracy of two or more diagnostic tests, and to identify and provide information on factors (covariates) that affect a test's diagnostic accuracy. Such a review summarizes the sensitivity and specificity of a test, and sometimes other measures as well, such as predictive values, likelihood ratios, ORs, or summary receiver operating characteristic (SROC) curves, and investigates where existing variation in results comes from.

Diagnostic accuracy reviews use the Quality Assessment of Diagnostic Accuracy Studies (QUADAS-2) tool to assess the quality of included studies in terms of risk of bias and concerns regarding the applicability over four domains, including patient selection, index test, reference standard, and flow and timing. Descriptive statistics of individual studies, such as sensitivity, specificity, positive likelihood ratio (LR), negative LR, and/or the diagnostic odds ratio (DOR), can be calculated, thus a descriptive forest plot, a SROC plot, or a plot of sensitivity *vs.* 1-specificity can be derived and presented.

A key issue for DTA review is to investigate the potential sources of heterogeneity. The threshold effect is a noticeable feature of DTA, which means the correlation observed between sensitivity and specificity by varying the threshold for a positive test result. The threshold effect is the most obvious source of heterogeneity in a DTA review. Several methods have been developed to explore the threshold effect. Statistically speaking, Spearman's correlation analysis is recommended to detect the potential threshold effect by assessing a linear correlation between the sensitivity and false-positive rate (i.e., 1-specificity). If a significant correlation exists, with a correlation coefficient of 0.6 or higher, the threshold effect can be regarded as substantial. Therefore, the SROC curve is appropriate to summarize the diagnostic accuracy.

The Moses-Littenberg method is the simplest model for deriving a SROC in meta-analysis of diagnostic tests, which is based on fixed-effects model, but could not provide estimates of the heterogeneity between studies. The Moses-Littenberg model fits a straight regression line to the logits of sensitivity and 1-specificity of each study, and uses the estimated intercept and slope in a form of back-transformed values to construct the SROC curve. Although this method is convenient for less mathematically or statistically complex meta-analyses, it ignores correlation between sensitivity and specificity, does not account for variability between studies, and does not optimally weight studies as well.

A SROC curve also can be obtained using a bivariate model or a hierarchical summary ROC (HSROC) model. These models take into account potential threshold effects and the correlation between sensitivity and specificity, and they are currently the most statistically rigorous and recommended methods for dealing with a threshold effect. Both models produce a HSROC curve as well as summary points of sensitivity and specificity, together with their confidence and prediction region. They directly estimate HSROC parameters such as accuracy (α_i), threshold (θ_i), and shape parameter (β) as random effects variables, which enables direct construction of a HSROC curve. If SROC curves are assumed to have the same shape (i.e., parallel curves), differences in test performance can be expressed as the relative diagnostic odds ratios (rDORs) comparing the DOR of one group of studies to that of another. The fit of alternative models (effect of adding or removing covariate terms from the bivariate or HSROC model) can be assessed using statistical tests to compare models with and without covariate terms. Covariates to be investigated should be prespecified with a clear justification for their selection.

25.5.2. *Network meta-analysis*

Conventional meta-analysis on the treatment effects of new drugs or interventions is conducted on the effect size based on pairwise head-to-head direct comparison, but in many cases, results from direct comparisons are relatively limited. Network meta-analysis (NMA), also known as multiple treatment comparison (MTC) or multiple treatment meta-analysis (MTM), is a popular way to combine evidence on multiple studies (usually randomized trials) comparing multiple treatments (or other interventions). There are two specific types of NMA, one is adjusted indirect treatment comparison (ITC), and another is mixed treatment comparison meta-analysis (MTC).

The introduction of the adjusted indirect treatment comparison (ITC) method, first proposed by Bucher *et al.* (1997), was developed with the odds ratio (OR) as the measure of treatment effect, and was specifically designed for the indirect comparison of A versus C when direct evidence of A versus B and B versus C was available (Figure 25.7.1). However, this model can only be applied to data generated from two-arm trials involving simple indirect comparison of three treatments. Later, an indirect treatment comparison technique, known as network meta-analysis, was developed by Lumley *et al.* to compare two treatments in the situation where an indirect comparison between two treatments of interest can be obtained through more than one common comparator or linking treatment. For example, if trials have separately compared treatment A to B, treatment C to B, treatment D to B, treatment B to E, and treatment F to E, one can incorporate results from trials in which the common comparator is B, as well as trials in which the common comparator is E (Figure 25.7.2). Thus, more than one common treatment can be used to conduct an indirect comparison between two treatments. The key feature of network meta-analysis using Lumley's model is a series of sequential ITC with unclosed loops.

Mixed/multiple treatment comparison meta-analysis (MTC or MTM), introduced by Lu and Ades, provides an even more sophisticated method for quantitatively addressing both direct and indirect comparisons of several competing interventions. MTC model has usually been done in a Bayesian framework with the aim of strengthening inference concerning the relative efficacy of two treatments by including both direct and indirect comparisons of these treatments. The key characteristic of MTC model lies in its underlying closed loops, and allows the synthesis of direct and indirect evidences simultaneously (Figure 25.7.3).

In general, as defined by the International Society for Pharmacoeconomics and Outcomes Research (ISPOR), NMA is a comparison of the effectiveness of two or more treatments, and categorizes the comparison type as MTC if the network geometry shows a closed loop and ITC if it does not.

Before conducting NMA, three major assumptions, similarity, homogeneity, and consistency, should be checked. Similarity assumption means that the selection of trials to compose the NMA should be based on rigorous criteria and thus studies should be similar. Besides study population, design, and outcome measures, trials must be comparable on effect modifiers to obtain an unbiased pooled estimate. Effect modifiers are study and patient characteristics (e.g. age,

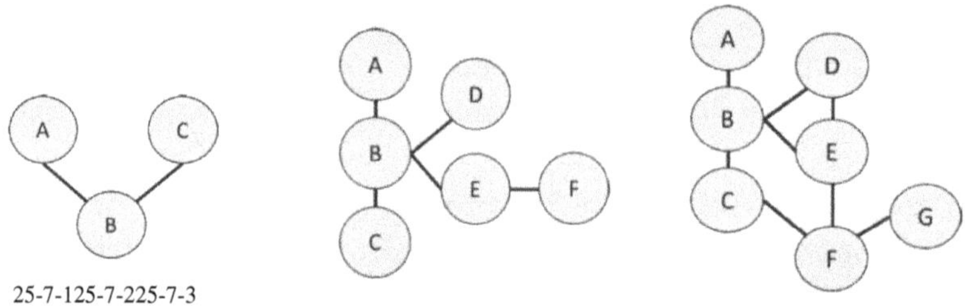

25-7-125-7-225-7-3

Adjusted indirect treatment comparison (ITC) Network meta-analysis Mixed treatment comparison (MTC)
simple indirect comparison series of ITC with unclosed loops with closed loops

Figure 25.7 Network diagrams and Examples of networks geometries

disease severity, duration of follow-up...) that are known to influence treatment effect of interventions. Imbalanced distribution of effect modifiers between studies can bias comparisons, resulting in heterogeneity and inconsistency. Homogeneity assumption means that there must be no relevant heterogeneity between trial results in pairwise comparisons. As with pairwise meta-analyses, homogeneity should be examined using standard procedures such as forest plots and measures of heterogeneity, with defining criteria established in advance. Depending on the size of the network, however, this may be a very lengthy process, as all possible combinations of two interventions must be included. Consistency assumptions means that there must be no relevant discrepancy or inconsistency between direct and indirect evidence, and some procedures have been developed for examining consistency. The results of examination of similarity, homogeneity, and consistency must be handled appropriately. If there has been a major violation of any of these assumptions, this may even mean that no worthwhile indirect comparison can be performed.

NMA can be performed within either a frequentist or a Bayesian framework. Similar to traditional pairwise meta-analysis, NMA can utilize the fixed-effect or the random effects model. Since most of NMA has indirect, multiple comparisons, Bayesian framework seems logically more valid and reliable, and 60–70% of NMA studies have taken a Bayesian approach. However, if the prior probability is not established in the study hypothesis, Bayesian analysis poses many limitations for ordinary researchers using NMA because the problem of establishing prior probability is rather more complex than the problem of testing the research hypothesis, that is, the original purpose of the analysis. After making several model-based choices, diagnostic processes must be undertaken to verify whether the model was appropriate. These approaches must assess heterogeneity and inconsistency, two assumptions underlying any NMA that are highly influential to the results. Methods of identifying and dealing with these issues are explored extensively in the NMA literature.

It is important to publish NMA results clearly and completely. Displaying the network, presenting relative effects and rank probabilities are an important part of reporting NMA results. There are several statistical programs available that can implement the various steps required to carry out a NMA. Frequentist models can be implemented using commercial programs such as SAS and STATA.

25.6. Common software for meta-analysis

25.6.1. *RevMan*

RevMan (Review Manager) is the software developed by The Cochrane Collaboration, which is used for preparing and maintaining Cochrane Reviews, and free for Cochrane authors and academic use. RevMan facilitates preparation of protocols and full reviews. It can also directly perform meta-analysis of the data entered, and present the results graphically.

The latest major version is RevMan 5.3, the next generation of online review-writing software, RevMan Web will be available soon. In addition to reviews of studies of the effects of healthcare interventions, we can use RevMan to write reviews of diagnostic test accuracy studies, reviews of studies of methodology and overviews of reviews.

Working with RevMan requires no programming. With the help of RevMan User Guide or online assistance available, we can easily conduct a meta-analysis step by step. Taking the systematic review of the intervention as an example, the main steps include: ① Creating a new review; ② Adding the basic information of the included studies, including each study's ID, year the study was conducted, other characteristics of studies, and the risk of bias table for each study; ③ Generating risk of bias graph and risk of bias summary; ④ Data analysis: first choosing data types, statistical methods, analysis models, effect measures and other parameters, then entering and calculating data, and figures and graphs can be generated (forest plot, summary of findings, funnel plot); ⑤ Performing sensitivity analysis and subgroup analysis when necessary.

The process of conducting a review for diagnostic accuracy test with RevMan is similar to the review of interventional trials. The QUADAS-2 tool can be implemented in RevMan for the assessment of methodological quality. RevMan can calculate sensitivity and specificity, plot study data in a ROC plane and draw a summary ROC curve for descriptive and exploratory purposes. It also includes the creation of new systematic reviews, the addition of basic information for included studies, input of research data, parameter settings and data analysis, output of forest plot with combined sensitivity and specificity analysis results and the output of SROC curve. However, RevMan cannot directly combine the "positive likelihood ratio" and "negative likelihood ratio" indicators of the diagnostic test.

25.6.2. *Stata*

Stata is a powerful and small statistical analysis software that enables users to analyze, manage, and produce graphical visualizations of data. It is primarily used in the fields of economics, biomedicine, and political science to examine data patterns. Stata's capabilities include data management, statistical analysis, graphics, simulations, regression, and custom programming. It also has a system to disseminate user-written programs that lets it grow continuously. Stata allows users to modify, add or publish ADO (ActiveX Data Objects) program files written in macro language and download them for free. Many of Stata's advanced statistical functions are implemented in this way.

Stata 16 offers the new suite of commands, meta, to perform meta-analysis. It's one of the most exciting new features in Stata 16-which was released in June, 2019. The new suite is broad, complete, and one of its strengths is its simplicity. Stata's meta command offers full support for meta-analysis from computing various effect sizes and producing basic meta-analytic summary and forest plots to accounting for between-study heterogeneity and potential publication bias.

Using Stata's new meta-analysis suite, we can easily summarize results from multiple studies, including estimate an overall effect size, present results in a forest plot, explore heterogeneity via subgroup meta-analysis or meta-regression, evaluate small-study effects and publication bias, produce a funnel plot, test formally for funnel-plot asymmetry, assess publication bias using the trim-and-fill method and perform cumulative meta-analysis.

25.6.3. *The R language*

R is a programming language and free software environment for statistical computing and graphics supported by the R Foundation for Statistical Computing. The R language is widely used among statisticians and data miners for developing statistical software and data analysis. R provides a wide variety of statistical (linear and nonlinear modeling, classical statistical tests, time-series analysis, classification, clustering, ...) and graphical techniques, and is highly extensible. Today, R is one of the most popular and powerful statistical analysis software available. Many of the advanced statistical analysis functions of the R software are implemented by downloading and installing various extension packages, and are continuously updated. The R programming language is known as the omnipotent of meta-analysis. Almost all meta-analysis methods can be implemented by R software, including individual patient data (IPD) meta-analysis, network meta-analysis, heterogeneity and publication bias test, forest plot, funnel plot, etc. See the appendix of this book for an introduction to the R language.

25.6.4. *WinBUGS/OpenBUGS*

The classical meta-analysis methods are based on frequentist methods for statistics. They revolve around estimating unknown parameters along with confidence intervals, and performing statistical tests with a null hypothesis (the P-value). Bayesian methods can be considered as an alternative to the classical approach to statistical analysis. The Bayesian paradigm provides in a very natural way a method for data synthesis from all studies by incorporating model and parameter uncertainty. Results of Bayesian analyses have an appealing interpretation, and they readily allow more complex models to be fitted to meta-analysis datasets, but they require specialized software and require specification of a prior distribution for each parameter.

WinBUGS (Bayesian Analysis Using Gibbs Sampling) is a versatile package that has been designed to carry out Markov chain Monte Carlo (MCMC) computations for a wide variety of Bayesian models, which is developed by the Institute of Bio-statistics in University of Cambridge, England. OpenBUGS is an open source version of WinBUGS. The main steps for Gibbs sampling with WinBUGS/OpenBUGS include data input, assignment of initial parameter value, model compilation, and update. After the Gibbs sampling converges, the mean, standard deviation, 95% confidence interval, and median of the parameter posterior distribution can be obtained. In recent years, Bayesian meta-analysis with WinBUGS/OpenBUGS, especially for network meta-analysis, has been greatly developed. For the specific principles and usage of WinBUGS/OpenBUGS, interested readers can refer to related books.

25.6.5. *Open Meta-Analyst*

Open Meta-Analyst (OMA) is a very powerful free open source software currently maintained by the Evidence-based Practice Center (EPC) of the School of Public Health of Brown University. EPC aims to provide high-quality evidence for AHRQ's clinical decision making and health policy development, which is one of the 12 centers selected and funded by the Agency for Healthcare Research and Quality (AHRQ). OMA offers not only random-effects model or fixed-effect model for meta-analysis of dichotomous variable, continuous variable, and diagnostic accuracy tests, but also Bayesian meta-analysis, cumulative meta-analysis and meta-regression.

25.7. Reporting the results of a meta-analysis

Ideally, according to the PRISMA checklist (Preferred Reporting Items for Systematic Reviews and Meta-Analyses, http://www.prisma-statement.org/), the results of a meta-analysis are as follow:

(1) Study selection: give numbers of studies screened, assessed for eligibility, and included in the review, with reasons for exclusions at each stage, ideally with a flow diagram.
(2) Study characteristics: for each study, present characteristics for which data were extracted (e.g., study size, PICOS, follow-up period) and provide the citations.
(3) Risk of bias within studies: present data on risk of bias of each study and, if available, any outcome level assessment.
(4) Results of individual studies: for all outcome (benefits or harms) considered, present, for each study: (a) simple summary data for each intervention group (b) effect estimates and confidence intervals, ideally with a forest plot.
(5) Synthesis of results: present results of each meta-analysis done, including confidence intervals and measures of consistency.
(6) Risk of bias across studies: present results of any assessment of risk of bias across studies.
(7) Additional analysis: give results of additional analyses, if done (e.g., sensitivity or subgroup analyses, meta-regression

The following is a brief report of the results of the Example 25.1 meta-analysis.

To quantitatively assess whether inhaled nitric oxide (NO) is effective in patients with ALI/ARDS, a risk ratio (RR) is used as a measure of treatment effect to perform a meta-analysis of the 9 RCTs included, comparing in-hospital mortality in the NO and control groups. The result of homogeneity test indicates the heterogeneity between studies is not statistically significant. Therefore, fixed-effect model is used to pool the effect size. The point of combined RR is estimated to be 1.104, i.e., on average, inhaled NO increases the risk of death in patients with ALI/ARDS by 10.4%. However, the 95% Confidence Interval of the combined RR is (0.938, 1.30), including 1, which means that the combined RR is not statistically significant. The result of the meta-analysis suggests inhaled NO does not improve survival and may cause harm in patients with ALI/ARDS.

25.8. Case analysis

Meta-analysis of cholesterol-lowering intervention therapy on reduction of the risk of death from coronary heart disease

To investigate whether cholesterol-lowering interventions can reduce the risk of death from coronary heart disease, Smith DG *et al.* collected 34 RCTs. See Table 25.8 for basic information. The interventions in the trial group include drug intervention, dietary intervention and surgical intervention. The patient types are divided into primary prevention, secondary prevention and other three types. Primary prevention is mainly for patients without cardiovascular disease. Secondary prevention is mainly for patients with existing cardiovascular disease. Non-primary prevention or non-secondary prevention is listed as the other. Try to perform meta-analysis of the data in Table 25.8.

(1) First, the heterogeneity test is performed, let y_i $=ln(\mathrm{OR}_i)$, weight of each study are calculated. Then, calculate the$Q$statistic and I^2 statistic using equation (25-4), (25-5), $Q = 88.23$, $P <$ 0.0001, and $I^{2=}$62.6%, indicating that there is heterogeneity between the studies, and the random effects model is adopted.
(2) Calculate the adjusted weight w_i^* by D-L method using equation (25-16).
(3) From equations (25-25) and (25-26), the combined OR is 0.89, the 95% CI is (0.78, 1.02), which contains 1. Therefore, it is not yet considered that cholesterol lowing interventions can reduce the risk of death from coronary heart disease.

Please discuss:

(1) Is the above meta-analysis method appropriate? Is the conclusion accurate? why?
(2) How to conduct a meta-analysis on the above information?

Table 25.8 Total mortality data from 34 RCTs investigating the effect of cholesterol-lowing interventions#

Trial	No. patients in treatment arm (n_{1i})	No. patients in control arm (n_{2i})	Total deaths in treatment (a_i)	Total deaths in control arm (c_i)	Odds ratio (OR_i)	95% CI for OR_i	Weight (w_i)	Adjusted w_i^*	Intervention	Patient type
1	204	202	28	51	0.48	0.29–0.79	14.98	7.43	Diet	Secondary
2	285	147	70	38	0.93	0.59–1.47	18.54	8.21	Drug	Secondary
3	156	119	37	40	0.62	0.36–1.04	13.83	7.14	Drug	Secondary
4	88	30	2	3	0.23	0.04–1.22	1.36	1.25	Drug	Secondary
5	30	33	0	3	0.14	0.01–2.89	0.43	0.41	Drug	Other
6	279	276	61	82	0.66	0.45–0.97	26.25	9.44	Drug	Secondary
7	206	206	41	55	0.68	0.43–1.08	18.26	8.16	Diet	Secondary
8	123	129	20	24	0.85	0.45–1.63	9.20	5.66	Diet	Secondary
9	1080	1015	111	113	0.98	0.74–1.29	50.03	11.39	Diet	Secondary
10	427	143	81	27	1.00	0.62–1.61	16.64	7.82	Drug	Secondary
11	244	253	31	51	0.58	0.36–0.94	16.45	7.78	Drug	Secondary
12	50	50	17	12	1.61	0.68–3.81	5.18	3.83	Drug	Secondary
13	47	48	23	20	1.33	0.60–2.97	5.98	4.25	Drug	Secondary
14	30	60	0	4	0.21	0.01–3.95	0.44	0.43	Surgery	Secondary
15	5552	2789	1025	723	0.65	0.58–0.72	326.57	14.11	Drug	Secondary
16	424	422	174	178	0.95	0.73–1.25	51.51	11.46	Diet	Primary
17	199	194	28	31	0.86	0.50–1.50	12.69	6.82	Diet	Secondary
18	350	367	42	48	0.91	0.58–1.41	19.79	8.45	Drug	Secondary
19	79	78	4	5	0.80	0.22–2.88	2.32	2.01	Drug	Secondary
20	1149	1129	37	48	0.75	0.49–1.16	20.36	8.55	Drug	Primary

(*Continued*)

Table 25.8 (*Continued*)

Trial	No. patients in treatment arm (n_{1i})	No. patients in control arm (n_{2i})	Total deaths in treatment (a_i)	Total deaths in control arm (c_i)	Odds ratio (OR_i)	95% CI for OR_i	Weight (w_i)	Adjusted w_i^*	Intervention	Patient type
21	221	237	39	28	1.59	0.94–2.68	14.15	7.22	Diet	Secondary
22	54	26	8	1	3.11	0.51–18.83	1.18	1.10	Diet	Secondary
23	71	72	5	7	0.72	0.23–2.29	2.89	2.42	Drug	Secondary
24	4541	4516	269	248	1.08	0.91–1.29	121.91	13.15	Diet	Primary
25	421	417	49	62	0.76	0.51–1.13	23.98	9.13	Surgery	Secondary
26	94	94	0	1	0.33	0.01–8.20	0.37	0.36	Drug	Secondary
27	311	317	19	12	1.63	0.79–3.37	7.25	4.86	Drug	Secondary
28	1906	1900	68	71	0.95	0.68–1.34	33.70	10.26	Drug	Primary
29	2051	2030	44	43	1.01	0.66–1.55	21.52	8.75	Drug	Primary
30	6582	1663	33	3	2.43	0.81–7.31	3.16	2.60	Drug	Primary
31	5331	5296	236	181	1.31	1.07–1.59	98.72	12.83	Drug	Primary
32	48	49	0	1	0.33	0.01–8.39	0.37	0.36	Drug	Other
33	94	52	1	0	1.68	0.07–42.10	0.37	0.36	Drug	Secondary
34	23	29	1	2	0.73	0.09–5.99	0.87	0.82	Drug	Secondary

Note: 0.5 has been added to every cell of every 2 × 2 table to allow for the arms of trials with 0 events.

Source: Smith GD, Song F, Sheldon TA. Cholesterol lowering and mortality: the importance of considering initial level of risk. BMJ, 1993,306(6893):1648.

25.9. Computer experiment

Lab 25-1 Meta-analysis using RevMan.

25.10. Frequently asked questions and summary

25.10.1. *Frequently asked questions*

1. What is the difference between meta-analysis and systematic review?

A systematic review is a scientific tool, as well as a form of research that provides a summary of medical research on a specific clinical question, using explicit methods to search, critically appraise, and synthesize the all relevant findings systematically. It is particularly useful in bringing together a number of separately conducted studies, sometimes with conflicting findings, and synthesizing their results.

The methods used to review many studies aims to limit bias or assumptions in health topics, allowing us to have greater confidence for drawing conclusions in medicine.

Systematic reviews can be used to establish whether scientific findings are consistent and generalizable across populations, settings, and treatment variations, or whether findings vary significantly by particular subgroups. Moreover, the explicit methods used in systematic reviews limit bias and, hopefully, will improve reliability and accuracy of conclusions.

Following a systematic review, data from individual studies may be pooled quantitatively and reanalyzed using established statistical methods. This technique is called meta-analysis. Therefore, every meta-analysis should be based on an underlying systematic review, but not every systematic review leads to a meta-analysis. Meta-analysis may or may not be a subset of systematic review depending on the nature of the studies included in the review, and whether the studies are similar enough so that combining their results is meaningful.

Systematic reviews and meta-analyses of randomized controlled trials (RCTs) are considered to be evidence of the highest level in the hierarchy of research designs evaluating effectiveness of interventions.

2. When performing the meta-analysis, effect size can be combined via fixed-effect model or random effects model. Which model should we use?

In the fixed-effect analysis, we assume that the true effect size is the same in all studies, and the summary effect is our estimate of this common effect size. In the random-effects analysis, we assume that the true effect size varies from one study to the next, and that the studies in our analysis represent a random sample of effect sizes that could have been observed. The summary effect is our estimate of the mean of these effects. The standard error of the summary effect and (it follows) the confidence intervals for the summary effect are wider under the random-effects model than under the fixed-effect model.

The selection of a model must be based solely on the question of which model fits the distribution of effect sizes, and takes account of the relevant source(s) of error. In general, it makes sense to use the fixed-effect model if two conditions are met. First, we believe that all the studies included in the analysis are functionally identical. Second, our goal is to compute the common effect size of the identified population, and not to generalize to other populations. By contrast, when the researcher is accumulating data from a series of studies that had been performed by researchers operating independently, it would be unlikely that all the studies were functionally equivalent. Typically, the subjects or interventions in these studies would have differed in ways that would have impacted on the results, and therefore we should not assume a common effect size. Therefore, in these cases the random-effects model is more easily justified than the fixed-effect model.

The strategy of starting with a fixed-effect model and then moving to a random-effects model if the test for heterogeneity is significant is a mistake, and should be strongly discouraged.

3. How to assess, and how to address the heterogeneity?

It is natural for effect sizes of studies collected in a meta-analysis to vary between the studies because of sampling variability. However, when this variation exceeds the levels that could be explained by sampling variation, it is referred to as the between-study heterogeneity.

Between-study heterogeneity may arise for different reasons and is generally divided into two types: clinical and methodological. Clinical heterogeneity is the variability in the intervention strategies, outcomes, and study participants. Methodological heterogeneity is the variability in the study design and conduct. Statistical heterogeneity refers to the cases when the variability between the observed effects cannot be explained by sampling variability alone. It arises when the true effects in each study are different and may be the result of clinical heterogeneity, methodological heterogeneity, or both. In what follows, we refer to statistical heterogeneity simply as heterogeneity.

How to assess heterogeneity? Forest plots are useful for visual examination of heterogeneity. Its presence can be evaluated by looking at the plotted confidence intervals, which are represented as horizontal lines on the plot. Heterogeneity is suspected if there is a lack of overlap between the confidence intervals. We can also test for heterogeneity more formally by using Cochrane's homogeneity test, Q statistic I^2 statistic.

There are several strategies to address heterogeneity when it is present. Here are some of the recommendations.

(1) Explore heterogeneity: Subgroup analyses and meta-regression are commonly used to explore heterogeneity. For such analyses to be proper, we must prespecify upfront (before meta-analysis) the study attributes you would like to explore. Often, meta-analysts are already familiar with the studies, so the genuine pre-study specification may not be possible. In that case, we should use caution when interpreting the results. Once heterogeneity is established, its exploration after the fact is viewed as data snooping and should be avoided.
(2) Using random-effects model: After careful consideration of subgroup analysis and meta-regression, we may consider a random effects meta-analysis to account for the remaining unexplained between-study heterogeneity.
(3) Exclude studies: generally, we should avoid excluding studies from a meta-analysis because this may lead to bias. We may consider doing this in the presence of a few outlying studies when

the reasons for the outlying results are well understood and are unlikely to interfere with research objectives. Even then, we still need to perform sensitivity analysis and report both the results with and without the outlying studies.

(4) Do not perform a meta-analysis: in the presence of substantial variation that cannot be explained, we may have to abandon the meta-analysis altogether. In this case, it will be misleading to report a single overall estimate of an effect, especially if there is a disagreement among the studies about the direction of the effect.

4. How to identify and control publication bias?

Publication bias occurs when the studies selected for a scientific review are systematically different from all available relevant studies, which typically arises when non-significant results are being under-reported in the literature.

The funnel plot is frequently used to explore publication bias. It is a scatter plot of the study-specific effect sizes versus measures of study precision. The asymmetry of funnel plot may be caused by factors other than publication bias such as a presence of a moderator correlated with the study effect and study size or, more generally, the presence of substantial between-study heterogeneity. Graphical evaluation of funnel plots is useful for data exploration but may be subjective when detecting the asymmetry. Statistical tests provide a more formal evaluation of asymmetry of funnel plot. Regression-based tests (Egger method), and a nonparametric rank-based test (Begg method) are commonly introduced to test for the asymmetry of funnel plot. These two tests explore the relationship between the study specific effect sizes and study precision. The presence of the asymmetry of the funnel plot is declared when the association between the two measures is greater than what would have been observed by chance.

However, tests for asymmetry of funnel plot are not able to estimate the impact of this bias on the final meta-analysis results. The non-parametric trim-and-fill method provides a way to assess the impact of missing studies because of publication bias on the meta-analysis. It evaluates the amount of potential bias present in meta-analysis and its impact on the final conclusion. This method is typically used as a sensitivity analysis to the presence of publication bias.

To reduce publication bias, meta-analysis should emphasize the complete collection of all studies, including unpublished negative findings, results from registered clinical trial, conference papers, dissertations and other grey literature. We can also contact the original researcher and ask them for relevant information as much as possible. In addition, extensive sample studies may, in most cases, approach the average of all studies (both published and unpublished). Therefore, in the sensitivity analysis, it should be compared whether the combined effect value of the extensive sample studies is consistent with the total combined effect value, which is also helpful to judge whether there is publication bias.

25.10.2. *Summary*

1. Meta-analysis is a systematic quantitative review and synthesis of the results from studies that have independently evaluated similar or equivalent interventions and outcomes. The most common application of meta-analysis is to combine the results of inconclusive clinical trials with the purpose of increasing the sample size and thereby conferring increased power to the statistical testing of treatment effects. Other important goals of meta-analysis include situations where published studies have showed contradictory results, or when a more accurate estimate of the treatment effect need to be obtained, or for the analysis of particular subgroups of patients for whom the results of clinical trials have not yet provided conclusive evidence..
2. To conduct a high-quality meta-analysis, adequate planning and the careful preparation of a study protocol are essential. The description of the study methods and procedures, especially the explicit inclusion and exclusion criteria, rigorous quality assessment of the included studies, must be comprehensive, and the presentation of study findings must be especially clear.

3. This chapter introduces standard meta-analysis methods for dichotomous data and continuous data. The summary measures of treatment effect for dichotomous variable data may be the odds ratio (OR), the risk ratio (RR) and the risk difference (RD). The summary measures of treatment effect for continuous data may be weighted mean differences (WMD) or the standardized mean difference (SMD). If the heterogeneity test does not reject H_0, fixed-effects model is generally used; if H_0 is rejected, the random-effects model can be selected. The meta-analysis methods of the fixed-effect model include the inverse variance method, the Mantel-Haenszel method, etc. The reciprocal variance method uses the reciprocal of the variance as the weight, and obtains the weighted estimate of the combined effect, which can be applied to the meta-analysis of various types of data. The random effects model can adopt the D-L method.
4. Meta-analysis is primarily an observational study, and each step of the meta-analysis may be biased. When reporting the results of a meta-analysis, various biases should be analyzed and discussed, especially the impact of publication bias on the outcome.
5. With the development of evidence-based medicine, meta-analysis methods are increasingly valued by medical professionals. It must be noted that the types of data in medical research are diverse, and the meta-analysis methodology itself is continually evolving. Moreover, the meta-analysis of a certain problem may need to be supplemented, updated, and re-evaluated with the development of medical research. Therefore, the results of the meta-analysis must be interpreted very carefully.

Think and Practice

I. Best Choice

1. Regarding to meta-analysis, which of the following statements are incorrect? ( )
   A. Meta is essentially an observational study, so there may exist different kinds of biases B. In meta-analysis, suppose heterogeneity test rejects H_0, fixed-effect model should be used to combine

effects C. When pooling bi-categorized variable data, OR and RR values were usually transformed to natural logarithm before combining the effects D. The basic idea of meta-analysis is to increase sample size, improve test efficiency and quantitatively evaluate the average effect by combining similar studies

The DerSimonian-Laird method is generally used in meta-analysis of random-effect model to combine effects

2. For continuous variable data based meta-analysis, if measurement units of included study are different, use ( ) as the effect index.
   A. Standardized mean difference B. Mean difference C. Standardized regression coefficient D. Standardized P value E. Risk difference
3. The statistic used in the heterogeneity test is ( )
   A. F statistic B. Q statistic C. t statistic D. H statistic E. Z statistic
4. The following graph is a forest map of a meta-analysis. The results of the meta-analysis are incorrectly described as ( )
   A. The effect index of this meta is the mean difference, so the invalid line in forest map is 0 B. The meta-analysis includes six studies, each of which has no statistical significance in point estimate and 95% CI C. The combined effect index of the meta-analysis is −1.77, and 95% CI does not contain 0 so the meta-analysis results have statistical significance D. The heterogeneity test result of this meta-analysis is p = 0.0006. So random-effect model should be used to merge effects E. The heterogeneity index I^2 = 77% of the meta-analysis indicates that there is significant heterogeneity among the included studies.

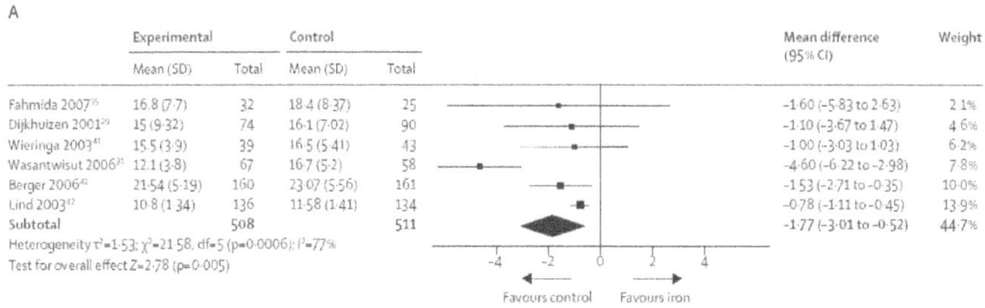

5. Regarding to publication bias, which of the following is incorrect? ( )
   A. The funnel diagram can be used to roughly determine whether there is publication bias B. Collect unpublished negative research results as much as possible can reduce publication bias C. Implement the registration system of clinical trials and promote transparency of clinical trials can effectively reduce publication bias. D. Publication bias often underestimates the combined effect when meta-analysis incorporates small sample studies. E. The basic idea of the funnel diagram is that the accuracy of incorporating research effects increases with the increase of the sample size.

II. Thinking question

1. What are the basic steps of meta-analysis?
2. In meta-analysis, suppose there is obvious heterogeneity among the included studies, how to deal with it?
3. What are the common biases of the meta-analysis?

III. Calculating question

1. Table 25.9 shows the results of seven clinical trials completed between the 1970s and 1980s on aspirin in reducing the risk of death after myocardial infarction. Try to use fixed-effect model and random-effect model to merge the effects, and give the point estimates and interval estimates of the combined effects. Then compare the combined effect values of these two methods.
2. To compare the preventive effect of sodium fluoride (NaF) toothpaste and sodium monofluorophosphate (SMFP) toothpaste on dental caries, the number of newly-added decayed, missing or filled teeth score (DFMS) after using 2–3 years later, is used as the evaluation measurement of the preventive effect of dental caries. Nine RCTs meeting the inclusion criteria are collected. Table 25.10 is the basic information of these nine studies and try to do a meta-analysis on them.

Table 25.9 Seven randomized clinical trials of aspirin in reducing the death risk after myocardial infarction

	aspirin		placebo	
Study	Death number	Illness case number	Death number	Illness case number
1	49	615	67	624
2	44	758	64	771
3	102	832	126	850
4	32	317	38	309
5	85	810	52	406
6	246	2267	219	2257
7	1570	8587	1720	8600

Table 25.10 Basic information of nine RCTs on NaF toothpaste and SMFP toothpaste for caries prevention

	NaF group			SMFP group		
Study	Cases (n1i)	The mean of newly-added DMFS ($\bar{x}_{1i}$)	Standard deviation (s1i)	Cases (n2i)	The mean of newly-added DMFS ($\bar{x}_{2i}$)	Standard deviation (s2i)
1	134	5.96	4.24	113	6.82	4.72
2	175	4.74	4.64	151	5.07	5.38
3	137	2.04	2.59	140	2.51	3.22
4	184	2.70	2.32	179	3.20	2.46
5	174	6.09	4.86	169	5.81	5.14
6	754	4.72	5.33	736	4.76	5.29
7	209	10.10	8.10	209	10.90	7.90
8	1151	2.82	3.05	1122	3.01	3.32
9	679	3.88	4.85	673	4.37	5.37

References

[1] Petitti, DB. *Meta-Analysis, Decision Analysis, and Cost-Effectiveness Analysis: Methods for Quantitative Synthesis in Medicine*. 2nd ed. New York, NY: Oxford University Press; 2000.

[2] Dickersin, K, Berlin, JA. Meta-analysis: state-of-the-science. *Epidemiol Rev.* 1992; 14: 154–176.

[3] Hunter, JE, Schmidt, FL. *Methods of Meta-Analysis: Correcting Error and Bias in Research Findings.* Newbury Park, CA: Sage Publications; 1990.
[4] Egger, M, Smith, DG. Meta-analysis: bias in location and selection of studies. *BMJ.* 1998; 316: 61–66.
[5] Higgins, JP, Jackson, D, Barrett, JK, *et al.* Consistency and inconsistency in network meta-analysis: concepts and models for multi-arm studies [J]. *Res Synth Methods.* 2012; 3(2): 98–110.

Xuyu Zhou, Xinrui Wang

CHAPTER 26

TIME SERIES

Time series analysis provides a mathematical model for dynamic data to reveal the law of development and change of variables quantitatively or describe the internal quantitative relationship among variables from a dynamic perspective. In medical researches, events are dynamically observed at regular intervals (often equidistant). Due to the involvement of random factors, the measurements at those time points are random variables. Such random variables (or the observed values) arranged in time order are called time series. For example, both the incidence of influenza among children somewhere (Table 26.1) and the amount of antibiotics produced by a pharmaceutical company (Table 26.2) constitute the time series data respectively.

26.1. Descriptions of time series

26.1.1. *Decomposition of time series*

The measured time series usually contain certain properties, which are generally considered to consist of three kinds of properties.

(1) Trend: With the progress of time (or the change of an ordinal variable), the series show monotonous rising or falling, even flat. The slope may vary in different stages.
(2) Seasonal fluctuation: In a broad sense, seasonality is the periodicity of a series. In a narrow sense, seasonality refers to the periodicity of a series that changes with the year, quarter, month, or week of the calendar.

(3) Irregular variation: It's the random disturbance integrated on regular variation and is pervasive in time series observations.

The above three properties of time series are generally integrated together according to the addition principle or the multiplication principle (by logarithmic transformation, the latter can also meet the pre-conditions of the additive model). Taking the time series satisfying the additive model as the example, after reasonable functional transformation, they can be decomposed into three parts, which are the trend part T_t, the seasonal part S_t and the irregular part I_t, as the following

$$X_t = T_t + S_t + I_t, \quad t = 1, 2, \ldots, \tag{26-1}$$

It is one of the important tasks of time series analysis to decompose these three parts from the time series. The trend and seasonal components of the time series can be expressed by specific functions. After the trend and seasonal terms being excluded, the time series appear as stationary process. The historical value in a stationary time series often contains the information of future value, which provides a basis for using historical measurements $x_1, x_2, \ldots, x_n$ to predict the future level x_{n+1} of the concerned variable. For example, the monitored results of $PM_{2.5}$ in air within 100 days are used to predict the level of $PM_{2.5}$ on the 5th day. It is usually called the prediction with the lead time $l = 5$.

26.1.2. *Autocorrelation function and autoregressive model*

Autocorrelation function (ACF) r_k is the measurement of the correlation degree and direction between the series of observed values at any time and the series itself with k units of shift. This shifting distance is often called lag, with lag $0, 1, 2, \ldots$ The corresponding sequence of correlation coefficients constitute the ACF. r_k can be obtained from any given time series,

$$r_k = \frac{\sum_{t=1}^{n-k}(x_t - \bar{x})(x_{t+k} - \bar{x})}{\sum_{t=1}^{n}(x_t - \bar{x})^2} \tag{26-2}$$

which is the value of sample autocorrelation function (SACF) from a time series with lag k.

In practical analysis, it is assumed that after normalization with zero as the mean (pretreatment of the whole time series, minus its own mean), time series x_t is only correlated to the observed values in the recent p periods, then the time series can be expressed by the following model

$$x_t = \varphi_1 x_{t-1} + \varphi_2 x_{t-2} + \cdots + \varphi_p x_{t-p} + a_t \tag{26-3}$$

It is known as an autoregressive (AR) model of order p, abbreviated AR(p), where $\varphi_i (i = 1, 2, \ldots, p)$ is the AR coefficient, a_t is the error term (i.e., the residual).

For a time series satisfying the AR model of order p, the AR coefficients can be obtained by solving the following simultaneous equations,

$$\begin{cases} r_1 = \varphi_1 + \varphi_2 r_1 + \varphi_3 r_2 + \varphi_4 r_3 + \cdots + \varphi_{p-1} r_{p-2} + \varphi_p r_{p-1} \\ r_2 = \varphi_1 r_1 + \varphi_2 + \varphi_3 r_1 + \varphi_4 r_2 + \cdots + \varphi_{p-1} r_{p-3} + \varphi_p r_{p-2} \\ \cdots \\ r_p = \varphi_1 r_{p-1} + \varphi_2 r_{p-2} + \varphi_3 r_{p-3} + \varphi_4 r_{p-4} + \cdots + \varphi_{p-1} r_1 + \varphi_p \end{cases} \tag{26-4}$$

where $r_i (i = 1, 2, \ldots, p)$ is the i-th value of the ACF.

26.1.3. *Partial ACF*

When construct a model for time series, a parsimonious pattern is preferred. For an AR model of order p, it is usual to start with a lower order number until the residual series meets the requirements (see white noise in Section 26.4.4). The process of attempt is just like the forward strategy in multiple regression analysis, and we could successively obtain the model $x_t = \varphi_1 x_{t-1} + a_t$, $x_t = \varphi_1 x_{t-1} + \varphi_2 x_{t-2} + a_t$, $x_t = \varphi_1 x_{t-1} + \varphi_2 x_{t-2} + \varphi_3 x_{t-3} + a_t, \ldots,$ $x_t = \varphi_1 x_{t-1} + \varphi_2 x_{t-2} + \varphi_3 x_{t-3} + \cdots + \varphi_p x_{t-p} + a_t$, etc. In the first, second, third, and the p-th regression model, the highest order coefficient is defined as partial autocorrelation function (PACF), denoted by $\varphi_{11}, \varphi_{22}, \varphi_{33}, \ldots, \varphi_{pp}$.

For a time series that can be modeled based on previous historical information, its ACF and PACF will approach 0 when the lag k is large enough. There are usually two kinds of performance, (1) tail off: after a few lags, the absolute value of the ACF/PACF gradually decreases into the confidence interval of zero. (2) cut off: after a few lags, the absolute value of the ACF/PACF decreases sharply into the confidence interval of zero.

26.1.4. *Stationarity of time series*

The stationary time series is the concrete realization of the stationary stochastic process. The so-called stationary process is the process in which the statistical properties do not vary over time. Mainly reflected in that the series may keep good similarity after shifting a truncated time series by any distance.

Preprocessing can be attempted when the time series presents non-stationary. Common and effective methods include ordinary difference, seasonal difference, and logarithmic transformation.

(1) Ordinary difference. Difference is a transformation of the original series. It may eliminate the non-stationarity of the series if the mean shifts from time to time. Let the original series be Z_t, then the difference between adjacent values

$$\nabla Z_t = Z_t - Z_{t-1}$$

constitutes a new time series. It is the first difference of the original series, also known as the difference series with the first-order.

Example 26.1. The following time series is a changing stock of a pharmaceutical company. Try to transform it to a stationary series.

As shown in Figure 26.1(a), the mean value of each period of the stock changes dramatically. After ordinary difference, the stationarity of the series in Figure 26.1(b) is greatly improved.

(2) Seasonal difference. If seasonal components are included in the series, seasonal difference can be used to eliminate the influence from seasonality. Let the seasonal length be S, for the series Z_t,

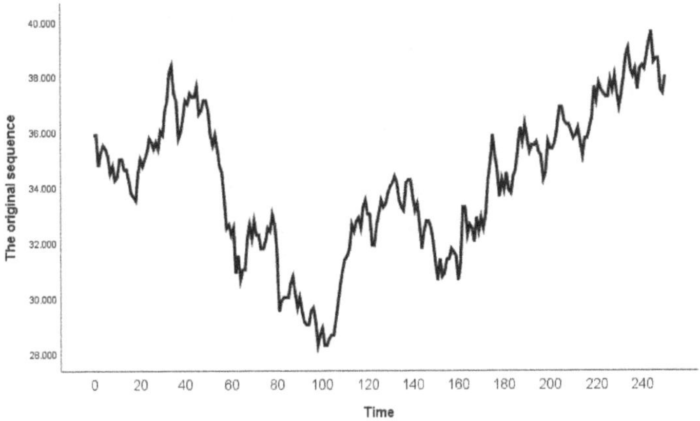

(a) Before difference

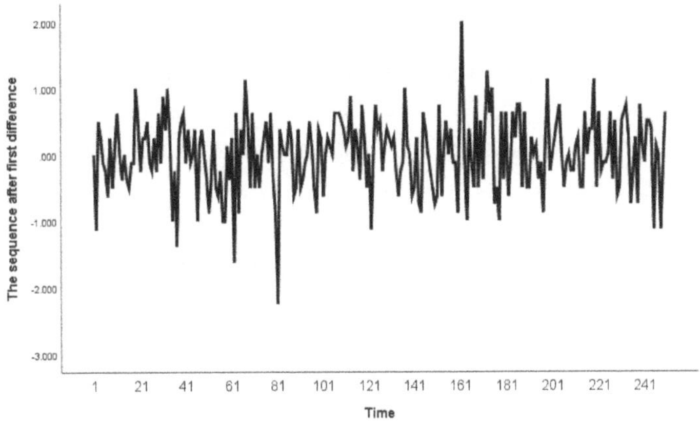

(b) After difference

Figure 26.1 Elimination of the non-stationarity with mean shift by the first-order difference

the seasonal difference is

$$\nabla_S Z_t = Z_t - Z_{t-S}$$

For example, if the season length $S = 4$, that is, there are 4 seasons in a year, for the time series of which measuring frequency is quarterly and the fluctuation includes annual periodicity, the seasonal difference transformation $\nabla_4 Z_t = Z_t - Z_{t-4}$ can eliminate the periodicity.

(3) Logarithmic transformation. When time series show different variability in different time periods, logarithmic transformation $Y_t = \log X_t$ can be taken to generate new time series, and the non-stationarity in the degree of variation can be modified.

Example 26.2. The following is a surveillance data on the incidence of influenza among children in a province. Try to transform it to a stationary series.

The time series in Table 26.1 is the surveillance data of the incidence of influenza among children in a province. As shown in Figure 26.2(a), the degrees of variation in the beginning and final stages are greater than that in the middle part of the series. After logarithmic transformation, the non-stationarity in the degree of variation shown in Figure 26.2(b) is greatly modified. The series has obvious annual periodicity, $S = 12$, and the processing results show better stationary properties after further seasonal difference, as shown in Figure 26.2(c).

Whether the time series is stationary can be judged by the following methods.

Table 26.1 The incidence of influenza among children in a city for 17 years (%)

	Month											
Year	1	2	3	4	5	6	7	8	9	10	11	12
1990	3.88	5.35	11.91	19.73	36.80	68.05	96.37	112.00	93.28	49.36	17.97	5.28
1991	3.74	2.61	7.24	16.75	25.66	40.54	73.43	91.84	53.00	25.55	10.77	3.24
1992	2.01	1.97	4.01	6.99	11.47	15.76	20.10	24.79	17.21	11.24	4.95	1.90
1993	0.89	1.20	2.28	2.87	4.72	7.94	12.95	17.40	9.48	8.61	3.76	1.68
1994	1.05	0.88	1.56	2.18	3.84	7.27	9.91	11.74	13.65	7.94	4.00	2.15
1995	0.54	1.37	2.33	2.04	3.28	7.15	9.15	11.58	7.91	5.26	2.36	1.34
1996	0.65	0.27	0.80	1.44	2.59	4.03	6.09	6.12	5.49	3.97	2.72	1.14
1997	0.46	0.57	0.60	1.26	1.73	3.27	4.79	5.31	4.48	3.10	1.52	0.72
1998	0.23	0.28	0.44	1.01	1.57	2.76	3.54	3.67	2.50	2.06	1.01	0.34
1999	0.26	0.18	0.24	0.44	0.78	1.54	1.96	2.65	2.54	1.70	0.62	0.28
2000	0.24	0.21	0.29	0.59	0.59	1.22	2.15	4.81	6.20	4.07	1.33	0.30
2001	0.24	0.10	0.27	0.54	1.84	3.94	7.87	8.63	10.99	6.56	1.27	0.17
2002	0.13	0.17	0.21	0.92	2.43	7.18	20.47	18.91	25.19	14.52	4.12	0.33
2003	0.23	0.36	0.59	1.64	5.87	12.58	29.00	28.96	21.42	20.34	3.01	0.31
2004	0.13	0.33	0.68	2.12	3.77	8.41	16.90	27.28	32.24	39.72	9.34	1.11
2005	0.23	0.26	0.46	1.19	2.88	7.94	18.56	56.25	65.13	68.04	18.17	2.90
2006	0.41	0.36	0.67	2.12	6.62	18.82	45.18	105.54	137.17	151.42	95.16	8.32

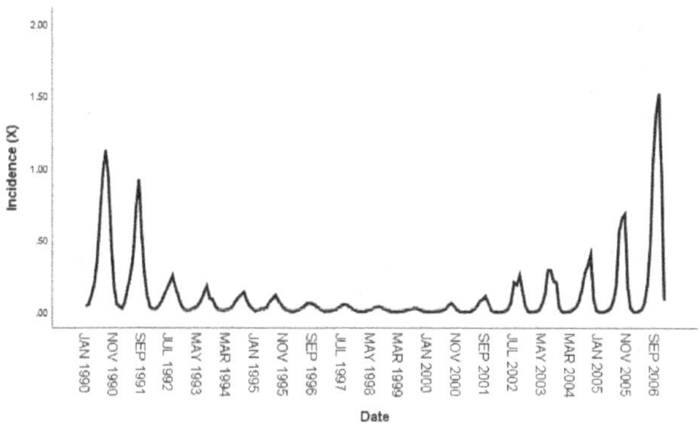

(a) Original series

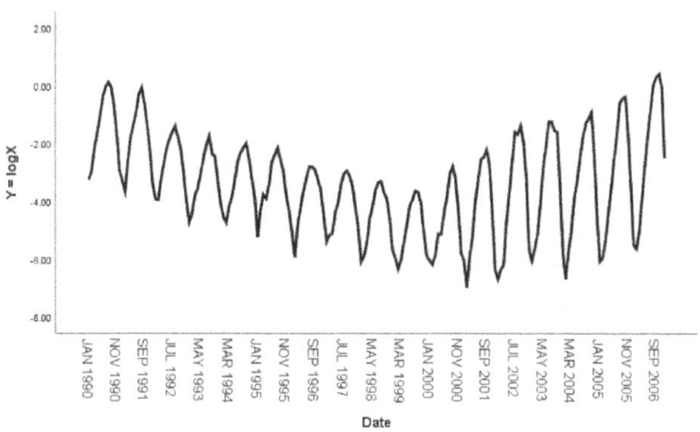

(b) After logarithmic transformation

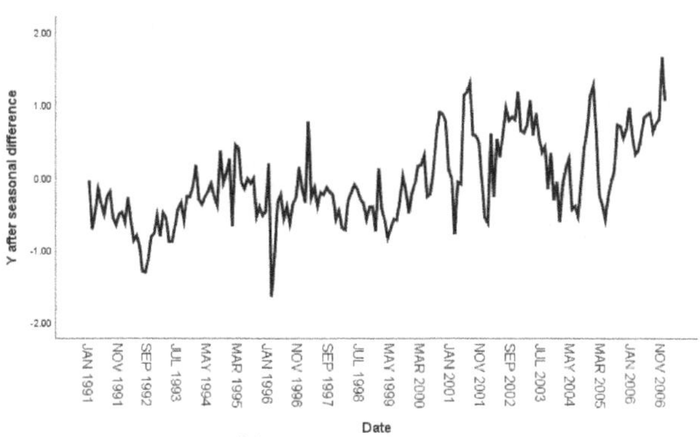

(c) After seasonal difference

Figure 26.2 Elimination of the non-stationarity and periodicity of heterogenous variability by logarithmic transformation and seasonal difference respectively

(1) Testing by data graph. Plot the time series in the $t - X_t$ two-dimensional coordinate system to check whether there is periodicity or tendency. If periodicity and trend are not obvious, the series is considered stationary.

Both Figures 26.1(b) and 26.2(c) belong to stationary time series.

(2) Testing by the ACF and PACF. If the ACF and PACF of a time series do not tail off nor cut off, the series is non-stationary. For example, if the decline (or periodic decline) of the ACF or PACF is with a very slow speed, this indicates that there may be a trend or periodicity in the series.

The ACF in Figure 26.3(a) is neither tailing off nor cutting off, this indicates that the series is non-stationary although the PACF in

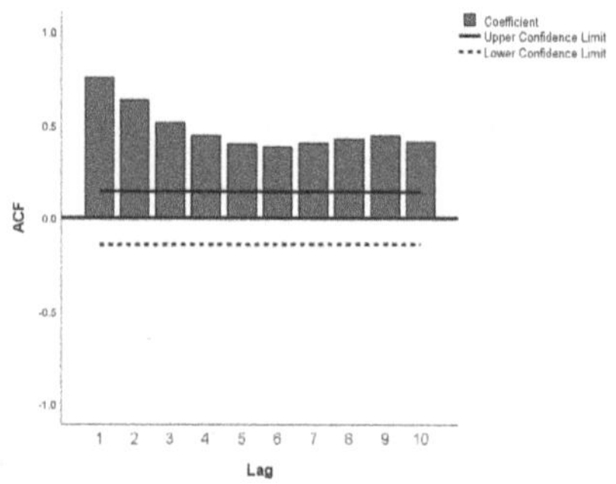

(a) ACF of the non-stationary series in Figure 26.2(a)

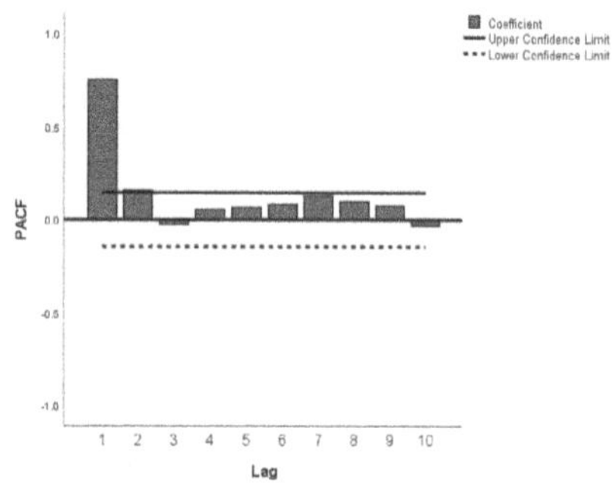

(b) PACF of the non-stationary series in Figure 26.2(a)

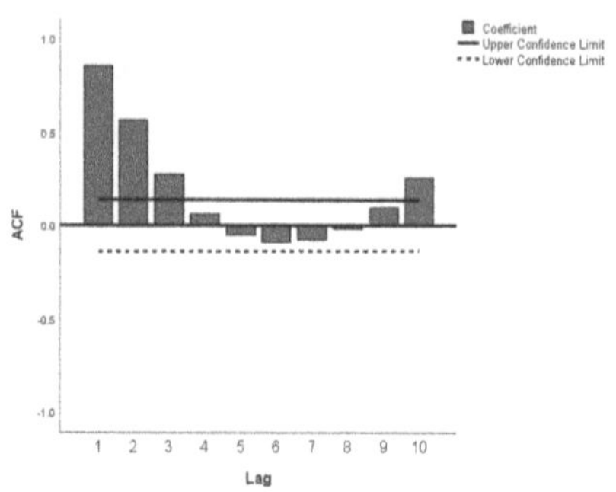

(c) ACF of the stationary series in Figure 26.2(c)

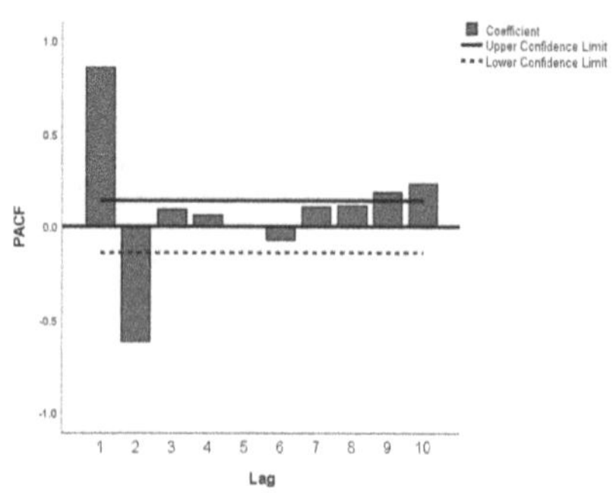

(d) PACF of the stationary series in Figure 26.2(c)

Figure 26.3 Judging stationarity of the series by ACF and PACF

Figure 26.3(b) is cutting off. The ACF is tailing off in Figure 26.3(c) and the PACF is cutting off in Figure 26.3(d), these indicate that the corresponding time series is stationary.

In addition, the stationarity test method also includes the latent root test, parametric test, run test, and so on.

26.2. Exponential smoothing

For influencing the future level of events, the newly observed value is more valuable than the early observed value, so the newly observed value should have a higher weight than the early observed value when predicting. Based on this logic, exponential smoothing is used to make a prediction by giving different weights to the new and early observations.

26.2.1. *Typical example*

Example 26.3. The time series of the production amount of an antibiotic in a pharmaceutical company are shown in Table 26.2, with an average of 355.19 thousand boxes. Use exponential smoothing to predict the production amount in January 1989.

26.2.2. *Statistical analysis*

The general formula for exponential smoothing prediction is

$$S_t = \alpha x_t + (1 - \alpha) S_{t-1} \tag{26-5}$$

where, S_t: smoothing value on the time point t ($t > 0$);
α: smoothing coefficient (range $0 < \alpha < 1$);
x_t: the actual observation on the time point t.

Table 26.2 The production amount of an antibiotic in a pharmaceutical company in 1988

Month	1	2	3	4	5	6	7	8	9	10	11	12
Quantity	371.5	267.4	372.4	368.2	349.4	362.8	420.9	380.4	385.6	335.0	338.5	306.6

For the time series data in Table 26.2, the estimation on the next time point can be obtained through repeated iteration.

Let $\alpha = 0.2$, the estimation process is as follows

$$
\begin{aligned}
S_1 &= 355.19 \\
S_2 &= 0.2 \times x_1 + 0.8 \times S_1 \\
&= 0.2 \times 371.5 + 0.8 \times 355.19 = 359.17 \\
S_3 &= 0.2 \times x_2 + 0.8 \times S_2 \\
&= 0.2 \times 267.4 + 0.8 \times 359.17 = 340.82 \\
&\cdots
\end{aligned}
$$

The predicted value in January 1989 is 349.21 (thousand boxes), which is summarized in Table 26.3.

26.2.3. *Determination of smoothing coefficient α*

In the prediction model (26-5), when the value of α is too small, the predicted value cannot closely track the new changes in the series; when the value of α is too large, the prediction model pays severe attention to the new random interference, which may also lead to poor prediction. In practice, multiple levels of values α are tried in software (such as SPSS) for selection, and the model with the minimum prediction error is selected as the best one.

26.3. ARIMA models

As mentioned above, the ACF and PACF are indices to describe the correlation between pieces of observations within the time series. On this basis, Box and Jenkins (1970) proposed the ARIMA model that summarizes the internal correlation of time series, which is a relatively mature time series modeling scheme.

26.3.1. *Typical example*

Example 26.4. Table 26.4 shows the incidence of cholangiocarcinoma in a city for 20 years. Fit an appropriate ARIMA model and perform predictions.

Table 26.3 Prediction of the production amount of an antibiotic in a pharmaceutical company by exponential smoothing (Unit: thousand boxes)

1988												1989
Jan.	Feb.	Mar.	Apr.	May	Jun.	Jul.	Aug.	Sept.	Oct.	Nov.	Dec.	Jan.
355.19	359.17	340.82	347.13	351.35	350.96	353.33	366.84	369.55	372.76	365.21	359.87	349.21

Table 26.4 The incidence of cholangiocarcinoma in a city for 20 years (1/10,000)

Year t	Incidence x_t	Year t	Incidence x_t
1	4.20	11	3.63
2	5.80	12	5.18
3	6.90	13	7.11
4	7.62	14	8.26
5	5.57	15	7.96
6	3.34	16	6.78
7	2.00	17	5.07
8	1.70	18	5.04
9	2.02	19	6.02
10	2.71	20	7.61

26.3.2. *Statistical analysis*

Time series modeling has three stages: identification, estimation, and diagnosis.

(1) Model identification is to select an existing model to describe the sequence according to the characteristics of time series, and then determine the number and types of parameters selected into the model, as well as their combination. In this process, the commonly used method is to plot the series and its ACF and PACF to find out the potential trend in the series, consider removing the trend through data transformation, and dealing with periodicity.

(2) Parameter estimation is to estimate the parameters in the model and test the hypothesis to make the model fit the actual data.

(3) Model diagnosis is to test the goodness of fit between the model and the actual data. The reliability of the model can be evaluated by the standard error calculated based on the residual, the confidence interval of the predicted value, etc. If it is not suitable, the model should be re-searched by returning to the first stage.

26.3.3. *Structure of ARIMA models*

The ARMA model is also known as the Box–Jenkins model. There are three basic patterns: the AR model, the moving average (MA) model, and the autoregressive and moving average (ARMA) model. When the series is stationary, the general expression of the model is

$$\begin{aligned} y_t = \varphi_1 y_{t-1} + \varphi_2 y_{t-2} + \cdots + \varphi_p y_{t-p} + a_t - \theta_1 a_{t-1} \\ - \theta_2 a_{t-2} - \cdots - \theta_q a_{t-q} \end{aligned} \tag{26-6}$$

where p and q are the orders of AR and MA, respectively, and the corresponding parameters $\varphi_1, \varphi_2, \ldots, \varphi_p$ and $\theta_1, \theta_2, \ldots, \theta_q$ are the coefficients of AR and MA respectively, $a_t, a_{t-1}, \ldots, a_{t-q}$ are random perturbation introduced in the period $t, t-1, \ldots, t-q$, which constitute the residual series.

By differencing, if a non-stationary time series can be transformed to a stationary one, the model adopted here is known as autoregressive integrated moving average (ARIMA) model. The ARIMA model is often expressed as ARIMA (p, d, q), where d is the order of difference.

26.3.4. *Establishment of ARIMA model*

For the time series, which include only a single measurement, its model form can be determined by the chart of functions ACF and PACF. Generally, the difference between the first p PACF value $\varphi_{11}, \varphi_{22}, \ldots, \varphi_{pp}$ and zero is statistically significant (the absolute value is greater than $1.96/\sqrt{N}$, where N is the significant sequence length), that is, the PACF cuts off at lag p, while the ACF tails off, suggesting that the time series should be fitted with the model AR (p). On the contrary, the difference between the first q ACF value $r_1, r_2, \ldots, r_q$ and zero is statistically significant (the absolute value is greater than $1.96/\sqrt{N}$, where N is the effective sequence length), that is, the ACF cuts off at lag p, while the PACF tails off, suggesting that the time series should be fitted with the model MA (q). When both ACF and PACF tail off, ARMA (p, q) model should be considered. For non-stationary time series, ARIMA (p, d, q) model can be used for fitting, where d is the order of ordinary difference.

For the time series with seasonal components, the seasonal difference can be used to eliminate the seasonality.

(1) Parameter estimation of the model

The sample ACF value r_k can be calculated from the series itself, and the relationship between the sample ACF and the AR coefficient $\varphi_1, \varphi_2, \ldots, \varphi_p$ of the model satisfies Equation (26-4). The parameter estimation can be easily completed with the knowledge of linear algebra, and the estimation of MA coefficient can be obtained by solving simultaneous equations. Here we omit the procedure.

The above parameter estimation can be easily realized by corresponding modules in general statistical analysis software such as SPSS and SAS.

(2) Diagnostic test of the model

The diagnostic test of the model should at least include the following contents: (1) Stationarity and reversibility test. As mentioned earlier, stationarity requires that the statistical characteristics of a series remain stable over time, and invertibility means that the dynamic change information of a series can be expressed by historical values (rather than future values). When the stationarity and reversibility tests fail, it is feasible to adjust the difference order. (2) Residual series test. When the absolute value of the ACF of the residual series is less than $1.96/\sqrt{n}$ ($n = N - d$, which is the significant sample size for fitting after considering the differential operation), it is considered that the residual series no longer contains non-stochastic components for modeling, and the residual can be regarded as white noise (see Section 26.4.4 for its detail), indicating that the goodness of fit is ideal. Statistics $Q = n\sum_{k=1}^{m} r_k^2$ can also be constructed for the first m (m is usually 6∼12) ACF value r_k. Q approximately follows χ^2 distribution with the degree of freedom $(m-p-q)$, where p and q are the orders of AR and MA, n is the significant sample size (i.e., the significant sequence length). (3) Over-fitting test. The over-fitting test is carried out to eliminate the redundant parameters that imply no statistical significance.

26.3.5. *Statistical analysis*

According to the time series given by Example 26.4, ACF and PACF are obtained by SPSS software (see Experiment 26.1 in Section 26.7 for detail), as shown in Table 26.5.

It is easy to find that $1.96/\sqrt{20} = 0.438$. Therefore, ACF or PACF with absolute value greater than 0.438 is considered to be of statistical significance. As can be seen from Table 26.5, ACF tends to be tails off, while PACF cuts off after lag 2, so AR(2) model is considered to fit the original sequence. The model is in the form of

$$x_t = 5.195 + 1.495x_{t-1} - 0.813x_{t-2} + a_t$$

The residual sequence is shown in Table 26.6.

The results of the ACF of the residual sequence are shown in Table 26.7. The absolute values of all ACFs does not exceed 0.438, suggesting that the residual sequence no longer contain non-stochastic components for modeling. $Q = n\sum_{k=1}^{m} r_k^2 = 22 \times 0.25008 = 5.502 < \chi^2_{8,0.5} = 7.34$, suggesting that there is no statistical significance between residual sequence and white noise (see Section 26.4.4 for details), indicating that the model is ideal.

Table 26.5 Autocorrelation and partial autocorrelation functions of incidence time series

lag	ACF	PACF
1	0.770	0.770
2	0.368	−0.554
3	−0.016	−0.104
4	−0.229	0.095
5	−0.335	−0.262
6	−0.367	−0.094
7	−0.343	−0.015
8	−0.244	0.015
9	−0.091	0.024
10	0.031	−0.134

Table 26.6 Residual sequence a_t of incidence time series

t	a_t	t	a_t
1	−0.995	11	−0.432
2	1.425	12	0.304
3	−0.009	13	0.665
4	0.368	4	0.190
5	−1.864	15	−0.259
6	−0.444	16	−0.056
7	−0.117	17	−0.246
8	−0.228	18	1.321
9	−0.549	19	0.955
10	−0.581	20	1.056

Table 26.7 Autocorrelation function of residual sequence a_t after fitting incidence data with AR(2)

lag	ACF	lag	ACF
1	0.130	6	0.137
2	0.143	7	−0.076
3	−0.296	8	−0.176
4	0.155	9	−0.139
5	0.162	10	0.002

The model can be used to predict future incidence. The predicted incidence of next year is:

$$x_t = 5.195 + 1.495x_{t-1} - 0.813x_{t-2} + a_t = 8.13(/100,000)$$

26.4. Analysis of time series in frequency domain

The foregoing analysis methods are based on the assumption that the observations at different time points are correlated to each other. Modeling, prediction, and model evaluation are all based on the observations along with the time, which belongs to the analysis of time domain, short for time-domain analysis. Another perspective of statistical analysis is carried out in the field of frequency, which is called analysis in frequency domain or spectral analysis.

Time-domain analysis method and frequency-domain analysis method belong to two theoretical perspectives of the same dynamic sequence data. The time-domain characteristics of time series including only a unique variable are as Figure 26.1(a), the horizontal axis is time, and the vertical axis is the value of the variable. In time-domain, if the time series after shifting j units can always be highly correlated with the series itself, it means that the series is somewhat a periodic activity (with period T equal to j) in the time series; conversely, if the time series after shifting s units is always not correlated with the sequence itself, it means that the series does not include periodicity (with period T equal to s). Frequency-domain analysis of time series transforms the original dynamic sequence into a new space. The horizontal axis is a set of period lengths, and the vertical axis is the intensity of periodicity. The more closely correlated of time series pieces and its shifted pieces by j units, the stronger the periodicity corresponding to period $T = j$.

This new space is called frequency-domain space, because fluctuations with a period of 0.1 second (second may be other units of time) are often referred to as fluctuations with a frequency of 10 Hz. The concepts of period and frequency are related so closely that the graph of "activity intensity (vertical axis) — preset period (horizontal axis)" mentioned above is called the frequency-domain feature description of time series no matter what the horizontal axis is scaled — frequency or period. In the frequency-domain space, we can know the contributions of various periodicity in the synthesis of final time series. This graph of "activity intensity-preset period" is called a periodogram.

The periodogram of stationary sequence is the comprehensive expression of the statistical characteristics of its periodic components. For a practical time series, one or several periodic activities are critical, while the other periodicities can be neglected. By comparing the intensity of periodicity on each preset period in the periodogram, we can find out the location of specific periodic activity in the sequence, which is the critical output of spectral analysis. Since the periodogram is based on the time series data of sampling research, the periodogram itself is not smooth and needs to be smoothed by window function. The smoothed figure is called spectral density.

26.4.1. *Typical example*

Example 26.5. The original data of time series are shown in Table 26.1. Here we discuss the periodicity and spectral densities of it.

26.4.2. *Spectrum of time series*

As long as there are enough presupposed periodic elements, the fluctuation information contained in time series can be decomposed into sine/cosine waves with various periods and intensities. The periodogram and spectral densities obtained by spectral analysis method demonstrate the possible periodicity that may exist in the time series. In the study of the correlation between average evoked potential waveform and mental retardation, researchers collected the neuro-electricity waveform of normal children and children with Down's disease. Spectral analysis showed that there were differences between the two groups in the frequency range of 0–4 and 8–11 Hz. Thus, it ensure the possibility to judge children's intelligence based on the spectrum of evoked potentials.

Based on the original time series, periodogram estimate the information components of each periodic component (horizontal axis can also be frequency) directly. This estimation method is based on Fourier transform (see related mathematical references for details). While spectral density graph uses different window functions to estimate the information components of each periodic component (horizontal axis can be replaced by frequency, too) more reliably. Window which is too narrow will make the information of spectral peaks not well centralized, resulting in "leakage"; while window which is too wide will make two characteristic peaks close to each other "compromised," and the resolution of periodic analysis will be reduced. Therefore, it is necessary to choose a proper window width according to the final efficiency.

26.4.3. *Statistical analysis*

Given the data provided by Example 26.2, we can realize the spectral analysis by using "Forecasting function" of "Analysis module" in SPSS, which can be used to find the spectrum. The results of periodogram and spectral density are shown in Figures 26.4 and 26.5, respectively.

From Figures 26.4 and 26.5, we can see that the time series of influenza incidence in children have periodic activities with a period of 12 months. The peaks locating on a period of 12 months are significantly different from the background noise, which are called the characteristic peaks of the original time series. In addition, the interval between cold and summer alternation is about 6 months, which is also shown in Figures 26.4 and 26.5.

Periodic analysis is helpful to reveal the regular periodicity of patient incidence changing with time. If the periodicity of a suspicious risk factor coincides with module of the periodicity of the diagnosed number of patients, this suggests that the suspicious factor may be a significant pathogenic factor, so as to provide a reference for further laboratory research.

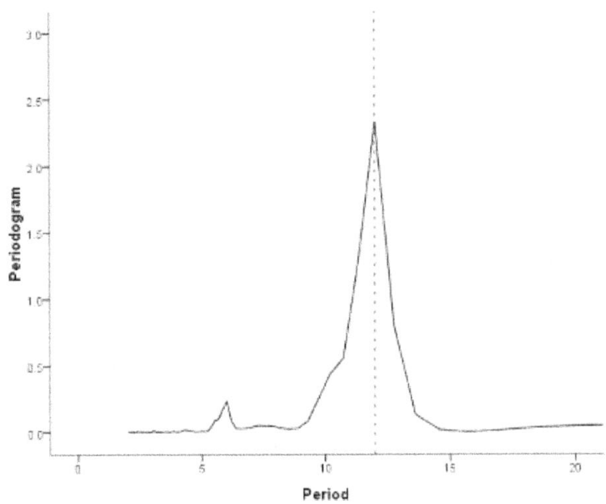

Figure 26.4 Periodogram of incidence of influenza monitoring sequence

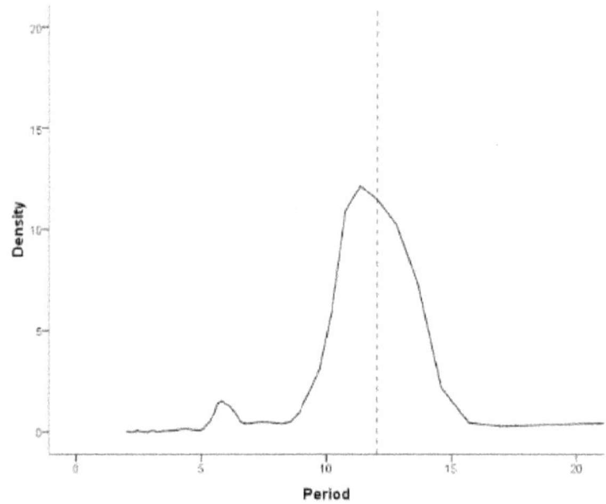

Figure 26.5 Spectral density of incidence of influenza monitoring sequence

26.4.4. *White noise*

White noise is a special time series. Let's intercept arbitrarily a fragment from the sequence. Wherever the intercepted fragment shifts to a new location, it will not correlated with the new fragment it covers. The shifting distance could not equal to 0. It is impossible to extract non-random information from such a sequence, and we can no longer expect any model to summarize the series.

In frequency-domain space, the white noise sequence has the uniform fluctuation intensity in each preset period. Just as white light contains the spectral components of red, orange, yellow, green, blue, and purple colored light in equal proportion, this sequence is called white noise sequence.

In dynamic data, there is interdependency or memorability between the observed values at different times of the sequence, and the information contained in it is the basis of mathematical modeling. On the contrary, white noise a_t is an ideal random sequence, theoretically "independent" and "memoryless."

When a model is used to fit time series, if the model is suitable, then the residual should be a white noise sequence, so the adaption test of the model becomes a test of the residual sequence. When a_t is not rejected as a white noise sequence, the model can be considered to be adapted to application; otherwise, the model fitting is not successful. Hypothesis tests should be conducted to determine whether a time series is white noise.

H_0: $a_1, a_2, \ldots, a_N$ is white noise.

When N is sufficiently large, the M components

$$\sqrt{N}\hat{\rho}_1(a), \sqrt{N}\hat{\rho}_2(a), \ldots, \sqrt{N}\hat{\rho}_M(a) \tag{26-7}$$

is approximated to a random variable independent of each other and subject to $N(0,\ 1)$. Therefore, testing the independence of $\{a_t\}$ is equivalent to testing whether the above M components are M independent random variables subject to $N(0,\ 1)$. Construct the statistic

$$Q = \sum \left(\sqrt{N}\hat{\rho}_j(a)\right)^2 = N\sum_{j=1}^{M} \hat{\rho}_j^2(a) \tag{26-8}$$

Q approximation obeys χ^2 distribution with degree of freedom $(M - p - q)$.

According to the given significance level α (usually α equal to 0.05), we can find the value of $\chi^2_\alpha(M - p - q)$ from the χ^2 distribution table. If $Q \leq \chi^2_\alpha(M - p - q)$, H_0 will not be rejected, which means $a_1, a_2, \ldots, a_N$ can be considered as a white noise sequence (the established model is adaptable). On the contrary, if H_0 is rejected, the established model is not adaptable, suggesting that more parameters should be included.

26.5. Repot writing

26.5.1. *Time-domain analysis*

The results needed to be reported for time-domain analysis of time series based on ARIMA model include:

(1) The pattern of ACF and PACF;
(2) The established mathematical model;
(3) Hypothesis testing of model parameters (the aim is to eliminate over-fitting);

(4) White noise test of residual sequences; (The aim is to ensure the retention of non-random components in residual sequences has been eliminated.)
(5) Forecasting future outcomes based on the model.

Take Example 26.4 for example. The report is as follows.

ARIMA model is constructed to the data of cholangiocarcinoma incidence. PACF cuts off at $k = 2$ and ACF tails off, thus AR(2) is preferred. The result is $x_t = 5.195 + 1.495x_{t-1} - 0.813x_{t-2} + a_t$. The hypothesis test to the coefficients either x_{t-1} or x_{t-2} shows $P < 0.001$, that means no redundant parameters are involved. The statistical inference shows the residual is white noise, $P > 0.5$, that means no more parameters are needed. We predict the incidence rate at $t = 21$ is 81.3 per million after input the observed values at $t = 19$ and $t = 20$.

26.5.2. *Frequency-domain analysis*

The results needed to be reported for frequency-domain analysis of time series include:

(1) Periodogram or spectral density.
(2) The reasonable explanation or the possible hint of characteristic peaks.

Take Example 26.2 for example. The report is as follows.

In Figure 26.4, the periodogram of influenza series is given. In Figure 26.5, the chart of spectral density is given. There is a primary peak at $T = 12$ and a secondary peak at $T = 6$, that means the activity of influenza is mainly with a periodicity 12, while the similarity among the series also exists with a periodicity 6. In practice the hypothesis to these peaks are also needed. Here we omit this procedure.

26.6. Case discrimination

Case 26.1: Based on the data of PM2.5 concentration ($\mu g/m^3$) observed continuously for 5 years in a city, the ARIMA model was established. The original data is a time series consisting of the mean of weekly PM2.5 concentration. After modeling, the white noise test of the residual sequence shows that $P < 0.20$, suggesting that there is no non-random component for modeling in the residual sequence. Therefore, it can be considered that the ARIMA model has a good ability for prediction. Do you think this interpretation is reasonable? Why?

26.7. Computer experiments

Experiments 26.1: Analyze the data by analysis in time domain to Example 26.4 with SPSS24.0

Experiments 26.2: Analyze the data by spectral analysis to Example 26.2 with SPSS24.0

26.8. Frequently asked questions and summary

26.8.1. *Frequently asked questions*

1. For a time series fitted by the ARMA (p, q) model, do the parameters of the AR part and the MA part of the model have to have p and q items respectively?

Answer: No. After fitting the time series using the ARMA (p, q) model, even if the AR coefficients of order p and the MA coefficients of order q have statistical significance, redundant AR coefficients and MA coefficients may still appear in the lower order part. Those coefficients need to be identified and removed through hypothesis testing. When many items are removed, the model is called sparse coefficient model.

2. How to set the sampling interval if we want to accumulate data that meets the requirements of time series analysis in practical work? What is the minimum sequence length requirement?

Answer: The requirement for the length of real data series is mainly related to the periodic characteristics that researchers focus on. If we do not want to omit the periodic feature of length T, the sampling interval should not be greater than $T/2$. If the maximum period of interest to researchers is $T_{\max}$, the empirical requirement is that the length of the data sequence should not be less than $5 \times T_{\max}$. For example, if an infectious disease has an 11-year pandemic, the length of data collection should be more than 55 years.

26.8.2. *Summary*

1. Time series analysis establishes appropriate mathematical models based on the regularly dynamic observed data to describe the development and evolution characteristics of events, and tries to predict the future levels.
2. Time series analysis methods include time-domain analysis and frequency-domain analysis. Time-domain analysis directly calculates the observed data and examines the relationship between current values and historical values. Assuming that the rule of correlation is relatively stable in a certain period of time in the future, the future levels can be predicted based on the information currently obtained. Frequency-domain analysis uses mathematical transformation (such as Fourier transform) to obtain the information components of each period (or frequency components) which are decomposed from total information. If the level of information component is different from that of noise somewhere, and the difference is statistically significant, the periodic components are regarded as the characteristics of time series. Periodogram or spectral density are the main tools for frequency-domain analysis.
3. If the model established for real-time series is adaptable, then the residual sequence after modeling should not be a sequence containing any non-random components, but only a white noise.

Think and Practice

I. Briefly Answered Questions

1. Take time-domain analysis as an example to illustrate the main purpose and steps of time series analysis.
2. Is the result of time-domain analysis instructive to frequency-domain analysis? Are the results of frequency-domain analysis

helpful to time-domain modeling? Please collect time series data by yourself and try to answer the above questions in the process of analysis.

3. What is the purpose of difference and seasonal difference? How to realize these two transformations?

II. Calculation and Analysis

1. The sample observations of a sequence are as follows. Please discussed the stationary of the sequence. If the sequence is not stationary, what measures should be taken to make the sequence stationary?

   2.5, 2.8, 3.5, 5, 6, 7.5, 9, 10.5, 12, 14, 15.5, 17, 19, 21, 22, 24, 25, 26, 28, 29, 30, 32, 34, 35, 36, 37, 38, 39, 38, 39.5, 40, 41, 40.5, 42, 43, 42.5, 43.5, 45, 46, 45, 46.5, 48.5, 48, 49, 48, 49.5, 49, 49.5, 50, 52, 51, 52, 53, 54

2. A general hospital has recorded the income of the medical examination center quarterly, as shown in Table 26.8.

Table 26.8 Income of a medical examination center in a hospital from 1991 to 1999 (Unit: RMB yuan)

t	x_t	t	x_t	t	x_t
1	2,575,800	13	2,953,430	25	3,329,890
2	2,606,680	14	2,986,450	26	3,361,130
3	2,639,000	15	3,017,050	27	3,392,070
4	2,671,000	16	3,048,120	28	3,423,520
5	2,702,380	17	3,079,180	29	3,455,050
6	2,733,890	18	3,109,000	30	3,487,140
7	2,765,840	19	3,143,240	31	3,516,750
8	2,796,710	20	3,171,630	32	3,550,370
9	2,829,000	21	3,205,110	33	3,580,560
10	2,859,800	22	3,235,900	34	3,611,470
11	2,892,200	23	3,266,950	35	3,644,170
12	2,921,900	24	3,297,650	36	3,674,310

Please use the original data to find the sample ACF and the sample PACF, and discuss:

(1) Is this sequence stationary?
(2) What model is suitable for describing this sequence?
(3) Estimation of parameters for the established models.
(4) Fulfill the hypothesis testing of the established model.

3. Table 26.9 shows the time series consisting of the number of sunspot bursts from 1770 to 1869. Please obtain the periodogram and spectral densities of this time series.

Table 26.9 Sunspot number from 1770 to 1869

101	82	66	35	31	7	20	92	154	125	85	68	38	23	10	24	83	132	131	118
90	67	60	47	41	21	16	6	4	7	14	34	45	43	48	42	28	10	8	2
0	1	5	12	14	35	46	41	30	24	16	7	4	2	8	17	36	50	62	67
71	48	28	8	13	57	122	138	103	86	63	37	24	11	15	40	62	98	124	96
66	64	54	39	21	7	4	23	55	94	96	77	69	44	47	30	16	7	37	74

Jinxin Zhang

CHAPTER 27

STRUCTURAL EQUATION MODEL

Structural equation modeling (SEM) is a method that integrates measurement and analysis. It examines latent constructs that are not directly observable using analysis of observed variables to estimate measurement error and evaluate the validity of the relationships modeled. In SEM, structural models are constructed to explore the relationship between latent variables. SEM has been widely used in psychology, sociology, behavioral science, and medicine in recent decades. This chapter introduces the process of SEM analysis and illustrates this process using specific cases.

27.1. Summary

27.1.1. *Analysis of chronic heart failure patient-reported outcomes*

Example 27.1. Patient-reported outcomes (PRO) constitute an important endpoint index that measures patient treatment efficacy. To investigate the relationship between reported outcomes and symptom dimensions of patients with heart failure, a multicenter questionnaire survey was conducted of 207 patients with heart failure using the patient-reported outcomes instrument for chronic heart failure (CHF-PROM). Table 27.1 shows the structure of the CHF-PROM. The physiological domain contains three dimensions and 16 items. The psychological domain contains four dimensions

Table 27.1 Structure of CHF-PROM

Domains	Dimensions	Variables	Num of items	Items
Physiology	Somatization	SOM	8	PHD1-, PHD2-, ..., PHD7-, PHD8-
	Appetite Sleep	APS	4	PHD9-, PHD10-, PHD11-, PHD12-
	Independent	IND	4	PHD13, PHD14, PHD15, PHD16
Psychology	Anxiety	ANX	8	PSD1-, PSD2-, ... PSD7-, PSD8-
	Depression	DEP	6	PSD9-, PSD10-, ..., PSD13-, PSD14-
	Fear	FEA	3	PSD15-, PSD16-, PSD17-
	Paranoia	PAR	4	PSD18-, PSD19-, PSD20-, PSD21-
Society	Support	SUP	5	SOD1, SOD2, SOD3, SOD4, SOD5
	Utilization	UTI	3	SOD6, SOD7, SOD8
Treatment	Compliance	COM	2	TRE1, TRE2
	Satisfaction	SAT	8	TRE3, TRE4, ..., TRE9, TRE10
	Effect of drug	EOD	2	TRE11, TRE12-

Note: "-" indicates reverse scoring.

and 21 items. The social domain comprises two dimensions and eight items. The therapeutic domain contains three dimensions and 12 items. Taking somatization symptoms in the physiological domain as an example, Table 27.2 shows the wording of each item.

In Table 27.1, the items are observed variables and the dimensions are latent variables. To investigate the relationship between somatization in the physiological domain and anxiety, depression, fear, and paranoia in the psychological domain in patients with heart failure, the above variables were used as latent variables and each item was used as an observed variable. A SEM was constructed to analyze the relationship between the observed variables and corresponding latent variables, as well as the structural relationship between different latent variables.

Table 27.2 CHF-PROM somatization items

1. Do you feel short of breath?	Never	Occasionally	About half of the time	Often	Always
2. Do you breathe faster than ordinary people?	Never	Occasionally	About half of the time	Often	Always
3. Do you feel chest tightness?(after day/night sleep)	Never	Occasionally	About half of the time	Often	Always
4. Do you have a cough?	Never	Occasionally	About half of the time	Often	Always
5. Do you have expectoration?	Never	Occasionally	About half of the time	Often	Always
6. Do you have a pallor?	Never	Occasionally	About half of the time	Often	Always
7. Is your lips purple?	Never	Occasionally	About half of the time	Often	Always
8. Do you have distension or pain?	Never	Occasionally	About half of the time	Often	Always

Depending on the research purpose and collected data, these relationships can be analyzed in terms of the following three aspects:

(1) Evaluation of the structural model validity: Whether the physical, psychological, and related dimensions of the scale have been effectively measured.
(2) Association study: Construction of a SEM to evaluate causal relationships and correlations between dimensions.
(3) Model evaluation: Evaluation of the model fit.

27.1.2. *Basic concepts*

The general SEM can be divided into two submodels: a measurement model and a structural model. The measurement model defines relations between the observed and latent variables. The measurement model, then, represents the confirmatory factor analysis (CFA) model described earlier in that it specifies the pattern by which each measure loads on a particular factor. In contrast, the structural model defines relations between the latent variables. A similar path analysis method is used to establish the structural relationships between the latent variables.

27.1.2.1. *Variable concepts and types*

Observed variable: An observed variable (manifest variable) is the variable measured in the data collection process, such as the scale item "Do you have a cough?"

Latent variable: A latent variable is measured by its connections to observed variables. Latent variables, such as depression or paranoia, cannot be directly measured.

Endogenous variable: An endogenous variable is a dependent variable that is explained by other variables. This category includes endogenous observed variables and endogenous latent variables.

Exogenous variable: An exogenous variable is a variable that can affect endogenous variables, including exogenous observed variables and exogenous latent variables.

27.1.2.2. *Confirmatory factor analysis*

Factor analysis and principal component analysis are data summary methods that reduce the dimensionality of a data set. Starting from the multiple correlations between items, factor analysis identifies the latent variables underlying the correlations, and uses these latent variables to explain the relationship between the original index variables. The two main types of factor analysis are exploratory factor analysis (EFA) and CFA. In EFA, factors are revealed from the relations among variables; the term "factor analysis" usually refers to this method. (See Chapter 24 for details.)

In CFA, the data are used to confirm a theoretical predetermined factor structure. In other words, in CFA, the researcher knows which factor will load on an observed variable. In EFA, the latent variables emerge from the observed variables. In contrast, CFA can be used to confirm the number of factors on a previously validated scale with the collected data. The difference is that CFA allows correlations between latent variables, whereas EFA requires potential variables to be independent. CFA is widely used in many research fields, such as sociology, psychology, behavioral research, education, management, and medicine. It is the most powerful method with which to evaluate the structural validity of a scale or test. The mathematical model of CFA constitutes the measurement model of SEM. Several CFA processes, such as theoretical model specification, parameter estimation, evaluation, modification, and interpretation, are similar to the SEM process.

27.1.2.3. *Structural equation modeling*

The general SEM model can be divided into two submodels: a measurement model and a structural model. The measurement model defines the relations between the observed and latent variables. When a SEM is used to analyze a problem, a path diagram should also be constructed. Figure 27.1 shows the path diagram for the first measurement model and describes the relationship between exogenous latent variables ξ (such as "somatization") and their indicators X. Figure 27.2 shows the path diagram for the second measurement model and represents the relationship between endogenous latent variables η and their indicators Y. Figure 27.3 shows the path diagram for the structural model and describes the structural relationship between exogenous latent variables ξ and endogenous latent variables η. Figure 27.4 shows the complete path diagram for the SEM and provides an intuitive illustration of the relationships between variables.

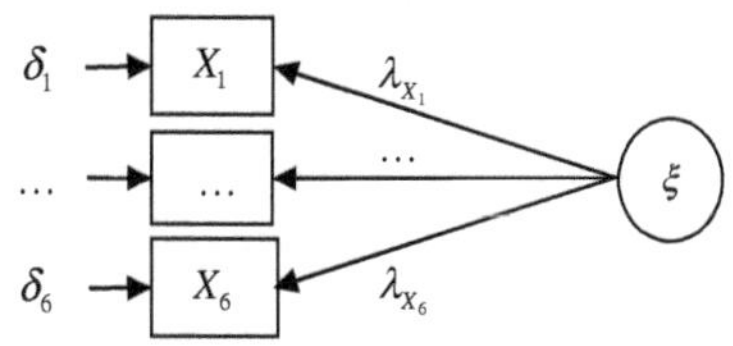

Figure 27.1 Measurement model I path diagram

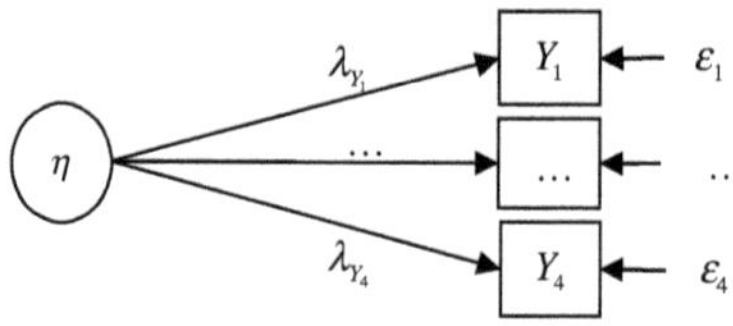

Figure 27.2 Measurement model II path diagram

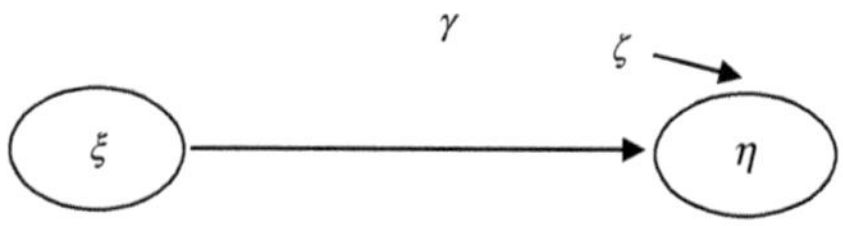

Figure 27.3 Structural model III path diagram

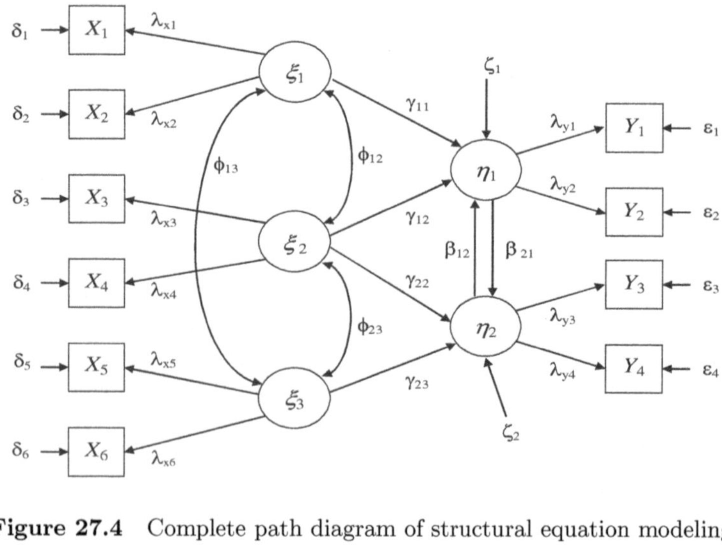

Figure 27.4 Complete path diagram of structural equation modeling

A single arrow between two variables indicates that a variable (start point) directly affects another variable (end point); a double arrow (curve) between two variables indicates that they are related, but that the relationship is probably not direct. As SEM is based on covariance matrix modeling, it is also called covariance structure modeling (CSM).

Table 27.3 The meaning of common icons in path diagrams of structural equation modeling

Icons	Meaning
○	Exogenous latent variable ξ and endogenous latent variable η
□	Exogenous indicators X and endogenous indicators Y
→ □	Measurement error of exogenous indicators X, expressed by δ
□ ← ○	The regression path of indicators to latent variable, whose coefficient is similar to factor load
□ ←	Measurement error of endogenous indicators Y, expressed by ε
○ ← ○	The influence of exogenous latent variable ξ on endogenous latent variable η
○ ←	Use ξ to predict the residual error of η, denote ζ

27.2. Basic idea of structural equation modeling

The purpose of SEM is to assume causality and correlation between variables according to existing knowledge, and then to verify, modify, and explain these associations based on data.

27.2.1. *Mathematical expression of the model*

Figure 27.4 shows the matrix equation and mathematical expression of the corresponding SEM.

$$X = \Lambda_X \xi + \delta \qquad \begin{aligned} X_1 &= \lambda_{X_1}\xi_1 + \delta_1 \\ X_2 &= \lambda_{X_2}\xi_1 + \delta_2 \\ X_3 &= \lambda_{X_3}\xi_2 + \delta_3 \\ X_4 &= \lambda_{X_4}\xi_2 + \delta_4 \\ X_5 &= \lambda_{X_5}\xi_3 + \delta_5 \\ X_6 &= \lambda_{X_6}\xi_3 + \delta_6 \end{aligned} \qquad (27\text{-}1)$$

$$Y = \Lambda_Y \eta + \varepsilon \qquad \begin{aligned} Y_1 &= \lambda_{Y_1}\eta_1 + \varepsilon_1 \\ Y_2 &= \lambda_{Y_2}\eta_1 + \varepsilon_2 \\ Y_3 &= \lambda_{Y_3}\eta_2 + \varepsilon_3 \\ Y_4 &= \lambda_{Y_4}\eta_2 + \varepsilon_4 \end{aligned} \qquad (27\text{-}2)$$

$$\eta = B\eta + \Gamma\xi + \zeta \qquad \eta = y\xi + \zeta \qquad (27\text{-}3)$$

Equations (27-1) and (27-2) are measurement models and equation (27-3) is a structural model.

X is the vector composed of exogenous observed variables of the order $q \times 1$.
Y is the vector composed of endogenous observed variables of the order $p \times 1$.
ξ is the vector composed of exogenous latent variables of the order $n \times 1$.
η is the vector composed of endogenous latent variables of the order $m \times 1$.
δ is the vector composed of measurement error of X.
ε is the vector composed of measurement error of Y.
Λ_x is the regression coefficient (factor loading) matrix of X to ξ of the order $q \times n$.
Λ_y is the regression coefficient (factor loading) matrix of Y to η of the order $p \times m$.
Γ is a coefficient matrix of ξ in the $m \times n$ order structural relationship.
ζ is the vector of the error composition of the structural equation between ξ and η of the order $m \times 1$.
B is the coefficient matrix of η in the structural relation of the order $m \times m$, and B is the non-singular matrix with 0 diagonal elements.

In a SEM, X and Y are usually used to represent exogenous and endogenous indicators, respectively. ξ and η are used to represent exogenous and endogenous latent variables, respectively. δ and ε respectively represent the measurement errors of X and Y in the model. ζ is the residual of the structural equation. β and γ respectively represent the effect between endogenous variables and the effect of exogenous variables on endogenous variables. $\Phi, \Psi, \theta_\varepsilon$ and θ_δ respectively represent the covariance matrix of ξ, η, ε, and δ. Σ represents the population variance–covariance matrix of $Z = (Y^T, X^T)^T$.

27.2.2. *Model assumptions*

To achieve parameter estimation, the model is usually required to meet these assumptions:

(1) The mean value of measurement error δ of X is 0, and the variance is constant. It is not related to ξ, and each δ is independent.
(2) The mean value of measurement error ε of Y is 0, and the variance is constant. It is not related to η, and each ε is independent.
(3) The mean value of the structural error ζ is 0, and the variance is constant. It is not related to ζ, and each ζ is independent.
(4) There is no correlation between δ, ε and ζ.

27.3. SEM modeling steps

The SEM modeling steps generally occur as outlined in the following five basic steps: model specification, model identification, model estimation, model evaluation, and model modification.

27.3.1. *Model specification*

The measurement model and/or the structural model are based on prior research and theory. These comprise a literature review to substantiate the selection of observed variables as indicators of latent variables, and the theory behind testing the relations among the latent variables in a structural model. There are three main types of model specification:

(1) Strictly confirmatory (SC): This refers to the theoretical model of the relationship between the variables based on prior knowledge, to confirm whether the theoretical model fits the actual sample data. This type of analysis is rare.
(2) Alternative models (AM): In this type of model specification, the researcher proposes several theoretical models about the relationship between the same set of variables. The fit between each model and the same sample data is tested and the optimal model selected according to the advantages and disadvantages of the fit.
(3) Model generating (MG): This type of model specification is used when the researchers are unsure about the structural relationship between variables. One or more theoretical models are first put forward to check whether these models fit the sample data well. Models that fit poorly are analyzed and corrected based on

prior knowledge, and the same sample data or other sample data are used to retest the modified model until an optimal model is produced. This method of analysis is more common.

Once a model is established, all model parameters must be estimated based on sample data. There are three types of model parameters that are important in SEM analyses: free, fixed, and constrained. Free parameters are estimated based on measured data; fixed parameters are set to 0 between variables that are considered irrelevant based on prior knowledge; and constrained parameters are usually set to a certain value or a value equal to other free parameters in the model. For example, if two indicators (X_1, X_2) have the same action intensity on latent variable (ξ), then the parameter (λ_1) between one of them (such as X_1) and ξ can be set as a free parameter, whereas the parameter (λ_2) between X_2 and ξ can be set as equal to λ_1, at which time λ_2 is a constrained parameter. Fixed and constrained parameters can save the degrees of freedom of the model.

Based on prior knowledge, Example 27.1 can be constructed as follows.

$\xi_1, \xi_2, \eta_1, \eta_2$ and η_3 are somatization, depression, fear, anxiety, and paranoia, respectively. X and Y are scores on observed variable items; δ and ε are the corresponding errors of X and Y.

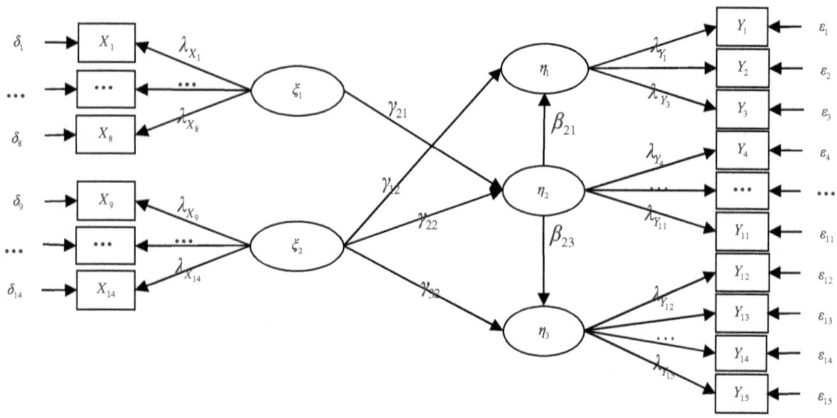

Figure 27.5 Theoretical model of Example 27.1

27.3.2. *Model identification*

Model identification involves the calculation of the sample matrix and the population matrix. The sample matrix is the consistency estimate of the corresponding population matrix, and the population matrix is a function of the model parameters. Therefore, a set of sample matrices (usually the variance–covariance matrix of the observed variables) is selected to form the vector S, and the population matrix constitutes the vector σ. The vector θ is composed of the parameters, and the vector equation $S = \sigma(\theta)$ can be obtained. $\sigma(\theta)$ is the population matrix as a function of θ, which is called the matrix structure in SEM. The parameters can be estimated by solving the equation $S = \sigma(\theta)$. Model identification involves considering whether each free parameter estimated from the model data can obtain a unique solution from the sample matrix. If we can find the unique solution of the parameter from the model, the parameter is identifiable. If all unknown parameters (free parameters) in the model are identifiable parameters, the model is an identification model.

In SEM, the degree of freedom is the difference between the number of independent elements in the variance–covariance matrix (S) and the number of free parameters in the model. Assume that p and q are the number of observed variables X and Y, respectively. If the number of free parameters is t, then

$$df = \frac{1}{2}(p+q)(p+q+1) - t$$

$df = 0$ indicates a saturated model; that is, all parameters are estimated. This is also called a just-identified model. $df > 0$ indicates an over-identified model; this type of model specifies fewer paths or variable relations, but the model-implied (reproduced) variance matrix is close to the sample covariance matrix. The order and rank condition are other matrix features that indicate that a model is identified, which implies that parameters can be estimated.

In SEM, there is no simple set of sufficient conditions that can be used as a basis for model identification. However, there are two necessary conditions to consider:

(1) Non-negative degrees of freedom represent a necessary condition for model identification.
(2) A measurement scale must be established for each latent variable in the model.

There are two ways to establish the measurement scale for a latent variable: one is to set the variance of the latent variable to 1; that is, the latent variable is standardized and has a standardized scale. Second, any factor loading λ of the observation indicator of the latent variable can be set to 1.

Even if the above two conditions are met, the problem of model identification will occur. Free parameters can usually be fixed or constrained to solve this problem.

27.3.3. *Model estimation*

The SEM estimation process is different from that of traditional statistical methods. Instead of trying to minimize the difference between predicted values and observed values in the sample, it aims to minimize the difference between the sample variance–covariance and the theoretical variance–covariance implicit in the model $(S - \Sigma(\theta))$ (residual of the SEM). There are three main estimation methods and fit function types in SEM: unweighted least squares (ULS), maximum likelihood (ML), and generalized least squares (GLS). The use of each estimation approach is based on the minimization of the corresponding fit function.

27.3.4. *Model evaluation*

After obtaining the parameter estimation, the model fit should be evaluated. This should be based on the following two aspects:

(1) Rationality of parameter estimation and hypothesis testing

Assuming that the model is specified correctly, the estimated parameter values should have the correct sign. The following signs are some indicators that the model is set incorrectly or the input matrix lacks sufficient information: the variance is negative, the absolute value of the correlation coefficient is greater than 1, the covariance or the correlation matrix is a non-positive definite matrix. In addition, a t-test of 0 is required for each free parameter.

(2) Model evaluation and selection of fit indices

The evaluation of the overall fit of the model is mainly based on the fit index (this is an abbreviation of "goodness of fit" statistic). There are many indices to evaluate the model fit. These indices can be roughly divided into four categories: absolute fit index, relative fit index, information criteria index, and parsimony fit index. The different categories of fit indices are shown in Table 27.4.

The values of the multinomial fit indices should be reported in the SEM results, and the degree of model fit comprehensively evaluated. Given the same degree of fit, the simplest model should be selected; that is, the fewer the model parameters, the better.

27.3.5. *Model modification*

During the process of hypothesis testing, a given model may not fit the data. The researcher should be guided to make changes by the residual values in the residual matrix, the modification index (MI), or theory. It is not recommended to change the structural model by adding or deleting a path unless additional theory substantiates the structural model modification. Generally, the measurement model will require the addition of an error covariance term between observed variables, which is sufficient to provide a better data-to-model fit.

For model modification, please refer to MacCallum's suggestions:

(1) Before describing a problem with the structural model, it is necessary to solve any problems with setting error variance of the measurement model and avoid any error identification problems of the measurement model, so that the structural model's parameter estimation and related information are more meaningful.
(2) Because estimation of SEM uses complete information technology, only one modification can be made at a time, and any modification will affect the estimation of other parameters.

Table 27.4 Fit indices and model fit criteria

Fit indices	Model-fit criteria
Absolute fit index (AFI)	
Goodness of fit index (GFI)	0 to 1. Value greater than 0.9 reflects a good fit
Adjusted goodness of fit index (AGFI)	0 to 1. Value greater than 0.9 reflects a good fit
Root mean square error of approximation (RMSEA)	Value greater than 0.05 reflects a good fit, 0.08 $\sim$ 0.10 reflects a general fit, and greater than 0.10 reflects a poor fit.
Root mean square residual (RMR)	0 to 1. Value less than 0.05 reflects a good fit
χ^2/df	Value less than 3 reflects a good fit
Relative Fit Index (RFI)	
Normed fit index (NFI)	0 to 1. Value greater than 0.9 reflects a good fit
Non-normed fit index (NNFI)	Value greater than 0.9 reflects a good fit
Incremental fit index (IFI)	Value greater than 0.9 reflects a good fit
Comparative fit index (CFI)	0 to 1. Value greater than 0.9 reflects a good fit
Information criteria index	
Akaike information criterio (AIC)	Compares values in alternative as small as possible
Consistent Akaike Information Criterio (CAIC)	Compares values in alternative models as small as possible
Expected cross validation index (ECVI)	Compares values in alternative models as small as possible
Parsimony fit index	
Parsimony goodness of fit index (PGFI)	Value greater than 0.9 reflects a parsimony fit
Parsimony fit index (PNFI)	Value greater than 0.9 reflects a parsimony fit

(3) The modification process should first add meaningful parameters. If necessary, reduce the meaningless parameters.

(4) The modification of the model should be guided by practical theories instead of relying only on the information provided by sample data.

Many SEM statistical software packages provide an MI. When a single fixed parameter or constrained parameter is released as a free parameter, the MI reflects the reduction of χ^2 caused by the new model fit. When fitting data using a theoretical model, we always hope that the model is also suitable for similar sample data from other sources. If the model is repeatedly modified according to specific sample data, the goodness of fit may decline when the resulting model is used to fit other sample data; this is called "overfitting." Therefore, some scholars suggest that the model should be cross-validated. In practice, if a larger sample can be obtained, it can be divided into two: half of which is used to fit the model and the other half used to modify the model.

27.4. Application of structural equation modeling

27.4.1. *Confirmatory factor analysis*

Example 27.2. CFA was used to evaluate the structure and validity of the psychological domain of the CHF-PROM instrument using data from 207 individuals (To assess instrument consistency, a reliability evaluation is required, such as Cronbach's α coefficient. Please refer to Chapter 10 for the evaluation method). The psychological domain of the CHF-PROM contains 21 items. These can be divided into four dimensions (i.e., four potential factors) to construct a multifactor model. The data file 27-1.csv is retrieved and the measurement model is constructed using R software (see computer Experiment 27.1 for the program). The results of the ML estimation and the partial fit indices of the evaluation model's overall fit are shown in Table 27.5.

The path diagram of SEM displayed differently in LISREL, AMOS, MPLUS, EQS, and other software programs. Figure 27.4 shows the traditional LISREL pattern, and Figure 27.6 and Figure 27.7 (below) show the path diagram generated by R software.

Table 27.5 indicates that the non-standard solutions of all items are statistically significant. The CFA standard solution in Figure 27.6 shows that the largest factor loading on the first latent variable in

Table 27.5 CFA maximum likelihood estimation of the CHF-PROM psychological domain

Latent variables (Dimensions)	Observed variables (Items)	Factor loads	SE	z	Error variance
ANX	PSD1	1.000			1.499
	PSD2	1.227	0.205	5.982	0.807
	PSD3	0.637	0.180	3.538	1.801
	PSD4	0.562	0.168	3.351	1.621
	PSD5	0.551	0.174	3.174	1.791
	PSD6	1.001	0.184	5.438	0.985
	PSD7	1.225	0.208	5.894	0.903
	PSD8	1.060	0.203	5.227	1.341
DEP	PSD9	1.000			0.654
	PSD10	1.273	0.149	8.557	0.628
	PSD11	1.206	0.133	9.086	0.381
	PSD12	1.171	0.138	8.458	0.567
	PSD13	1.074	0.164	6.544	1.334
	PSD14	0.992	0.135	7.322	0.772
FEA	PSD15	1.000			0.596
	PSD16	1.304	0.132	9.867	0.299
	PSD17	1.135	0.120	9.486	0.387
PAR	PSD18	1.000			0.127
	PSD19	0.937	0.064	14.599	0.271
	PSD20	0.997	0.067	14.872	0.285
	PSD21	0.539	0.087	6.162	0.797
Fit Indices	$\chi^2 = 460.555$, $df = 182$			RMSEA = 0.086	
	AIC = 11881.165			NFI = 0.778	
	IFI = 0.853			CFI = 0.851	

the psychological domain, anxiety, was for item PSD2; therefore, this item is the best measure of anxiety. The largest factor loading on the second latent variable, depression, was for item PSD11; therefore, this item is the best measure of depression. The largest factor loading on the third latent variable, fear, was for item PSD16; this item is the best measure of fear. The largest factor loading on the fourth latent variable, paranoia, was for item PSD18, and this is the best measure

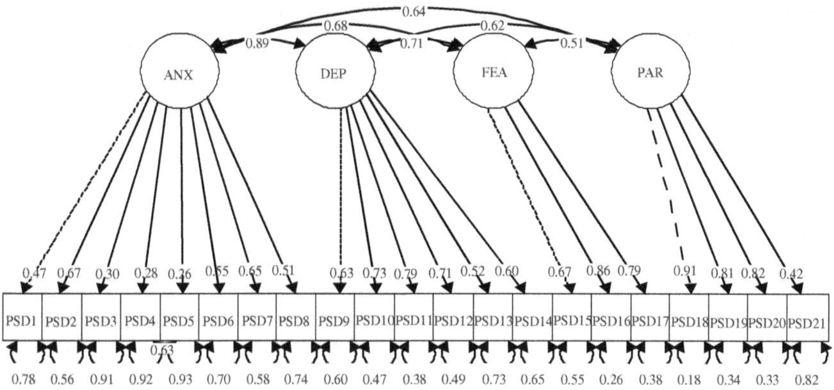

Figure 27.6 Standardized CFA path diagram of the CHF-PROM psychological domain

of paranoia. There were strong positive correlations among the four latent variables.

27.4.2. *Structural equation modeling analysis*

Example 27.3. The relationships between somatization, anxiety, depression, fear, and paranoia in patients with heart failure were investigated. In the SEM shown in Figure 27.5, anxiety (ANX), fear (FEA), and paranoia (PAR) are endogenous latent variables. Somatization (SOM) and depression (DEP) are exogenous latent variables. Data are in the file 27-2.csv and R software was used to build the models (see the computer program test 27-2). ML estimation was used for model fitting. The results are shown in Table 27.6 and Table 27.7.

Table 27.6 shows the results of the measurement model. The factor loadings of the first items for each latent variable are set to 1. The results show that each item is statistically significant. The estimation results of the structural model are shown in Table 27.7 and indicate that the model fits well. Figure 27.7 is the standard solution; a detailed explanation is shown in the results report. In the process of model fitting, it was found that the PHD4-PHD5MI was

Table 27.6 Maximum likelihood estimation of the measurement model for the physical and psychological domains of patients with heart failure

Measurement model	Latent variables (Dimensions)	Observed variables (Items)	Factor loads	SE	z	Error variance
Model I	SOM	PHD1	1.000			0.680
		PHD2	0.888	0.114	7.818	0.854
		PHD3	0.796	0.115	6.930	1.144
		PHD4	0.480	0.108	4.426	1.415
		PHD5	0.520	0.112	4.643	1.482
		PHD6	0.516	0.089	5.833	0.816
		PHD7	0.519	0.107	4.836	1.342
		PHD8	0.287	0.104	2.765	1.447
Model II	DEP	PSD9	1.000			0.655
		PSD10	1.278	0.149	8.562	0.624
		PSD11	1.204	0.133	9.051	0.385
		PSD12	1.169	0.139	8.430	0.569
		PSD13	1.077	0.165	6.548	1.331
		PSD14	0.994	0.136	7.317	0.771
Model III	ANX	PSD1	1.000			1.497
		PSD2	1.236	0.205	6.033	0.795
		PSD3	0.678	0.181	3.736	1.777
		PSD4	0.683	0.174	3.936	1.556
		PSD5	0.678	0.179	3.780	1.723
		PSD6	0.990	0.182	5.431	0.992
		PSD7	1.185	0.203	5.831	0.942
		PSD8	1.071	0.203	5.282	1.329
Model IV	FEA	PSD15	1.000			0.598
		PSD16	1.305	0.133	9.844	0.301
		PSD17	1.140	0.120	9.481	0.384
Model V	PAR	PSD18	1.000			0.126
		PSD19	0.936	0.064	14.611	0.272
		PSD20	0.996	0.067	14.889	0.285
		PSD21	0.536	0.087	6.137	0.798

large (MI = 115.9); the two items were cough and somatization, so the modification was carried out (see Experiment 27.2 program). It should be noted that prior knowledge should be used when revising the model to avoid overfitting.

Table 27.7 Maximum likelihood estimation of structural equation modeling for the physiological and psychological domains of patients with heart failure

	Structure coefficient	Standard error	z
SOM–ANX	0.122	0.054	2.237
DEP–ANX	0.807	0.148	5.462
ANX–FEA	0.206	0.223	0.924
DEP–FEA	0.577	0.227	2.537
DEP–PAR	0.340	0.243	1.400
ANX–PAR	0.452	0.254	1.781
Fit indices	$\chi^2 = 799.894$, $df = 368$ AIC = 17006.445 IFI = 0.817		RMSEA = 0.075 NFI = 0.706 CFI = 0.813

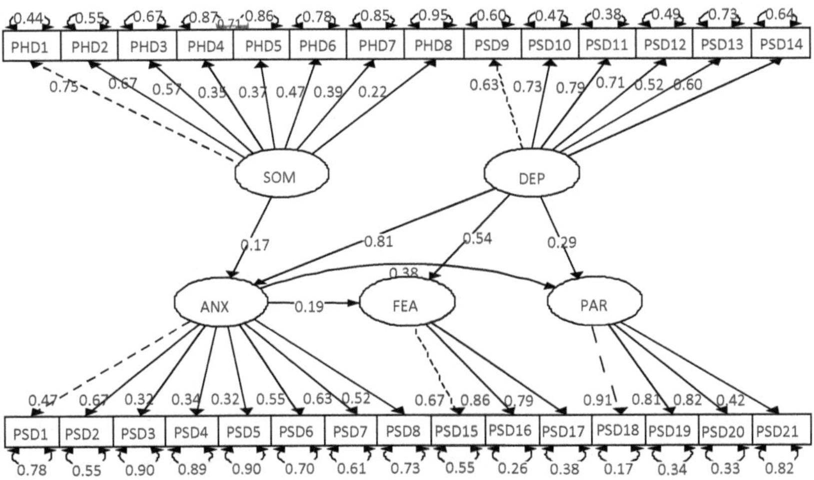

Figure 27.7 The standardized path diagram of structural equation modeling for physiological and psychological domains

27.5. Results report

The analysis results of the SEM should contain the following:

(1) The purpose of using the SEM.
(2) Determination of the exogenous latent variables and endogenous latent variables in the analysis.

(3) Check of whether the data meet the preconditions of the SEM.
(4) Method of fitting the SEM.
(5) Mention of whether there are missing data values and how to handle these.
(6) The final model and the statistics that reflect the model fit.
(7) The path diagram of the standardized SEM.
(8) Finally, a table is used to summarize the results of the inductive analysis. The following statistics are included in the table: estimated values of structural coefficients, standard deviations of structural coefficients, standardized structural coefficients, values, squared residuals, and model fit indices.

Example 27.1: A brief summary of the analysis results

To explore the relationship among different latent variables in the physiological and psychological domains of heart failure patients, we take anxiety (ANX), fear (FEA), and paranoia (PAR) as endogenous latent variables (η), and take somatization (SOM) and depression (DEP) as exogenous latent variables (ξ). We then construct a SEM. Table 27.7 shows the main results of the final model.

All items in the measurement model are statistically significant, and the goodness of fit measures indicate that the structural model fits the data well. In Figure 27.7, all the standardized path coefficients are positive: anxiety-somatic symptoms 0.17, anxiety-depression 0.81, fear-depression 0.54, paranoid-depression 0.29, fear-anxiety 0.19, and paranoia-anxiety 0.38. The indirect effects of depression on fear and paranoia are 0.15 and 0.30 respectively, indicating mediation effects of anxiety on fear and paranoia. According to the causal relationships among different variables in the model, targeted measures can be taken to improve the patients' psychological states and scores.

27.6. Case discrimination

Case 27.1 To explore the relationship between the physiological and psychological dimensions of heart failure patients, change the path direction of the theoretical model diagram constructed

Table 27.8 Maximum likelihood estimation results of adjusted structural equation modeling

	Structural coefficient	Standard error	z
ANX–SOM	0.673	0.156	4.321
FEA–ANX	0.432	0.104	4.162
PAR–ANX	0.342	0.084	4.074
ANX–DEP	0.664	0.155	4.289
FEA–DEP	0.207	0.086	2.401
PAR–DEP	0.073	0.069	1.060
Fit indices	$\chi^2 = 800.140$, $df = 368$		RMSEA = 0.075
	AIC = 17006.692		NFI = 0.706
	IFI = 0.816		CFI = 0.813

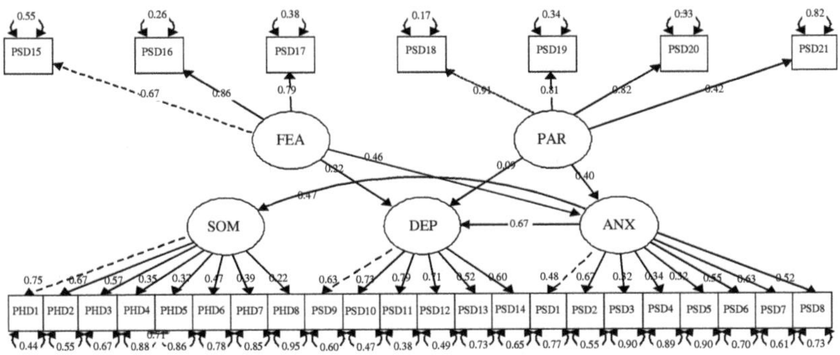

Figure 27.8 Standardized path diagrams of structural equation modeling in physiological and psychological domains

in Figure 27.5 to adjust somatization (SOM), anxiety (ANX), and depression (DEP) as the endogenous latent variables (η) and fear (FEA) and paranoia (PAR) as the exogenous latent variables (ξ), comparing the results of the SEM above. The data in data file 27-3.csv were analyzed using R software and ML estimation was used to fit the model. The results of the structural model are shown in Table 27.8.

Compare the difference between the diagram of SEM constructed after changing the path direction (Figure 27.8) and the SEM based on the theoretical model (Figure 27.7).

27.7. Computer experiments

Exp 27.1 R software is used to implement Example 27.2: CFA.

Fitting the CFA model, reporting the main results, and appending the path diagram. Item reliability and scale validity were evaluated using factor loadings and a goodness of fit index.

Exp 27.2 R software is used to implement Example 27.3: SEM.

Fitting the SEM, reporting the main results, and appending the path diagram. Item reliability and scale validity were evaluated using factor loadings and a goodness of fit index. Statistical significance between latent variables and the model fit were evaluated using structural coefficients and a goodness of fit index.

27.8. FAQ and summary

27.8.1. *FAQs*

(1) What are the sample size requirements for SEM?

To obtain stable, reliable, meaningful results and accurate parameter estimates, the use of SEM requires a large sample size. This is because (1) SEM estimates the parameters according to the asymptotic theory; to satisfy the assumptions of consistency and normal distribution, the sample must be large enough; (2) when the sample is small, the statistics fitted by the model are tested in terms of their deviation from the χ^2 distribution; (3) as sample size increases, the covariance estimation is more accurate, and more reliable SEM results are obtained. When the sample size is large, all types of fit indices, distributions, tests, and their efficacy will be meaningful and a reasonable model evaluation can be carried out.

There are no standard rules for sample size, but the needs of sample representativeness, model estimation, and model evaluation are generally considered. Stevens (1996) suggests that the sample size should be at least 15 times the number of observed variables or indicators. In practice, it is best to avoid as far as possible a SEM analysis with less than 200 cases, as the analysis results will be unstable and inaccurate. If the sample size is insufficient, it is recommended to choose a more robust estimation method, such as the S-B adjustment method or bootstrap resampling to estimate the SEM for small samples and non-normal data.

(2) What should be done if the data do not obey the multivariate normal distribution?

SEM analysis generally requires data to follow a multivariate normal distribution. When the normality assumption is violated, the results of SEM analysis must be questioned. Therefore, when writing research papers, the data distribution characteristics and the hypothetical test results should be presented. It is impossible to judge the distribution characteristics of the data owing to the lack of original data for each variable, particularly when the researchers use a matrix as the input data. In these cases, it is even more important to explain that the distribution type is a normal distribution or a multivariate normal distribution. When the data violate distribution assumptions, researchers are more likely to reject models that are actually well constructed, or to assume that individual estimation parameters are not 0, increasing the type I error of statistical inference.

Four methods can be used to process non-normal data: (1) variable transformation. After variable transformation, the interpretation of estimated parameters should be conducted according to the new measurement. The factor loadings obtained are different from the factor loadings of the original non-normal observation variables, so it is generally not recommended to use the transformed variables for research purposes; (2) the standard deviation of the statistics and parameters is tested using an adjusted model based on the normal theory, such as the S-B adjustment method; (3) nonparametric estimation methods, such as Browne's asymptotically distribution free method; (4) bootstrap resampling.

(3) How to choose the overall evaluation criteria of the model?

Model evaluation comprises two aspects: parameter evaluation and overall goodness of fit evaluation. An ideal fit index should have the following characteristics: (1) it is not affected by the sample size;

(2) complex models should contain penalties (to produce a model with more free parameters); (3) it is sensitive to an incorrectly constructed model. Table 27.4 lists some commonly used fit indices. Although there are many fit indices, none provide a perfect test of whether the theoretical model has good fit. The NNFI, CFI, AGFI, RMSEA and other indices are relatively widely used. Bollen suggests that it is better to report results by combining multiple indices rather than relying on a single index.

27.8.2. *Summary*

(1) The general SEM model can be divided into two submodels: a measurement model and a structural model. The measurement model defines relations between the observed and latent variables. The structural model defines relations among the latent variables.
(2) SEM variable types: endogenous variables and exogenous variables. Latent variables and observed variables can be categorized as endogenous variables and exogenous variables. Endogenous variables are affected by the action of variables in the model, and are dependent variables in the causal model; exogenous variables affect other variables in the model, and are independent variables in the causal model. Usually, X and Y are used to represent exogenous observed variables and endogenous observed variables, and ξ and η are used to represent exogenous latent variables and endogenous latent variables.
(3) The SEM modeling steps generally occur as outlined in the following five basic steps: model specification, model identification, model estimation, model evaluation, and model modification. The SEM is based on theories and constructs to form hypotheses to be tested and then fitted with data.
(4) Sample requirements: a larger sample size will increase the model reliability. Generally, the ratio of the number of sample cases to the estimated parameters in the model should be at least 10:1. If the data deviate from normality, the ratio should reach 15:1.
(5) Results report: standardized coefficients. The results of all parameter estimates are presented in a standardized form, and

the standardized values of the parameters are between −1 and 1, which is easy to understand.

Think and Practice

1. Best Choice

(1) Which of the following statements about SEM is wrong? ( )
A. The measurement model reflects the relationship between observed variables and latent variables. B. The structural model reflects the structural relationships between latent variables. C. SEM is also called path analysis. D. SEM can analyze direct and indirect effects. E. SEM is based on a covariance matrix, so it is called a covariance structure model.

(2) Which of the following statements about latent variables is wrong? ( )
A. They can be measured using a set of correlated observed variables. B. They are divided into endogenous latent variables and exogenous latent variables. C. They are divided into continuous latent variables and discrete latent variables. D. Latent variables can also be directly measured. E. Latent variables can represent hypothetical constructs.

(3) Which of the following statements about CFA is correct? ( )
A. CFA can evaluate content validity. B. CFA can be used to evaluate construct validity. C. CFA can evaluate discriminant validity. D. CFA can evaluate predictive validity. E. CFA can evaluate nomological validity.

(4) Which of the following statements about the fit index selection criteria is wrong? ( )
A. When χ^2/df less than 3, the model has good fit. B. When RMSEA less than 0.05, the model has good fit. C. The closer NNFI is to 1, the better the fit. D. The closer AGFI is to 1, the better the fit. E. Only one indicator is used to test the SEM fit, and the results of multiple indicators do not need to be reported.

(5) Which of the following is correct about SEM model modification? ( )
A. Model modification should be guided by practical theories. B. Model correction should first remove statistically insignificant

parameters. C. Multiple parameters can be modified simultaneously. D. Model modification is based mainly on the information provided by the sample. E. Model modification needs to be repeated until a good fit is achieved.

2. Questions for Reflection

(1) What is the basic idea behind a SEM?
(2) What is the basic flow of SEM fitting?

3. Question on Calculation

With the "Patient-Reported Outcome scale with heart failure" as the data background, the data in the social and therapeutic domain of patients with heart failure (see 27-4. csv for SPSS database) were applied. Taking treatment compliance and satisfaction as endogenous latent variables and social support as exogenous latent variables, the SEM was constructed and interpreted.

References

[1] Yanbo, Z, *et al. Latent Varible Analysis (in Chinese).* Higher Education Press; 2009.
[2] Jietai, H, Zhonglin, W, Zijuan, C. *Structural Equation Model and its Applications (in Chinese).* Beijing: Educational Science Press; 2004.
[3] Haozheng, Q. *Structural Equation Model: Theory, Technology and Application of LISREL (in Chinese).* Taiwan: YehYeh Book Gallery; 2003.
[4] Jing, T, Jiangping, X, Xiaojuan, H, Qinghua, H, Yanbo, Z. CHF-PROM: validation of a patient-reported outcome measure for patients with chronic heart failure. *Health Qual Life Outcomes.* 2018; 6: 51. https://doi.org/10.1186/s12955-018-0874-2
[5] John, CL. *Latent Variable Models: An Introduction to Factor, Path and Structural Analysis.* New York, NY: Lawrence Erlbaum Associates; 1998.
[6] Bollen, KA. *Structural Equations with Latent Variables.* New York, NY: Wiley; 1989.
[7] MacCallum, RC, Rozhowski, M. Model modifications in covariance structure analysis: the problem of capitalization on chance. *Psychol Bull.* 1992; 111(3): 490–504. https://doi.org/10.1037/0033-2909.111.3.490

Yanbo Zhang

CHAPTER 28

MULTI-LEVEL MODEL

As mentioned in the previous sections, an important assumption in conventional regression model is that the observed outcomes of individuals are mutually independent. But in practice, due to subjective or objective factors, there are often some similar characteristics among observed individuals in a certain range of time or space so that outcomes of individuals are no longer independent and appear to have a hierarchical structure. Under such circumstance, analyzing through a conventional regression model may lead to a biased result. Multi-level models, such as random intercepts model, random slopes model and two-level logistic regression model, introduced in this chapter are more appropriate in dealing with this kind of data.

28.1. Introduction

Various terms of multi-level models have been used in literatures, such as *random coefficient models*, *hierarchical linear models*, *mixed-effects*, or *mixed models*. Although these models may differ in terms of computational algorithms, application conditions or study domains, they are all suitable for dealing with hierarchical or non-independent data.

28.1.1. *Characteristics of multi-level data*

Hierarchy is a common phenomenon in nature, thus, it is naturally full of multi-level data in society. For example, body mass index (BMI) is a response variable to study influencing factors of obesity in a province. Due to the differences in economic level, dietary habits, natural environment and health care resources among different districts/counties in the province, the degree of obesity could be relatively close, and the BMI variation could be small within the same district/county; while as the degree of obesity tends to be different in different districts/counties, hence the BMI variation is comparatively significant among different districts/counties. Obvious hierarchy exists, namely, "district/county-individual." The district/county is defined as high-level, namely the level-2 unit, while individual as low-level, that is, level-1 unit. In this case, observed outcomes of individuals are no longer completely independent.

Multi-level models are powerful tools for dealing with hierarchical data. The hierarchical structure that low-level units are nested in high-level units assumes individual characteristics similar in the same high-level unit, but different among multiple high-level units. The observed individual data clustered in the same high-level unit can also be measured as intra-class correlation in statistics. And heterogeneity exists among different high-level units. The independence assumption of all individual data by most traditional statistical methods cannot be met by this type of data, so that most conventional methods are not appropriate to use anymore. Multi-level models stem from the characteristic of hierarchical structure and evaluate the impact of high-level units on the relationship between explanatory variables and response variable of low-level units.

Multi-level models are also suitable for repeated measurement data, such as child growth study, which repeatedly measures children's growth indicators such as height and weight during their growth process. There is a correlation between the heights of the same child in different periods so that the measurements are not independent, instead, a certain growth pattern exists. It appears to be a hierarchical structure of "individual-growth period" in the analysis where each individual is viewed as a high-level unit and each measurement is viewed as a low-level unit.

Multi-level models are more appropriate compared with traditional regression models for data with hierarchical structure, as they include high-level units and low-level units simultaneously in the same model. However, they also have some limitations, such as the complexity of models with many parameters, a larger sample size needed to ensure the robustness of estimation, and potential biased estimation due to insufficient sample size of low-level.

28.1.2. *Case study*

Example 28.1. To investigate influence factors of maternal hospital delivery cost in a certain area, 27 districts/counties in the area were randomly sampled and 52,557 maternal hospital delivery cases from 2015 to 2017 were collected from the medical record homepage database, including hospital delivery cost, hospitalization day, maternal age, delivery mode, etc. The data are shown in Table 28.1. The hierarchical relationship between district/county and the maternal is shown in Figure 28.1.

Table 28.1 52,557 maternal hospital delivery data in a certain area

ID	Code of districts/counties	Hospital stay day	Age groups	Delivery mode	Delivery cost (RMB)
2816	3	5	4	0	2027.33
3706	3	3	1	0	4995.06
7360	3	3	4	0	1050.03
⋮	⋮	⋮	⋮	⋮	⋮
179,744	88	5	4	1	4108.17
179,889	88	5	1	1	4786.99
180,093	88	4	3	1	4736.38

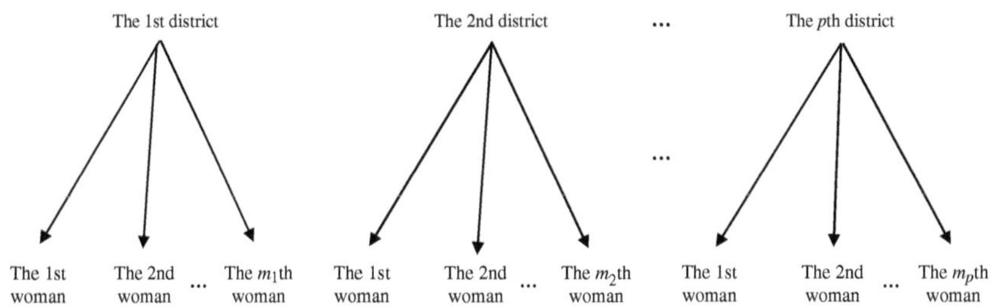

Figure 28.1 Hierarchical relationship between districts/counties and the maternal.

Table 28.2 Assignment of variables

Variables	Definition and assignment
Response variable	
Hospital delivery cost in logarithm; *lgcost*	Continuous variable
Explanatory variables	
Variables of districts/counties	
Type of districts/counties; *place*	0 Non-minority areas 1 Minority areas
Variables of individuals	
Hospitalization day; *days*	Continuous variable
Age grouping (year); *agegroup*	0 < 20 1 25∼ 2 30∼ 3 35∼ 4 20∼24
Ethnic; *ethnic*	0 Ethnic Han 1 Minority
Year; *year*	0 2017 1 2016 2 2015
Type of hospital; *hospital*	0 General hospital 1 Specialized hospital 2 Maternity and child health hospital 3 Community or township hospital
Admission situation; *severity*	0 Critical 1 Emergency 2 General
Delivery mode; *delivery*	0 Cesarean section 1 Natural delivery
Complication; *complication*	0 Yes 1 No
Surgical operation; *surgery*	0 Yes 1 No
Data structure	
Individual level; *id*	Level-1
District/County level; *county*	Level-2

Because of variability in economic level, hospital delivery accessibility and medical level in different districts/counties, the medical services gained by maternal individuals in the same district/county tend to be homogeneous, while the medical services in different districts/counties are heterogeneous. In theory, the data have a hierarchical structure, with the district/county the level-2 unit and the maternal individuals the level-1 unit. Relevant variable assignments are shown in Table 28.2.

28.2. Random intercepts model

A random intercepts model is the simplest form of multi-level models. It can not only help us understand the multi-level model better, but also lay the basis of fitting more complex model.

In statistics, the concepts of *fixed effects* and *random effects* would be referred when explaining the impact of a factor. If researchers are not interested in extrapolation of treatment effects and all treatments of interest are involved in the design, each factor of treatment can be considered to have a fixed effect. If the treatment groups are only a random sample selected from a population, the information obtained from current dataset needs to be generalized to that population, the random effects of treatment factors should be considered.

As shown in Example 28.1, if researchers only care about whether there is a difference in hospital delivery cost among the 27 districts/ counties in the study region, the factor for each district/county, should be added into the model as fixed effect. However, the 27 districts/ counties in the study is just a random sample of all the districts/ counties in this region. And researchers are concerned about not merely the difference of hospital delivery costs among the 27 districts/ counties, but also the overall situation of the region represented by these randomly sampled districts/counties. Statistical inferences can be made for the population based on the sample of the 27 districts/ counties. At this moment, the district/county's impact on hospital delivery costs should be considered as random effects.

Generally speaking, the construction of a statistical model is an exploration process that should consider both the analysis objective and the theoretical basis. It is generally recognized that fitting multi-level models should start at zero model, and then successively add the potential explanatory variables on different levels and their cross-level interactions. Therefore, this section will introduce the two-level random intercepts model in this order through Example 28.1.

28.2.1. *Zero model*

There is an apparent two-level hierarchical structure in Example 28.1, with the maternal individuals at level-1 and district/county at level-2. Due to the positive skew distribution of hospital delivery cost, the value of hospital delivery cost has been transformed into logarithm (*lgcost*). Then, we can fit a two-level linear model as

$$y_{ij} = \beta_{0j} + e_{0ij}, \quad \beta_{0j} = \beta_0 + u_{0j} \qquad (28\text{-}1)$$

where, $i = 1, 2, \ldots, n_j$ indicating the level-1 unit — the maternal individual, while $j = 1, 2, \ldots, J$ referring to the level-2 unit — district/county. β_{0j} is the intercept that represents the mean estimator of response variable y at the baseline in the jth district/county. Various values of β_{0j} in different districts/counties indicate that it is a random variable at the district/county-level. β_0 is the average intercept that represents the overall mean estimator of y_{ij}. u_{0j} is the difference between β_{0j} and β_0, which is a random variable without direct measurement, and also called the *latent variable*. It reflects the random effect of the jth district/county on y and usually assumed as a Normal variable $u_{0j} \sim N(0, \sigma^2_{u_0})$. Therefore, u_{0j} is also called the level-2 *residual error term*, that is, the random error of level-2 unit. The random parameter $\sigma^2_{u_0}$ is the variance of u_{0j}, which reflects the variation of *lgcost* among districts/counties. Thus, the multi-level model provides information of the population area by taking the mean estimates of these districts/counties as a random variable and estimating its random effect u_{0j} and random coefficient $\sigma^2_{u_0}$. e_{0ij} is the level-1 unit's random residual error term and usually assuming that $e_{0ij} \sim N(0, \sigma^2_{e_0})$. In addition, the model assumes that the residuals of level-1 and level-2 are mutually independent, that is, $\mathrm{Cov}(u_{0j}, e_{0ij}) = 0$.

It shows that the response variable y_{ij} can be expressed as the sum of the fixed part β_0 and the random part $(u_{0j} + e_{0ij})$, where β_0 describes the fixed effects and the variances of the random part, $\sigma^2_{u_0}$ and $\sigma^2_{e_0}$, describe the random effects in the model.

The variance of the response variable can be written as

$$\mathrm{Var}(y_{ij}) = \mathrm{Var}(\beta_0 + u_{0j} + e_{0ij}) = \mathrm{Var}(u_{0j} + e_{0ij}) = \sigma^2_{u_0} + \sigma^2_{e_0} \tag{28-2}$$

According to Formula (28-2), the total variance of y_{ij} is decomposed into two components, the inter-class or class-level variance, $\sigma^2_{u_0}$, and the intra-class or individual-level variance, $\sigma^2_{e_0}$. The inter-class variance reflects the part that could be explained by the class-level variables in the total variation of y_{ij}, while the intra-class variance reflects the part explained by the individual-level variation. Thus, the above-mentioned model is called the *variance component model*,

Table 28.3 Parameter estimates of the zero model for hospital delivery cost

Parameter	Estimate	SE	Z value	P value
Fixed parameter				
β_0	3.5101	0.0286	122.759	<0.001
Random parameter				
σ^2_{u0}	0.0219	0.0060	3.632	<0.001
σ^2_{e0}	0.0413	0.0003	162.065	<0.001
−2*loglikelihood	−18,231.998			

in which the total variation of the response variable is decomposed into different levels in corresponding to the data structure and fully embodying the basic ideas and characteristics of the multi-level models.

The model (28-1) does not contain any explanatory variable except for the intercept, so that the model is also called *zero model*, *empty model*, or *random intercepts model*.

Based on the data of Example 28.1, parameter estimates of the zero model are shown in Table 28.3.

According to Table 28.2, the response variable has two variance components: the inter-class variance σ^2_{u0} and the intra-class variance σ^2_{e0}. Wald test is performed on the inter-class variance (i.e., the district/county-level variance) as follows,

$$W = \left(\frac{0.0219}{0.0060}\right)^2 = 13.3225.$$

Compared with the χ^2 distribution critical value with 1 degree of freedom, the P value is less than 0.001. It is said that the mean of *lgcost* is different among different districts/counties and there is an inter-class heterogeneity or intra-class correlation in the data, indicating that it is appropriate to use a multi-level model. The similarity of variables within a group can be measured by the *intra-class correlation* coefficient (ICC or ρ).

$$\rho = \frac{\sigma^2_{u0}}{\sigma^2_{u0} + \sigma^2_{e0}} = \frac{0.0219}{0.0219 + 0.0413} = 0.347,$$

which indicates that 34.7% of the total variation of *lgcost* is caused by the variation among districts/counties.

In Example 28.1, ρ represents the proportion of the variance of *lgcost* in different districts/counties to the total variance, which actually reflected the clustering or similarity of *lgcost* of pregnant women in the same district/county. If ρ is close to 0, it indicates that the data do not have a hierarchical structure and the variation at district/county-level can be ignored. In other words, there is no clustering of maternal *lgcost* in a district/county and the model is simplified into fixed effect model. Otherwise, the existence of variation in different counties cannot be ignored.

From the introduction above, the zero model can be used to estimate the inter-class and intra-class variance, and further calculate the index reflecting the similarity or clustering of the measurements in the same class. The multi-level models are necessary only if there is a substantial intra-class relationship in the data. Thus, a zero model lays the foundation of further constructing multi-level models.

28.2.2. *Two-level random intercepts model*

After initially confirming the existence of intra-class correlation and the justification of multi-level model through the zero model, explanatory variables can be further added into the model to explore the impacts of these variables on the dependent variable.

For the two-level structure of the data in Example 28.1, the random intercepts model can be written as

$$\begin{aligned} y_{ij} &= \beta_{0j} + \beta_1 x_{ij} + e_{0ij}, \\ \beta_{0j} &= \beta_0 + u_{0j}, \end{aligned} \tag{28-3}$$

where the hypothesis and statistical meaning of these symbols are basically consistent with the zero model, except for β_1 and x_{ij}. The intercept β_{0j} indicates the mean estimate of y at the baseline in the jth district/county when all continuous explanatory variables are 0 and all categorical explanatory variables are the reference. The quantity β_1 is the regression coefficient of the explanatory variable x, which does not change corresponding to the change of level-2 unit. The quantity x_{ij} is the observed value of explanatory variable that can not only be a *contextual variable* of level-2, such as the district/county variable in Example 28.1, like whether the district/county being a minority area, but also be an individual characteristic variable of level-1, such as hospitalization days, maternal age, and delivery mode. This is also one of the advantages of multi-level models over traditional model.

Model (28-3) can be further written as

$$y_{ij} = (\beta_0 + \beta_1 x_{ij}) + (u_{0j} + e_{0ij}). \tag{28-4}$$

The response variable y_{ij} in model (28-4) can be expressed as the sum of the fixed part $(\beta_0 + \beta_1 x_{ij})$ and the random part $(u_{0j} + e_{0ij})$. The parameters β_0 and β_1 quantify the fixed effects of the model, while the variances of the random part σ_{u0}^2 and σ_{e0}^2 describe the random effects in the model. Compared with the zero model, this model has the same random effect terms. In addition, it includes fixed effect covariates.

From model (28-3), it is not difficult to find that, except for e_{0ij} existing in all linear models, only the intercept β_{0j} is set to have a random effect so that model (28-3) is called a *random intercepts model*, and the zero model can be regarded as a special case of this model. Under the condition of existence of intra-class correlation or inter-class heterogeneity of the data justified by the zero model, explanatory variables at high-level are logically needed to explain the variation. Therefore, those explanatory variables of level-2 should be initially included to extend the zero model. The number of contextual variables in the model should not be more than the number of level-2 units. Because of the limited interpretation of contextual variables, the explanatory variables of level-1 have to be included for further controlling the effects of individual characteristics on the response. The principles and methods of variable inclusion are same as that of multiple linear regression, which will not be repeated here.

On the basis of the zero model in Example 28.1, the level-2 variable, "*place*," is included first, that is, whether the district/county is a minority county. The model is written as

$$y_{ij} = \beta_0 + \beta_1 place_j + u_{0j} + e_{0ij}. \tag{28-5}$$

After adding the *place* variable, the model estimates are shown in model I in Table 28.4. Wald test for σ^2_{u0} is significant with $P < 0.001$, indicating that the means of *lgcost* are different in different districts/counties. The fixed part β_0 in the model indicating the mean estimate of *lgcost* in minority areas is 3.4537. The quantity β_1 is the regression coefficient of the *place* variable that indicates that the mean estimate of *lgcost* in non-minority areas is 0.1501 higher than that in minority areas ($P < 0.001$).

After the inclusion of the contextual variable, variance estimate of district/county-level is 0.0164 which is somehow smaller than 0.0219 in the zero model. It indicates that a small part of inter-class variation is explained by the contextual variable (district/county). However, the individual-level variance does not change compared with that in zero model, which indicates that the district/county-level variable cannot explain the intra-class variation.

After continuous variable inclusion and selection based on model (28-5), the final model (28-6) is determined, and its estimates are shown in model II in Table 28.4.

$$\begin{aligned} y_{ij} = \beta_0 &+ \beta_1 place_j + \beta_2 days_{ij} + \beta_3 agegroup_{ij} \\ &+ \beta_4 year_{ij} + \beta_5 hospital_{ij} + \beta_6 severity_{ij} \\ &+ \beta_7 delivery_{ij} + \beta_8 complication_{ij} + \beta_9 surgery_{ij} + u_{0j} + e_{0ij} \end{aligned} \quad (28\text{-}6)$$

In model II, the mean estimate of *lgcost* is 2.9652 when all categorical variables are at the baseline level. When other variables are controlled, the mean estimate of *lgcost* in non-minority areas is 0.1340 higher than that in minority areas. With each additional day of hospital stay, the mean estimate of *lgcost* increase by 0.0172. The remaining coefficients are interpreted similarly. According to the results of Formula (28-6) and Table 28.4, the regression coefficient of each explanatory variable is fixed in the random intercepts model, which indicates that the impacts of explanatory variables on *lgcost* are consistent among districts/counties; while the mean estimates of intercept of the same explanatory variable vary among different districts/counties.

Table 28.4 Parameter estimates of random intercepts model

Parameter	Zero model	Model I	Model II
Fixed parameter			
β_0(*intercept*)	3.5101(0.0286)	3.4537(0.0313)	2.9652(0.0209)
β_1(*place*)			
Minority areas			
Non-minority areas		0.1501(0.0512)	0.1340(0.0338)
β_2(*days*)			0.0172(0.0003)
β_3(*agegroup*)			
20∼ 24			
<20			−0.0023(0.0020)
25∼			0.0097(0.0012)
30∼			0.0167(0.0017)
35∼			0.0220(0.0022)
β_4(*year*)			
2015			
2016			0.0150(0.0018)
2017			0.0016(0.0019)
β_5(*hospital*)			
Community hospital			
General hospital			0.2896(0.0024)
Specialized hospitals			0.2211(0.0034)
Maternal and child health Hospital			0.1622(0.0028)
β_6(*severity*)			
General			
Emergency			0.0426(0.0020)
Critical			0.1177(0.0094)
β_7(*delivery*)			
Natural delivery			
Cesarean section			0.2561(0.0014)
β_8(*complication*)			
No			
Yes			0.0756(0.0029)
β_9(*surgery*)			
No			
Yes			0.0412(0.0018)
Random parameter			
$\sigma^2_{u_0}$	0.0219(0.0060)	0.0164(0.0046)	0.0071(0.0020)
$\sigma^2_{e_0}$	0.0413(0.0003)	0.0413(0.0003)	$0.0140(8.64 \times 10^{-5})$
−2*loglikelihood	−18,231.998	−18,239.383	−75,045.991

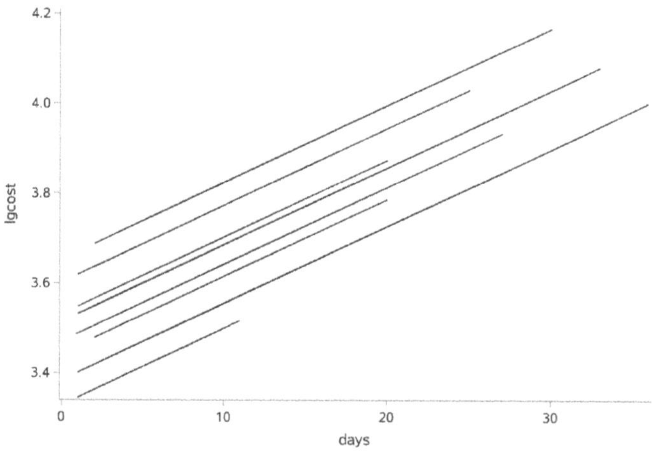

Figure 28.2 Illustration diagram of the random intercepts model between *lgcost* and *days*.

Take the relationship between *lgcost* and hospital stay days for example, use the model II in Table 28.4 and fix other variables, the characteristics of the random intercepts model are illustrated in Figure 28.2 where different districts/counties have the same slope but different intercepts. (For graphical clarity, only 8 of the 27 districts/counties are drawn in the graph.)

28.2.3. *Hypothesis testing of model parameters*

Three methods can be adopted to test the hypotheses about model parameters.

(1) Wald test. The null hypothesis is $H_0 : \beta = 0$, and the W statistic is written as

$$W = \left(\frac{\hat{\beta} - 0}{\hat{\sigma}_\beta} \right)^2.$$

If H_0 is true, the W statistic follows a χ^2 distribution with 1 degree of freedom. When testing several parameters at the same time, the W follows a χ^2 distribution where the degrees of freedom are the number of parameters to be tested.

(2) Likelihood ratio test. The null hypothesis is $H_0 : \lambda_0 = \lambda_1$, and the log-likelihood ratio statistics or deviance statistics is written as

$$D_{01} = -2\ln\lambda_0 - (-2\ln\lambda_1)$$

where, $-2\ln\lambda_1$ and $-2\ln\lambda_0$ are the minus twice the natural logarithm of the likelihood of two nested models (such as the zero model and the model with covariates), respectively. If H_0 is true, D_{01} follows a χ^2 distribution with q degrees of freedom where q is the difference between the number of parameters in the two models.

(3) Establish separate and joint confidence intervals (CIs) of parameters for hypothesis testing.

The results of the three test methods are generally similar.

Taking model I in Table 28.4 for example, the coefficient estimate of district/county variable in non-minority areas is 0.1501 with standard error being 0.0512. The W statistics is

$$W = \left(\frac{0.1501}{0.0512}\right)^2 = 8.5945, \quad P < 0.001,$$

which suggests that the mean estimate of *lgcost* of maternal in non-minority areas is 0.1501 higher than that in minority areas. Meanwhile, from zero model to model I, the deviance decreases from −18,231.998 to −18,239.383. The deviance statistics is

$$D_{01} = -18231.998 - (-18239.383) = 7.385,$$

with the degree of freedom $q = 4-3 = 1$ so that we can get $P < 0.001$ according to the χ^2 distribution, which is statistically significant and say that the model is better than the zero model after including the *place* variable. This result is consistent with the Wald test mentioned above. When multiple covariates are added simultaneously, the deviance statistic reflects the joint effect of those covariates on the model fitting. For example, comparing with model I and model II, the deviance is

$$D_{12} = -18239.383 - (-75045.991) = 56806.608.$$

According to the χ^2 distribution with the degree of freedom $q = 19 - 4 = 15$, we can get $P < 0.001$, which mean that model II added with more variables is better than model I.

When the sample size is large enough, the hypothesis test methods for fixed parameters can also be used for random parameters. Although Wald test is used when testing the variance of district/county-level in zero model in Table 28.2, the likelihood ratio test is better than Wald test for linear models.

28.2.4. *Model assumption and diagnosis*

For the random intercepts model, the basic assumption is that the level-2 residual u_{0j} and level-1 residual e_{0ij} are both normally distributed and mutually independent, that is, their covariance is 0.

The model assumption can be roughly checked by the residual plot. Based on the model (28-6), the standardized residual normal score plots are shown in Figures 28.3 and 28.4 with the standardized residual of *lgcost* of maternal being vertical axis and its normal score being horizontal axis.

The residual normal score plot of the individual-level and district/county-level are both approximately to be a straight line, which confirm the normal assumption of level-1 and level-2 residuals in the model mentioned above.

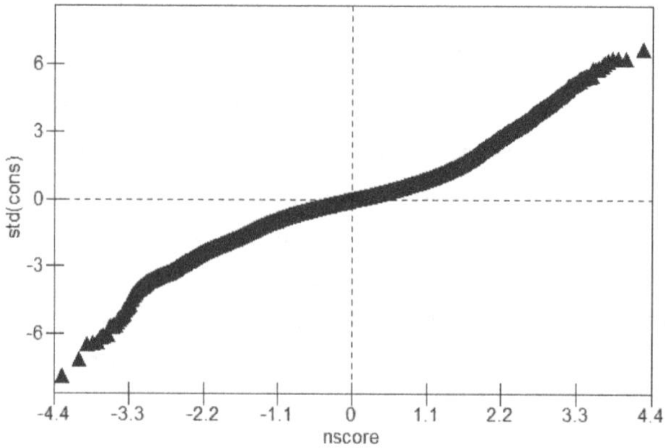

Figure 28.3 The standardized residual normal score plot of level-1 unit.

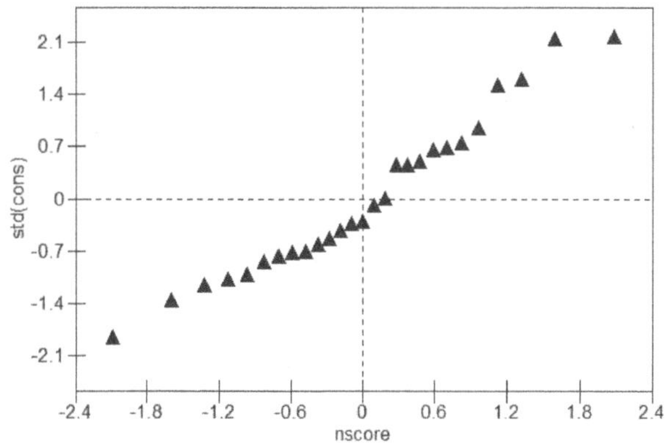

Figure 28.4 The standardized residual normal score plot of level-2 unit.

28.3. Random slopes model

In the random intercepts model, we are assuming that the random effects of high-level units are only the varying intercepts, while the regression coefficients of low-level explanatory variables are fixed. In fact, the effects of low-level explanatory variables on response variable may vary in different high-level units. Therefore, the *random slopes model* or *random coefficient model* in this section is an extended version of random intercepts model which is targeted at the hierarchical data that the regression coefficients of the low-level explanatory variables varying among different high-level units.

28.3.1. *Model establishment and parameter estimation*

Example 28.2. Now we take the two-level data of hospital delivery costs discussed in Example 28.1 as an example to illustrate the basic structure and hypothesis of the random slopes model. In Table 28.4, the estimated coefficient (slope) of hospitalization days on hospital delivery costs in model II implies that *lgcost* would increase by 0.0172 units with each additional day of hospital stay. For the different kinds of admitted patients in each district/county and different fee scales in each day, it is possible that the estimated slope varies from district/county to district/county. Thus, it is necessary to assume that the slope is a random variable with a distribution at district/county-level. This provides the realistic basis for fitting a random slopes model.

The general form of the random slopes model can be expressed as follows,

$$\begin{aligned} y_{ij} &= \beta_{0j} + \beta_{1j}x_{ij} + e_{0ij}, \\ \beta_{0j} &= \beta_0 + u_{0j}, \quad \beta_{1j} = \beta_1 + u_{1j}. \end{aligned} \tag{28-7}$$

Except for the random term β_{1j}, all the parameters in the model are consistent with the random intercepts model. In Formula (28-7), the random variables β_{1j} are the regression coefficients of x_{ij} whose estimates vary among level-2 units. This indicates that the effect of explanatory variable x_{ij} on response y_{ij} varies with the change of level-2 units. The average slope β_1 represents the average change of y with respect to x over all j units at level-2, that is, the average effect estimate of x_{ij} on y_{ij}. The random variables u_{1j} reflect the difference between β_{1j} and β_1, which are always assumed that $u_{1j} \sim N(0, \sigma_{u_1}^2)$.

Model (28-7) can be further expressed as:

$$y_{ij} = (\beta_0 + \beta_1 x_{ij}) + (u_{0j} + u_{1j}x_{ij} + e_{0ij}). \tag{28-8}$$

Model (28-8) is expressed as the sum of the fixed part $(\beta_0 + \beta_1 x_{ij})$ and the random part $(u_{0j}+u_{1j}x_{ij}+e_{0ij})$. The fixed effect is described by the mean, which determines the average regression line over the all subjects with the average intercept β_0 and slope β_1. The random effects in the model are described by variance, which reflects the relationship between the variation of the response y_{ij} and the covariate x_{ij} at individual-level.

Different from the ordinary multiple linear regression model, multi-level models have different residual terms at different levels. We refer the e_{0ij} as the level-1 residuals which denote intra-class variation and the u_{0j} and u_{1j} as the level-2 residuals which denote inter-class variation of β_{0j} and β_{1j}, respectively. The following assumptions are made for the model (28-8):

$$\begin{aligned}
&e_{0ij} \sim N(0, \sigma_{e_0}^2),\\
&E(u_{0j}) = \mathrm{E}(u_{1j}) = 0,\\
&\mathrm{Cov}(u_{0j}, e_{0ij}) = 0, \mathrm{Cov}(u_{1j}, e_{0ij}) = 0,\\
&E(\beta_{0j}) = \beta_0, \mathrm{Var}(\beta_{0j}) = \mathrm{Var}(u_{0j}) = \sigma_{u_0}^2,\\
&E(\beta_{1j}) = \beta_1, \mathrm{Var}(\beta_{1j}) = \mathrm{Var}(u_{1j}) = \sigma_{u_1}^2,\\
&\mathrm{Cov}(u_{0j}, u_{1j}) = \sigma_{u01}.
\end{aligned}$$

where, $\sigma_{e_0}^2$ is the variance of the level-1 residuals. $\sigma_{u_0}^2$ refers to the variance of β_{0j}, the mean estimate of y_{ij}, which is also called the variance of intercepts. And $\sigma_{u_1}^2$ refers to the variance of the slope β_{1j}. σ_{u01} is the covariance of the above intercept and slope deviations which reflects their correlation. The covariance matrix of the level-2 random coefficients u_{0j} and u_{1j} can be written as Ω_2.

$$\Omega_2 = \begin{pmatrix} \sigma_{u_0}^2 & \sigma_{u01} \\ \sigma_{u01} & \sigma_{u_1}^2 \end{pmatrix}$$

When given the fixed effect estimate and the explanatory variable x_{ij}, the variance of the dependent variable in model (28-8) is

$$\begin{aligned}
\mathrm{Var}(y_{ij}|\beta_0, \beta_1, x_{ij}) &= \mathrm{Var}(u_{0j} + u_{1j}x_{ij} + e_{0ij})\\
&= \sigma_{u_0}^2 + 2\sigma_{u01}x_{ij} + \sigma_{u_1}^2 x_{ij}^2 + \sigma_{e_0}^2.
\end{aligned}$$

It is not difficult to see that the random slopes model has a composite residual structure, which is related to the value of x_{ij}. This compound random variance leads to the heteroscedasticity of the model and makes the ordinary least square method not appropriate for the multi-level modeling.

In the multi-level models, the fixed regression coefficient is a constant, while the random regression coefficient varies among level-2 units, which can be interpreted as the interaction effect between level-2 units and explanatory variables. Therefore, the regression coefficient of level-2 explanatory variables must be fixed, while the coefficient of level-1 explanatory variables can be either fixed or random.

For the same data, the likelihood ratio test of two nested models can be used to determine whether the random slopes model is more appropriate than the random intercepts model. Assuming that model 1 is a random intercepts model and model 2 is a random slopes model, $-2\ln\lambda_1-(-2\ln\lambda_2)$ follows a χ^2 distribution with 2 degrees of freedom if the null hypothesis is true. Another method is generalized Wald test that if the joint null hypothesis $\sigma^2_{u_1}=0$ and $\sigma_{u_{01}}=0$ is true, the Wald statistic follows a χ^2 distribution with 2 degrees of freedom, while the degree of freedom is 1 when only one of the null hypothesis is true.

Theoretically, it is possible that both the intercepts and slopes of all level-1 explanatory variables can be random, which is also known as the *random effects model* in some literatures. However, with increasing number of random slopes at level-1, the number of level-2 residual variance and covariance parameters will increase greatly and may cause model estimation unstable, not converging and the like. Therefore, before fitting a random slopes model, we should firstly determine which slopes of explanatory variables in the model are being specified as random slopes according to the objective of the analysis, data characteristics, and our experience. Then, perform a hypothesis testing for corresponding variance in the covariance matrix of level-2 residuals to verify the existence of random slopes. In practice, if both fixed and random coefficients of level-1 explanatory variables exist in the same model, then it is called *mixed effect model* in some literatures.

In multi-level models, if the coefficient of x_{ij} is random, which refers to $\sigma^2_{u_1}\neq 0$, then the intra-class variation exists and the relationship between x_{ij} and y_{ij} is influenced by some contextual variables so that further exploration is needed to dig out those variables. In a model expression, it means that there is an interaction effect between level-2 contextual variables and level-1 explanatory variables. Apart from the interaction effects of different variables in multiple regression model, this effect comes from different level's interaction so that it can be said as *cross-level interaction* or *micro-macro interaction*. The main difference between model (28-8) and the model with cross-level interaction is only in the fixed part.

The interpretation of main effect and interaction effect in multi-level models is consistent with that in ordinary linear model. It is important to note that, as with ordinary linear model, when the interaction effect is statistically significant, the main effect must be remained in the model no matter whether it is statistically significant or not.

28.3.2. *Results on model fitting*

In Example 28.1, in order to explore the influencing factors of hospital delivery costs, we specified the slope of hospital stay days being a random variable based on the random intercepts model. The results are shown in random slopes model I in Table 28.5.

According to the results in Table 28.5, the random coefficients σ_{u0}^2 ($P < 0.001$) and σ_{u2}^2 ($P < 0.001$) of the random slopes model I indicate that both intercept and slope vary among districts/counties, that is, due to the variation in different districts/counties, the number of hospital stay days has different impact on *lgcosts*. Meanwhile, compared with the random intercepts model II, the value of $-2\ln\lambda$ in the random slopes model I decreases from $-75,045.991$ to −81,322.200, $P < 0.001$, so that the random slopes model I is better fitting the data than the random intercepts model II.

In order to illustrate the influence of the variable district/county on the relationship between hospital stay days and hospital delivery cost, cross-level interaction of district/county types and hospital stay days can be further included in the model. The results are shown in random slopes model II in Table 28.5.

Comparing the results of random slopes model I and model II, we can find that the value of $-2\ln\lambda$ decreases from −81,322.200 to −81,344.344, $q = 1$, $P < 0.001$. It can be considered that the random slope model II is a better fit to the data than the random slope model I.

In the random slopes model II, when all categorical variables are at their reference level, the mean estimate of *lgcost* β_0 is 2.8916. When other variables are held constant, the mean estimate of *lgcosts* for those aged 25–29, 30–34, 35 and over are 0.0089, 0.0147 and 0.0186 higher than that for the maternal aged from 20 to 24, respectively;

Table 28.5 Parameter estimates for random slopes model

Parameters	Random intercepts model II	Random slopes model I	Random slopes model II
Fixed parameters			
β_0 (*intercept*)	2.9652(0.0209)	2.9414(0.0261)	2.8916(0.0246)
β_1 (*place*)			
Minority areas			
Non-minority areas	0.1340(0.0338)	0.1239(0.0316)	0.2589(0.0340)
β_2 (*days*)	0.0172(0.0003)	0.0239(0.0033)	0.0335(0.0028)
β_3 (*agegroup*)			
20∼ 24			
<20	−0.0023(0.0020)	0.0007(0.0019)	0.0007(0.0019)
25∼	0.0097(0.0012)	0.0089(0.0012)	0.0089(0.0012)
30∼	0.0167(0.0017)	0.0147(0.0016)	0.0147(0.0016)
35∼	0.0220(0.0022)	0.0186(0.0020)	0.0186(0.0020)
β_4 (*year*)			
2015			
2016	0.0150(0.0018)	0.0157(0.0017)	0.0157(0.0017)
2017	0.0016(0.0019)	0.0049(0.0018)	0.0049(0.0018)
β_5 (*hospital*)			
Community or township health center			
General hospital	0.2896(0.0024)	0.2972(0.0023)	0.2973(0.0023)
Specialized hospitals	0.2211(0.0034)	0.2258(0.0033)	0.2258(0.0033)
Maternal and child health hospital	0.1622(0.0028)	0.1710(0.0027)	0.1710(0.0027)
β_6 (*severity*)			
General			
Emergency	0.0426(0.0020)	0.0360(0.0019)	0.0360(0.0019)
Critical	0.1177(0.0094)	0.0882(0.0089)	0.0882(0.0089)
β_7 (*delivery*)			
Natural delivery			
Cesarean section	0.2561(0.0014)	0.2514(0.0013)	0.2514(0.0013)
β_8 (*complication*)			
No			
Yes	0.0756(0.0029)	0.0737(0.0028)	0.0737(0.0028)
β_9 (*surgery*)			
No			
Yes	0.0412(0.0018)	0.0352(0.0017)	0.0352(0.0017)

Table 28.5 (*Continued*)

Parameters	Random intercepts model II	Random slopes model I	Random slopes model II
β_{10}(*days* × *place*)			
Hospitalization days × Minority areas			
Hospitalization days × Non-minority areas			−0.0260(0.0045)
Random parameters			
σ^2_{u0}	0.0071(0.0020)	0.0140(0.0051)	0.0096(0.0027)
σ_{u02}		−0.0015(0.0006)	−0.0006(0.0003)
σ^2_{u2}		$0.0003(8.34 \times 10^{-5})$	$0.0001(3.52 \times 10^{-5})$
σ^2_{e0}	$0.0140(8.64 \times 10^{-5})$	$0.0124(7.65 \times 10^{-5})$	$0.0124(7.65 \times 10^{-5})$
−2*loglikelihood	−75,045.991	−81,322.200	−81,344.344

the mean estimate of *lgcost* for emergency and critical maternal are 0.0360 and 0.0882 higher than that for the maternal with general admission; the mean estimate of *lgcost* of the cesarean section maternal is 0.2514 higher than that of natural delivery; the mean estimate of *lgcost* of the maternal with complications is 0.0737 higher than that without complications; the mean estimate of *lgcost* of the maternal with surgical operation is 0.0352 higher than that without surgical operation. In minority areas, the mean estimate of *lgcost* increases by 0.0335 with each additional day of hospitalization; while in non-minority areas, the mean estimate of *lgcost* increases by 0.0335 − 0.0260=0.0075 with each additional day of hospitalization.

Similarly, according to the random slopes model II, when other variables are fixed, we can discuss the relationship between the *lgcost* and hospitalization days and illustrate the characteristics of the random slopes model in Figure 28.5. It shows that the slop and intercept vary from district/county to district/county (For graphical clarity, only 8 out of 27 districts/counties are selected for drawing). The hypothesis test of the model is same as that in the section of "random intercepts model."

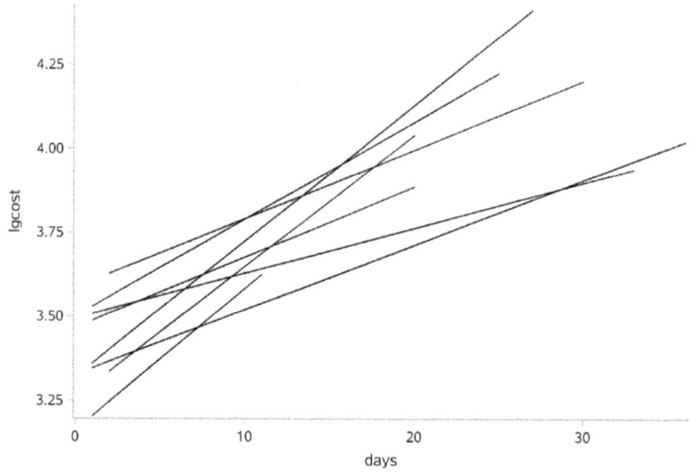

Figure 28.5 Regression lines of *lgcost* on hospitalization days for 8 district/county.

28.4. Multi-level logistic regression

In both the random intercepts model and random slopes model mentioned above, the response variable is continuous. In fact, there exists a huge number of inherently hierarchical categorical data in observational and experimental researches. The hierarchical structure could be natural or artificial. For instance, in the teratogenic test, pregnant rats were test subjects, and they were randomly divided into two groups: one group was given suspicious teratogens treatment and the other was a blank control, respectively. After delivery, the occurrence of malformation among the offspring of the two groups was observed and analyzed. In the experiment, there is a clear hierarchical structure, "maternal rat-offspring rat," which is also known as "the effect of litter," because of that the genetics, length of pregnancy, metabolic environment of teratogens, and the like factors have the same impact on one litter. Thus, the probability of malformation occurrence within one litter tends to be similar, while the probability between litters tends to be different. This means that the probability of malformation among each pup in the experiment is not completely independent.

Such case also exists in the survey research. For example, to investigate prevalence of chronic diseases of residents in a province, 14 districts/counties were randomly selected; in each district/county, 5 sub-districts/townships were randomly selected; in each sub-district/township, 2 communities/villages were selected; and in each community/village, 60 households were randomly selected; permanent residents of each household were surveyed. The survey data have an obvious hierarchical structure (sub-district → community → household → individual). Residents from the same district/county, sub-district, community, household bear some similarity or aggregation in terms of economic level, geographical environment, lifestyle, and health service utilization. In other words, the individual observations are non-independent each other in nature. If the outcome is binary variable (positive or negative, occurring or not), traditional statistical methods would ignore the hierarchy within the data so that underestimate the standard error of the estimators and lead to false positive. Multi-level logistic regression model can decompose the random error term in the traditional model into several levels corresponding to the data hierarchy so as to make the random error more pure and provide the possibility of fitting well the hierarchical data.

28.4.1. *Basic principles and methods*

If our response variable in an experiment is binary and coded as whether the event occurring or not, the multi-level model known as *multi-level generalized linear model* would be adopted.

Now a two-level binary case is used as an example to illustrate the two-level logistic regression.

(1) Basic form of two-level logistic regression.

The basic form of two-level logistic regression is

$$\begin{aligned} \text{logit}(P_{ij}) &= (\beta_0 + u_{0j}) + \beta_1 x_{ij} \\ u_{0j} &= \beta_{0j} - \beta_0, u_{0j} \sim N(0, \sigma_{u0}^2) \end{aligned} \tag{28-9}$$

$$\text{Var}(P_{ij}) = \frac{\delta\pi_{ij}(1 - \pi_{ij})}{n_{ij}} \tag{28-10}$$

In Formula (28-9), β_1 is the parameter of treatment effect, which is also known as the fixed effect parameter. u_{0j} is the difference between β_{0j} and β_0, which is also known as the random effects or high-level residuals. σ^2_{u0}, the variance of u_{0j}, is known as the parameter of random effects measuring the difference of logit(P) among high-level units. The larger the σ^2_{u0} is, the stronger clustering within a high-level unit is. However, if $\sigma^2_{u0} = 0$, the model degenerates to a single-level logistic regression model.

σ^2_{u0} is the only random parameter that needs to be estimated in the model, which is called random intercepts model or the variance component model as introduced previously.

Both CI estimation and Wald test above mentioned are valid for the two-level logistic regression model.

(2) Scale parameter δ

δ in Formula (28-9) is a scale parameter. If the response variable followed a binomial distribution, the scale parameter should be 1 or close to 1. That is, when the fixed effect parameter β and random effect parameter σ^2_{u0} are determined, the variance estimate of response variable is $\pi_{ij}(1 - \pi_{ij})/n_{ij}$.

When fitting a model, if the assumption of binomial distribution is true, we can set the scale parameter δ be 1. Otherwise, the null hypothesis will be tested.

(3) Assessing high-level effect

When practically fitting a logistic model, two methods should be considered to justify whether there is a high-level effect: a statistical test for the random parameter σ^2_{u0}; and a measure of *variance partition coefficient* (VPC), which is the proportion of high-level variance to the total variance. When the response variable is continuous, the VPC is equivalent to the ICC. Taking the two-level variance component model as an example, the VPC indicates the ratio of the level-2 variance to the total variance, $\sigma^2_{u0}/(\sigma^2_{u0} + \sigma^2_{e0})$. However, when the response variable is a discrete variable, VPC and ICC are not equivalent. Taking the binomial data, for example, the level-1 variance depends on the values of the explanatory variables in the model, so that there is no simple way to calculate the VPC. Goldstein *et al.* proposed several methods for estimating VPC of discrete response data, including model linearization method, simulation method, binomial linear simulation method, and latent variable method. For the binomial distribution data, the level-1 variance of the two-level random intercepts model can be approximated by $\sigma_{e_0}^2 \approx \pi^2/3$. While the estimation of VPC for the random slopes model is more complicated, one may refer to the relevant literatures.

28.4.2. *Case study*

Now the health service survey data are taken as an example to further illustrate the application of the multi-level logistic regression model for binary data in research.

Example 28.3. A survey on a chronic disease was conducted in rural areas of a province. 2100 households in 70 communities/villages of 35 townships were selected, where a total of 4926 people aged 15 and above were surveyed. The purpose of the survey was to explore the influencing factors of the chronic disease in rural areas of the province.

Taking whether respondents suffered from chronic disease within 6 months as the response variable, the binary two-level logistic model is applied taking on account of the hierarchically structured data.

The assignment of all variables is shown in Table 28.6. Categorical variables such as gender, marital status, employment status, and education level are included in the form of dummy variable. Age is segmented and also included in model as dummy variables.

SPSS 25.0 is used for statistical analysis. The households are the level-2 units and the individuals are the level-1 units. A two-level logistic variance component model is fitted with scale parameter δ set to be 1. The results of zero model are shown in Table 28.7.

The level-2 variance is statistically significant ($P < 0.001$), suggesting household clustering in the outcome data, so that the hierarchical structure cannot be ignored. In the two-level model, the potential factors that may impact on the prevalence of chronic

Table 28.6 Assignment of variable

Variables	Definition and assignment
Response variable	
Chronic disease condition within 6 months; *chronic*	0 No 1 Yes
Explanatory variables	
Demographics	
Gender; *gender*	1 Male 2 Female
Age; *age*	1 15–24 2 25–44 3 45–64 4 ≥65
Marital status; *marriage*	1 Unmarried 2 Married 3 Divorced/windowed
Educational level; *edu*	1 Illiterate/semi-illiterate 2 Primary 3 Secondary or higher
Employment; *occup*	1 Employed 2 Retired 3 Student 4 Unemployed
Family status	
Impoverished households; *poverty*	1 No 2 Yes
Data structure	
Individual level; *id*	Level-1
Household level; *family*	Level-2
Township level; *town*	Level-3

Table 28.7 Estimates of two-level logistic zero model

Parameter	Estimate	*SE*	*Z* value	*P* value
Fixed parameter				
β_0	−0.782	0.037	−21.119	<0.001
Random parameter				
$\sigma^2_{u_0}$	0.674	0.086	7.831	<0.001
δ	1.000	0.000	—	—

diseases of rural residents are included. After variable selection, the parameter estimates are shown in Table 28.8.

Results in Table 28.8 show that the main factors affecting the prevalence of chronic diseases among rural residents in the province are *gender*, *impoverished*, *age*, and *employment status*. After adjusting for other covariates and comparing to the counterparty,

Table 28.8 Estimates of two-level logistic component variance model on chronic disease prevalence

Parameter	Estimate	*SE*	*Z* value	*P* value	*OR*	95% CI of *OR*
Fixed part						
intercept	−4.291	0.384	−11.162	<0.001	—	—
poverty	0.422	0.124	3.401	0.001	1.53	(1.20, 1.94)
gender						
Male						
Female	0.300	0.076	3.959	<0.001	1.35	(1.16, 1.57)
age						
15∼						
25∼	1.509	0.387	3.898	<0.001	4.52	(2.12, 9.66)
45∼	3.198	0.382	8.368	<0.001	24.48	(11.58, 51.77)
65∼	3.892	0.390	9.979	<0.001	49.01	(22.82, 105.26)
occup						
Employed						
Retired	1.039	0.165	6.284	<0.001	2.83	(2.05, 3.91)
Student	−0.112	0.678	−0.166	0.869	0.89	(0.23, 3.35)
Unemployed	0.562	0.125	4.499	<0.001	1.75	(1.37, 2.24)
Random part						
σ_{u0}^2	0.509	0.091	5.624	<0.001	—	—
δ	1.000	0.000	—	—	—	—

the residents of *impoverished*, *female*, *more aged*, *retired*, and *unemployed* are more likely to suffer from chronic diseases.

Then we take the explanatory variable as an example to illustrate the relationship between the parameters and the odds ratio (*OR*). The estimated *OR* of chronic-disease prevalence in the 25–44 age group is $e^{\hat{\beta}_2} = e^{1.509} = 4.52$, which means that the risk of chronic disease in 25–44 age group is 4.52 times as high as that in 15–24 age group. The 95% CI of *OR* is $e^{\hat{\beta}_2} \times e^{\pm 1.96 \times SE}$, that is, $e^{\hat{\beta}_2 \pm 1.96 \times SE} = e^{1.509 \pm 1.96 \times 0.387} = (2.12, 9.66)$.

As there still exists higher level structure (township-level), three-level model could be further considered.

It should be noted that the estimated coefficients of covariates in the model above are fixed. If we want to take the random effects into account as well, the model would be built with random slopes that is so-called random slopes model. That is, the effects of the low-level covariates on the response variable are different among the high-level units. The basic structure and hypothesis of random slopes model are illustrated below based on two-level model.

$$\text{logit}(P_{ij}) = (\beta_0 + u_{0j}) + (\beta_1 + u_{1j})x_{ij} = \beta_{0j} + \beta_{1j}x_{ij},$$
$$\begin{pmatrix} u_{0j} \\ u_{1j} \end{pmatrix} \sim MN(0, \Omega), \Omega = \begin{pmatrix} \sigma_{u0}^2 & \sigma_{u01} \\ \sigma_{u01} & \sigma_{u1}^2 \end{pmatrix}. \qquad (28\text{-}11)$$

As shown in Formula (28-11), the difference between random slopes model and random intercepts model is the additional term β_{1j}. In variance component model, the coefficient of x_{ij} is a fixed value β_1, while in random coefficient model, it is assumed that the effect of x_{ij} randomly varies among different level-2 units with its random effect u_{1j} following a normal distribution with mean 0 and variance $\sigma_{u_1}^2$. If the random effect of slope μ_{1j} and the random effect of intercept u_{0j} have a covariance, $\sigma_{u_{01}}$ would be applied to measure it.

28.4.3. *Method for parameter estimation*

The variance/covariance of the random effects at level-1 and level-2 could often be estimated by maximum likelihood (ML) method. ML has some properties of large sample size. ① Consistency: With the increase of sample size, the ML estimate gradually approaches the true value of the parameter. ② Asymptotic normality: The ML estimate shows an approximate normal distribution centered on the true value of the parameter, which makes the statistical hypothesis test possible. ③ The estimated likelihood function can be used to evaluate the model fitting and comparison. Typically, there are two kinds of ML methods for estimating multi-level model parameters, ML and restricted maximum likelihood (REML) which is also called "maximum residual likelihood method." When the number of level-2 units is not too large, the estimation of level-1 residual variance $\sigma_{e_0}^2$ by ML and REML are similar, but the REML estimate of level-2 residual variance/covariance has smaller bias. Thus, the REML method is preferable when there is only a small sample size at high-level.

Moreover, the parameters can also be estimated by the methods of iterative generalized least squares (IGLS) (Goldstein H, 1991, 1986) or restricted iterative generalized least squares (RIGLS) (Goldstein H, 1989). When the random effects of the model follow a multi-variate normal distribution at each level, the IGLS is equivalent to the ML, and the RIGLS is equivalent to the REML. There are some other methods for parameter estimation — Fisher scoring (Longford, 1993) which was proved to be equivalent to IGLS by Raudenbush in 1994; and the generalized estimating equations (GEE) proposed by Zeger and Liang in 1986, etc. With the development of Markov chain Monte Carlo (MCMC) method, especially Gibbs sampling, full Bayes method has become more feasible in calculation, which improves the parameter estimation in small sample size situation.

28.5. Report writing

An analysis report of multi-level model mainly contains: ① analysis objectives; ② model construction and variable selection; ③ explanation for the clustering effect of high-level units; ④ Summary table for regression coefficient estimates and its standard error, test statistics and P value. OR and its 95% CI are needed when the response variable is categorical variable.

Take Example 28.3 for instance, results of a two-level logistic regression model are reported as follows.

A cross-sectional study was conducted to investigate the influence factors of chronic diseases prevalence in rural area of a province. Demography and disease information of 4926 residents aged 15 and above in this area was collected, and a two-level logistic regression model was fitted.

The parameter estimates of the two-level logistic regression model were shown in Table 28.8. It indicated that there was a family aggregation effect for chronic diseases. Poor families, gender, age, and employment status were the influence factors of chronic diseases among rural residents in the region. After keeping other influence factors constant, the estimated OR of poverty families was 1.52 with 95% CI of 1.20 $\sim$ 1.94 compared with non-poverty families. Compared with male, the estimated OR of female was 1.35 with 95% CI of 1.16 $\sim$ 1.57. For the age group, compared with 15 $\sim$ 24 years old, the estimated OR of 25 $\sim$ 44 years old, 45 $\sim$ 64 years old, and 65 years old and above were 4.52, 24.48, and 49.01 with 95% CIs of 2.12 $\sim$ 9.66, 11.58 $\sim$ 51.77, and 22.82 $\sim$ 105.26 respectively. Compared with employment, the estimated OR for retirement and unemployment were 2.83 and 1.75 with 95% CIs of 2.05 $\sim$ 3.91 and 1.37 $\sim$ 2.24, respectively.

28.6. Case discrimination

Case 28.1: In order to understand the impact of psychological stress (X) on academic performance (Y), 4059 students from 65 schools were randomly selected for analysis. The researchers proposed two different approaches: ① In terms of the schools, the average psychological stress score and average academic performance of students in each school were calculated, and then the relationship between them was estimated by the ordinary linear regression method. ② In terms of the students, the school was set as dummy variable, and the model of the relationship between psychological pressure and academic performance was fitted for each school.

Please discriminate the above two approaches and evaluate their rationality. If both are inappropriate, please propose a reasonable approach.

28.7. Computer experiments (See exp28-1 to exp28-3 in digitized resource)

Experiment 28.1: Using SPSS to fit a random intercepts model for Example 28.1.

To learn the operational process of fitting a random intercepts model, understand the model structure, and explain the results of fixed and random effects.

Experiment 28.2: Using SPSS to fit a random slopes model for Example 28.2.

To learn the operational process of fitting a random slopes model, understand the model structure, compare operational processes between random intercepts model and random slopes model, and explain the results of fixed and random effects.

Experiment 28.3: Using SPSS to fit a two-level logistic regression model for Example 28.3.

To learn the operational process of fitting a two-level logistic regression model and explain the results.

28.8. Frequently asked questions and summary

28.8.1. *Frequently asked questions*

1. What kind of data should be analyzed by multi-level models?

Answer: When there is a hierarchical structure in data, that is, the effect of low-level units on the response variable is aggregated in a high-level unit, the multi-level models should be used. The estimation method of traditional regression model is based on the assumption that individual observations are mutually independent, which is not true when the data has a clustering effect at high-level. Therefore, traditional regression model may result in unreliable results. However, by multi-level models considering the relationship between high-level units and low-level units one can obtain more pure random residuals of low-level units, which is more appropriate for statistical analysis.

2. How to determine the clustering effect in a dataset?

Answer: There are usually two ways to determine the clustering effect of data. First, the ICC measures the proportion of variance among high-level units to the total variance, which reflects the correlation or clustering of low-level units within the same high-level unit. The closer to 1 its value is, the stronger the hierarchical structure of the data is; inversely, the closer to 0 the value is, the weaker the clustering effect of low-level units is. Second, the random parameter σ_{u0}^2 in multi-level models represents the variance component of high-level units. A statistically significant result from the hypothesis testing of σ_{u0}^2 suggests a non-ignorable clustering effect on the data incorporating with subject-matter knowledge.

3. What is the main difference between the random intercepts model and random slopes model?

Answer: The main difference between the random intercepts model and the random slopes model is whether the coefficient of the explanatory variable is fixed or not. The coefficient of explanatory variable in the random intercepts model is fixed, indicating that the relationship between the response variable and explanatory variable is the same among all high-level units. The coefficient of explanatory variable in the random slopes model changes randomly, indicating that the relationship between response variable and explanatory variable changes randomly among different high-level units, that is, each high-level unit might have its own slope.

28.8.2. *Summary*

1. A multi-level model takes the hierarchical structure of data into account so that it is more reasonable and reliable than the traditional regression model. The important feature of multi-level data is the hierarchical structure that makes low-level measurements nest within high-level units.
2. The random intercepts model is the simplest form of the multi-level models where the coefficients of explanatory variables are fixed, which indicates that the relationship between response variable and explanatory variables are the same among different high-level units. The ICC reflects the degree of clustering of low-level units within their high-level units. The closer to 1 the value is, the stronger the hierarchical structure of the data is; inversely, the closer to 0 the value is, the weaker the clustering effect of low-level units is.
3. If the coefficient of explanatory variable x_{ij} in the random intercepts model is a random variable, then the model is a random

coefficient model, which means that each high-level unit has its own intercept and slope, indicating that the relationship between response variable and the explanatory variable changes randomly among high-level units.

4. When the response variable of hierarchical data is a categorical variable, the multi-level model of categorical variable can be applied with appropriate nonlinear link functions according to the type of response variable. Commonly, when the response variable follows a binomial distribution, the link function logit can be used, which results in multi-level binary logistic regression model.

Think and Practice

I. Questions for Reflection

1. How to choose the random intercepts model or the random slopes model to perform a statistical analysis?
2. What are the meaning of the variances of level-2 units and level-1 units, respectively? What is the difference?

II. Questions on Calculation

1. Example 18.4 in Chapter 18, 16 rats of the same species and month age were randomly divided into two groups. Two kinds of feeds A and B were provided in the same environment and weight measurement was regularly conducted in order to analyze the influence of the two kinds of feeds on the body weight changes of rats (see data in data28-3).
   (1) Can the data be analyzed using a multi-level model? If so, what are the level-1 units and level-2 units, respectively?
   (2) Referring to Figure 18.4, in what form should the *time* variable be incorporated into the multi-level models?
   (3) Please fit a two-level random intercepts model and explain the results.
2. A provincial government wants to learn about the factors influencing the health services utilization of rural residents. A multi-stage stratified sampling method was performed to select 1666 residents

aged 15 years and over from 1003 households of 70 communities/villages in 35 townships/districts. Residents' health services utilization was reflected by whether the residents who reported illness within 2 weeks had seen a doctor (see data in data28-4).

(1) What is the hierarchy of the data?
(2) What are the factors influencing the patients seeing doctor within 2 weeks?

Juying Zhang, Min Yang

CHAPTER 29

ITEM RESPONSE THEORY

Item response theory (IRT) was originated in the field of psychological and educational measurement, belonging to the domain of measurement. Since IRT was presented in the middle of the 20th century, a set of mature models have been established, including unidimensional model, multi-dimensional model, non-parametric model, etc. These models have been widely used in the field of measurement. However, due to the complexity of the models and parameter estimation, application of IRT in other fields is limited, especially in biomedical fields. The purpose of this chapter is to introduce IRT briefly, so as to promote the application of IRT in biomedical research.

29.1. Introduction

In research with scales as instrument, sum score or weighted sum score of each item based on classical test theory (CTT) is considered as a measurement of the outcome. The weighted sum method is intuitive and easy to be understood. However, in some situations, CTT may miss some important information, such as the differences between items.

Example 29.1. In a sampling survey on older adults' disability, researchers used the scale of activity of daily living (ADL) as the instrument. The independence of the older adults on dressing, eating, transferring, walking, bathing, and toileting were investigated. An item was scored 1 (independence) when the participant could

Table 29.1 Response patterns on each ADL item of older adult, which has a sum score of 4

ID	Eating	Dressing	Transferring	Walking	Bathing	Toileting	Sum	Z-score[a]
1	0	0	1	1	1	1	4	−1.025
2	1	0	0	1	1	1	4	−1.354
3	0	1	1	0	1	1	4	−1.025
4	1	0	1	0	1	1	4	−1.255
5	0	1	0	1	1	1	4	−1.147
6	0	1	1	1	0	1	4	−1.147
7	1	0	1	1	0	1	4	−1.354
8	1	1	0	1	0	1	4	−1.446
9	1	1	1	0	0	1	4	−1.354
10	0	1	1	1	1	0	4	−1.147
11	1	0	1	1	1	0	4	−1.354
12	1	1	1	1	0	0	4	−1.446

[a]Bayes expected a-posteriori estimation of latent trait ("ability") by fitting a 2-parameter logistic model.

accomplish the task independently, and otherwise, it was scored 0 (disability). Then the independence of participant was measured with sum of the 6-item scores. A higher sum score indicates a stronger independency. Otherwise, lower sum score indicates a weaker independency and more serious disability. A total of 10,000 older adults were surveyed. The results showed that participants with sum scores of 0, 1, 2, 3, 4, and 5 accounted for 5.44%, 1.13%, 1.2%, 1.13%, 1.71%, and 2.15%, respectively. However, further analysis found that there were 12 response patterns with a sum score of 4 in the survey data (see Table 29.1 for details). Generally speaking, a loss of lower limb function has a greater impact on the quality of life of older adults than a loss of upper limb function. For older adults with a sum score of 4, the condition of losing independency on eating and dressing (ID = 1) is different from the condition of losing that on bathing and toileting (ID = 12) in nature. Obviously, the sum of scores cannot distinguish this difference. Then, what method should be used? Based on the latent trait theory, IRT can solve this problem.

Further analysis found that, roughly speaking, the independence proportions according to every ADL items were lower in participants

Table 29.2 The proportions of independence on each ADL items corresponding to different sum scores of older adults

Sum score	Number of the elderly	Eating	Dressing	Transferring	Walking	Bathing	Toileting
0	544	0.000	0.000	0.000	0.000	0.000	0.000
1	113	0.796	0.088	0.035	0.080	0.000	0.000
2	120	0.942	0.683	0.100	0.200	0.033	0.042
3	113	0.885	0.664	0.575	0.451	0.080	0.345
4	171	0.988	0.871	0.754	0.649	0.263	0.474
5	215	0.977	0.902	0.930	0.693	0.651	0.847
6	8724	1.000	1.000	1.000	1.000	1.000	1.000

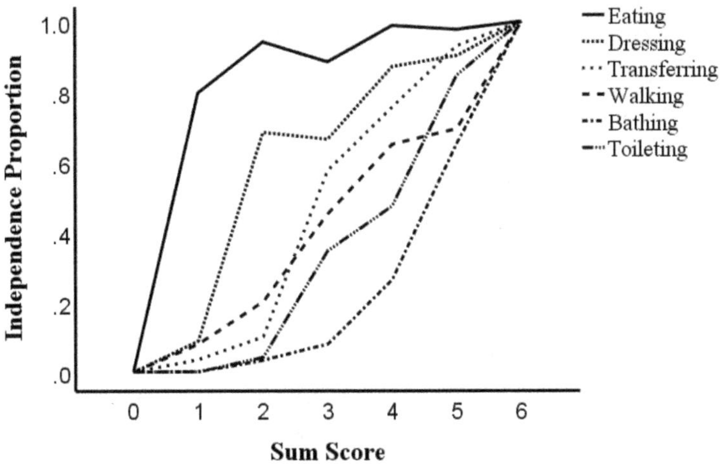

Figure 29.1 The relationship between proportion of independence on each ADL item and the sum score of older adults

with lower sum scores, as shown in Table 29.2. Figure 29.1 shows that the independence proportion of older adults on each ADL item can be expressed with a function of the sum score. If the sum score is regarded as a latent trait of older adults, then the response of older adult on each ADL item might be a non-linear function of the latent trait.

Under the theoretical framework of IRT, the "ability" of the examinee to be tested is regarded as a latent trait. The response of examinee on each item is regarded as a function of both of the item characteristic and the examinee's latent trait, which is called item characteristic function.

The item characteristic curve (ICC) in Figure 29.2 indicates that the relationship between the examinees' response and their latent trait appears to be an ascending s-shaped curve in theory. The basic idea of IRT is to describe the ICC with a mathematical model. Figure 29.2 shows the theoretical ICCs of eating, dressing and bathing after fitting the data in Example 29.1 with Rasch model in IRT.

The original IRT model had two assumptions: unidimensionality and local independence. The unidimensionality assumption requires that the scale measures a single trait of the examinees only that the responses to all items depend on a same latent trait. The local independence assumption requires that the item responses are independent each other given the latent trait of the examinee. The multidimensional IRT developed in late 1970s, which can be fitted when

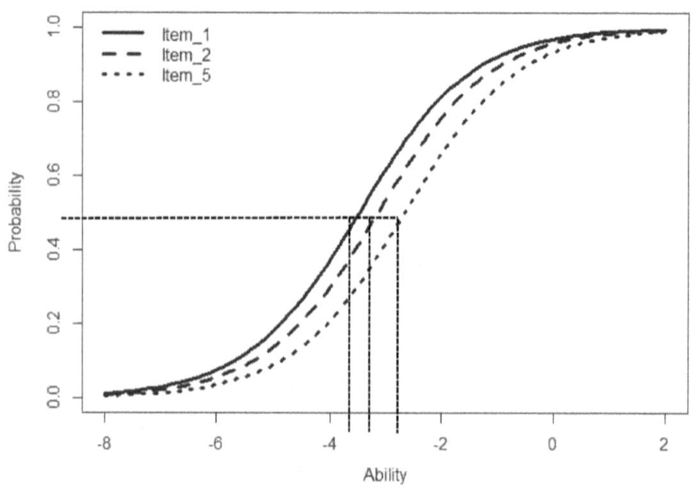

Figure 29.2 The item characteristic curves (ICCs) of eating (Item_1), dressing (Item_2), and bathing (Item_5) based on single-parameter model

multiple latent traits are needed to respond to items, does not need to satisfy unidimensionality assumption.

29.2. Common IRT models

Item characteristic function, which expresses the relationship between the response, item characteristic, and the examinee's latent trait, is called item response model. According to the categories of item, the basic IRT models can be divided as dichotomous model, ordinal model, and polytomous model. The dichotomous model is applicable to 0/1 scoring items such as correct or incorrect, whether or not, yes or no. The ordinal model is suitable for scoring items with several ordinal options (such as Likert form). The polytomous model is suitable for items with nominal options, but it is rarely used in biomedical research. According to the number of item characteristic parameters contained in the model, the basic IRT models can be classified as single-parameter, 2-parameter, and 3-parameter models. There are normal-ogive model, logistic model, probit model, and other popular models in applications. In the following sections, we would introduce the dichotomous and ordinal logistic models.

29.2.1. *Dichotomous logistic model*

The response of examinee j on item i is denoted by a random variable X_{ij}. For a dichotomous item, there are two options, such as correct and incorrect. It is convenient to code them as 1 for correct ($X_{ij} = 1$) and 0 for incorrect ($X_{ij} = 0$). The examinee's latent trait is presented by a parameter $\theta \in (-\infty, +\infty)$. The probability of correct on item i is usually presented as $P_i(\theta)$.

29.2.1.1. *Single-parameter model*

The probability of correct on item i is shown in Formula (29-1). There is only one parameter "difficulty" in the model, which is also called Rasch model.

$$P_i(\theta) = \frac{e^{(\theta-\beta_i)}}{1 + e^{(\theta-\beta_i)}} \tag{29-1}$$

The difficulty parameter is presented by $\beta_i \in (-\infty, +\infty)$, which is also called location parameter. β_i is the point on the latent trait scale when an examinee has a probability 0.5 of correct on the item (the inflection point of ICC). As shown in Figure 29.2, the difficulty parameters of "bathing," "dressing," and "eating" are −2.67, −3.15, and −3.48, respectively. It can be deduced that the probability of independence on "bathing" is 0.5 for an older adult with "ability" of −2.67. While the probability of independence on "eating" is 0.5 for an older adult with independence of −3.48. In other word, the difficulty parameter of "bathing" is higher than that of "eating." So, compared with "eating," "bathing" is a harder thing for older adults.

29.2.1.2. *2-Parameter model*

Comparing the three ICCs in Figure 29.2, we can find that except at both ends, the three curves are parallel. But Figure 29.1 indicates that the proportion of independence on 6 items against the sum score are not parallel. Therefore, another item parameter should be introduced to indicate the unparallel relationships, so that the probability of correct on item i is modified as Formula (29-2). This IRT model is called 2-parameter dichotomous logistic model, where the item parameter $\alpha_i \in (0, +\infty)$ denotes the discrimination power of item i with a name of discrimination parameter.

$$P_i(\theta) = \frac{e^{\alpha_i(\theta-\beta_i)}}{1 + e^{\alpha_i(\theta-\beta_i)}} \tag{29-2}$$

The value of α_i is proportional to the slope of the tangent to the ICC at the inflection point. α_i indicates the power of discrimination among examinees with different values of the latent trait, which is also called scale parameter. Generally, a good item has a larger discrimination parameter, but it is seldom larger than 2.5.

The data in Example 29.1 was fitted with a 2-parameter dichotomous logistic model. The ICCs of "bathing," "dressing," and "eating" were not parallel (see Figure 29.3). "Eating" had a least discrimination parameter of 1, and "Bathing" had a largest discrimination parameter of 2.5.

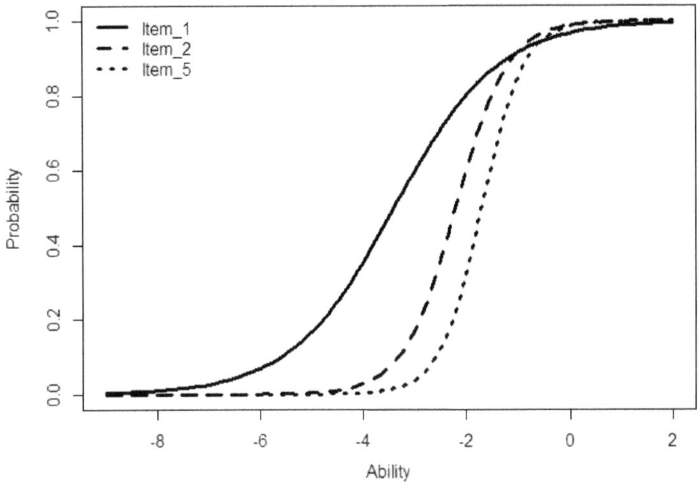

Figure 29.3 The ICCs of eating (Item_1), dressing (Item_2), and bathing (Item_5) based on 2-parameter model

The Akaike information criterion (AIC) and Bayesian information criterion (BIC) are commonly used to select optimal model. Model with a smaller AIC and BIC is selected as the optimal model. The AIC and BIC values were 18899.43 and 18942.69, respectively, when 2-parameter logistic model was fitted to the data in Example 29.1. For the data in Example 29.1, the 2-parameter logistic model was better fitted than the single-parameter model (AIC = 24975.92, BIC = 25019.18). The estimated values of "ability" (latent trait) for older adults were shown in Table 29.1. The "ability" of older adults with ID = 1 and with ID = 12, whose sum scores both were 4, were −1.025 and −1.446, respectively. The older adult with ID = 12 had a worse "ability" in terms of independence than ID = 1. Obviously, IRT can discriminate the difference among participants even with the same sum score.

29.2.1.3. *3-Parameter model*

In single-parameter model and 2-parameter model, for an examinee with an extremely low latent trait value ($-\infty$), the probability of correctly responding an item (or choosing "1") is 0, so the lower limit of ICC is 0. But in real world, an examinee with extremely low latent trait, may still respond correctly on the item by guessing. In this case, a guessing parameter, which is usually denoted by $c_i \in (0, 1)$, needs to be introduced to indicate the probability of "correct" totally by guessing. Obviously, c_i is the height of the lower asymptote of the ICC so that it is also called asymptotic parameter. The model shown in Formula (29-3) is called 3-parameter logistic model.

$$P_i(\theta) = c_i + (1 - c_i)\frac{e^{\alpha_i(\theta-\beta_i)}}{1 + e^{\alpha_i(\theta-\beta_i)}} \tag{29-3}$$

The data in Example 29.1 were fitted with 3-parameter model, and the ICCs of "eating," "dressing," and "bathing" were shown in Figure 29.4. The guessing parameter of "eating," "dressing," and "bathing were 0.1, 0, and 0, respectively. AIC and BIC were 18,932.22 and 18,975.49, respectively, which were worse than those of the 2-parameter logistic model. It showed that for the data in Example 29.1, the 3-parameter model was not an optimal one.

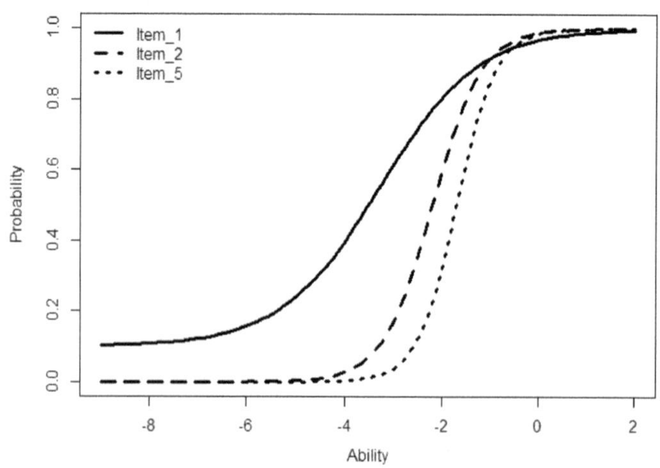

Figure 29.4 The ICCs of eating (Item_1), dressing (Item_2), and bathing (Item_5) based on 3-parameter model

29.2.2. *Ordinal logistic model*

The ordinal logistic models in IRT include partial credit model, generalized partial credit model, and graded response model (GRM). The following would only introduce the commonly used GRM.

Example 29.2. To assess the health status of older adults, 290 older adults were investigated with a physical function scale. The physical function scale consists of 5 items (named P1–P5, respectively), each of them has 5 graded options. Part of the data is shown in Table 29.3. Here we take item P1 as an example to introduce the GRM.

Let $X = 0, 1, \ldots, 4$ denotes the score on item P1, and higher score indicates better physical function. Based on the dichotomous models discussed above, X can be dichotomized as followings.

X is dichotomized as $\{0\}$ and $\{1,2,3,4\}$, and then the first item characteristic function for P1 based on 2-parameter model can be

Table 29.3 Part of the data on physical function of older adults

ID	P1	P2	P3	P4	P5	Sum	Z-score[a]
1	0	0	1	1	0	2	−2.485
2	0	1	1	1	0	3	−2.148
3	0	0	2	2	0	4	−1.951
4	0	1	0	4	0	5	−2.202
5	1	2	1	2	0	6	−1.580
6	1	1	1	2	0	5	−1.810
7	0	2	0	2	0	4	−2.199
8	0	0	1	1	0	2	−2.485
9	3	1	1	1	0	6	−1.602
10	2	0	2	3	2	9	−0.890
11	1	0	1	2	1	5	−1.925
12	0	3	1	3	0	7	−1.571
13	3	0	1	1	0	5	−1.924
14	1	2	2	4	0	9	−0.869
15	3	2	2	3	0	10	−0.303

[a]Bayes expected a-posteriori estimation of latent trait by fitting a GRM.

defined as:

$$P_1^*(\theta) = P(X \geq 1|\,\theta) = \frac{e^{\alpha(\theta-\beta_1)}}{1+e^{\alpha(\theta-\beta_1)}}$$

X is dichotomized as {0,1} and {2,3,4}, then the second item characteristic function for item P1 can be defined as:

$$P_2^*(\theta) = P(X \geq 2|\,\theta) = \frac{e^{\alpha(\theta-\beta_2)}}{1+e^{\alpha(\theta-\beta_2)}}$$

In a similar way, the third and fourth item characteristic functions for item P1 can be defined as:

$$P_3^*(\theta) = P(X \geq 3|\,\theta) = \frac{e^{\alpha(\theta-\beta_3)}}{1+e^{\alpha(\theta-\beta_3)}}$$

$$P_4^*(\theta) = P(X \geq 4|\,\theta) = \frac{e^{\alpha(\theta-\beta_4)}}{1+e^{\alpha(\theta-\beta_4)}}$$

The ICCs corresponding to above four functions are shown in Figure 29.5.

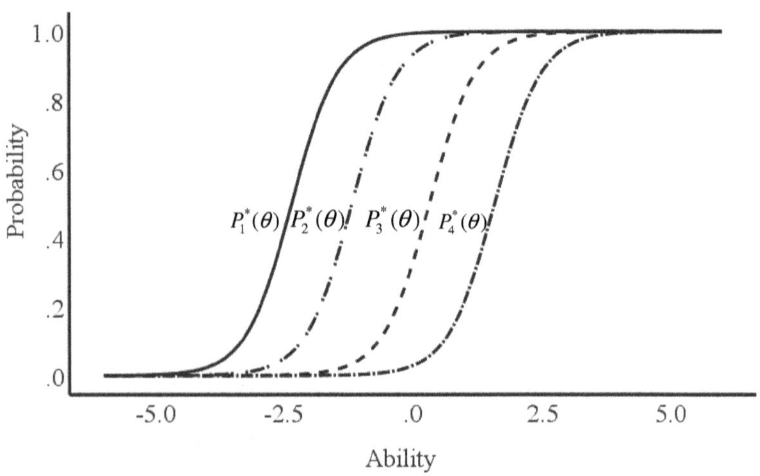

Figure 29.5 Four-item characteristic curves for item P1

It is obvious, $P_0^*(\theta) = P(X \geq 0) = 1$. The probabilities of scoring 0, 1, 2, 3, 4 on item P1 are presented as follows:

$$P_0(\theta) = 1 - P_1^*(\theta)$$
$$P_1(\theta) = P_1^*(\theta) - P_2^*(\theta)$$
$$P_2(\theta) = P_2^*(\theta) - P_3^*(\theta)$$
$$P_3(\theta) = P_3^*(\theta) - P_4^*(\theta)$$
$$P_4(\theta) = P_4^*(\theta)$$

According to $P_0(\theta)$, $P_1(\theta)$, $P_2(\theta)$, $P_3(\theta)$, and $P_4(\theta)$, the probability curves of scoring 0, 1, 2, 3, 4 on item P1, which are usually called category response curves (CRCs) of GRM, can be drawn (see Figure 29.6).

For a Likert item in which the response categories graded, 2-parameter GRM is commonly used. Based on the above analysis, the item category function for an m grades item can be expressed as Formula (29-4), where $\beta_{ik}(\beta_{ik} \leq \beta_{ik+1}, k = 1, 2, \ldots, m-2)$ refers to the difficulty threshold of an examinee responding with $\geq k$ other

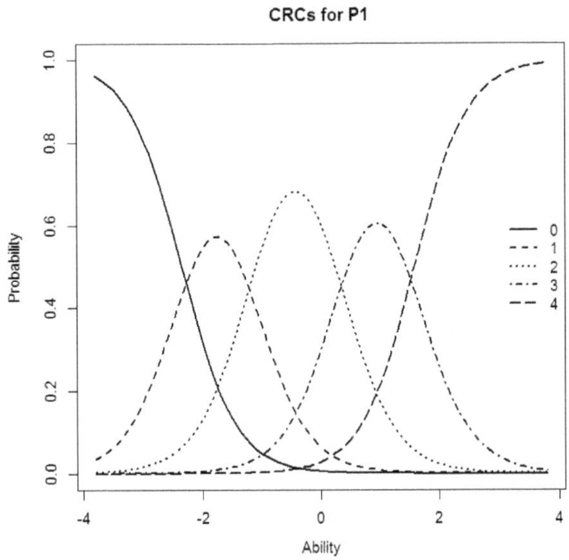

Figure 29.6 Category response curves (CRCs) of item P1

than $\leq k-1$ on item i. In GRM, there is one discrimination parameter and $m-1$ difficulty threshold parameters for each item.

$$P_{ik}(\theta) = \begin{cases} 1 - \dfrac{e^{\alpha_i(\theta-\beta_{ik+1})}}{1+e^{\alpha_i(\theta-\beta_{ik+1})}}, & k=0 \\ \dfrac{e^{\alpha_i(\theta-\beta_{ik})}}{1+e^{\alpha_i(\theta-\beta_{ik})}} - \dfrac{e^{\alpha_i(\theta-\beta_{ik+1})}}{1+e^{\alpha_i(\theta-\beta_{ik+1})}}, & k=1,2,\ldots m-2 \\ \dfrac{e^{\alpha_i(\theta-\beta_{ik})}}{1+e^{\alpha_i(\theta-\beta_{ik})}}, & k=m-1 \end{cases} \tag{29-4}$$

29.2.3. *Other IRT models*

All the models mentioned above require the data to meet the assumption of unidimensionality, and the abilities of examinees are independent and identically distributed. But, the modern IRT models developed recently have not been limited by these basic assumptions. When unidimensionality is not assumed, the multi-dimensional IRT model can be used alternatively. When examinees come from different groups and there is a cluster effect, multi-level IRT model could be considered. Non-parametric IRT does not need a model and draws CRCs directly, so it is increasingly favored by researchers. Due to limited space, these models are not covered in detail here.

29.2.4. *Measuring error in IRT*

In IRT, the measuring error of an item and a scale is assessed by information function. The information function of an item represents the amount of information contributed by the item when evaluating the latent trait of the examinee. The larger the value of the information function is, the greater the contribution of the item to latent trait estimation of the examinee will be. Otherwise, the contribution is smaller. The information function of item i is presented as Formula (29-5).

$$I_i(\theta) = \frac{[P_i'(\theta)]^2}{P_i(\theta)(1-P_i(\theta))} \tag{29-5}$$

For a dichotomous 3-parameter logistic model, the item information function can be expressed by Formula (29-6), which is determined by both the item characteristic parameters and the subject latent trait. For single-parameter model (the guessing parameter is 0 and the discrimination parameter is 1), when the difficulty parameter of the item is equal to the latent trait of the subject, the item information function reaches the maximum value.

$$I_i(\theta) = \frac{a_i^2(1-c_i)}{(1+e^{\alpha_i(\theta-\beta_i)})(c_i+e^{\alpha_i(\theta-\beta_i)})} \quad (29\text{-}6)$$

$P_i'(\theta)$ is the derivative of $P_i(\theta)$ to θ. It reflects the rate at which the probability $P_i(\theta)$ of responding correctly changes with latent trait θ.

The information function of a scale is defined as the sum of the information function of all items, as shown in Formula (29-7).

$$I(\theta) = \sum_{i=1}^{q} I_i(\theta) = \frac{1}{Var(\theta)} \quad (29\text{-}7)$$

It can be deduced that the estimation error of the latent trait is smaller as the scale information function is larger. Therefore, the reliability of a scale can be assessed by mean value of the scale information function.

29.3. Real data analysis

29.3.1. *Problems to be solved*

For the examinees in Example 29.2, the problems are as follows.

(1) What are the characteristics of the scale and items (parameters on difficulty and discrimination, and information function)?
(2) How is the quality of life (latent trait) of patients or healthy people?
(3) How is the reliability of the scale for estimating the quality of life of patients or healthy persons?

29.3.2. *Model selection*

To fit an unidimensional IRT model, the unidimensionality and local independence should be assumed. The unidimensionality assumption requires that only the latent trait that the scale aims to assess is dominant among all minor factors that might affect the response. The principal component analysis and factor analysis are commonly used methods to check the unidimensionality assumption. Reckase demonstrated that unidimensionality could be assumed when the total variance explained by the first component (or factor) is not less than 20%. The result of principal component analysis for data in Example 29.2 demonstrates that the unidimensionality might be held, since the first component accounts for 56.0% of the total variance.

The local independence assumption refers to that the response on an item is not correlated with the responses on other items given the trait. In general, the unidimensionality assumption is correlated with the local independence assumption. If the unidimensionality assumption is confirmed, it is not necessary to investigate the local independence assumption again.

The 5 items in Example 29.2 are all Likert items, so GRM is appropriate.

29.3.3. *Parameter estimation*

The examinees' latent trait and the parameters of item characteristic in IRT models are estimated simultaneously, which beyond the capacity of traditional parameter estimation methods such as maximum likelihood and least squares. More complex estimation methods are required for IRT models. People have proposed several methods, among which joint maximum likelihood estimation, marginal maximum likelihood estimation, Bayes estimation, Markov chain Monte Carlo (MCMC) estimation, and conditional estimation are commonly

Table 29.4 Estimates of characteristic parameters for the 5 items in Example 29.2

Item	$\hat{\beta}_1$	$\hat{\beta}_2$	$\hat{\beta}_3$	$\hat{\beta}_4$	$\hat{\alpha}$
P1	−2.339	−1.168	0.328	1.584	2.230
P2	−2.091	−1.243	0.356	1.480	2.507
P3	−2.961	−1.776	0.135	1.125	2.977
P4	−5.360	−2.765	−1.315	0.687	1.196
P5	−2.011	−0.862	0.371	1.301	1.388

used. It is not surprise that these methods are complex and difficult. Due to space constraints, this chapter would not elaborate them in detail.

Specialized software for IRT analysis includes BILOG, MULTILOG, RUMM, NOHARM, etc. Professor Haiqi Dai in Jiangxi Normal University, China, also developed a software for IRT analysis: ANOTE. Besides, in recent years some R packages for IRT analysis have been developed, such as ltm, catR, mirt, etc. The characteristic parameters of items in Example 29.2 were estimated by marginal maximum likelihood estimation with R package "ltm." The estimators were shown in Table 29.4 and the CRCs of the 4 items were shown in Figure 29.7. The Bayes expected a-posteriori

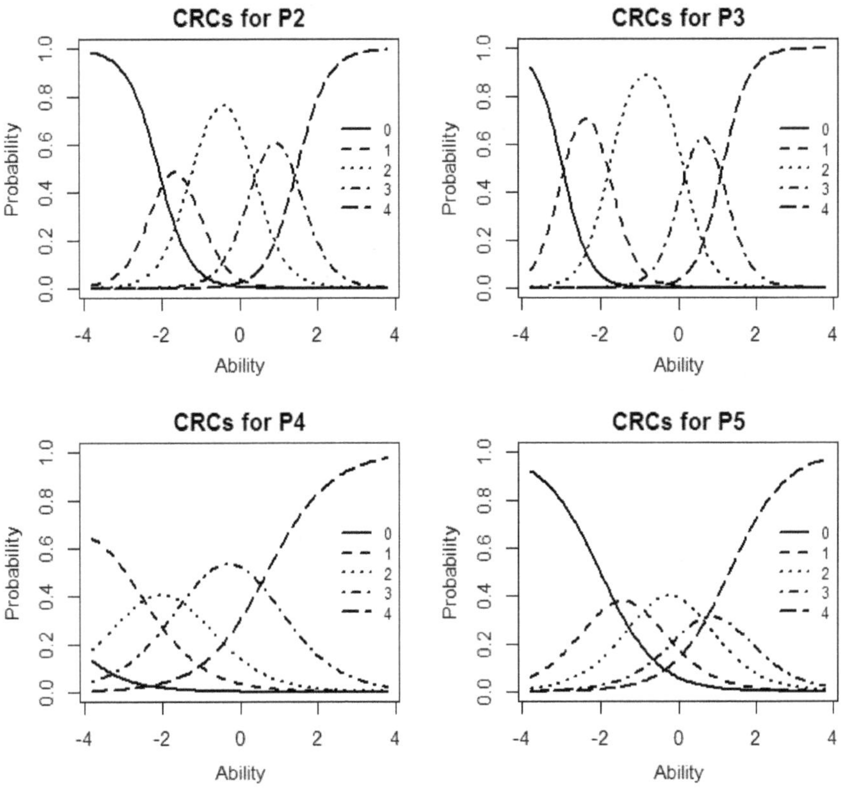

Figure 29.7 The CRCs of item P2, P3, P4, and P5

Table 29.5 Descriptive statistics of 290 older adults' physical health estimators

Minimum	P25	Median	Mean	P75	SD	Maximum
−2.486	−0.544	−0.014	−0.002	0.577	0.909	1.991

estimation of older adults' physical health were obtained simultaneously. Part of older adults' estimated physical health (Z-score) were shown in Table 29.3. The estimated physical health of the 2 older adults with ID = 3 and ID = 7, whose sum scores both were 4 but had different response patterns, were −1.951 and −2.199, respectively. The descriptive statistics of 290 older adults' physical health (estimated latent trait) were shown in Table 29.5. AIC and BIC value for GRM fitting to data in Example 29.2 were 3460.31 and 3552.06, respectively.

29.4. Application of IRT

29.4.1. *Application of IRT in biomedicine*

Since it was proposed, IRT has been mainly applied in the fields of psychology and education. The application in biomedicine began at the end of the 20th century. For example, Haley and McHorney used IRT to evaluate the unidimensionality of physical function domain in SF-36. They also established a repeatable scoring criterion with Rasch model, which was proved to be more accurate than sum scoring of Likert items. IRT is mainly applied in the following aspects in biomedicine.

1. Testing construct validity and reliability of the scales

Given a scale with several domains, one may fit an IRT model for the whole scale ignoring the domains; meanwhile, one may fit IRT models for different domains respectively. Then comparing the goodness of fit between these 2 approaches, if the goodness of fit of the second approach is better than that of the first approach, it is concluded that different domains measure different aspects of the trait and the construct validity is fine. Otherwise, the construct validity of the scale is not good.

The information function can be used to test the reliability of a scale. The mean of the information function of the scale is called the average information content. Larger the average information content is, smaller the measurement error is, and then it can be concluded that the reliability of the scale is good. Noerholm *et al.* proved that the model fit was good when 2-parameter models were fit to different domains of WHOQOL-BREF respectively, whereas the model fit was not good when a single 2-parameter model was fit to all the items as a whole. It indicated that different domains of WHOQOL-BREF measured different aspects of quality of life, so they concluded that WHOQOL-BREFF had good construct validity.

2. Scaling individuals

IRT based scores represent an optimal scaling of individuals on the trait. The latent trait estimated by IRT can be used as the measurement for the examinee, which is more accurate than the conventional sum of item scores. For the assumption that the latent trait follows $N(0, 1)$, the estimated latent trait by IRT should be converted by a linear transformation $Z \times 100 + 50$, such that the average score after transformation is around 50.

3. Testing measurement bias or differential item functioning (DIF)

DIF refers to the situation that different populations (gender, age, country, etc.) with the same potential trait have a different responses on an item. IRT can be applied to test DIF by comparing the parameters of an item for different groups with same potential trait. Most scales in biomedical research are rooted in certain cultural background and have cultural differences. Therefore, DIF analysis is necessary when comparing the scale data with different cultural backgrounds.

4. Computerized adaptive test (CAT)

Under the theoretical framework of IRT, the information function of the item represents the measurement error. The measurement error is smaller as the information function is larger. The estimation error of latent trait reaches the minimum value when the scale composed of the items that make the information function reach the maximum value. According to the examinee's responses on the former items, the computer selects the subsequent items that make the information function reach the maximum value, and then estimates the examinee's latent trait according to all of his or her responses. Such a process is called CAT. CAT has been widely used in various disease diagnosis and health outcome measurement.

5. Development and modification of scales

In the process of scale development and modification, the items are selected by IRT statistics such as difficulty parameter, discrimination parameter, and item information function. The information functions of the scales with different item combinations are calculated firstly; then the combination with least number of items and largest information function is selected as the final scale. When developing new scales or revising existing scales, the items displaying DIF would normally be revised or discarded.

29.4.2. *Cautions in application*

1. Assumptions of unidimensionality and local independence must be satisfied for unidimensional IRT models.

There are unidimensional models and multi-dimensional models in IRT. While constrained by space, this chapter only introduces the unidimensional models. The unidimensionality and local independence of data must be tested before fitting a unidimensional model. Only when the data satisfy the assumptions of unidimensionality and local independence, the unidimensional IRT models could be tried to estimate the item characteristic parameters and examinee's latent trait. Otherwise multi-dimensional models should be tried.

2. Initial values in parameter estimation

Parameter estimation in IRT usually uses algorithms of iteration, which needs to set up the initial values for the item characteristic parameters and examinee's latent trait. The statistical packages for IRT analysis usually have default initial values. Generally, after iterations, the estimators can reach the converge criterion and are less affected by the initial values. In case of the estimations inconsistent with the professional knowledge, the initial values could be judged to get reasonable estimators hopefully under the condition that the assumption unidimensionality and local independence are verified.

29.5. Report writing

In general, the report for the analysis based on IRT should include the followings:

(1) Objectives
(2) The model assumptions of IRT
(3) The goodness of fit
(4) The estimates of subjects' latent trait

Report for Example 29.2

Objectives: To evaluate the health status of 290 elderly people interviewed with a physiological scale.

The model assumptions: The result of principal components analysis showed that 56.0% of the total variance was explained by the first component so that the unidimensionality assumption was considered to be satisfied.

The goodness of fit: The AIC and BIC were 3460.31 and 3552.06, respectively.

The estimates of examinees' latent trait: The estimated physical health ("Z-score") of 15 elderly people were shown in Table 29.3; and the descriptive statistics of the elderly physical health were shown in Table 29.5.

29.6. Case discrimination

Case 29.1 A researcher fitted a Rasch model to a data set of ADL scale, of which the response options comprised 5-categories (1 denotes no limitation, 5 denotes total limitation). For Rasch model is a dichotomous model, the researcher converted each ADL item into 4 dichotomous items, such as Item1_1–Item1_4 for Item 1 (see Table 29.6). In such a way, each item can get 4 difficulty parameters, which can be considered as the difficulty thresholds of 0–1, 1–2, 2–3, 3–4, respectively, and the 4 difficulty thresholds should be monotone increasing. However, the 4 difficulty parameters were not monotone increasing for some items in fact. For example, the 4 difficulty parameters of item 1 were 4.5, −4.68, 0.87, and 1.4, respectively. To avoid this problem, the researcher combined the categories 1, 2, 3, and 4 to make the item be a dichotomous item with 2 response options (0, 1–4), and then fitted the combined data with the dichotomous logistic model. Please comment on this study.

Case 29.2 A researcher used EQ-5D scale (see Tables 29.7 and 29.8) to evaluate older adults' health status. The data were fitted with GRM and the estimated Z-scores for health status of older adults were shown in Table 29.8. The one with ID = 11 had the best health status, while the one with ID = 1 had the worst health status. Please comment on this study.

Table 29.6 Convert Items 1–4 dichotomous items

Item1	Item1_1	Item1_2	Item1_3	Item1_4
0	0	0	0	0
1	1	0	0	0
2	1	1	0	0
3	1	1	1	0
4	1	1	1	1

Table 29.7 EQ-5D scale

Under each heading, please tick the One box that best describes your health TODAY.

E1 MOBILITY	(1) I have no problems in walking about	☐
	(2) I have some problems in walking about	☐
	(3) I am confined to bed	☐
E2 SELF-CARE	(1) I have no problems with self-care	☐
	(2) I have some problems in washing or dressing myself	☐
	(3) I am unable to wash or dress myself	☐
E3 USUAL ACTIVITIES (e.g., work, study, homework, family, or leisure activities)	(1) I have no problems with performing my usual activities	☐
	(2) I have some problems with performing my usual activities	☐
	(3) I am unable to perform my usual activities	☐
E4 PAIN/ DISCOMFORT	(1) I have no pain or discomfort	
	(2) I have moderate pain or discomfort	☐
	(3) I have extreme pain or discomfort	☐
E5 ANXIETY/ DEPRESSION	(1) I am not anxious or depressed	☐
	(2) I am moderately anxious or depressed	☐
	(3) I am extremely anxious or depressed	☐

Table 29.8 Responses on ED-5D scale and estimated health status of 11 older adults

ID	E1	E2	E3	E4	E5	Sum score	Z-score	Order
1	1	1	1	1	1	5	−1.547	1
2	1	2	1	1	1	6	−1.207	2
3	1	1	1	3	1	7	−1.190	3
4	3	2	1	1	1	8	−0.106	5
5	1	2	2	2	2	9	−0.682	4
6	3	3	1	2	1	10	0.355	6
7	3	3	1	3	1	11	0.660	7
8	3	3	1	3	2	12	0.952	8
9	3	3	3	3	1	13	1.353	9
10	3	3	3	3	2	14	1.669	10
11	3	3	3	3	3	15	1.842	11

29.7. Computer experiments

Experiment 29.1 Fit a dichotomous single-parameter logistic model

Experiment 29.2 Fit a dichotomous 2-parameter logistic model

Experiment 29.3 Fit a dichotomous 3-parameter logistic model

Experiment 29.4 Fit a GRM

29.8. Frequently asked questions and summary

29.8.1. *Frequently asked questions*

1. What should we do when the assumptions of unidimensionality and local independence are not satisfied?

If the assumptions of unidimensionality and local independence are not satisfied, the unidimensional IRT model cannot be used. In fact, besides the unidimensional model, there are multi-dimensional models, which could be considered.

2. What is the difference and relationship between IRT logistic model and logistic regression?

The difference:

(1) The independent variable X in Logistic regression is an observable variable (explicit variable), while there is no independent variable in IRT logistic model. In other words, independent variable is an unobservable latent variable in IRT Logistic model.
(2) Logistic regression results in a single equation, while IRT logistic model results in a set of equations, where the number of equations equals to the number of items in the scale.

The relationship:

When the latent trait of examinees are known and the item characteristic parameters are to be estimated, the IRT logistic model is just logistic regression.

3. What are the advantages and limitations of IRT and CTT?

	Advantages	Limitations
CTT	It is simple and easy to be understood. The sum of the scores of all items is an estimated value of the examinee's latent trait. The parameters of difficulty and discrimination are easy to calculate as well.	The item parameters depend on the examinees' latent trait. CTT's model assumptions require parallel measurements, which can hardly be met in real world.
IRT	The latent trait and item parameters are invariant. The concept of measurement precision is more reasonable because the measurement reliability is related to both the latent trait and the item parameters.	The models are more complex. The estimation of latent trait and item parameters is more troublesome and needs specialized computer software for analysis.

4. In application, how to choose from single-parameter, 2-parameter, and 3-parameter models?

The single-parameter model is relatively simple. However, unidimensionality and local independence, zero probability of guessing and all items having same discrimination degree are assumed. Few scales meet so many assumptions as a whole, especially the assumption of same discrimination parameter. The guessing probabilities of items used in biomedical research can be ignored. The 2-parameter model is commonly used in biomedicine, for no restriction on discrimination parameter. The 3-parameter model compass relatively more information on items, but the parameter estimation is more complex.

For items with guessing parameters of 0, fitting a 3-parameter models will increase AIC and BIC values instead. According to the target latent trait measured by the scale, one can preliminarily judge whether the guessing parameter is 0 or not and choose an optimal model incorporating with AIC and BIC values.

29.8.2. *Summary*

1. IRT is a theory based on latent trait. It uses a nonlinear function to depict the relationship between examinees' response on an item, item's characteristics and examinees' latent trait.
2. Common used IRT models include 3/2/single-parameter dichotomous logistic models, GRMs, and so on. There are both difference and relationship between logistic models in IRT and logistic regression.
3. The assumptions of unidimensionality and local independence should be satisfied when one wants to fit a unidimensional IRT model. In application, the model assumptions and the initial values in parameter estimation should be paid more attention to.
4. The IRT models use information function to present measurement error. The larger the information function value, the smaller the measurement error. Item's information function is determined by both the item parameters and the latent trait of examinees. For single-parameter model, when the latent trait of the examinee is equal to the difficulty parameter of the item, the item information function gets the maximum value.

Think and Practice

I. Questions for Reflection

1. Which IRT models are commonly used? For what data should they be applied to respectively?
2. What are the main assumptions for IRT models?

II. Question on Calculation

A researcher assessed health status of 106 adult females with a scale consisted of 5 Likert items. The responses were shown in Table 10.9 in Chapter 10 of this book. Try to fit a GRM to the data and estimate the difficulty and discrimination parameters of these 5 items; then draw the CRCs and calculate the mean and standard deviation of the 106 females' health status.

Yaofeng Han

CHAPTER 30

STATISTICS FOR GENETICS

Recent developments in molecular genetics provide opportunities for genetic research on complex traits in humans. Many human diseases, such as insulin-dependent diabetes, hypertension and schizophrenia, are considered to have genetic effects. Gene mapping is extremely important for etiological studies and may lead to better treatments. The main goal of human disease genomics research is to reveal the genetic mechanism of complex genetic diseases. Complex diseases, such as diabetes, obesity, osteoporosis, hypertension, cardiovascular diseases, are generally determined by a variety of genetic and environmental factors and their interactions. Genetic epidemiology studies try to seek to elucidate the role of genetic and environmental factors in the occurrence of disease in population. The surge in the field of genetic epidemiology has been accompanied by the increasing developments of statistical methods. In this chapter, we focus on genetic association analysis, including some basic concepts, population-based and family-based association analysis.

30.1. Basic concepts

30.1.1. *Genetic terminology*

1) Gene and locus. In the human somatic cell, there are 23 pairs of chromosomes, including 22 pairs of autosomes and one pair of sex chromosomes. Females have two of the same kind of sex chromosome (XX), while males have two distinct sex chromosomes with different in shape and size (XY). The chromosomes determine the cell differentiation, cell function and the development of the human body, behavior and intelligence. The observable trait is called **phenotype**, such as height, weight, blood type and disease status. **Gene**, a molecular unit of heredity, is a functional part of DNA, which determine various biological traits. It is estimated that there are about ten thousand nuclear genes in human beings. Each gene has its specific location in the chromosome, called **locus**.

2) Polymorphism. The locus sometimes represents a perceptive DNA marker or a DNA fragment with polymorphism. Any of the alternative forms of a gene that may occur at a given locus are termed as alleles. Alleles are often denoted by letters or numbers, such as A, a, B, b, 1, 2 or 3. In a diploid cell of an individual, the pair of alleles at a locus is referred to as the **genotype**, such as A/a or Aa (the "/" can be omitted). The individual with identical alleles is called a **homozygote**, such as AA or aa. The individual with different alleles is called a **heterozygote**, such as Aa. A gene may have multiple alleles. An example of **multiple allelism** that occurs in humans is that of ABO blood type. The blood types exist as three alleles, which are represented as I^A, I^B and I^O. I^A and I^B are co-dominant, and both of them are dominant to the recessive I^O allele. There are four phenotypes (A, B, AB, or O) and six possible genotypes for the ABO blood groups. The phenotype depends upon the genotype, but can also be influenced by environmental factors. If someone has blood type A, their genotype is either AA or AO for Blood type A. Similarly, someone who is blood type B could have a genotype of either BB or BO. Someone with blood type AB must have both the A and B alleles. The genotype must be AB. Someone with blood type O must have genotype OO.

The proportion of alleles at a locus in a population is called as the **gene frequency**; for example, $P(A) = 0.3$ means that 30% of alleles at this locus in this population are A. The total of gene frequencies of all different alleles at a certain locus is 1. The genotypic frequency is the proportion of individuals carrying a certain genotype in a population. For example, $P(Aa) = 0.3$ means that 30% of individuals in the population carried the genotype Aa.

3) Genetic markers. Gene mapping is the sequential allocation of loci to a relative position on a chromosome. There are landmarks in genetic maps known as **genetic markers**. The more markers there are on a genetic map, the more likely it is that at least one marker will be located close to a disease gene. Several commonly used types of markers include restriction fragment length polymorphisms (RFLP), variable number of tandem repeat polymorphisms (VNTR), microsatellite polymorphisms, and single nucleotide polymorphisms (SNPs, pronounced "snips"). SNPs are the most common type of genetic variation among people. **SNPs** are specific nucleotide sites in the human genome where it is possible to have two (or even three or four) different nucleotides (A, T, C, or G) at a specific position on a chromosome. In humans, most SNPs are biallelic (e.g., C and T). As a result, the possible genotype values in the population are CC, CT and TT. A SNP with two alleles C and T is shown in Figure 30.1. At a specific site, some persons have nucleotide C, whereas other persons have T. SNP is a kind of high-density genetic marker. SNPs occur

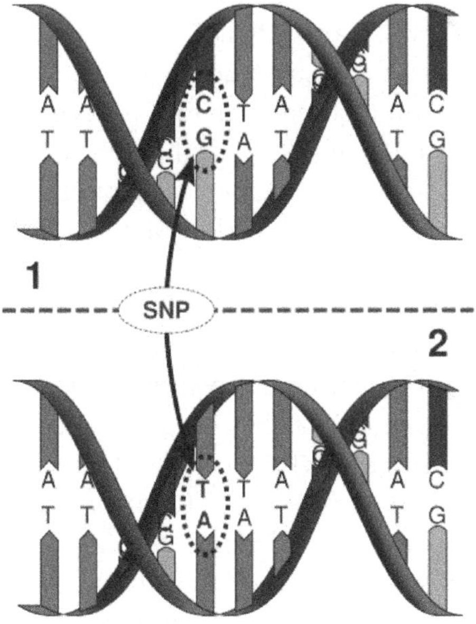

Figure 30.1 Single nucleotide polymorphism (SNP)

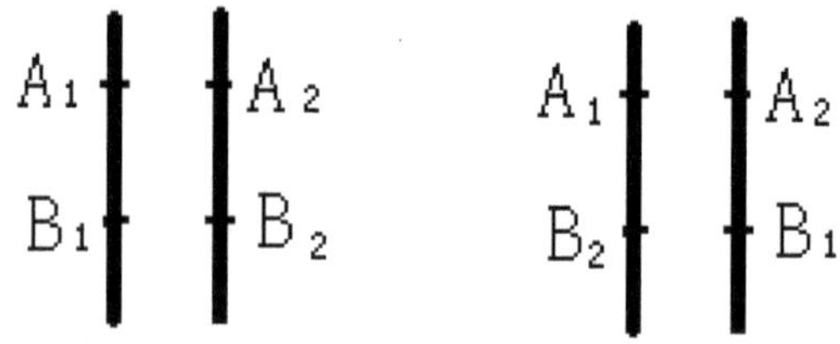

Figure 30.2 Both haplotype pairs A_1B_1/A_2B_2 and A_1B_2/A_2B_1 can fit observed genotypes A_1/A_2 and B_1/B_2

once in every 300 nucleotides on average, and about 10 millions of SNP sites have been identified in humans.

4) Haplotype. Haplotype is a contraction of the term haploid genotype. A **haplotype** consists of the alleles at closely linked loci on the same chromosome that tend to be inherited together from a single parent. When chromosome origin for each allele is unknown, multiple haplotype pairs can fit observed genotype. As shown in Figure 30.2, an individual is heterozygote in both loci on a chromosome, with genotype A_1/A_2 and B_1/B_2 respectively. Then the phase is ambiguous, and the haplotype pairs might be A_1B_1/A_2B_2 or A_1B_2/A_2B_1. Haplotyping refers to the reconstruction of the unknown true haplotype configurations from observed data. Family information can help determine phase at many markers. Still, many ambiguities might not be resolved. Some statistical methods, including EM (expectation-maximization) algorithm and MCMC (Markov Chain Monte Carlo), were developed for haplotyping.

5) Linkage and recombination. From Mendel's second law, if two genetic loci are on different chromosomes, the transmission of alleles at one locus is independent of that at another locus (the recombination rate $\theta = 1/2$). However, if the two genetic loci are close together, the alleles that are paternal or maternal in origin tend to transmit together to an offspring. This phenomenon is called as **linkage**. Chromosomal **crossover** is the exchange of genetic material between homologous chromosomes that results in recombinant chromosomes. When the alleles in an offspring haplotype at two markers derive

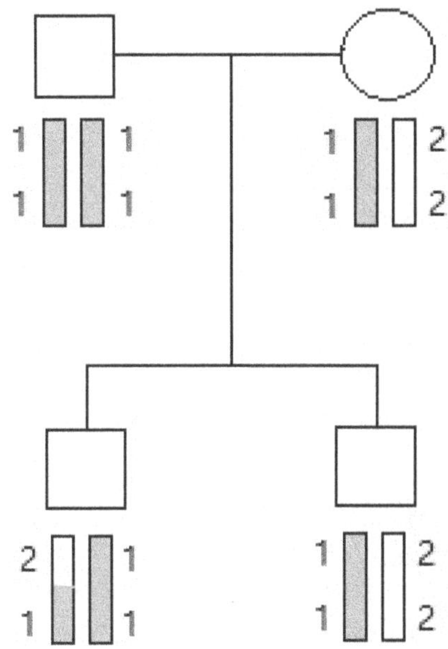

Figure 30.3 A recombination in the offspring haplotype 21

from different parental chromosomes, the event is called a **recombination**. For example, there is a recombination in the offspring haplotype 21 in Figure 30.3. The further apart two points on the chromosome are, the higher probability that a crossover and recombination happens. Recombination probability termed recombination fraction θ, can be estimated by distance between two points. The recombination fraction for two linked loci is less than 1/2.

6) Hereditary mode. The penetrance function is the set of probability distribution functions for the phenotype given the genotype (s). Suppose we know that a disease is caused by a single major gene that exists within the population in two alleles: d, the wild type or normal allele, and D, the mutant or disease susceptibility allele. The prevalence of the individuals with genotype DD, Dd or dd is called penetrance of DD, Dd or dd, denoted by f_{DD}, f_{Dd}, f_{dd}, $(1 \geq f_{DD} \geq f_{Dd} \geq f_{dd} \geq 0)$ respectively. The penetrance is actually conditional prevalence, i.e. $P(\text{Affected}|\text{genotype})$. When the population is in H-W equilibrium, the prevalence will be

$$P_A = P(\text{Affected}) = q^2 f_{DD} + 2q(1-q)f_{Dd} + (1-q)^2 f_{dd}$$

where q is the frequency of allele D.

The hereditary mode is determined by the penetrances. If $1 \geq f_{DD} = f_{Dd} > f_{dd} \geq 0$, it's called dominant hereditary mode, and complete dominant mode in the special case when $f_{DD} = f_{Dd} = 1, f_{dd} = 0$. Similarly, its recessive hereditary mode if $1 \geq f_{DD} > f_{Dd} = f_{dd} \geq 0$, and complete recessive mode in the special case when $f_{DD} = 1, f_{Dd} = f_{dd} = 0$.It's called additive if $1 \geq f_{DD} \geq f_{Dd} \geq f_{dd} \geq 0$, $f_{Dd} = \frac{1}{2}(f_{DD} + f_{dd})$, and called multiplicative if $1 \geq f_{DD} \geq f_{Dd} \geq f_{dd} \geq 0$, $f_{Dd} = \sqrt{f_{DD} f_{dd}}$.

To infer the hereditary mode, we should collect the pedigree and segregation information. The segregation analysis is common used to infer the hereditary mode. The inferences are based on the segregation information derived from the collected pedigree data. The details are ignored here.

30.1.2. *Hardy-Weinberg equilibrium*

Random mating is defined as that any female has the same chance of mating with any male. Accordingly, the probability of mating type is the product of female genotypic frequency and male genotypic frequency; for example $P\{AA \times Aa\} = P(AA)P(Aa)$. Assuming that a locus has two possible alleles, i.e., A and a, the frequencies of allele A and allele a are:

$$P(A) = p, \quad P(a) = q = 1 - p$$

If three genotype frequencies for this pair of alleles in certain generation of a population are

$$P(AA) = p^2, \quad P(Aa) = 2pq, \quad P(aa) = q^2 \tag{30-1}$$

Then, under random mating, there will no change in either the allele or the genotypic frequencies in the next generation. This is an equilibrium status in the population. A special name is given to this equilibrium: it is called a Hardy-Weinberg equilibrium (HWE). In a large, random mating population, and no immigration, no selection and no mutation, the allele and genotypic frequencies are constant from generation to generation. In genetic analysis, Pearson χ^2 test is used to test the hypothesis of Hardy-Weinberg Equilibrium. The test statistic

$$\chi^2 = \sum \frac{(O-E)^2}{E} \tag{30-2}$$

is chi-square distributed with v = (number of genotype-Number of alleles) degrees of freedom, under HWE.

In equation (30-2), O is the observed genotypic count. E is the expected genotypic count. For the locus with two possible alleles and under the hypothesis of HWE, the expected frequencies of genotype AA, Aa, aa in a random sample with n individual are np_A^2, $2np_Ap_a$, np_a^2. The allele frequency p_A, p_a can be estimated by

$$\hat{p}_A = \frac{2n_{AA}+n_{Aa}}{2n}, \quad \hat{p}_a = \frac{2n_{aa}+n_{Aa}}{2n} \tag{30-3}$$

where n_{AA}, n_{Aa}, n_{Aa} are the observed number of individuals with genotype AA, Aa and aa respectively.

Example 30.1. In a genetic study of hypertension, 197 individuals were randomly sampled from a population. The sample frequencies of genotype AA, Aa, and aa of angiotension-converting enzyme (ACE) are 26, 93, and 78, respectively. To test if this population is in HWE or not, we calculate

$$\hat{p}_A = \frac{2n_{AA}+n_{Aa}}{2n} = 0.368, \quad \hat{p}_a = \frac{2n_{aa}+n_{Aa}}{2n} = 0.632$$

Under the null hypothesis of HWE, the expected frequencies of genotype AA, Aa, aa

$$197 \times 0.368^2 = 26.68,\ 2 \times 197 \times 0.368 \times 0.632 = 91.63,$$
$$197 \times 0.632^2 = 78.69$$

Then

$$\chi^2 = \frac{(26-26.68)^2}{26.68} + \frac{(93-91.63)^2}{91.63} + \frac{(78-78.69)^2}{78.69} = 0.0439, \quad v = 1$$

$P = 0.8346$, and conclude the null hypothesis of HWE.

30.2. Linkage equilibrium (LD) and haplotype block

30.2.1. *Linkage equilibrium*

If the alleles of two loci are randomly combined, these two loci are called in linkage equilibrium. Suppose that in a population, allele A occurs with frequency $P(A)$ at one locus, while at a different locus allele B occurs with frequency $P(B)$. Let $P(AB)$ be the frequency of the AB haplotype. When the two loci are in linkage equilibrium, $P(AB) = P(A)P(B)$. The level of linkage disequilibrium between A and B can be quantified by the coefficient of LD, which is defined as $D = P(AB) - P(A)P(B)$. $D = 0$ means linkage equilibrium between two loci. When both loci have only two alleles A, a, and B, b, respectively, then $D = P(AB) - P(A)P(B) = P(a)P(b) - P(a)P(b) = -P(Ab) + P(A)P(b) = -P(aB) - P(a)P(B)$, and

$$P(AB) = P(A)P(B) + D, \quad P(Ab) = P(A)P(b) - D,$$
$$P(aB) = P(a)P(B) - D, \quad P(ab) = P(a)P(b) + D.$$

It's easy to show the LD coefficient D also satisfies

$$D = P(AB)P(ab) - P(Ab)P(aB) \tag{30-4}$$

Besides D, the common measures of LD include D' and r^2. D' is defined as

$$D' = \frac{|D|}{D_{\max}} = \begin{cases} \dfrac{D}{\min\{P(A)P(b),\, P(a)P(B)\}}, & \text{if } D > 0 \\ \dfrac{-D}{\min\{P(A)P(B),\, P(a)P(b)\}}, & \text{if } D < 0 \end{cases} \tag{30-5}$$

where $D_{\max}$ represents the upper bound on D. D' is also called normalized LD coefficient since $D' \in [0, 1]$. Values of D' that are close to 1 indicate high levels of LD, while values close to 0 suggest low LD. $D' < 1$ if all four possible haplotypes are observed in the sample. In the special case when $D' = 1$, i.e. at least one haplotye has 0 frequency, we say the two loci is complete LD. The most useful LD measure is

$$r^2 = \frac{D^2}{P(A)\,P(a)\,P(B)P(b)} \tag{30-6}$$

We can show r is actually Pearson correlation coefficient of allelic value between the loci. The two loci is called perfect LD if $r^2 = 1$. We can test LD by using a test statistic

$$\chi^2 = \frac{ND^2}{P(A)\,P(a)\,P(B)P(b)} = Nr^2, \tag{30-7}$$

where N is two times of sample size, since each individual provides two haplotypes. The statistic follows chi-square distribution with $v = 1$ degrees of freedom under linkage equilibrium. It is actually Pearson χ^2 statistic.

Example 30.2. To detect the LD of two linked SNPs, 387 individuals were genotyped and summarized in Table 30.1.

As shown in Table 30.1, $P(SNP2 = 1/1 \mid SNP1 = 1/1) = 96.9\%$, $P(SNP2 = 1/2 \mid SNP1 = 1/2) = 92.7\%$, and $P(SNP2 = 2/2 \mid SNP1 = 2/2) = 92.5\%$. That means alleles 1 of the two SNPs is tend to combine together. To obtain LD coefficient, we need the frequency of haplotypes. Several haplotyping softwares, including Haplo and Phase, can help us to reconstruct the underlying haplotypes from observed genotype data. The estimated frequencies via Phase for haplotypes 11, 12, 21, and 22 are 0.417445, 0.019537, 0.010544, and 0.552475 respectively. By (30-4)$\sim$(30-7), we have $D = 0.2304$, $D' = 0.9562$, $r = 0.9388$, $\chi^2 = 682.283$, $P < 0.001$. Therefore, we say the two SNPs are LD.

Table 30.1 Joint sample distribution of two SNP genotypes

	SNP2			
SNP1	1/1	1/2	2/2	合计
1/1	124 (96.9%)	4 (3.1%)	0(0.0%)	128 (100%)
1/2	9 (5.0%)	166 (92.7%)	4 (2.2%)	179 (100%)
2/1	0(0.0%)	6 (7.5%)	74 (92.5%)	80 (100%)
Total	133 (34.4%)	176 (45.5%)	78 (20.2%)	387 (100%)

30.2.2. *Haplotype blocks and tag SNP*

The chromosomal regions with strong LD, hence only a few recombinations, were termed haplotype blocks. The length of haplotype blocks was variable, with some extending more than several hundred Kb. These blocks are separated by hotspots, regions in which recombination events are more likely to occur. A haplotype block usually contains only a small number of distinct haplotypes. For example, a haplotype block with six SNPs might have only three or four haplotypes observed. The haplotype blocks cannot be directly observed, and they must instead be statistically inferred, such as the method via confidence interval of D', four gametes principle, etc. The inferred haplotype blocks in the centromeric region of chromosome 15 in Tibetans is shown in Figure 30.4. The paired LD measures $100r^2$ are shown in the boxes.

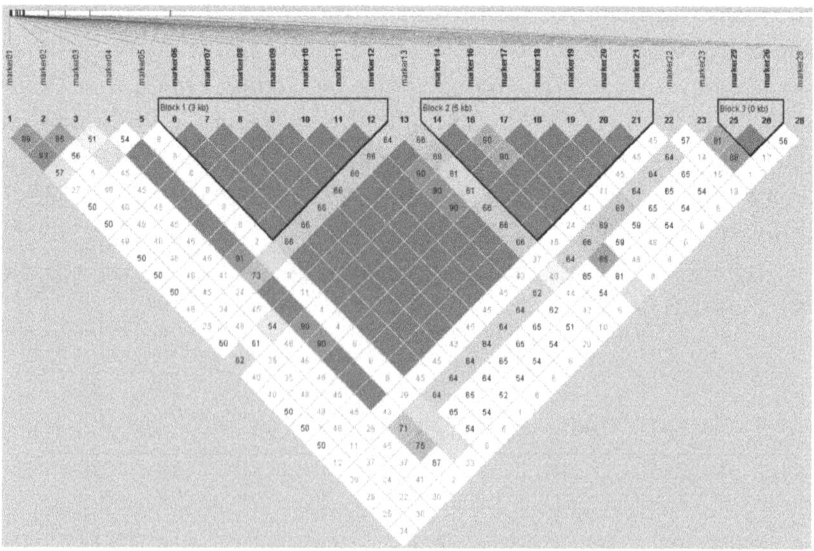

Figure 30.4 LD matrix and haplotype blocks in the centromeric region of chromosome 15 in Tibetans

From: Huang W, Li C, Labu, *et al.* High resolution linkage disequilibrium and haplotype maps for the genes in the centromeric region of chromosome 15 in Tibetans and comparisons with Han population. Chinese Science Bulletin, 2006, 51(5):542–551.

In general, alleles tend to be more correlated within LD blocks than across LD blocks. To reduce redundancies, we can determine the smallest subset of SNPs that characterizes the variability in the region of high LD, a process referred to as SNP tagging. A tag SNP is a representative SNP in a region of high LD that represents a haplotype. Sequencing the whole genome of each individual in a study sample is often too costly. Genotyping arrays used for genome-wide association studies (GWAS) are based on tagging SNPs. As a subset of all of the SNPs in the genome, tag SNPs can be extremely useful for testing the association without genotyping all of the SNPs.

30.3. Population-based association analysis

Genetic association studies aim to detect association between one or more genetic polymorphisms and a trait. Once an allele of a gene is over represented in a case population relative to the control, it may be established that such an allele of the gene is associated with the studied disease. Population-based case-control design and family-based designs such as the case-parent triad design is often used for genetic association studies.

30.3.1. *Population-based case-control design*

Association can be demonstrated, if it exists, by comparing allele frequencies at the marker locus in random samples of unrelated patients and controls. Therefore, genetic association studies can use population-based case-control design. In this simple case, familiar methods such as χ^2 tests of association, Cochran-Armitage trend test and logistic regression can be used.

Pearson χ^2 test statistic

$$\chi^2 = \sum \frac{(O-E)^2}{E}$$

where O is "observed count," and E is "expected count." There are two kinds of χ^2 tests, genotype-based χ^2 test and allele-based χ^2 test. The tests are executed using a contingency table analysis with rows representing binary disease status and columns representing the g

observed genotype classes or k observed allele classes respectively. So the genotype-based χ^2 test compares genotype frequencies, and the allele-based χ^2 test compares allele frequencies at the marker locus in random samples of unrelated cases and controls. It's assumed there is an additive or multiplicative allele effect on the disease susceptibility in allele-based χ^2 test. Both tests assume Hardy-Weinberg equilibrium holds in the combined sample of cases and controls. When H_0, no association between the marker and affection status of a particular disease, holds, genotype-based and allele-based χ^2 statistics have an asymptotic χ^2 distribution with g-1 and k-1degrees of freedom (df) respectively. For biallelic markers, genotype-based and allele-based χ^2 statistics are asymptotically χ^2 distributed with $df = 2$ and $df = 1$ respectively.

Example 30.3. In a genetic association study of diabetes, random samples of unrelated 366 diabetes patients and 390 normal subjects were recruited. The genotyping results for a candidate single nucleotide polymorphism (SNP) marker are shown in Table 30.2.

The genotype-based χ^2 test statistic

$$\chi^2 = \sum \frac{(O-E)^2}{E} = 11.268,$$

$df = 2$, $P = 0.004$. Therefore there is significant difference in the genotype distribution between case and control groups, and association between diabetes and the SNP marker is suggested. Furthermore, we can calculate the odds ratio (OR) values for

Table 30.2 Genotype frequencies for 366 diabetes patients and 390 normal subjects

	Genotype			
Group	11	12	22	Total
Case	107	198	61	366
Control	159	181	50	390

Table 30.3 Allele frequencies for 366 diabetes patients and 390 normal subjects

	Allele		
Group	1	2	Total
Case	412* (56.28%)	320 (43.72%)	732 (100%)
Control	499 (63.97%)	281 (36.03%)	780 (100%)

Note: *412 = 2*107 + 198, similar for other cells.

genotype 12 and 22, with 11 as reference level, are 1.626 and 1.813 respectively.

The allele-based contingency table is shown in Table 30.3. In similar way, we calculate $\chi^2 = 9.325$ with $df = 1$ and $P = 0.002$. The OR value for allele 2 relative to 1 is $OR = 1.379$. The results suggest the significant difference of allele frequency distribution between case and control group.

The general genotype-based χ^2 test is performed regardless of the underlying hereditary mode. If the genotype risks are additive, the genotype-based χ^2 test will not be as powerful as allele-based χ^2 test which is tailored to this scenario, because of smaller sample size and larger degree of freedom. If allele 1 is assumed a risk allele for a biallelic marker, one way to improve power to detect dominant (or recessive) risks is to count heterozygotes with genotype 1/2 into homozygotes with genotype 1/1 (or 2/2 respectively) since the heterozygotes have same risk with homozygote 1/1 (or 2/2 respectively). And then a 2×2 table rather than 2×3 table is constructed and a Pearson 1-df test can be applied.

For complex traits, it is widely thought that heterozygote risk is constrained to lie within the range defined by the two homozygote risks, that is $f_{AA} \geq f_{Aa} \geq f_{aa}$, where A is risk allele. So the widely used dose-response model, the Cochran–Armitage trend test (also known as just the Armitage test) is also used for testing a marker for association with a disease locus. The table for Armitage test is set up as Table 30.4.

Table 30.4 Genotype distribution for case and control groups

	Risk allele count			
Group	0	1	2	Total
Case	r_0	r_1	r_2	R
Control	s_0	s_1	s_2	S
Total	n_0	n_1	n_2	N

Cochran-Armitage trend test Statistic is given as

$$Z = \frac{\sum_{i=0}^{2} t_i(Sr_i - Rs_i)}{\sqrt{\frac{RS}{N}\left[\sum_{i=0}^{2} t_i^2 n_i(N - n_i) - 2\sum_{i=0}^{1}\sum_{j=i}^{2} t_i t_j n_i n_j\right]}} N(0,1) \tag{30-8}$$

or

$$\chi_{CA}^2 = Z^2 \sim \chi_1^2 \tag{30-9}$$

under H_0, where t_0, t_1, t_2 are pre-specified weights for 3 genotypes according to the hereditary mode. For example, the additive allele effect model describes the linearity of the genotype–phenotype relationship for the binary trait, and t_0, t_1, t_2 can be coded as 0, 1, and 2. Similarly, $(t_0, t_1, t_2) = (0, 1, 1)$ and (0,0,1) for dominant and recessive model respectively. The linear trend test statistic corresponding to additive model with $(t_0, t_1, t_2) = (0, 1, 2)$ is

$$Z = \frac{\sqrt{N}[N(r_1 + 2r_2) - R(n_1 + 2n_2)]}{\sqrt{RS[N(n_1 + 4n_2) - (n_1 + 2n_2)^2]}} \tag{30-10}$$

The linear trend test for the data from Table 30.2 shows $Z = 3.128$ and $p = 0.0018$.

30.3.2. *Association analysis in presence of the effects of covariates*

In presence of the effects of covariates, stratified χ^2 test or logistic regression can used to detect and control their effects. Stratified χ^2 test can be used when there only exist few categorical covariates.

The most common used method is logistic regression, and Chapter 20 gives the details.

In theory, one can analyze several covariates in the logistic-regression. The allele-based and genotype-based model can be fitted in logistic regression just by regarding the marker as ordinal and categorical variable respectively.,

$$\ln\left(\frac{\pi_i}{1-\pi_i}\right) = \begin{cases} \beta_0 + \beta_M Z_{(M)i} + \sum_j \gamma_j X_{ij}, & \text{allele-based model} \\ \beta_0 + \beta_{Mm} Z_{(Mm)i} + \beta_{MM} Z_{(MM)i} + \sum_j \gamma_j X_{ij}, & \\ & \text{genotype-based model} \end{cases} \tag{30-11}$$

where the subscript i means the ith individual, $\pi_i = P(Y_i = 1)$ is the probability of being affected, X_{ij} is the jth covariate, and Z_i is the coding variable of the three genotypes of the marker as shown in the following Table 30.5.

The above allele-based model is in fact an additive model. The dominance (or recessive) model can also be fitted in logistic regression, simply by coding (*mm*, *Mm*, *MM*) as (0, 1, 1) (or 0, 0, 1, respectively).

Logistic regression of disease status can be performed on several genes and all covariates simultaneously. When the markers are tight closed and in strong linkage disequilibrium, haplotype-based model can be applied.

Table 30.5 Coding variables in logistic model

	Allele-based model	Genotype-based model	
Genotype	$Z_{(M)i}$	$Z_{(Mm)i}$	$Z_{(MM)i}$
mm	0	0	0
Mm	1	1	0
MM	2	0	1

30.3.3. *Genome-wide association study (GWAS)*

Genome-wide studies (GWAS) are studies of common genetic variation across the entire human genome designed to identify genetic associations with observed traits. GWAS were made possible by the availability of chip-based microarray technology for assaying one million or more SNPs. Because genome-wide association studies examine SNPs across the genome, they represent a promising way to study complex common diseases in which many genetic variations contribute to a person's risk.

The most common design of GWAS is case-control design. This method obtains DNA from people with a particular disease (cases) and unaffected controls, and identifies SNPs where one allele is significantly more common in cases than controls. Several traditional statistical methods were described above for testing for an association between a SNP and a binary trait, such as χ^2 test, Cochran-Armitage trend test, and logistic regression. Figure 30.5 presents a Manhattan plot from a GWAS study. The plot shows on the y-axis

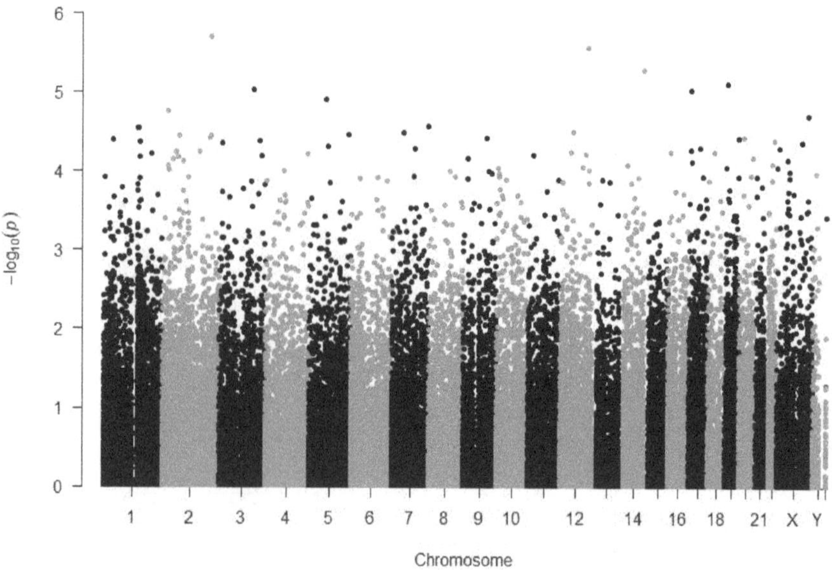

Figure 30.5 Manhattan plot

the negative log-base-10 of the p value for each SNP in the genome (along the x-axis).

In a GWAS analysis, each SNP is tested for association with the phenotype. Therefore, hundreds of thousands to millions of tests are conducted, each one with its own false positive probability. Testing multiple hypotheses can result in an inflation of the error rate, which we want to control. Multistage designs have been proposed as one way of handling this multiple testing issues. The number of genotyped SNPs is reduced at each stage of the design, so that genome-wide significance is achieved step-by-step. In addition, several methods, including false discovery rate (FDR) control and resampling-based methods, have been developed to address this multiple testing problem.

30.3.4. *Population structure analysis*

The association between disease and genotype might be attributable to a confounding variable. When the confounding variable has been measured in the study, it is relatively straightforward to deal with the problem during analysis. The classical method is by stratification or logistic regression. An important issue in case–control studies of disease-marker association is the possibility of confounding by unmeasured population stratification or admixture. The term population stratification is used to refer to the phenomenon in which a population consists of subgroups within which there is random mating but between which there is little mixing. Admixed populations are populations formed by the recent admixture of two or more ancestral populations. When cases and controls are sampled from a population that contains two or more subpopulations, a false positive result can arise if both rates of disease and allele frequencies differ by subpopulation. We focus on genomic control (GC), principal components analysis (PCA), and multidimensional scaling (MDS) to deal with unknown population structure in case–control association studies.

The approach GC is proposed by Devlin and Roeder (1999), who suggested that the effect of admixture and stratification is to inflate the 1 df Cochran-Armitage test statistics by a constant factor λ. In the presence of population stratification, the association test statistics T_i is $\lambda\chi^2$ distributed under the null hypothesis of no association. The degree of inflation λ is dependent on the nature of the structure and sample size, and it can be estimated by $\hat{\lambda} = median(T_i)/0.4549$. Therefore, the adjusted test statistics

$$T_i^a = \frac{T_i}{\hat{\lambda}} \tag{30-12}$$

is χ^2 distributed with 1 degree of freedom under the null hypothesis.

The approach PCA has become a standard tool for detecting population structure. Suppose we have M markers and n individuals. Let G_{is} be the number of variant alleles for marker s, individual i. Thus for autosomal data we have the value of G_{is} is 0, 1 or 2. The normalized version of G_{is} is given by

$$X_{is} = \frac{G_{is} - \bar{G}_s}{\sqrt{2\hat{p}_s(1-\hat{p}_s)}}$$

where $\bar{G}_s = \frac{1}{2n}\sum_{i=1}^n G_{is}, \hat{p}_s = \frac{1}{2n}\sum_{i=1}^n [I(G_{is}=1) + 2I(G_{is}=2)] = \frac{1}{2n}\sum_{i=1}^n G_{is} = \frac{1}{2}\bar{G}_s$. Then we obtain the $n \times n$ covariance matrix $\psi = [\psi_{ij}]$

$$\psi_{ij} = \frac{1}{M}\sum_{s=1}^{M} X_{is}X_{js} = \frac{1}{M}\sum_{s=1}^{M} \frac{(G_{is}-\bar{G}_s)(G_{js}-\bar{G}_s)}{\bar{G}_s(1-\bar{G}_s/2)}$$

We then compute an eigenvector decomposition of ψ. Eigenvectors corresponding to large eigenvalues are exposing nonrandom population structure. To control for population stratification, a popular method is to adjust for the 10 top principal components (PCs) in the logistic regression models used to association tests.

The approach MDS is also called principal coordinate analysis (PCoA). The idea is to provide a low-dimensional representation of the data that captures information on the variability between individuals across markers. Briefly, the aim of MDS is to fit the data into a lower dimensional space (coordinate system) such that the pairwise distances between individuals are similar to the original distances (in the higher dimensional space.) MDS thus begins by defining a measure of similarity between all pairs of individuals. Let G_{is} be the number of variant alleles for marker s, individual i. The similarity between two individuals is then defined as the distance between the respective vectors of G_{is}. The obtained $n \times n$ similarity matrix is denoted by $D = [d_{ij}]$. Let $A = [a_{ij}] = [-d_{ij}^2/2]$. Then bi-directional normalized matrix is given by $B = [b_{ij}] = [a_{ij} - \bar{a}_{i\cdot} - \bar{a}_{\cdot j} + \bar{a}_{\cdot\cdot}]$. We then compute an eigenvector decomposition of B. Then k eigenvectors corresponding to k large eigenvalues are selected to be a k-dimensional space, and we therefore represents n individuals in the lower space as $\tilde{X} = [\tilde{x}_{ij}]_{n \times k}$. They can be regard as covariates in logistic regression for adjusting the propulsion structure.

30.4. Family-based association analysis

The association between a disease and a genetic marker can arise from confounding by underlying stratification and admixture (substructure) within the population. Population stratification can occur in case-control or other population-based designs. It's important to make comparisons between cases and controls, as far as possible, within homogeneous subpopulations. Family-based designs have been proposed to counteract confounding due to population stratification.

30.4.1. *Transmission disequilibrium tests (TDT)*

The best-known of the family-based design is the case-parent triad design. The case-parent triad design and transmission disequilibrium tests (TDT) proposed by Spielman (1993) suggested to collect case-parent trios. Alleles or genotypes transmitted to affected individuals are compared with untransmitted alleles or genotypes, providing a control sample that is inherently matched to the case sample with regard to population structure. TDT also has the advantage that it does not require data either on multiple affected family members or on unaffected sibs.

Suppose that we have a sample of n case-parent trios. In these families there will be a total of $4n$ parental marker alleles, $2n$ of which are transmitted and $2n$ of which are not transmitted. An over-transmitted allele among the affected indicates that a disease-susceptibility locus for a trait of interest is linked and associated with

Table 30.6 Combinations of transmitted and non-transmitted marker alleles from $2n$ Parents to n affected children

	Non-transmitted allele		
Transmitted allele	M	m	Total
M	n_{11}	n_{12}	n_{1+}
m	n_{21}	n_{22}	n_{2+}
Total	n_{+1}	n_{+2}	$2n$

the marker locus. The data on marker alleles in the affected children can be set up as in Table 30.6.

In Table 30.6, n_{11} (or n_{22}) is the number of homozygous parents with genotype MM (or mm respectively). The transmitted allele from homozygous parent is same with the non-transmitted allele n_{12} (or n_{21}) is the number of heterozygous Mm parents who transmit M (or m respectively) and do not transmit m(or M respectively) to the affected offspring. TDT suggests the association exists if significant difference observed between n_{12} and n_{21} TDT proposed by Spielman is also referred to as McNemar's χ^2 test,

$$\chi^2 = \frac{(n_{12} - n_{21})^2}{n_{12} + n_{21}} \tag{30-13}$$

Note that only the data from heterozygous parents should be used in the test since the homozygous parents provide no information about the transmission disequilibrium.

Example 30.4. The data for this study were from Spielman *et al.* (1993) and assembled from 94 families with two or more IDDM (insulin-dependent diabetes mellitus) children. The candidate marker is the region of tandem-repeat DNA (5' flanking polymorphism [5'FP]) adjacent to the insulin gene on chromosome 11p. The heterozygous parents transmitted 124 alleles (78 class 1 alleles and 46 class X alleles) to their diabetic offspring.

So here n_{11}, n_{22} are 78 and 46 respectively when TDT is used, the difference observed is highly significant;

$$\chi^2 = \frac{(n_{12} - n_{21})^2}{n_{12} + n_{21}} = \frac{(78 - 46)^2}{124} = 8.26,$$

with degree of freedom $df = 1$, and $p = 0.004$. This finding suggests that the 5′ FP contributing to IDDM susceptibility.

TDT has been extended to a marker locus with more than two alleles (Spielman *et al.*, 1996; Sham PC, 1995). For the TDT in the general case when the marker have m ($m \geq 2$) alleles, the transmitted/non-transmitted tale is shown as Table 30.7.

n_{ij} in Table 30.7 is the number of parents with genotype ij who transmit i and do not transmit j to the affected offspring. Sham (1995) pointed out the test of symmetry which tests the symmetry of the TDT table can be used to detect the transmission disequilibrium. The statistic

$$T_s = \sum_{i<j} \frac{(n_{ij} - n_{ji})^2}{n_{ij} + n_{ji}} \tag{30-14}$$

is asymptotically χ^2 distributed with $df = m(m-1)/2$, under H_0. In the special case when $m = 2$, T_s is just the TDT statistic proposed by Spielman.

Table 30.7 Combinations of transmitted and non-transmitted m marker alleles from $2n$ Parents to n affected children

	Non-transmitted allele				
Transmitted allele	1	2	...	m	Total
1	n_{11}	n_{12}	...	n_{1m}	n_{1+}
2	n_{21}	n_{22}	...	n_{2m}	n_{2+}
...	...	...	...	...	...
m	n_{m1}	n_{m2}	...	n_{mm}	n_{m+}
Total	n_{+1}	n_{+2}	...	n_{+m}	$2N$

Table 30.8 TDT table for 154 parents from 77 trios

	Non-transmitted allele			
Transmitted allele	1	2	3	Total
1	9	17	22	48
2	18	20	13	51
3	19	23	13	55
Total	46	60	48	154

Example 30.5. In the association study in the German population between NTD(neural tube defect) and gene Mthfr (Methylenetetrahydrofolate reductase) (Stegmann *et al.*, 1999). 77 affected-parent trios were collected. The TDT table was set up as Table 30.8.

$$T_s = \sum_{i<j} \frac{(n_{ij} - n_{ji})^2}{n_{ij} + n_{ji}} = \frac{(18-17)^2}{18+17} + \frac{(22-19)^2}{22+19} + \frac{(23-13)^2}{23+13} = 3.026$$

And $p = 0.388$. Therefore no association for the marker Mthfr is concluded.

30.4.2. *Family-based association test*

There is a particular problem in classical TDT for late-onset traits, since parents of affected may be deceased at the time of diagnosis. In this case of missing parents in late-onset disease, unaffected siblings may be used as controls. Martin *et al.* (2000) proposed the pedigree disequilibrium test (PDT) which combines the TDT and sib-TDT into a test for general pedigrees. It splits a pedigree into a list of all case–parent trios and discordant sib pairs. Then for a specific pedigree, we can calculate

$$D = \frac{1}{N_T + N_S} \left(\sum_{j=1}^{N_T} X_{T_j} + \sum_{j=1}^{N_s} X_{s_j} \right)$$

where N_T and N_S are the total number of trios and discordant sib pairs, X_{T_j} is the number of transmissions of allele M minus the number of its non-transmissions, and X_{s_j} is the number of copies of allele

M in the affected sib minus the number in the unaffected. After computing this measure for each pedigree of $i = 1,\ldots,$ N pedigrees, we have $D_1, D_2, \ldots, D_N$. The PDT statistic

$$T = \frac{\sum_{i=1}^{N} D_i}{\sum_{i=1}^{N} D_i^2} \tag{30-15}$$

is asymptotically χ^2 with 1 degree of freedom under null hypothesis of no association.

To deals with a variety of different pedigree structures, Lake *et al.* (2000) provided a family-based association approach (FBAT).Let T_{ij} be the trait value of person j in pedigree i, and X_{ij} denote some coding of its genotype. The score statistic S is defined as $S = \sum_{i=1}^{N} \sum_j T_{ij} X_{ij}$, and the test statistic

$$T = [S - E(S)]\,[var(S)]^{-1}\,[S - E(S)] \tag{30-16}$$

is asymptotically χ^2 with 1 degree of freedom for a biallelic marker under null hypothesis of no association.

30.5. Results reporting

Generally, report on genetic association analysis includes the following aspects:

(1) Information of the markers in the analysis.
(2) Objective and statistical method.
(3) Summary of the results.

For example, to detect the association between immunoglobulin A (IgA) nephropathy and marker C2180T located in the 3' untranslated region (UTR) in Megsin gene, 151 case-parent trios were collected and entered into analysis (Table 30.9).

According to the data from Table 30.9, the transmitted/non-transmitted allele cross table for TDT analysis are showed in Table 30.10.

$$\chi^2 = \frac{(95 - 68)^2}{95 + 68} = 4.472, P = 0.034$$

Table 30.9 Genotype counts of transmissions in 155 case-parent trios

	Affected offspring genotype		
Mating type	CC	CT	TT
CC × CC	19		
CC × CT	4	4	
CC × TT		7	
CT × CC	36	30	
CT × CT	15	15	6
CT × TT		10	7
TT × TT			2

Table 30.10 Transmitted/non-transmitted allele counts from 310 trios

	Non-transmitted allele		
Transmitted allele	C	T	Total
C	119	95	214
T	68	28	96
Total	187	123	310

The results show that there is association between the marker C2180T and IgA nephropathy.

30.6. Case analysis

In a case-control study to detect the association between marker L and diabetes, 299 patients and 341 healthy persons were selected, including 179 males and 461 females. The genotyping information are shown in Table 30.11.

The difference between the gender distributions of case group and control group is not significant since

$$\chi^2 = \sum \frac{(O-E)^2}{E} = 0.667, \quad \text{df} = 1, \quad P = 0.414$$

Table 30.11 Genotype and gender frequencies

	Male			Female		
	MM, Mm	mm	Total	MM, Mm	mm	Total
Case	43	36	79	165	55	220
Control	53	47	100	130	111	241
Total	96	83	179	295	166	461

Table 30.12 Genotype frequencies

	Genotype		
	MM, Mm	mm	Total
Case	208	91	299
Control	183	158	341
Total	96	83	179

Therefore, we conduct genetic association analysis on a single combined table (Table 30.12).

The Pearson χ^2 test statistic

$$\chi^2 = \sum \frac{(O-E)^2}{E} = 16.943, \quad \text{df} = 1, \quad P < 0.001$$

Then the association between marker L and diabetes is concluded. Please identify the key flaws in the analysis.

30.7. Computer experiments (see electronic resources from exp30.1 and exp30.2

Experiment 30.1 Test of H-W equilibrium. The data used in the test for Hard Weinberg equilibrium analysis is from Example 30.1. Learn how to use EXCEL to conduct HW equilibrium test, based on the formula (30-1)~(30-3)

Experiment 30.2 TDT analysis. The data used in the analysis is from Example 30.4. Learn how to use SPSS to do TDT analysis.

30.8. FAQs and Summary

30.8.1. *FAQs*

(1) What is the difference between linkage and linkage disequilibrium?

Linkage and linkage disequilibrium are different. Linkage generally refers to the physical state of being linked due to the chromosomal organization of the genome. Linkage is the physical proximity of the loci. Linkage disequilibrium (LD) refers to the presence of a statistical association between allelic variants. It is the non-random association of alleles at different loci which may or may not be due to linkage.

(2) How to select "best" model from candidate models?

There are allele-based, additive, dominant, recessive and general genotype-based models in the association analysis. Akaike information criterion (AIC) or Bayesian information criterion(BIC) can be used in model selection from a set of candidate models, given data. The AIC or BIC for a model is usually written in the form [-2logL + kp], where L is the likelihood function, p is the number of parameters in the model, and k is 2 for AIC and log(n) for BIC. The model with the lowest AIC or BIC is preferred.

(3) What are the main advantages of population-based and family-based methods for association analysis?

Population-based and family-based methods are very useful tools in genetic association studies. Population-based association studies are typically performed using unrelated cases and controls. Population stratification can cause spurious associations, although the analytic methods are simple and classical for population-based case and control designs. Family-based designs require specialized analytic methods, but they have distinct advantages. Family designs allow for control of population stratification. Another advantage is that only family-based data will potentially exhibit genotyping errors in the form of Mendelian inconsistencies.

30.8.2. *Summary*

In this chapter, we give some basic genetic terminologies in the first session, such as gene, locus, chromosome, polymorphism, allele, genotype, phenotype, Marker, Haplotype, Hardy-Weinberg Equilibrium, hereditary mode, dominant, recessive, additive, multiplicative, penetrance, linkage, etc. In the second session, we introduce linkage disequilibrium (LD), the construction of haplotype block and SNP tagging. In the next two sessions, we present genetic association methods for population-based case and control designs and family-based designs, including χ^2 test and logistic regression, GWAS, population structure analysis, TDT, PDT, FBAT, etc.

Think and Practice

Questions for Reflection

1. What are the Hardy-Weinberg equilibrium and linkage equilibrium?
2. Can we conduct Pearson χ^2 test to detect LD of the two SNPs based on the data shown in Table 30.1 in Example 30.2?
3. When the hereditary mode of a specific disease is known, how can we use the information to improve the power in the χ^2 test and logistic regression methods in population-based case and control designs.

Calculation questions

1. For a random mating population with proportions (0.25, 0.10, 0.65), (0.30, 0, 0.70) or (0, 0.60, 0.40) for a marker's genotype AA, Aa, please estimate the genotype proportions in next generation respectively.
2. Test whether genotype proportions in following four populations are in Hardy-Weinberg equilibrium or not and calculate the equilibrium proportion for those non-H-W populations: (0.5, 0, 0.5); (0.36, 0.15, 0.49); (0.09, 0.10, 0.81); (0.45, 0.45, 0.10).
3. Please show the LD coefficient r for two biallelic markers is just Pearson correlation.

4. For the biallelic marker, please show the statistic in (30-7) to test LD is actually Pearson χ^2 statistic.

References

[1] Balding, DJ, Bishop, M, Cannings, C. *Handbook of Statistical Genetics.* 3rd ed. John Wiley & Sons, Ltd; 2008.

[2] Bickeböller, H, Clerget-Darpoux, F. Statistical properties of the allelic and genotypic transmission/disequilibrium test for multiallelic markers. *Genet Epidemiol.* 1995; 12(6): 865–870. https://doi.org/10.1002/gepi.1370120656

[3] Clayton, DG. A generalization of the transmission/disequilibrium test for uncertain-haplotype transmission. *Am J Hum Genet.* 1999; 65: 1170–1177. https://doi.org/10.1086/302577

[4] Fang, JQ. *Medical Statistics and Computer Experiments (in Chinese).* 4th ed. Beijing: Shanghai Science and Technology Press; 2012.

[5] Foulkes, AS. *Applied Statistical Genetics with R.* New York, NY: Springer; 2009.

[6] Gabriel, SB, Schaffner SF, Nguyen H, *et al.* The structure of haplotype blocks in the human genome. *Science.* 2002; 296: 2225–2229. https://doi.org/10.1126/science.1069424

[7] Huang, W, Li, C, Labu, *et al.* High resolution linkage disequilibrium and haplotype maps for the genes in the centromeric region of chromosome 15 in Tibetans and comparisons with Han population. *Chinese Sci Bull.* 2006; 51(5): 542–551. https://doi.org/10.1007/s11434-006-0542-5

[8] Li, YJ, Du, Y, Li, CX, *et al.* Family-based association study showing that immunoglobulin a nephropathy is associated with the polymorphisms 2093C and 2180T in the 3′ untranslated Region of Megsin Gene. *J Am SocNephrol.* 2004; 15: 1739–1743. https://doi.org/10.1097/01.ASN.0000130858.00688.46

[9] Martin, ER, Monks, SA, Warren, LL, Kaplan, NL. A test for linkage and association in general pedigrees: the pedigree disequilibrium test. *Am J Hum Genet.* 2000; 67: 146–154. https://doi.org/10.1086/302957

[10] Niu, T, Qin, ZS, Xu, X, Liu, JS. Bayesian haplotype inference for multiple linked single-nucleotide polymorphisms. *Am J Hum Genet.* 2002; 70: 157–169. https://doi.org/10.1086/338446

[11] Qin, ZS, Niu, T, Liu, JS. Partition-ligation-expectation-maximization algorithm for haplotype inference with single-nucleotide polymorphisms. *Am J Hum Genet.* 2002; 71: 1242–1247. https://doi.org/10.1086/344207

[12] Spielman, RS, McGinnis, RE, Ewens, WJ. Transmission test for linkage disequilibrium: the insulin gene region and insulin-dependent diabetes mellitus. *Am J Hum Genet.* 1993; 52(3): 506–516.

[13] Spielman, RS, Ewens, WJ. The TDT and other family-based tests for linkage disequilibrium and association [J]. *Am J Hum Genet.* 1996; 59: 983–989.

[14] Stegmann, K, Ziegler, A, Ngo, E. *et al.* Linkage disequilibrium of Mther genotypes 677C/T-1298A/C in the German population and association study in probands with neural tube defects (NTD). *Am J Med Genet.*

1999; 87(1): 23–29. https://doi.org/10.1002/(SICI)1096-8628(19991105)87:1⟨23::AID-AJMG5⟩3.0.CO;2-E

[15] Stephens, M, Smith, NJ, Donnelly, P. A new statistical method for haplotype reconstruction from population data. *Am J Hum Genet.* 2001; 68: 978–989. https://doi.org/10.1086/319501

[16] Wang, M, Ji, Z, Wang, S, *et al.* Mechanisms to protect the privacy of families when using the transmission disequilibrium test in genome-wide association studies. *Bioinformatics.* 2017; 33(23): 3716–3725. https://doi.org/10.1093/bioinformatics/btx470

Caixia Li

CHAPTER 31

STATISTICS FOR BIOINFORMATICS

Large amounts of biomedical data have been generated and collected due to the rapid development of molecular biology technology in recent decades, such as gene chip technology, next-generation sequencing, mass spectrometry, and chromatography, protein–protein interaction detection technology, new drug testing technology, etc. Modern life science and medical research have entered a high-throughput, large-scale era of omics study. In pace with the initiation of the Human Genome Project, Bioinformatics becomes a newly emerging interdisciplinary subject involving biology, statistics, and computer science, which focuses on storing, retrieving, and analyzing biological information by means of computers. Bioinformatics is one of the major frontier fields of life sciences and natural sciences today, and it is also one of the core fields and most dynamic fields of natural sciences in the 21st century. The GWAS study described in the previous chapter is a typical example of the application of statistical analysis techniques to bioinformatics research. We will start this chapter with an introduction to gene expression data generated by gene chip technology and high-throughput sequencing (HTS) technology, and further introduce how to think and solve bioinformatics problems from a statistical perspective.

31.1. Overview

The genome is regarded as the original blueprint of cells. For a gene to work, the corresponding mRNA is first transcribed according to the protein to be expressed. This procedure is called gene expression. When more proteins of a certain type are needed, more corresponding mRNAs are transcribed. Therefore, the abundance of mRNA in cells indicates the expression level of corresponding genes. Sometimes, we simply call it gene expression.

Cells contain the same genome information in a specific organism, but genes express differently among different tissues and at their different developmental stages. In a particular tissue, only about a third of the total number of genes are expressed simultaneously. Only genes that perform some basic functions in cells are expressed in all tissues. These genes are called housekeeping genes. On the other hand, many genes show different tissue-specific expression patterns. This means that they can be highly expressed in one type of cell and low or non-expressed in other cells. In multicellular organisms, different types of cells express different genes at different times, and the level of expression varies. Cell function is achieved through the regulation of gene expression.

Therefore, it is undoubtedly of great significance to study the expression level of all genes. The study of all transcripts is called transcriptome. Currently, gene chip technology (microarray) and transcriptome sequencing technology (RNA-Seq) are the two core technologies in transcriptome research. These techniques can measure mRNA abundance of thousands of genes simultaneously. Because mRNA degrades quickly, it is usually reverse transcribed into complementary DNA (cDNA) in the expression measurement.

31.1.1. *Gene chip technology*

Gene chip is a technology developed in the mid-1990s. The basic principle of gene chips is the complementary base-pairing hybridization of DNAs. A large number of DNA fragments (called probes) are arrayed onto a substrate, typically a glass slide or a silicon chip. Based on the principle of in situ hybridization (ISH), fluorescent labeled target cDNAs are applied on the chip to hybridize with the probes whose sequences are complementary to the cDNA sequences. The DNA fragments that do not hybridize to any probe are washed off.

The laser scanning confocal system is used to "read" the fluorescence intensities at each probe location, which record the expression levels of the genes represented by the probes. This technology can be used to profile the expression of genes in various physiological or pathological processes, such as metabolism, stress, canceration, and development. Due to the influence of background optical noise and non-specific hybridization on gene expression, data from these confounding sources need to be obtained simultaneously in the experimental process. Different manufacturers generally use their own technology platforms. The two most commonly used platforms are the dual-color fluorescent cDNA chip first developed by Brown and Botstein Laboratories in Stanford University and the high-density oligonucleotide microarray developed by Afymetrix Company.

The experimental flow chart of cDNA chip has been shown in Figure 31.1. A cDNA chip experiment consists of a pair of mRNA samples, one of which is the test sample and the other is the control sample. The two samples were first reverse transcribed into cDNA and labeled with different fluorescent dyes, usually red fluorescent

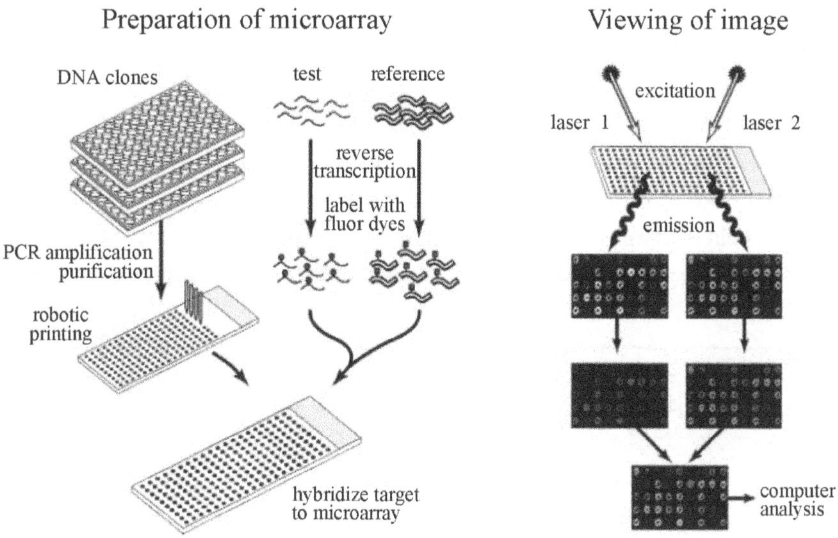

Figure 31.1 Flow chart of cDNA chip experiment (http://compbio.pbworks.com/)

dye Cyanine 5 (Cy5) and green fluorescent dye Cyanine 3 (Cy3), and then hybridized to the probes in equal proportion. After competitive hybridization, the fluorescent signals at each location on the chip can separately be detected by the confocal scanners. Local background noise outside the probe position on the substrate can also be detected. The ratio of red fluorescence intensity to green fluorescence intensity corrected by background signal at each location can be used as the relative abundance measurement of the corresponding nucleotide sequences.

The hybridization process of Affymetrix oligonucleotide chip is similar to that of the cDNA chip. The difference is that Affymetrix gene chips have higher density and shorter oligonucleotide probes. Each experiment of oligonucleotide chip contains only one sample. Because of the short probe sequence (usually consisting of 25 bases), multiple probes on the chip to represent a gene highly improves the specificity. The oligonucleotide chips generally use 11–20 pairs of probes to represent a gene (Figure 31.2), which are jointly called a probeset. Each pair of these probes contains a perfect match (PM) probe and a mismatch (MM) probe. The only difference in sequence between the two probes is based on the middle, whereas the rest are identical. PM probes are used to detect specific hybridization signals of targeted genes, while MM probes are used to detect non-specific hybridization signals.

Multiple limitations have been found in gene expression profile using gene chip technology. For instance, it can only detect the gene levels which correspond to the pre-customized probe sequences on the chip. The cross hybridization method may introduce heavy

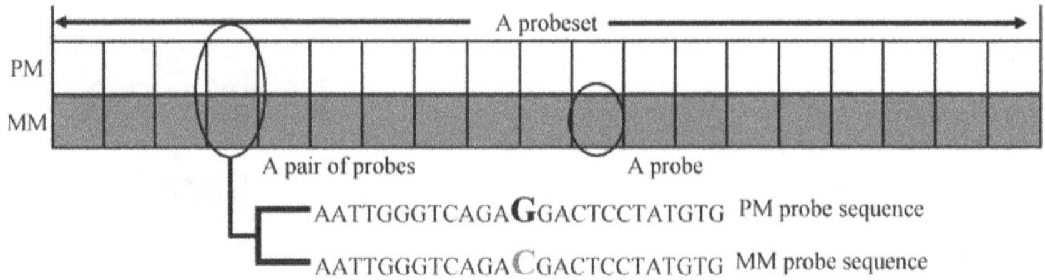

Figure 31.2 Illustration of Affymetrix gene chip probeset

background noise. It has limited detection range due to the background and signal saturation. In addition, it is hard to compare gene expression values when using different experimental approaches. Alternatively, direct sequencing and quantitative analysis of cDNA has been introduced.

31.1.2. *High-throughput sequencing*

In the early 1990s, Sanger sequencing was used for the sequencing of cDNA or expression sequence tag (EST) libraries. However, it has low throughput and is generally unable to quantify. Therefore, based on Sanger sequencing, scientists have developed serial analysis of gene expression (SAGE), cap analysis of gene expression (CAGE), massively parallel signature sequencing (MPSS), and so on. A large number of short sequences have been generated by these methods but many of them cannot be positioned on the reference genome because of lack of uniquely mapping information. There remain other issues, for example, the full transcriptome analysis cannot be performed or has a high cost, and the discrimination of the transcriptional isoforms is also problematic.

Since 2005, next generation sequencing (NGS) technologies, such as the Roche 454, Illumina Solexa, and ABI SoLiD, have been brought into existence. The number of sequencing reads produced by each technology platform ranges from millions to even billions, and the read lengths can be 30$\sim$400 base pairs, for which we called it HTS. NGS provides a new approach for transcriptome profiling with potential advantages including lower sequencing costs, higher read accuracy, and a larger volume of data. The application of NGS in transcriptome analysis is called RNA sequencing (RNA-Seq). The flow chart of RNA-Seq experiment has been shown in Figure 31.3 and a typical RNA-Seq experiment includes: long RNAs are first converted into libraries of cDNA fragments through RNA fragmentation; sequencing adapters are subsequently added to each cDNA fragment and a short sequence is obtained from each cDNA using HTS; the resulting sequence reads are aligned with the reference genome or transcriptome, and classified as exon, junction or other types.

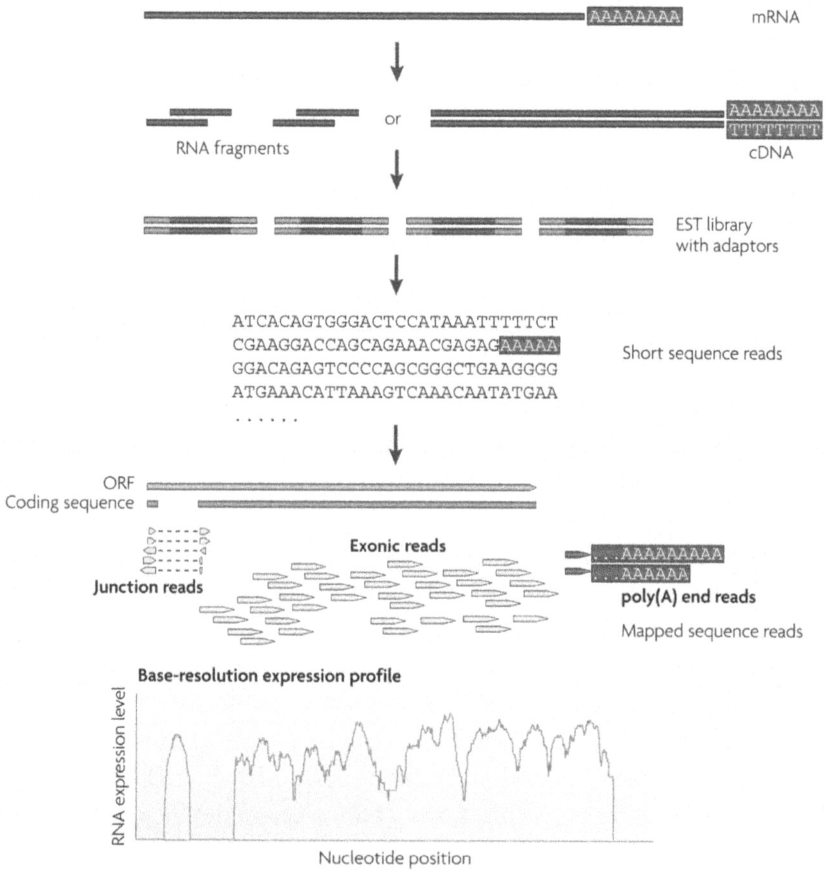

Figure 31.3 RNA-Seq experiment (Wang *et al.* (2009))

DNA sequencing technologies have continuously achieved an extraordinary advancement in the past 10 years. Third generation sequencing, such as single-molecule real-time (SMRT) sequencing developed by Pacific Bioscience and nanopore sequencing developed by Oxford Nanopore, has emerged since 2012. Compared with the previous technologies, their greatest feature is single-molecule sequencing, without the need for PCR amplification before sequencing. However, either using second or third generation sequencing can only analyze the average gene expression level of all the sampled cells. In recent years, single-cell RNA sequencing (scRNA-seq) has been proposed for transcriptome analysis of single cells. Namely, gene expression profiling analysis is always at the forefront of technological change.

31.2. Data preprocessing

31.2.1. *Preprocessing of gene chip data*

The data of gene chip expression profiles are derived from image signals, which can be further analyzed only after background adjustment, normalization, and expression value estimation. The purpose of background adjustment is to remove the effect of optical noise and nonspecific hybridization in the experiment. Normalization corrects for overall chip brightness and other factors that may affect expression intensity and reduces unwanted variation across chips, thereby makes measurements from different chips comparable. A gene on an Affymetrix oligonucleotide gene chip is represented by a set of probes, so it is necessary to combine the multiple probe intensities for each probeset to produce an expression value. Numerous statistical methods are available for every preprocessing phase. In this section, we introduce the robust multichip average (RMA) method recommended by Irizarryet *et al.* (2003) for Affymetrix gene chip data, which integrates convolution background adjustment, quantile normalization, and a model-based expression estimates.

Irizarry *et al.* (2003) proposed that only PM probe intensities were included into the expression estimation because the MM probe may also detect the specific hybridization signal. For the nth probeset, the signal intensity PM_{ijn} of the jth probe on the ith chip can be denoted as a background plus signal model with the form:

$$PM_{ijn} = bg_{ijn} + s_{ijn}, i = 1, \ldots, I;\ j = 1, \ldots, J;\ n = 1, \ldots, N$$

Here bg_{ijn} represents background signal caused by optical noise and non-specific hybridization and has a normal distribution $N(\mu_i, \sigma_i^2)$. The s_{ijn} represents real biological signal which has an exponential distribution $Exp(\lambda_i)$. Quantile normalization is applied to the signal intensity after background adjustment, namely s_{ijn}, to make the measurements comparable between chips. Briefly, it is assumed that the signal intensity of each chip has the same empirical distribution, then the quantile–quantile (QQ) plot of the normalized signal intensity distribution follows the I-dimensional identity line. Subsequently, the expression values at the gene level are estimated using the normalized intensities. To obtain an expression measure we assume that for each probeset, the background adjusted, normalized, and log transformed PM intensities, denoted with Y, follow a linear additive model

$$Y_{ijn} = \alpha_{in} + \beta_{jn} + \varepsilon_{ijn}$$

Here α_{in} represents the logarithmic expression level of the ith chip, β_{jn} represents a probe affinity effect, and ε_{ijn} represents an independent identically distributed error term with mean 0. For identifiability it is assumed that $\sum_j \beta_{jn}^2 = 1$ for all probesets. The model fitting gives the estimation $\hat{\alpha}_{in}$ of each gene expression level on the chip.

Example 31.1. Irizarry *et al.* (2003) used a set of dilution experiments to illustrate the feasibility and effectiveness of the RMA method. Two source of cRNA A (human liver tissue) and B (Central Nervous System cell line) were hybridized to human chip (HG-U95A) in a range of proportions and dilutions. Four samples containing 20 or 10μg cRNA of source A or source B can be obtained through the affydata package of R software. These samples were labeled with 20A, 20B, 10A, and 10B, respectively. Experiment 31.1 shows the R code for RMA. And Figure 31.4 provides the distribution of the signal intensity of the PM probes in a logarithm scale, which includes those values before and after background adjustment and quantile normalization. The upper part of the figure gives the MA plots, where

$$M = log_2(PM_{20A}) - log_2(PM_{10A})$$

$$A = \frac{log_2(PM_{20A}) + log_2(PM_{10A})}{2}$$

And the box plots of log_2(PM) of the four samples are shown in the lower part.

Before preprocessing, the LOESS curve significantly deviates from zero and several outliers are observed, which is shown at the

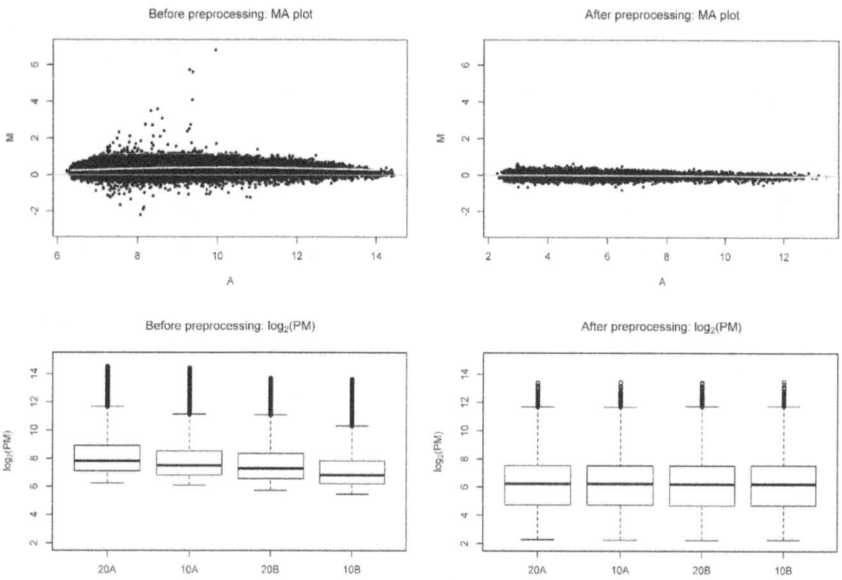

Figure 31.4 Changes of signal intensity before and after preprocessing using RMA method

top left of Figure 31.4. This indicates that there might be a "difference" in signal intensity between 20A and 10A samples. But after preprocessing, the LOESS curve almost overlaps with the horizontal line and the outliers disappear at the top right figure, which indicates that the background signal and dilution effect have been corrected. The box plots in the lower part of Figure 31.4 also provide similar evidence that RMA is a useful tool for preprocessing of Affymetrix gene chip data.

31.2.2. *Preprocessing of RNA-Seq data*

A high-throughput RNA-Seq approach offers a snapshot of the entire transcriptome profile without prior knowledge of a reference sequence. And the sequence information from this technology is also extracted from the imaging signals. According to the study design and sequencing platforms (e.g., Illumina HighSeq 2500), a large number of short RNA fragments will be generated, each of which is called a "read". Besides the sequence information from the sample, the sequencing data may also contain the primer or adaptor information. Moreover, the $3'$ or $5'$ end of the sequences may contain data with low sequencing quality, and some environmental or reagent contaminant sequences may also be included in the data. Therefore, quality evaluation and quality control is an essential process for analysis. FASTQC and MultiQC are commonly used tools for quality evaluation, and a lot of quality control software has been developed, including TrimGalore, Trimmomatic, NGSQC Toolkit, and PRINSEQ. Subsequently, we need to know where the "reads" come from and what roles they are playing. The utilities such as BWA, SOAP2, and Bowtie2 are applied to align them to some known reference genomes, such as human reference genomes, for the purpose to know their exact location and which genes they come from. This process is called sequence alignment or sequence mapping. According to the amount of "reads" aligned to each gene, the quantitative measurement of the gene expression can be obtained.

The best known pipeline to quantify the gene expression level is to use a feature counting tool, like HTSeq-count or featureCounts, to estimate the read count of each gene. However, this quantitative approach is biased by a couple of factors such as gene length, GC content, and sequencing depth. Therefore, the measurements obtained are not comparable between samples. For this reason, the read counts are normalized and reads per kilobase per million reads (RPKM) and other statistics like fragments per kilobase per million reads (FPKM) are commonly used for the measurement of gene expression. RPKM stands for the number of reads from a gene per thousand base lengths in every million reads, that is,

$$\text{RPKM} = \frac{Total\ gene\ reads}{Mapped\ reads\ (millions) * Gene\ length\ (kilobase)}$$

31.3. Bioinformatics data analysis

Digital image signals are preprocessed and summarized as measurements of gene expression that can be further analyzed. These data can be written in a two-way table, namely a matrix in Figure 31.5, where row i represents the i gene, column j corresponds to the j

Condition / Gene	C_1	C_2	$\cdots$	C_j	$\cdots$	C_n
G_1	x_{11}	x_{12}	$\cdots$	x_{1j}	$\cdots$	x_{1n}
G_2	x_{21}	x_{22}	$\cdots$	x_{2j}	$\cdots$	x_{2n}
$\vdots$			$\vdots$			
G_i	x_{i1}	x_{i2}	$\cdots$	x_{ij}	$\cdots$	x_{in}
$\vdots$			$\vdots$			
G_m	x_{m1}	x_{m2}	$\cdots$	x_{mj}	$\cdots$	x_{mn}

Figure 31.5 Matrix storage form of gene expression profiles

experimental condition (or sample), and each element x_{ij} denotes the measurement of gene i in experimental condition (or sample) j.

31.3.1. *Identification of differentially expressed genes*

In the data analysis of gene expression profile, researchers from biological or clinical fields usually focus on the differences in gene expression between different experimental groups. As a hypothetical test, the screening of differentially expressed genes is usually based on the statistical test of the P value. If the test statistic is continuous, the P value obeys the uniform distribution of [0,1] under the null hypothesis. Therefore, if the P value is relatively small (e.g., $P < 0.05$), then we have reason to reject the null hypothesis. According to the different research designs and the characteristics of data distribution, we can use parametric or non-parameter methods of group comparison or paired comparison for analysis. Here we introduce the permutation test and significance analysis of microarrays (SAM) methods for gene chip data development.

The principle of the permutation test is to construct test statistics according to research problems and use current samples to generate the theoretical sampling distribution of test statistics according to the principle of permutation and combination. If it is difficult to obtain the exact theoretical distribution, the approximate distribution can be obtained by using simulation sampling technology. The probability of obtaining current samples and more extreme samples from the distribution (that is, P value) can be calculated for statistical inference. Following is an example of the permutation test for comparing the mean values between two groups. The implementation steps are described as follows:

(1) Determine the hypothesis testing problem. H_0: $\mu_1 = \mu_2$ *vs.* H_1: $\mu_1 \neq \mu_2$; $\alpha = 0.05$.
(2) Construct test statistic D. The advantage of permutation test is that test statistic can be determined according to the test problem, without considering its theoretical sampling distribution. Assume that $D = X_1 - X_2$, and calculate the statistic D_{obs} of the current samples.
(3) Generating empirical sampling distribution Under the assumption of H_0, the empirical distribution of D is obtained by simulation. Assume that H_0 holds, meaning that the two groups come from the same population, when the sample size remains unchanged, any random grouping of the samples will result in two new groups of random samples of the same population, which is called a permutation sample. Based on this theory, the test statistic D of the sample can be obtained. Repeat *for* k (e.g., $k = 20{,}000$) times to obtain a number of permutation samples and the value of the test statistic D, thus generating the empirical sampling distribution of D.
(4) Calculate P value and make inference.

$$P = P(|D| \geq |D_{\text{obs}}|) = \frac{\text{Number of}\,|D| \geq |D_{\text{obs}}|}{k}$$

If P is less than a given value α, the null hypothesis would be rejected; otherwise, no conclusion can be reached.

Example 31.2. To study the difference of gene expression profiles among different subtypes of leukemia, Chiaretti *et al.* (2004) conducted an Affymetrix microarray experiment involving 128 patients with acute lymphoblastic leukemia (ALL). The estimated logarithmic expression level of the gene "34893_at" in 37 patients with BCR/ABL subtype and 42 patients with NEG subtype is shown in Table 31.1. We used the permutation test to compare the difference of the expression levels of the genes between the two subtypes.

Table 31.1 Estimation of expression level for gene "34893_at" in two subtypes of ALL study

ALL subtype	$\log_2$ (expression level)									
BCR/ABL	8.68	7.67	8.14	8.46	7.66	7.14	7.29	8.11	8.08	7.43
	7.51	7.66	7.84	7.80	8.30	8.35	8.03	7.93	7.31	7.70
	7.20	7.52	7.27	6.52	7.76	7.15	7.10	7.43	7.87	7.64
	8.01	7.40	7.97	7.77	9.06	7.43	8.00			
NEG	6.80	7.96	7.73	7.76	7.54	8.05	8.17	7.75	7.38	7.98
	7.52	6.77	7.56	7.79	7.05	7.19	7.69	6.79	7.77	6.39
	7.76	5.82	7.63	7.27	8.09	6.38	7.64	7.35	7.05	7.74
	7.43	7.64	7.27	7.53	7.08	8.56	6.97	7.05	8.19	7.84
	7.32	6.86								

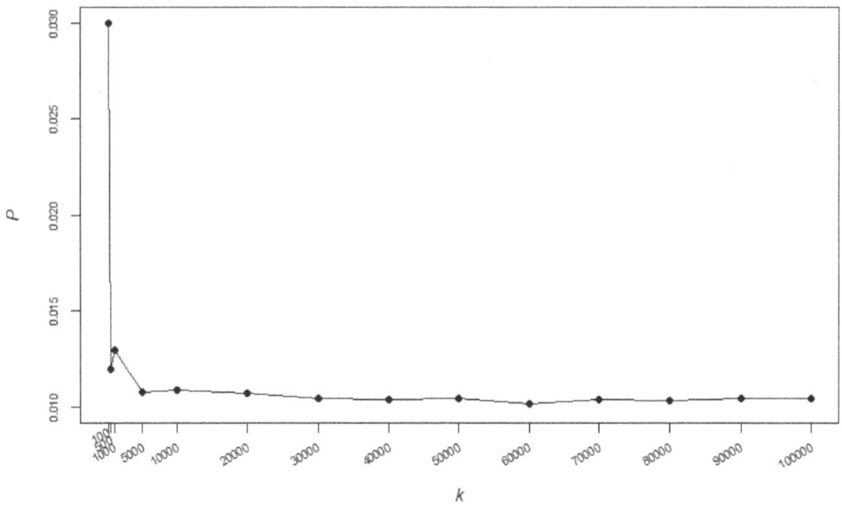

Figure 31.6 Comparison of sample means under different repetition times of permutation test

From Table 31.1, $\bar{x}_1 = 7.74$, $s_1 = 0.49$; $\bar{x}_2 = 7.43$, $s_2 = 0.54$.

Construct the difference between the mean of two samples as the investigative statistic D, then $D_{\text{obs}} = \bar{x}_1 - \bar{x}_2 = 7.74 - 7.43 = 0.31$.

Using R to calculate P value under different repeated sampling times, that is, $P(|D| \geq 0.31)$, and the variation of P value with repeated sampling times is shown in Figure 31.6.

From the simulation results, the fluctuation range of P value is larger when k is less; when k increases, the fluctuation range of P value gradually decreases, and when the number of simulations k reaches 20,000 or more, the P value tends to be stable, and finally stabilizes near 0.0104.

A statistical problem called "multiple testing" would occur when thousands of genes are tested simultaneously. To solve this problem, a direct solution is to control the cumulative type I error rate. Bonferroni correction is often used to correct type I errors. For example, when we compare data for m times at the α level simultaneously, the threshold of rejecting null hypothesis is adjusted to α/m in a single statistical test. However, this method is often conservative in screening differentially expressed genes. Benjamini and Hochberg provided a compromised solution, that is, to control the false discovery rate (FDR), which is achieved by controlling the expected value of the proportion of "false rejected null hypothesis" to "all rejected null hypothesis".

Example 31.3. Thirty-seven patients with BCR/ABL subtype and 42 patients with NEG subtype were selected as subjects in the ALL study. In order to find which of the 2391 genes were expressed differently between the two groups, the gene expression levels between the two groups were compared by permutation test. In order to control the accumulated type I errors, Bonferroni correction was performed for $\alpha = 0.05$, and the corrected threshold of type I error was $0.05/2391 = 0.00002$, as a result, 14 genes were screened out. Alternatively, if we try to control FDR and set the threshold to 0.05, 108 genes will be screened out (see Experiment 31.2). This example shows that Bonferroni correction method is more conservative than the FDR method.

Because of the cost of experiment and the difficulty of sample acquisition, many gene chip experiments only contain a small number of repetitive samples under each experimental condition. Therefore, it is difficult to obtain stable and reliable variance estimates for each gene expression level. Researchers consider using information on the expression level of all genes to estimate these variance, thus developing a number of test methods based on t-like statistics, of which the

SAM method is one of them. This method first calculates the relative differences of expression levels between groups of each gene i:

$$d_i = \frac{\bar{x}_{i1} - \bar{x}_{i2}}{s_i + s_0}$$

In theory, the distribution of d_i is independent of the level of gene expression in the case of low expression abundance, we can correct the problem of s_i being too small by adding a small normal quantity s_0 to the denominator, s_0 is determined by the "moving window" to minimize the coefficient of variation of the d_i value. In order to determine which genes have significant difference in expression level between groups, the theoretical sampling distribution of d_i is generated according to the principle of permutation test, and the FDR values of different gene expression levels between groups are estimated. Finally, the differentially expressed genes are obtained by adjusting the FDR value.

31.3.2. *Clustering and classification*

Finding differentially expressed genes from gene expression profiles is only the first step in the analysis of gene expression profiles. Through the analysis of gene expression patterns, the discovery of known and unknown gene functional modules and further study of gene co-regulation network are the higher research objectives. According to the understanding of gene expression rules and experimental grouping, the analysis methods can be divided into supervised learning and unsupervised learning. The former establishes classifiers for expression profiles based on known biological information of specific samples or genes, and then classifies and predicts the functions of genes. The latter clusters similar samples or genes by calculating and comparing the statistical distances of genes in expression profiles. In different chapters of this book, the commonly used classification methods are described in detail, such as linear discriminant and decision tree in Chapter 22, artificial neural network and support vector machine in Chapter 32, and clustering analysis in Chapter 23. This section gives an introduction to the two-way clustering methods commonly used in gene expression profile analysis.

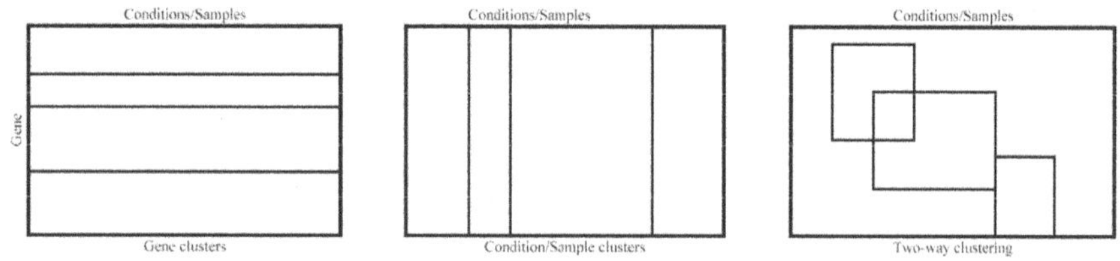

Figure 31.7 Basic ideas of two-way clustering

Gene expression data have a two-way correlation (gene direction or conditional direction). Traditional clustering methods can only cluster genes or conditions/samples in a single direction to find overall information on the gene expression matrix, while a large number of biological information may be hidden. In order to search for the hidden information in the data matrix, the concept of two-way clustering is proposed (Figure 31.7). Two-way clustering or bi-clustering is a method to find gene subsets and condition (or sample) subsets with strong similarity at the same time.

The simplest two-way clustering method is to cluster genes or conditions/samples separately and then aggregate them for display. A more complex method is to introduce a specific criterion and use an iterative algorithm to optimize the criterion. Lazzeroni and Owen (2002) proposed a two-way additive model called the plaid model. Assuming that there are K number of bi-directional classes, the plaid model can be expressed as:

$$x_{ij} = \mu_0 + \sum_{k=1}^{K} \rho_{ik}\theta_{jk}(\mu_k + a_{ik} + b_{jk}),$$

Among them, $\rho_{ik} \in \{0, 1\}$ stands for the bi-directional class of genes, $\theta_{jk} \in \{0, 1\}$ stands for the bi-directional class of conditions (or samples), μ_0 stands for the baseline value of gene expression, a_{ik} stands for the gene effect value, and b_{jk} stands for the conditional effect value. The plaid model obtains the estimation of each parameter by minimizing the error. Furthermore, Turner *et al.* (2003) adopted an iterative algorithm to automatically select the optimal number (K) of bi-directional classes, thus reducing the dependence on the prior knowledge of K.

Example 31.4. We studied 10 ALL1/AF4 patients and 5 E2A/PBX1 patients in ALL study. From all 12,625 probesets, we selected at least one group of 81 genes with an average expression value of more than 100 and a P value of less than 0.0002 in a two-sampled t-test for cluster analysis. Figure 31.8 shows the heat maps obtained by gene direction system clustering, sample direction system clustering and the two-way clustering using plaid model method. It can be seen that the two-way clustering method displays a more obvious pattern of the gene expression.

31.3.3. *Dimensionality reduction*

Gene expression profile data usually contain thousands of genes, and the expression level of each gene includes multiple duplicate samples, which can be very demanding for the traditional data visualization technology. If we can map data in a two-dimensional or at most a three-dimensional space, it will be easier to grasp the relationship between data and have a better intuitive understanding of the data. Therefore, we need to use dimension reduction methods, such as multidimensional scaling (MDS), principle component analysis (PCA), and singular value decomposition (SVD). MDS is a very important method used in expression profile analysis. Here we further elaborate its importance.

Assume that we were given the distance between sample points (such as correlation coefficient) in a high-dimensional space, using the MDS method, we can find the representatives of a group of data points in a low-dimensional space (such as two-dimensional space). These data will reflect the distance between two data points to an extend. Using a matrix composed of distances or dissimilarities between n objects as input data, MDS can show n points in a k-dimensional Euclidean space, and the distance between any two given points is as "close" as possible to the distance of thc input matrix. Many altered MDS algorithms have been generated to define the "proximity" between Euclidean distance and input distance between points. According to the different measurement scales of input data (i.e., distance or dissimilarity), MDS algorithm can be divided into metric MDS and non-metric MDS.

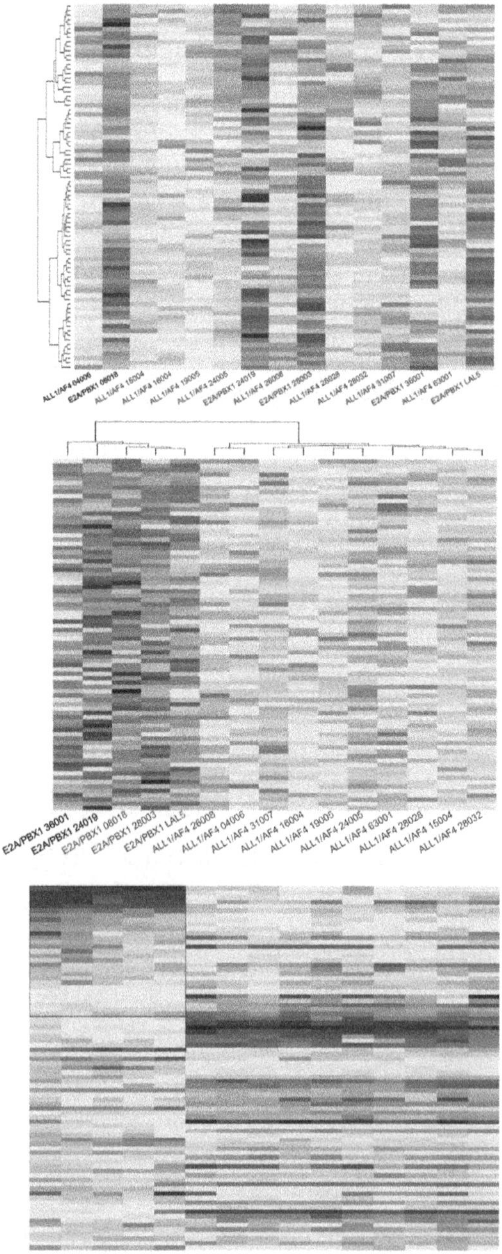

Figure 31.8 Cluster results of gene expression in ALL1/AF4 and E2A/PBX1 subgroups in the ALL study

The classical metric MDS algorithm uses the least square method to define proximity, which can be solved by eigenvalue decomposition of centralized inner product matrix of distance. The classical metric MDS algorithm has a good property that it has nested dimensions. In other words, the first two dimensions of its three-dimensional solution ($k = 3$) are also its two-dimensional solution ($k = 2$). Two statistics can be used to evaluate the goodness of fit of classical MDS algorithm: one is the ratio of the sum of the first k eigenvalues greater than zero to the sum of the absolute values of all eigenvalues; the other is the ratio of the sum of the first k eigenvalues greater than zero to the sum of all eigenvalues greater than zero. As for the number of k, as in how many dimensions should be used so that the points in the MDS graph can fully represent the input distance data, can be determined by using a screen plot. A common criterion is to select the dimension k that does not change the goodness of fit statistics significantly when compared with dimension $k + 1$ or higher.

Non-metric MDS algorithm has many forms according to different definitions of loss function. Assuming that we need to find a k-dimensional MDS relationship for n objects, we can minimize the following loss functions:

$$S^2 = \frac{\sum_{i \neq j} [d_{ij} - f(\delta_{ij})]^2}{\sum_{i \neq j} d_{ij}^2},$$

Among them, d_{ij} stands for the distance between data point i and j, while $f(\delta_{ij})$ stands for the monotone transformation function of observation distance δ_{ij}, and S is a "stress" function. For different loss functions, distance is given different relative importance. In some cases, we may want to preserve local similarity at the expense of losing partial long-distance relations, while in others, we may want to preserve overall relationships at the expense of losing partial information.

Dimension reduction may not get results with direct biological significance, and may even be difficult to explain. Therefore, it is undoubtedly more meaningful to select genes that account for a large proportion of observed variations for analysis directly. From this point of view, our aim is to find the part of the gene with the most variation in the sample. Gene shaving is used to obtain subjects of interest by searching several sets of genes with the smallest variation within a group and the largest variation among samples. Specifically, the gene shaving method searches for a series of gene subsets (S_k, k is the size of the subset), so that $\mathrm{var}_J(\sum_{i\in S_k} x_{iJ}/k)$ has the greatest value, in which,

$$Var_J\left(\frac{1}{k}\sum_{i\in S_k} x_{iJ}\right) = \frac{1}{n}\sum_{j=1}^{n}\left[\frac{1}{k}\sum_{i\in S_k}(x_{iJ}-x_i)\right]^2$$

In order to obtain the optimal solution, we need to traverse all gene subsets with the number k, which may be quite time-consuming. Hastie *et al.* (2000) obtained the approximate optimal solution of the function above by searching for the optimal weight vector, which greatly improves the computational efficiency.

31.4. Visualization of bioinformatics data

Visualization is an indispensable part of exploring, analyzing, and reporting data, which offers key insights into data issues, like goodness-of-fit and data quality, in ways that are meaningful and intuitive. High-throughput biological data create many challenges for visualization methods. The datasets are large and usually have very high dimension. In most cases, they are also related to a large number of known biological information, for example annotation information including the gene names and their loci and function details.

Given the importance of visualization methods for the comprehension of bioinformatics data, it is similarly important that good tools for producing plots and displays be readily available. This section focuses on the statistical graphs, tools, methods, and the biological interpretation commonly used in bioinformatics.

31.4.1. *Volcano plot*

In the field of statistics, the volcano plot is a type of scatter plots which can quickly identify the degree of numerical change from large-scale repetitive data. Its Y axis and X axis correspond to statistical

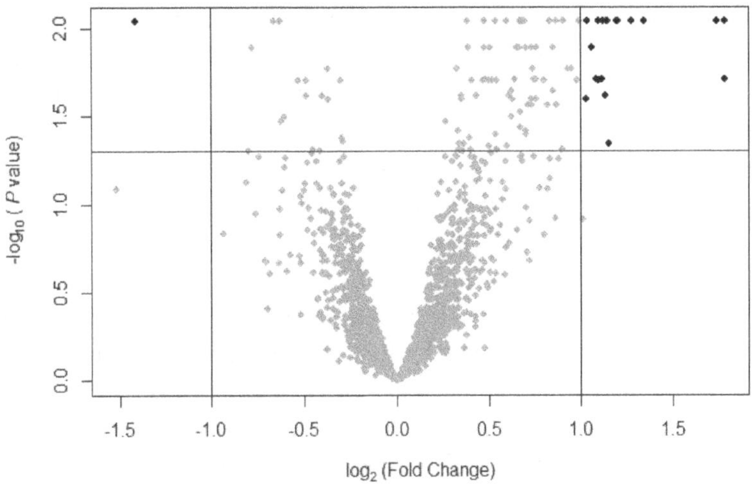

Figure 31.9 An example of volcano plot

significance and the change value of statistics respectively. Because it resembles the shape of a volcanic eruption, it is called a volcano plot. Volcano plots are particularly common in the analysis of omics experimental data. A volcano plot can place the P value of a statistical test together with the magnitude of the effect, making it more convenient to quickly identify the data points with greater effect and statistical significance.

Figure 31.9 shows the results of the identification of differentially expressed genes in 37 patients with BCR/ABL subtype and 42 patients with NEG subtype by permutation test. The figure shows P values and the magnitude of the effect together. The X-axis corresponds to the logarithm of between-group signal intensity ratio of the genes, that is, fold change, which represents the measurement effect. The Y-axis is the negative logarithm of the corresponding corrected P values. Black points represent genes with fold change >1 and FDR <0.05.

31.4.2. *Venn diagram*

The venn diagram, also known as the logic diagram, is a diagram that shows the overlapping relationship among different sets. Venn

Diagrams use points on the plane to represent elements in a set and closed curves to represent sets. Usually, a Venn diagram consists of several overlapping closed curves, which are generally represented by circles, and each circle represents a set. Points in closed curves represent elements in the sets, while points outside closed curves represent elements outside the sets. This way, it is easy to visualize the relationship between sets.

Venn diagrams are widely used in bioinformatics data analysis. For example, as can be seen from Figure 31.9, the results of screening differentially expressed genes by fold change and by permutation test may vary greatly. Each method has its own advantages and disadvantages, therefore it is difficult to determine which is better. Our purpose of screening differentially expressed genes is likely to be a kind of experimental verification using subsequent methods, etc. In this case, the requirements for controlling false positives in the screening results should be more stringent. Figure 31.10 shows the differentially expressed genes identified by five methods: fold change, permutation test, two-sample t-test, rank-sum test, and SAM. The screening criteria requires the fold change method of >2, while other in methods the adjusted FDR must be <0.05. The results show that 18 genes are found simultaneously by the five methods. Further validation

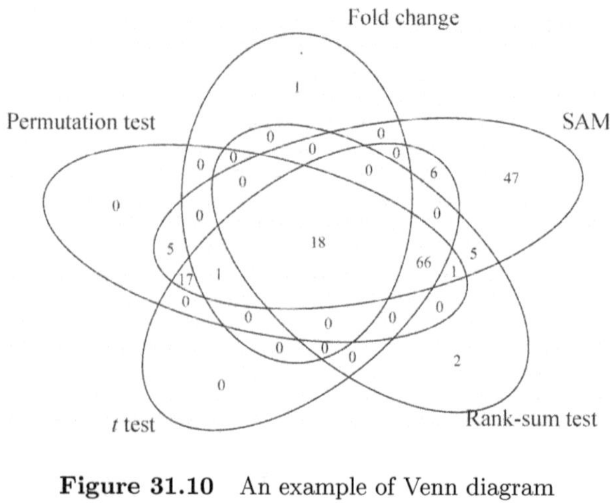

Figure 31.10 An example of Venn diagram

experiments on these 18 genes are more likely to achieve the expected results while saving costs.

31.4.3. *Heatmap*

The heatmap, or false color image, has had a long history since its first appearance. It shows the structure of data by rearranging rows and columns and annotating them. Eisen *et al.* (1998) were the first to use it on microarray data, now it has become a standard method for the visualization of this kind of data.

The heatmap is a kind of color grid graph in the form of a two-dimensional matrix, and its data also have the form of a two-dimensional matrix. The color of the square grid on the graph is determined by the input value corresponding to the matrix data. The order of rows and columns of a matrix can be rearranged independently. In general, rearranging rows and columns will help similar rows and columns to be placed adjacent to each other. Systematic clustering is the most commonly used sorting method, of course, other methods can also be used. If the systematic clustering is used for sorting, it is customary to show the tree graph of the systematic clustering on the graph. In most cases, some of the square areas on the graph have relatively uniform colors, which makes it easy for us to determine which rows (usually representing genes) and columns (usually representing samples) have similar expression values.

Here, we use the data from Case 31.4 once again to manifest an example of the application of a heatmap. Figure 31.11 is a two-way clustering map obtained by the systematic clustering of genes and conditions/samples. The results show that there are obvious differences in expression patterns of 81 genes between ALL1/AF4 and E2A/PBX1 subgroups. Through these genes, we can easily separate the two subgroups.

31.4.4. *Visualization of distance*

A large number of statistical analysis techniques (such as system clustering and classification and decision tree) can produce graphics such as tree structure diagrams that reflect the "distance" between

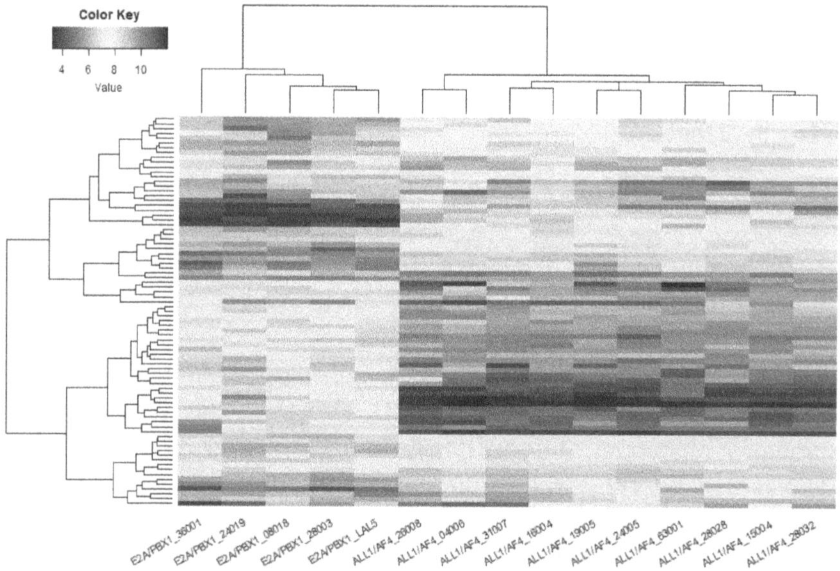

Figure 31.11 An example of heatmap

research objects. As a matter of fact, tree diagrams cannot be used for data visualization because they cannot necessarily reflect the structural relationship of the data. In many cases, they impose a structural relationship on the data, applying it on the interpretation of observed values could be precarious. For example, system clustering establishes a new distance between objects, which corresponds to the branch length of a tree structure diagrams.

Common distance visualization methods include principal component analysis (PCA) and MDS. Here we continue the introduction on MDS from the previous section, and to illustrate the visualization of distances. Take the data from ALL as an example. First, the gene expression values of samples are standardized, and then the Euclidean distance between samples is calculated as a measure of similarity between samples. We use three MDS algorithms to present the distance of the sample data. Since the input data are based on the differentially expressed genes selected by the two-sample t-test, as shown in Figure 31.12, the three algorithms show that the data are

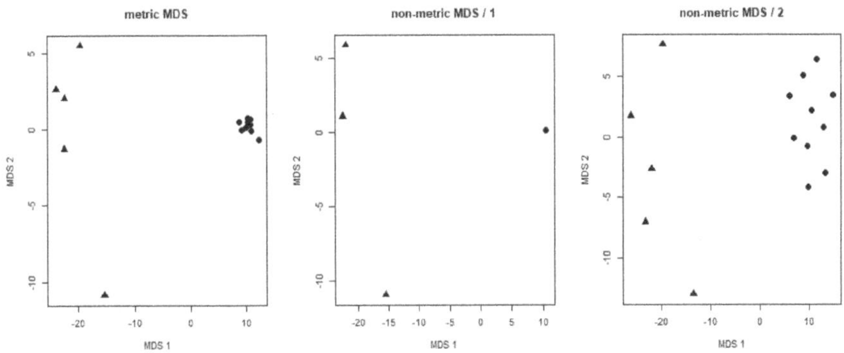

Figure 31.12 MDS illustration

well divided into two groups, and also that different MDS algorithms endowed different relative importance weights to the same distance between samples.

Although non-metric MDS is based on the analysis method of non-metric data, when the data in the distance matrix of quantitative scale is unreliable and the order of distance is reliable, the results obtained by non-metric method are closer to reality than those obtained by metric method.

31.4.5. *Plotting along genomic coordinates*

Some genetic defects associated with diseases, such as deletion or amplification, may induce the expression of adjacent genes on chromosomes, which prompts people to pay attention to the distribution of gene expression locations on chromosomes. Genomic DNA has a double-strand structure, one is called sense strand and the other is called anti-sense strand. Each strand contains the coding sequence of genes, so the visualization method will also reflect the distribution of genes on the double strand.

We still use the data of ALL as an example to show the genome coordinate map. Here, our aim is to understand the distribution of differentially expressed genes in two subtypes of ALL1/AF4 and NEG. ALL experiment is based on HG-U95Av2 chip, so we first

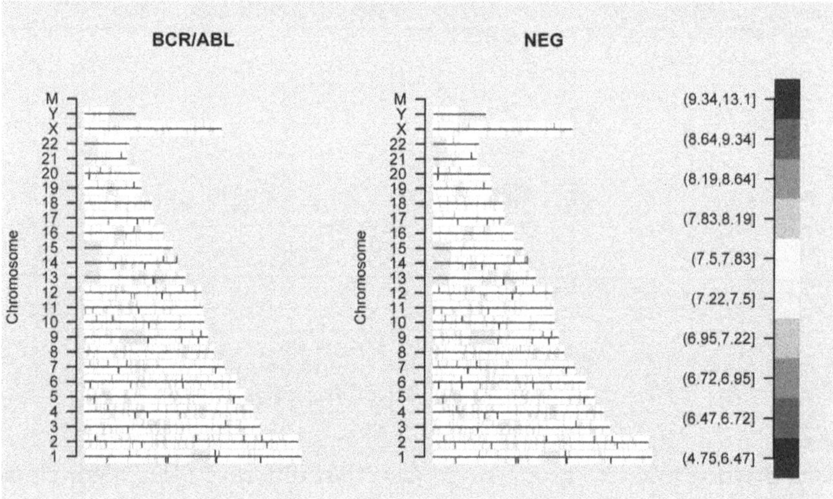

Figure 31.13 An example of coordinate map of the human genome

construct the distribution of all genes locations on the chip according to the chip information; then, we select 108 differentially expressed genes identified by FDR <0.05 in two subgroups. After that, mark the genes on the genome map according to the location of the selected genes; gene expression values are displayed by different colors, as shown in Figure 31.13.

In addition to the location information of genes, typical genomic experiments may also contain external annotated data obtained from public resource databases such as NCBI, Ensembl, and UCSC, or data from other experiments, which can be integrated into a genome coordinate map as needed, such as circos plot.

31.5. Report writing

Gene expression profiling is generally reported as follows:

(1) Study design and methods
(2) Data preprocessing
(3) Statistical analysis methods
(4) Statistical results (e.g., the test statistics and their P values)

The results in Example 31.3 can be reported as:

To identify genes associated with response to the genetic translocation BCR/ABL, we compared expression profiles (total 2391 genes) of B-lineage ALL from 37 patients with BCR/ABL and 42 patients with BCR/ABL negative. Permutation t-test with FDR cutoff of 0.05 was used to identify 108 genes deemed reliable predictors of response to the presence of BCR/ABL.

31.6. Discussion questions

Case 31.1: A comparative analysis of 37 ALL patients with expression of BCR/ABL fusion gene caused by chromosome translocation and 42 patients with negative expression of BCR/ABL fusion gene (NEG) was carried out. It concludes from a biological perspective that genes with larger fold changes (e.g., fold change >2) should be selected, while those with smaller fold changes, even those with statistically significant changes in expression levels, should be ignored. Please state your point of view and elaborate: What are the best criterion to use to decide whether a gene is significantly regulated? If fold change is applied as a criterion, will there be situations in which a fold change is statistically significant but not likely to be significant in a biological sense? If a conservative statistical correction (e.g., Bonferroni method) is applied but no genes are found to change significantly, is this biologically plausible?

31.7. Computer experiments

Experiment 31.1: Perform gene chip data preprocessing using data from Example 31.1.

Learn to use R software to describe and preprocess gene chip data.

Experiment 31.2: Identify the differentially expressed genes using data from Example 31.2 and compare the results obtained by different statistical methods using Venn diagram.

Learn to use R software to identify differentially expressed genes with different statistical methods.

31.8. Frequently asked questions and summary

31.8.1. *Frequently asked questions*

1. Which method is more susceptible to outliers, choose between permutation test and rank-sum test?

Permutation test and rank-sum test are both non-parametric methods, which do not depend on the hypothesis of data distribution. The permutation test rearranges the original sample to generate the theoretical sampling distribution of the test statistic where the numerical information is utilized, but instead the rank-sum test uses the ranks of each sample. Therefore, compared with rank-sum test, permutation test is more susceptible to outliers.

2. In the analysis of gene expression profiles, the clustering for genes or samples using different methods usually give inconsistent results. How could we make the choice?

If we have no prior information about those genes or samples and are performing exploratory analysis, the unsupervised learning method can be used. Numerous distance functions are available for the clustering and results obtained by different distances may not be the same. Therefore, the distance and clustering methods used should be documented. If the training set is available, the clustering approach can be selected according to the clustering effect of the training data. We can also select an appropriate clustering approach based on the expertise combined with results from previous research, for example having a search on GO database.

31.8.2. *Summary*

This chapter focuses on the common bioinformatics data analysis, namely the gene expression profile analysis. Two commonly used techniques for gene expression profiling are introduced: gene chip and RNA-seq. The original data produced by these two technologies both are image signals, so we first explained how to preprocess these data and generate the measurements of gene expression. Then, the statistical problems of gene expression profiling, such as differential expression analysis, clustering and classification, and their visualization, are discussed. This chapter summarizes the statistical methods applied in bioinformatics, where we emphasizes how to consider and solve bioinformatics problems from a statistical perspective and expands the application of statistics.

Think and Practice

I. Best Choice

1. The reason why gene chip data need to be normalized is ( ).
   A. Gene expression values are not normally distributed B. Some experiments use cDNA labeled with fluorescence, while others employ cDNA labeled with radioactivity C. The efficiency of dye incorporation may vary for different samples D. Housekeeping genes may be expressed as varying levels between samples E. None of the above
2. Among the following methods for identifying differentially expressed genes, it is impossible to calculate the P value of ( ).
   A. t-test B. Permutation test C. Fold change D. SAM E. None of the above

II. Questions for Reflection

1. Compare the advantages and disadvantages of gene chip and RNA-Seq in gene expression profiling.
2. What steps should one take while doing gene chip data preprocessing and RNA-Seq data preprocessing? Why?
3. Give a brief description of the common problems and statistical resolutions in gene expression profile analysis.

III. Programming

1. Download the cDNA chip data provided by Brooks *et al.* (2009) from http://www.public.iastate.edu/~dnett/microarray/sam3.0/. Use the "limma" package of R to do the following analysis:

   (a) Data preprocessing;
   (b) Feature genes identification.

(2) Based on the data in Experiment 31.2, complete the following exercises by using packages integrated in the Bioconductor project of R:

   (a) What genes are differentially expressed between the two groups of patients? Use different statistical methods and compare the results obtained via Venn diagram.
   (b) Where are these differentially expressed genes located in the human genome? Try to use the genome coordinate map to show the corresponding results.

Yu Liu, Juan Xu, Xia Li

CHAPTER 32

DATA MINING

Data mining is a complex process of extracting hidden information and knowledge from a large number of incomplete, noisy, fuzzy and random data. Data mining methods are widely derived from artificial intelligence, which integrates mathematics, statistics, computer technology, machine learning and other disciplines, and has grown up to be a hot technology in the era of massive data.

Data mining principles are usually complex and the algorithms are diverse. The top ten classic algorithms include C4.5 (for decision tree), k-Means (for clustering), SVM (support vector machine), Apriori (for association rule mining), EM (expectation maximization algorithm), PageRank (for web page ranking), AdaBoost (an iterative algorithm), kNN (K-nearest neighbor algorithm), Naive Bayes, and CART (classification and regression tree). Additional common data mining methods, such as linear discrimination and decision tree can be found in Chapter 22 and cluster analysis in Chapter 23. Here, this chapter only provides a brief introduction to the basic principles and software implementation for three methods of data mining: association rule mining, artificial neural network and support vector machine.

32.1. Association rules mining

Association rule mining (ARM) aims to identify interesting associations between variables and items in the dataset. ARM is also known as market basket analysis, which illustrates an important application scenario of the algorithm. The association between beer and diaper in Walmart supermarkets are a typical case of association rule mining.

Association rule technology has been extensively applied in various fields. When we browse commodities, for instance, online shopping platforms such as Amazon and Taobao Mall will prompt us "customers who buy this commodity also buy...". These cases are the most frequent application examples of association rules in our daily life.

Example 32.1. The UCI DB (http://archive.ics.uci.edu/ml/datasets.php) is a database for algorithm testing provided by University of California Irvine. A doctor downloaded the recurrence data of breast cancer, wherein researchers collected basic information from 286 breast cancer patients (Table 32.1). The doctor intended to find out some meaningful association rules so as to help predict recurrence of breast cancer.

Patients with recurrence-events of breast cancer (Class=recurrence-events) may usually accompany by some conditions such as a higher degree of malignancy (deg-malig=3). Then there may exist an interesting association between deg-malig=3 and Class=recurrence-events. We can adopt some quantitative indicators to measure the strength of these associations, and screen out the valuable association rules.

32.1.1. *Basic concepts*

(1) Transactions, items and item sets

Transaction is a record or observation in a database. The relationship between the item and item sets is very similar to that between element and sets in mathematics. For example, a commodity in the

Table 32.1 Variables in recurrence data of breast cancer

Variable name	Variable description	Variable value
Class	Recurrence or not (two categories)	no-recurrence-events, recurrence-events
age	Age of patients (9 groups)	10∼19, 20∼29, 30∼39, 40∼49, 50∼59, 60∼69, 70∼79, 80∼89, 90∼99
menopause	Menopause (three categories)	lt40, ge40, premeno
tumor-size	Tumor size (12 groups)	0∼4, 5∼9, 10∼14, 15∼19, 20∼24, 25∼29, 30∼34, 35∼39, 40∼44, 45∼49, 50∼54, 55∼59
inv-nodes	Number of invaded lymph nodes (13 groups)	0∼2, 3∼5, 6∼8, 9∼11, 12∼14, 15∼17, 18∼20, 21∼23, 24∼26, 27∼29, 30∼32, 33∼35, 36∼39
node-caps	Nodular cap or not (two categories)	yes, no
deg-malig	Degree of malignancy (three categories)	1, 2, 3
breast	Location of lump (two categories)	left, right
breast-quad	Quadrant of lump (5 groups)	left-up, left-low, right-up, right-low, central
irradiat	Radiotherapy or not (two categories)	yes, no

shopping basket is an item, and the collection of several items is an item set. Size of an item set represents the number of items contained in the item set, for example, {beer, diaper} is an item set with size=2.

(2) Association rule

An association rule is generally written in the form of A $\Rightarrow$ B. Where A is a prerequisite (left-hand-side, LHS), B is the corresponding associated outcome (right-hand-side, RHS), and $\Rightarrow$ represents the implicit relevance between A and B. For example, the association rule in basket analysis, Diaper $\Rightarrow$ Beer, indicates that consumers who purchase diapers tend to buy beer as well.

(3) Support, confidence and lift

Strength of an association rule can be evaluated by three indicators: support, confidence and lift. To clarify the meaning of these three concepts, let's look at a hypothetical example. Researchers collected disease information on 10,000 patients, of which 1,000 were individuals with diabetes, 2,000 with arteriosclerosis, 500 with hypertension, 800 with both diabetes and atherosclerosis, and 300 with both atherosclerosis and hypertension.

Support refers to the possibility of occurrence of {A, B} appearing in all item sets, namely the probability that both A and B are contained in the item sets. Then, we have support $(A \Rightarrow B) = P(A \cup B)$.

Support measures the quantity of an association rule. By setting the minimum support threshold, it is possible to eliminate meaningless rules with lower "shot rate" and preserve those implied by the more frequent item sets. When support of an item set {A, B} is greater than or equal to a predetermined support threshold, {A, B} can be defined as a frequent item set.

Defining support threshold is usually the first step to establish strong association rules. In the above example, support for {diabetes, arteriosclerosis} is 800/10000 = 8%, while support for {arteriosclerosis, hypertension} is 300/10000 = 3%. If the minimum support threshold is set to 5%, {diabetes, atherosclerosis} becomes the high-frequency item set, while {atherosclerosis, hypertension} is excluded.

Confidence is the conditional probability that item B appears in the transaction set that includes item A, namely confidence $(A \Rightarrow B) = P(B \mid A)$. Confidence measures the reliability of an association rule in terms of quality. Setting a minimum confidence threshold is the second step for screening strong association rules. In the above example, confidence of {diabetes, atherosclerosis} is 800/1000 = 80%, while confidence of {atherosclerosis, hypertension} is 300/2000 = 15%. When the minimum confidence threshold is set to 70%, {diabetes, arteriosclerosis} is retained and {arteriosclerosis, hypertension} is excluded.

Lift is the ratio of the possibility that item B appears in an item set including item A and without the condition that item A is in the same item set

$$\text{lift}(\text{A} \Rightarrow \text{B}) = \frac{P(B|A)}{P(B)} = \frac{confidence(\text{A} \Rightarrow \text{B})}{P(B)}$$

Lift can be understood as the degree to which the appearance of A promotes the "appearance rate" of B on the basis of the possibility of B's own occurrence. Similar to confidence, lift is also an indicator that measures the reliability of association rules and can be regarded as a supplement to confidence.

Larger lift with value ≥ 1 indicates greater A-to-B promotion and stronger association between A and B. In the above example, the lift of item sets {diabetes, arteriosclerosis} and {arteriosclerosis, hypertension} can be calculated as:

$$\text{lift}(\text{Diabetes} \Rightarrow \text{Atherosclerosis}) = \frac{800/1000}{2000/10000} = 4$$

$$\text{lift}(\text{Atherosclerosis} \Rightarrow \text{Hypertension}) = \frac{300/2000}{500/10000} = 3$$

In summary, the above association rules can be simply expressed as:

Diabetes ⇒ Arteriosclerosis [support=8%; confidence=80%; lift=4]

Arteriosclerosis ⇒ Hypertension [support=3%; confidence=15%; lift=3]

32.1.2. *Basic principles and algorithms*

Association rule mining usually consists of two steps: (1) screening out all high-frequency item sets that satisfy the minimum support threshold; (2) detecting all rules that satisfy the minimum confidence threshold of the high-frequency item sets. These thresholds for support and confidence are usually set manually based on the needs of data mining tasks.

The methods of mining high-frequency item sets mainly include Apriori algorithm, Eclat algorithm and FP-growth algorithm. Apriori is the most classic algorithm among these methods, with clear principle and convenient implementation, but relatively low efficiency.

In Apriori algorithm, multiple scans of the database are performed for calculating the support of each item set and identifying all frequent item sets to generate association rules. The first scan obtains the set L_1 for frequent 1-item sets; the kth $(k > 1)$ scan generates the set C_k of candidate k-item sets by the result of the k-1 scan, and also determines the support of elements in the set C_k; when the set C_k of candidate k-item sets turns out to be empty, the algorithm ends.

32.1.3. *Question analysis*

Let's go back to the breast cancer recurrence data in Example 32.1. The dataset was transformed into the transaction database. The first 10 records are shown in Table 32.2. Since we aimed to find out association rules that are meaningful for recurrence prediction of breast cancer, outcome B (right-hand-side, RHS) in the target association rules should be adjusted to recurrence of breast cancer (i.e., Class = recurrence-events).

In this case, we used Apriori algorithm to identify high-frequency item sets. By setting minimum support threshold as 0.01 and minimum confidence threshold as 0.50, we screened out a total of 1424 association rules (Figure 32.1). To screen out the association rules needed as possible, the support threshold is set to be smaller to retain more rules.

Table 32.3 lists the first three association rules in descending order by support, all of which show high confidence (>0.52) and lift (>1.78). These rules suggest that breast cancer patients with high malignancy, nodular cap, or high malignancy and carcinogenesis occurring in the left breast are more likely to relapse. Association rules with potential value can also be quickly screened out through ranking them in descending order by confidence or lift.

To further identify strong association rules, we could adjust the minimum support to 0.05 and the minimum confidence to 0.70. Only three association rules were finally screened out (Table 32.4). Readers can interpret the practical significance of these three association rules by themselves.

Table 32.2 The first 10 transaction records of breast cancer recurrence dataset

Observation	Transaction
1	{Class=no-recurrence-events, age=30~39, menopause=premeno, tumor.size=30~34, inv.nodes=0~2, node.caps=no, deg.malig=3, breast=left, breast.quad=left_low, irradiat=no}
2	{Class=no-recurrence-events, age=40~49, menopause=premeno, tumor.size=20~24, inv.nodes=0~2, node.caps=no, deg.malig=2, breast=right, breast.quad=right_up, irradiat=no}
3	{Class= no-recurrence-events, age= 40~49,menopause= premeno, tumor.size= 20~24, inv.nodes=0~2, node.caps=no, deg.malig=2, breast= left, breast.quad=left_low, irradiat=no}
4	{Class=no-recurrence-events, age=60~69, menopause=ge40, tumor.size=15~19, inv.nodes=0~2, node.caps=no, deg.malig=2, breast=right, breast.quad=left_up, irradiat= no}
5	{Class=no-recurrence-events, age=40~49, menopause=premeno, tumor.size=0~4, inv.nodes=0~2, node.caps= no, deg.malig=2, breast=right, breast.quad= right_low, irradiat= no}
6	{Class=no-recurrence-events, age=60~69, menopause= ge40, tumor.size=15~19, inv.nodes=0~2, node.caps= no, deg.malig=2, breast=left, breast.quad=left_low, irradiat=no}
7	{Class=no-recurrence-events, age=50~59, menopause=premeno, tumor.size=25~29, inv.nodes=0~2, node.caps=no, deg.malig=2, breast=left, breast.quad=left_low, irradiat=no}
8	{Class=no-recurrence-events, age=60~69, menopause= ge40, tumor.size=20~24, inv.nodes=0~2, node.caps=no, deg.malig=1, breast=left, breast.quad=left_low, irradiat=no}
9	{Class=no-recurrence-events, age=40~49, menopause=premeno, tumor.size=50~54, inv.nodes=0~2, node.caps=no, deg.malig=2, breast=left, breast.quad=left_low, irradiat=no}
10	{Class=no-recurrence-events, age=40~49, menopause=premeno, tumor.size=20~24, inv.nodes=0~2, node.caps=no, deg.malig=2, breast=right, breast.quad=left_up, irradiat= no}

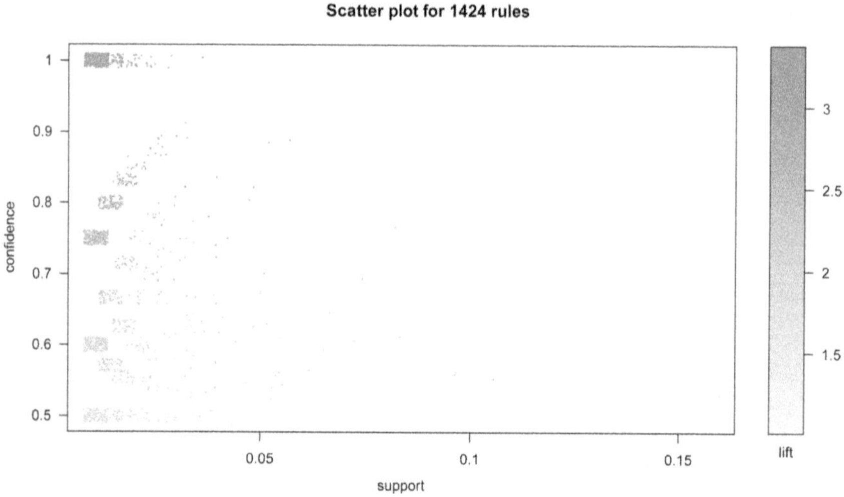

Figure 32.1 Visualization of the support, confidence, and lift for the 1424 association rules

Table 32.3 The first three association rules listed in descending order by support

Association rules	Support	Confidence	Lift	Frequency
{deg.malig=3}=> {Class= recurrence-events}	0.157343	0.529412	1.781315	45
{node.caps= yes} => {Class= recurrence-events}	0.108392	0.553571	1.862605	31
{deg.malig= 3, breast= left} => {Class= recurrence-events}	0.097902	0.560000	1.884235	28

Table 32.4 Association rules with support >0.05 and confidence >0.70

Association rules	Support	Confidence	Lift	Frequency
{node.caps=yes, deg.malig=3} => {Class=recurrence-events}	0.080420	0.766667	2.579608	23
{node.caps=yes, breast=left} => {Class=recurrence-events}	0.073427	0.700000	2.355294	21
{node.caps=yes, deg.malig=3, breast=left} => {Class=recurrence-events}	0.055944	0.888889	2.990850	16

32.2. Artificial neural network

Artificial neural network (ANN) is a research hotspot in the field of artificial intelligence since the 1980s. ANN is a man-made and functional realization aimed computing model by abstracting the human brain neuron network from the perspective of information processing. In the last decade, great progress has been made in the research of artificial neural networks, which provided successful solutions for various practical problems used to be difficult for modern computers in fields of pattern recognition, intelligent robots, automatic control, predictive estimation, biology, medicine and economy etc., with good intelligence characteristics.

Example 32.2. For the breast cancer recurrence data in Example 32.1, one physician intends to establish a neural network model to predict breast cancer recurrence. Readers can also compare the binary logistic regression model (see Chapter 20) with the neural network model in this section.

32.2.1. *Basic concepts*

The simplest artificial neural network model consisting of only one "neuron" (Figure 32.2) is taken as the example to introduce the structure of artificial neural networks and related basic concepts.

(1) Input layer: The input layer of the neural network is formed by the operation unit of the input observation data, such as the structural unit of the input variables x_1, x_2, x_3 and intercept term in the figure below.

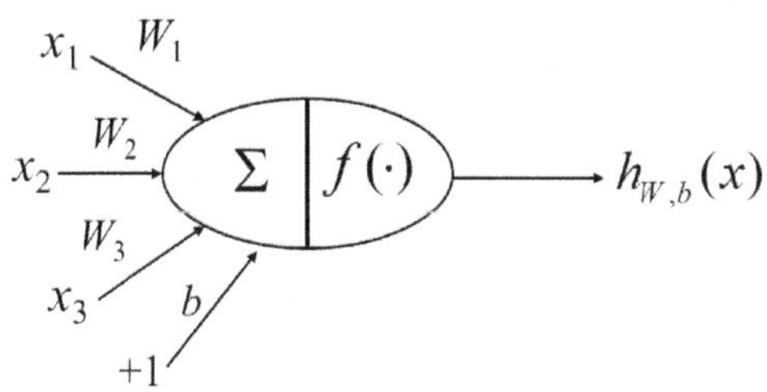

Figure 32.2 Basic structural pattern of artificial neurons

(2) Link weight: Link weight represents the connection between neurons. All connections in the neural network will have corresponding weights, which are usually transmitted in the form of weighted summation of input variables. The weight can be negative or positive, very small or very large, even zero. W_1, W_2, and W_3 in Figure 32.2 are the link weights corresponding to the input variables x_1, x_2, and x_3, respectively.
(3) Activation function: Also known as the conversion function, activation function is introduced to overcome the lack of expression ability of linear models, and usually tends to be monotonous and differentiable (we can use the gradient descent method to find out the extreme value) nonlinear function with the output value limited to a finite interval (e.g. [0, 1]). Activation function generally includes sigmoid function (sigmoid), hyperbolic tangent function (tanh), and linear correction unit (ReLu function), etc.
(4) Output layer: It is the target output of the neural network and can be a single or multiple output values. If the activation function $f(.)$ uses the sigmoid function

$$f(z) = \frac{1}{1+\exp(-z)}$$

Then the output value can be expressed as

$$h_{W,b}(x) = f(W^T x) = f\left(\sum_{i=1}^{3} W_i x_i + b\right)$$

In addition to input layer and output layer, a common neural network also includes hidden layers, which are the layers consisted of numerous neurons and connections between input layer and output layer. Hidden layers can be multiple, but customarily to be single in practice. The number of hidden layer nodes (neurons) is uncertain; and the more the number is, the higher degree of non-linearity the neural network shows. It is customary to select 1.2 to 1.5 times of the number of input nodes as the number of hidden layer nodes. The hidden layer is so-called "black box". Almost no one can understand how the activation functions in the hidden layer combine their variables in all cases. This is a typical case of computer substitute for human thinking.

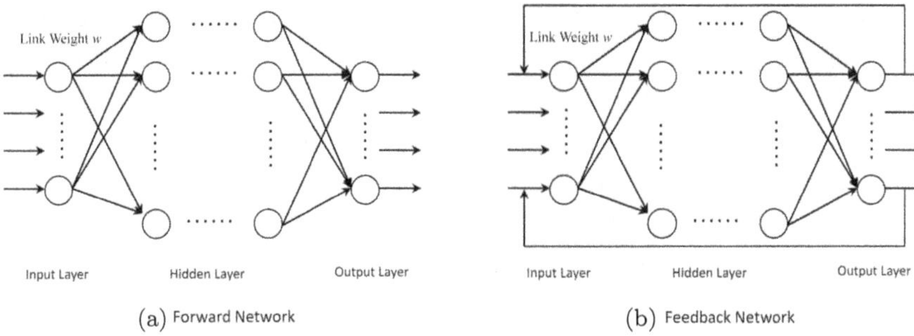

Figure 32.3 Two typical structural diagrams of neural networks

Neural networks can be divided into two types: forward network and feedback network (see Figure 32.3) according to different connection modes between neurons. The forward network consists of input layer, hidden layer and output layer; hidden layer can have several layers and each layer's neurons can only receive the output of the previous layer's neurons, such as multi-layer perceptron neural network, linear neural network and radial basis function neural network. The feedback networks have feedback connections from the output layer to the hidden layer (or input layer); therefore, input signals are transmitted back and forth between neurons, starting from a certain state, after several changes, gradually tending to a stable state or entering other states such as periodic oscillation. In contrast, forward network is more widely used for its simple structure and easy training.

32.2.2. *Basic principles and algorithms*

As seen above, artificial neural network is composed of large numbers of connected input and output nodes, which represent specific activation functions, as well as the connections between each two nodes that represent weighted values (i.e. link weight) of the signal through the network. The output of the network varies by connection mode, weight and activation function of the network. The learning process of most neural network models is to continuously adjust the weight parameters until the error between the model predictive output and the observed output of training samples is minimized.

The BP algorithm, with its full name of error back propagation algorithm, is the most successful and widely used neural network learning algorithm. The BP neural network is a multi-layer feed-forward neural network trained by sigmoid function and BP algorithm. BP algorithm essentially takes the square of the network error as the objective function and the gradient descent method to calculate the minimum value of the objective function.

BP algorithm includes two basic processes: forward propagation of signal and backward propagation of error, that is, the calculation process of the error output is performed from input to output, while the adjustment process of weights and thresholds is performed from output to input.

(1) In the forward propagation, the input signal acts on the output node through the hidden layer, and the output signal is generated by non-linear transformation. If the actual output does not match the expected output, the backward propagation of error will be processed.
(2) Backward propagation of error is the process of re-transmitting the output error layer by layer from hidden layers to input layers, and allocating the error to all units in each layer. The error signal obtained from each layer is used as the basis for further adjusting the weight of each unit. By adjusting the connection strengths and thresholds between input layer nodes and hidden layer nodes, and those between hidden layer nodes and output layer nodes, it makes the error decrease along the gradient direction. Once the network parameters (i.e. weight and threshold) corresponding to the minimum error are determined through repeated training, the learning process terminates.

32.2.3. *Example analysis*

Usually, data need to be pre-processed before building the neural network model: (1) dummy transformation of category variables; (2) standardization (or normalization) of numerical variable.

The most frequently used methods of data standardization are min-max standardization and Z-score standardization.

(1) Formula of min-max standardization:

$$x = \frac{x_k - x_{min}}{x_{max} - x_{min}}$$

where x_{min} and x_{max} are the minimum and maximum values of the sample data, respectively.

(2) Formula of Z-score standardization:

$$x = \frac{x_k - \mu}{\sigma}$$

where μ and σ are the mean and standard deviation of the sample data, respectively.

All variables in this example are categorical variables, so dummy transformation is needed. Dummy transformation for variable Class is shown in Figure 32.4. We can see that a new variable has been created for each category of the categorical variables. The process of dummy transformation creates a new dataset with 45 columns, including two output variables and 43 explanatory variables (input variables).

Since the breast cancer recurrence data in this case is relatively simple, a neural network model with a single hidden layer can be used. Our idea is to first randomly divide the dataset into training set and test set, then construct the basic model using the training set, and finally output the optimal model by continuous adjustments

Observation	*Class*
1	no-recurrence-events
2	no-recurrence-events
...	...
141	no-recurrence-events
142	no-recurrence-events
...	...
285	recurrence-events
286	recurrence-events

⟹

Observation	*no-recurrence-events*	*recurrence-events*
1	1	0
2	1	0
...	...	...
141	1	0
142	1	0
...	...	...
285	0	1
286	0	1

Figure 32.4 Dummy transformation for variable class in Example 32.2

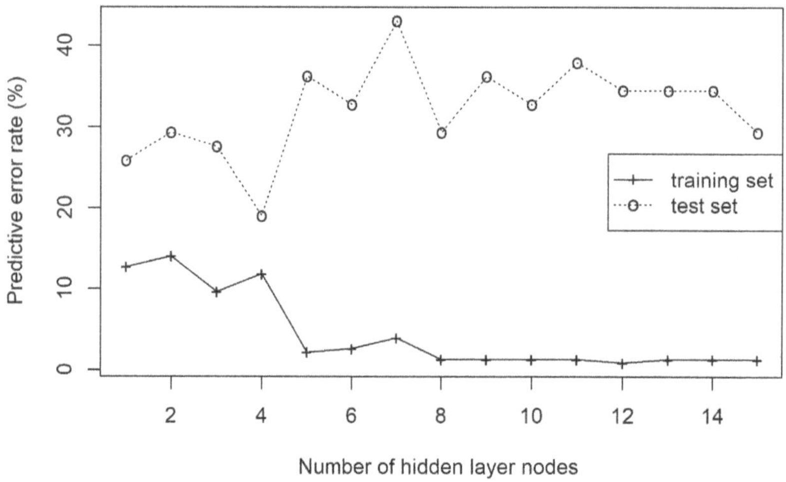

Figure 32.5 Predictive error rates of the neural network models with different number of hidden layer nodes

of modeling parameters according to the predictive performance in the test set. In this example, we randomly select 80% of the original dataset as the training set, and the remaining 20% as the test set (random seeds is set to 100).

Determining the number of hidden layer nodes is a key step of constructing a neural network model. Figure 32.5 shows the model performance on training set and test set with different number of nodes, in terms of error rate in prediction of breast cancer recurrence. It can be seen that when the number of nodes is 4, the model has the lowest predictive error rate in the test set; when the number of nodes is more than 5, the model shows excellent predictive ability in the training set but rapidly increasing error rate in the test set, suggesting poor generalization ability due to model over-fitting.

In summary, the number of hidden layer nodes should be set to 4, the single-layer forward neural network in this case can be expressed as 43-4-2. It means that the number of nodes in input layer, hidden layer and output layer is 43, 4 and 2, respectively, and the network model contains totally 186 weight parameters. The predictive results (confusion matrix) of the final neural network model in training set and test set are shown in Tables 32.5 and 32.6. The predictive error

Table 32.5 Predictive performance of breast cancer recurrence on training set

Observed classification	Predictive classification	
	No-recurrence	Recurrence
No-recurrence	160	3
Recurrence	24	41

Table 32.6 Predictive performance of breast cancer recurrence on test set

Observed classification	Predictive classification	
	No-recurrence	Recurrence
No-recurrence	38	0
Recurrence	11	9

rates in training set and test set are 11.8% and 19.0%, respectively, and most misclassifications turns to be identifying recurrence cases as no-recurrence cases.

Please note that since the initial weight used for iteration in the process of building a neural network model is randomly generated by the system, different models may be obtained even using the same parameter settings, thus resulting in some differences in the predicted results. In addition, model iteration may stop due to the limitation of default maximum number of iterations, so the final model obtained in this case will not be the optimal. Therefore, it is recommended to run the model multiple times during modeling optimization process, so as to choose the final evaluation model with the best fitting performance from all the generated models.

32.3. Support vector machine

Support vector machine (SVM) was first proposed by Corinna Cortes and Vapnik in 1995. It has many unique advantages in solving small sample, non-linear and high-dimensional pattern recognition. It is one of the hotspots in the field of machine learning. Support vector machine has been successfully implemented in various fields, such as handwritten numeral recognition, object recognition, speaker recognition and benchmark time series prediction test.

Example 32.3. Besides neural network model, SVM model could also be applied to predict the recurrence of breast cancer in Example 32.1.

32.3.1. *Basic concepts and principles*

The essence of machine learning is the process of establishing approximate models of research problems and making them approach to real models. The error between approximate model and real model is called risk, and the error between the real result and the predicted result of the approximate model of the sample data is called empirical risk. Traditional machine learning method constructs the learning model through minimizing the empirical risk. Structural risk includes empirical risk and confidential risk, wherein confidential risk indicates the predictive credibility of the model in unknown samples. SVM is a machine learning method that classifies and predicts linear and non-linear data based on the principle of minimum structural risk.

SVM methods can be divided into linear SVM and non-linear SVM. Linear SVM searches for the optimal separation hyperplane in the original space (see Figure 32.6). In the figure, circles and squares represent two types of samples, and an infinite number of hyperplanes can be found to completely separate all circles from those squares. Although the training errors are all equal to zero, there is no guarantees that these hyperplanes can perform equally well in unknown samples.

As seen in Figure 32.6, both decision boundaries B_1 and B_2 can accurately divide the training samples into their respective categories. Each decision boundary B_i corresponds to a pair of hyperplanes b_{i1} and b_{i2}. b_{i1} can be obtained by moving a hyperplane parallel to the decision boundary until approaching the nearest square; similarly, b_{i2} can be obtained by moving a hyperplane parallel

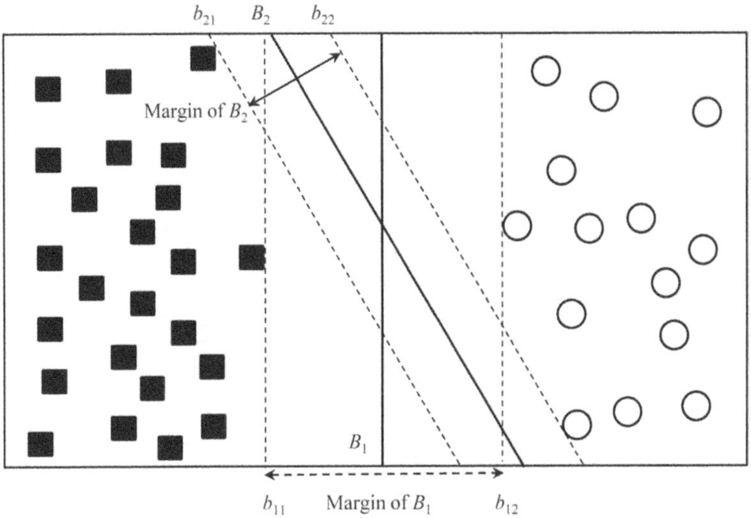

Figure 32.6 Margin of decision boundary

to the decision boundary until approaching the nearest circle. The distance between these two hyperplanes is defined as the classification margin. Obviously, the margin of B_1 is larger than that of B_2. In this example, B_1 is the maximal margin hyperplane of the training samples, which is also the optimal separating hyperplane that SVM is searching for. Sample observations that fall on the separating hyperplane are defined as support vectors.

If the margin is small, any slight perturbation of decision boundary may have a great impact on classification. Therefore, the classification with a smaller margin of decision boundary is more sensitive to over-fitting of the model, and its generalization ability on unknown samples is poor; if the margin increases, the distance between classes becomes larger, which will increase the classification accuracy of the corresponding hyperplane.

In order to solve the problem of linear inseparability of support vector machine, kernel functions are usually used to transform the original feature to improve the original feature dimension, and then construct linear SVM in high-dimensional space. This process mainly includes two steps: (1) transforming the original training sample

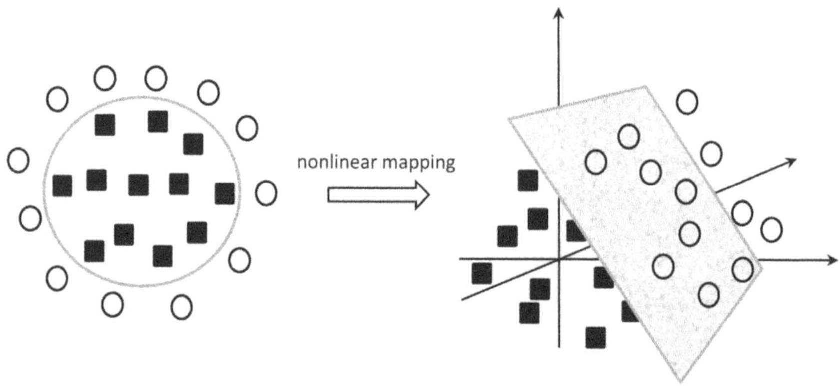

Figure 32.7 Constructing the optimal separating hyperplane in high-dimensional space through feature mapping

data into higher dimensional space through non-linear mapping; (2) searching for the maximum marginal hyperplane in the new space corresponding to the nonlinear separation hypersurface of the original space. Common kernel functions include linear kernel function, polynomial kernel function, radial basis kernel function (also known as Gaussian kernel function) and sigmoid kernel function. Figure 32.7 clearly shows the circles and squares that are linearly inseparable in a two-dimensional plane, which can be completely separated by a plane in three-dimensional space through nonlinear mapping.

32.3.2. *Example analysis*

Here we use the "e1071" package in R software to construct the neural network model. In order to facilitate the comparison with the neural network model in Example 32.2, we still randomly select 80% of the original data as training set, and the remaining 20% as test set (random seeds is also set to 100). Previous studies have shown that the radial basis kernel function has a high recognition rate and good performance, therefore, radial basis kernel function is used as the kernel function in SVM modeling process in this example.

In addition to the kernel function, there are another two important parameters in the process of SVM modeling: gamma and cost. (1) parameter gamma implicitly determines the distribution of data after mapping to a new feature space, thus affecting the shape of the separating plane. Elevated gamma values usually indicate increased number of support vectors; (2) parameter cost, also known as penalty factors, reflects the tolerance to the errors. Higher penalty factor suggests greater intolerance to errors, which may easily lead to over-fitting and poor generalization ability. On the contrary, excessively low penalty factor may result in under-fitting.

By comparing the classification error rates in test set of models trained using different parameters for gamma and cost, we can choose the optimal model parameters. Preliminary screening results demonstrate that when gamma is taken in $\{10^{-3}, 10^{-2}, 10^{-1}\}$ and cost is taken in $\{10^{-1}, 10^{0}, 10^{1}, 10^{2}, 10^{3}\}$, parameter combination of {gamma= 0.1, cost= 10} produces the smallest predictive error, with error rates of 8.77% and 25.86% in training set and test set, respectively (Table 32.7).

Through modeling adjustments using preliminarily selected parameters, we can easily have the predictive performance (confusion matrix) of the final SVM model in training set and test set, as shown in Tables 32.8 and 32.9. Compared with neural network model in the previous section, SVM model constructed in this case exhibits slightly worse classification performance in the test set.

Please note that the optimal modeling parameters shown in this example are only the condition after initial screening. Readers can make finer adjustments in more subtle parameters sets, e.g., taking

Table 32.7 Classification error rates (%) of SVM models using different parameters for gamma and cost

	gamma (training set)			gamma (test set)		
Cost	10^{-3}	10^{-2}	10^{-1}	10^{-3}	10^{-2}	10^{-1}
10^{-1}	28.51	28.51	28.51	34.48	34.48	34.48
10^{0}	28.51	28.51	19.74	34.48	34.48	31.03
10^{1}	28.51	21.49	8.77	34.48	31.03	25.86
10^{2}	22.81	17.54	1.32	31.03	27.59	36.21
10^{3}	22.81	7.02	1.32	27.59	27.59	36.21

Table 32.8 Predictive performance of breast cancer recurrence on training set

Observed classification	Predictive classification	
	No-recurrence	Recurrence
No-recurrence	16	1
Recurrence	19	46

Table 32.9 Predictive performance of breast cancer recurrence on test set

Observed classification	Predictive classification	
	No-recurrence	Recurrence
No-recurrence	36	2
Recurrence	13	7

gamma values from 0.1 to 1.0 and cost values from 1 to 10. In addition, model results presented here and Example 32.2 are sensitive to the random sampling, because they may vary as training set and test set change.

32.4. Results report

Results report forms for data mining are quite different due to complex and diverse methods and various output models. For example, association rule mining mainly adopts support, confidence and lift to describe the strength of association rules. Generally, when the purpose of data mining is classifying discrimination and regression forecast, model performance of classification or prediction (accuracy) in the test set should be explicitly reported.

1. Classifying discrimination: the classification accuracy (or error rate) of the object model in training set and test set.
2. Regression forecast: the root mean square error (RMSE) in the test set and the variation that can be explained by the model (R-square).

The following reports correspond to the results of two virtual examples respectively: (1) Train a neural network model to analyze 1000 chest CT images for diagnosis whether the subject has lung cancer or not; (2) Construct a support vector machine model to predict the annual average $PM_{2.5}$ concentration ($\mu g/m^3$) in urban areas through combining information of land use, green space, traffic and meteorological data around urban environmental monitoring stations, then assess the long-term health effects of $PM_{2.5}$.

The neural network model developed in this case shows an accuracy of 91.4% (640/700) and 86.7% (260/300) in lung cancer diagnosis for training samples of 700 CT images and testing samples of 300 CT images respectively.

The results of 10-fold cross-validation shows that our SVM model could explain 85% of the variation in annual $PM_{2.5}$ concentration ($R^2 = 85\%$), with a predictive RMSE (root mean squared error) of $5.5\,\mu g/m^3$.

32.5. Case analysis

Titanic dataset on the kaggle website (https://www.kaggle.com/c/titanic) collected passenger information (including whether survived or not) on the Titanic shipwreck. This dataset has been split into training set (891 records with known survival outcome) and test set (418 samples without given survival outcome). Some of these records are partially missing. The dataset mainly includes variables of PassengerId (passenger identifier), Survived (survival outcome: 0 = No, 1 = Yes), Pclass (ticket class: 1 = 1st, 2 = 2nd, 3 = 3rd), Name (passenger name), Sex (passenger gender), Age (passenger age), SibSp (number of siblings/spouses aboard the Titanic), Parch (number of parents/children aboard the Titanic), Ticket (ticket number), Fare (ticket fare), Cabin (cabin number) and Embarked (port of embarkation). We now aim to train a machine-learning model based on training set and then use this model to predict whether or not the passengers especially in test set survived the sinking of the Titanic. Researcher A plans to select Pclass, Sex, Age, SibSp, Parch and Fare as independent variables to establish a conventional binary logistic regression model, while researcher B intends to use all variables except Survived as input variables in a neural network model.

Questions:

(1) Can researcher A achieve a prediction of the survival status of passengers in the test set? What are the advantages and disadvantages of the logistic regression model compared to the data mining model?
(2) Is researcher B's practice appropriate? What adjustments should he make?

32.6. Computer experiment

Experiment 32.1. Using R software to implement association rule mining for Example 32.1. Students should learn to perform association rule mining based on Apriori algorithm using R software.

Experiment 32.2. Using R software to model artificial neural network for Example 32.2. Students should learn to implement ANN model using "nnnet" package in R software.

Experiment 32.3. Using R software to implement support vector machine for Example 32.3. Students should learn to perform SVM modeling using "e1071" package in R software.

32.7. Common questions and summary

32.7.1. *Common questions*

1. What are the differences and relations between data mining and statistical analysis?

Data mining is closely related to statistical analysis. The essence of data mining and statistical analysis is to explore and discover potential or unknown rules in data based on a certain theoretical framework. The main differences between data mining and statistical analysis include:

(1) Data collection: Statistical analysis collected the sample data (sample size is generally small) according to certain research design, while data mining usually includes the total population data (the amount of data is large).
(2) Data form: Statistical analysis usually deals with structural data, while the data form of data mining is relatively complex, such as voice, image and text.
(3) Theoretical basis: Statistical analysis is mainly based on mathematical theories such as probability theory and mathematical statistics, which usually requires rigorous hypothesis testing process and focuses on model construction; while data mining is mainly based on computer science and machine learning theory, which does not emphasize statistical testing, but focuses on algorithm implementation.
(4) Output of results: Parameter estimation results of statistical analysis are intuitive and easy to explain, putting emphasis on describing the quantitative correlation between explanatory variables and response variables. The modeling output of data mining is less interpretative, with its focus on the accurate prediction of output variables.

2. What shifts should be made in the concepts of data processing in big data era?

(1) From part (sample) to whole (population): all data can be included into our analyses rather than only the data obtained from random sampling;
(2) Focusing on efficiency rather than absolute accuracy: it will lead to greater insight and benefits when appropriately ignoring microcosmic accuracy of data analysis;
(3) More focus on correlation rather than causality: no longer keen on finding a causal relationship, but on identifying a correlation between things.

3. How to choose the appropriate methods for data mining?

In practical application, we mainly choose data mining methods according to the purpose of analysis. Generally, the application scenario of association rule introduced in this chapter is relatively clear. In most other cases, we can use several methods (e.g., random forest, artificial neural network, and support vector machine) to analyze the same data alternatively, and then select the optimal solution by comparing the performance of different mining methods.

32.7.2. *Summary*

1. Data preprocessing is the preprocessing of data before data analysis and data mining. It is necessary to perform data preprocessing, so as to improve data quality and make data mining process more effective. Data preprocessing mainly includes data cleaning (including outlier detection), data integration, data reduction and data conversion.
2. Association rule, also known as shopping basket analysis, is a data mining method that discovers the associations by analyzing the occurrence rules of variables (item sets). The key to association rule mining is to filter out high-frequency item sets that satisfy the conditions of support, confidence and lift. The main algorithms include Apriori, Eclat and FP-growth.
3. The output of neural network models varies by connection mode, weight parameters and activation function of the network. Activation functions generally include S-shaped curve function (sigmoid), hyperbolic tangent function (tanh) and linear correction unit (ReLu function).
4. To solve linearly inseparable problem of support vector machine, kernel functions are usually used to transform the original features to improve the original feature dimension, and then construct a linear SVM in high-dimensional space. Common kernel functions include linear kernel functions, polynomial kernel functions, radial basis kernel functions (also known as Gaussian kernel functions), and sigmoid kernel functions.

Think and Practice

I. Questions for Reflection

What are the basic ideas and processes of data mining methods such as artificial neural network and support vector machine?

II. Questions on Calculation

1. Dataset "data_liver.csv" describes the basic information and biochemical indicators from 579 patient records. Columns in the dataset are detailed in Table 32.10. Please randomly select 80% samples from the dataset and train a neural network model to predict whether a patient have liver disease or not. You should use the remaining 20% samples as the test set for evaluation of classification accuracy of the trained model.
2. Dataset "data_diabetes.csv"contains information on 768 female patients with diabetes aged over 21 years. Columns in the dataset are detailed in Table 32.11. Please use the whole dataset to train a support vector machine model (using cross-validation for model evaluation) to diagnostically predict whether a patient has diabetes or not. Please also compare whether data normalization has impacts on model predictive performance.
3. Dataset "data_chd.csv" contains the information of 25 patients with coronary heart disease (CHD) and 25 normal people in Example 22.1 (see Table 22.1 in Chapter 22). To predict whether

Table 32.10 Details of variables in dataset "data_liver.csv"

Columns	Variable description	Variable notes
Age	Age of the patient	Quantitative, years
Gender	Sex of the patient	Qualitative, Male or Female
Total_Bilirubin	Total bilirubin	Quantitative, mg/dL
Direct_Bilirubin	Direct bilirubin	Quantitative, mg/dL
Alkaline_Phosphotase	Alkaline phosphatase	Quantitative, IU/L
Alamine_Aminotransferase	Alanine aminotransferase	Quantitative, IU/L
Aspartate_Aminotransferase	Aspartate aminotransferase	Quantitative, IU/L
Total_Protiens	Total protein	Quantitative, g/dL
Albumin	Albumin	Quantitative, g/dL
Albumin_and_Globulin_Ratio	Albumin and globulin ratio	Quantitative
Liver_Disease	Patient with liver disease or not	Qualitative, 1: yes; 0: no

Table 32.11 Details of variables in dataset "data_diabetes.csv"

Columns	Variable description	Variable notes
Pregnancies	Number of pregnancies	Quantitative
Glucose	Blood glucose concentration	Quantitative, mg/dL
BloodPressure	Diastolic pressure	Quantitative, mm Hg
Skin Thickness	Skin thickness	Quantitative, mm
Insulin	Insulin	Quantitative, mU/L
BMI	Body mass index	Quantitative, kg/m^2
DiabetesPedigree Function	Heritability degree of diabetes	Quantitative
Age	Age	Quantitative, year
Outcome	Patient with diabetes or not	Qualitative, 1: yes; 2: no

a patient has CHD or not, please train an artificial neural network model and support vector machine (SVM) model respectively using the whole dataset. Is the predictive performance of ANN and SVM models better than linear discriminant model?

References

[1] Han J, Kamber M, Pei J. *Data Mining: Concepts and Techniques [M]*. 3rd ed. Burlington: Morgan Kaufmann Publishers; 2012.
[2] Tan P, Steinbach M, Kumar V. *Introduction to Data Mining [M]*. London: Pearson; 2005.
[3] Fan M, Fan H. *Introduction to Data Mining [M]*. Beijing: People's Posts and Telecommunications Press; 2011.
[4] Huang W, Wang Z. *Data Mining: R Language Practice [M]*. Beijing: Electronic Industry Press; 2014.

Yunquan Zhang, Yong Yu, Chuanhua Yu

Appendix A

Introduction for Statistical Software

APPENDIX A1

INTRODUCTION TO SPSS

SPSS, abbreviated from Statistical Package for Social Sciences, was developed by three graduate students at Stanford University in 1968, who founded the company under the name of SPSS that was acquired by IBM in 2009. After years of development, SPSS has become one of the most authoritative software on a global scale.

SPSS launched the first Windows version 4.0 in 1992 and, so far, it has evolved to version 25.0. The upgrade of SPSS is reflected in the following four aspects. First, the upgrade is based on the operating platform. For example, SPSS 7.0 is based on Windows 95, and SPSS 11.0 and above meet Windows XP. Second, it upgrades the function of data exchange and management. For example, SPSS 15.0 can read the data from most types of database. Third, it upgrades the output results, such as the continuously enhanced graphical function of the output results, which is the unique characteristic of SPSS. Fourth, it upgrades the function of statistical analysis, such as the added multiclass logistic analysis module of SPSS 9.0, statistical map module of SPSS 10.0, complex sampling module of SPSS 12.0, decision tree module of SPSS 13.0, linear structural equation module of SPSS 14.0, expanded programming function of SPSS 15.0, and added Bayesian statistics of SPSS 25.0. Compared with other international authoritative software, SPSS has the unique operation mode of menus and dialog boxes. Most operations can be completed with the mouse, so it is the most widely used statistical software for non-professional statisticians due to easy operation. Despite its constant upgrades, there is no major change in the content of its basic statistical analysis.

Considering the extensive users, this book chooses SPSS 25.0, but the content of this book is also applicable for the users of other versions.

A1.1. Major windows and functions

SPSS 25.0 has four major windows, namely Data Editor, Viewer, Syntax Editor, and Script Editor. This book introduces only the first three.

A1.1.1. *Data Editor*

Open Data Editor: Start SPSS, and Data Editor opens automatically; to create a new data file, click menu File/New/Data.

Data Editor can create new data files, and edit and display existing data files. It consists of Data View and Variable View, which are switched and displayed separately. Data View displays and edits values, while Variable View defines, displays, and edits variable features. SPSS 25.0 can open multiple data files at the same time.

A1.1.2. *Viewer*

Open Viewer: Start SPSS, and Viewer opens automatically with Data Editor; to open a new Viewer, click menu File/New/Output.

All statistical analysis results, including texts, graphics and tables, are displayed in Viewer. After the first SPSS process, the produced analysis result is automatically written in the opened Viewer. The subsequent analysis results of all SPSS processes are written in the Viewer of this result until a new Viewer is opened. Multiple Viewers can be operated at the same time, but only one Viewer is designated, that is, the analysis result is only written in the currently designated viewer.

Viewer consists of two views. The left view displays the output title, called title view, while the right view displays the specific output content of the statistical analysis including statistical graph, statistical table, and text description, called content view.

According to the three forms of output results, namely texts, graphics, and tables, Viewer has three editors, namely text editor, graph editor, and table editor. The output results can be edited by these activated (double click) editors.

A1.1.3. *Syntax Editor*

Open Syntax Editor: When the SPSS process is selected through the dialog box for the first time, click Paste, and Syntax Editor opens automatically, while the corresponding statements of this SPSS process are automatically written in this Syntax Editor; to open a new Syntax Editor, click File/New/Syntax.

In Syntax Editor, the SPSS process appears in the form of command statements. It can also edit the command statements of special processes that the dialog box operation cannot implement. All the command statements in Syntax Editor eventually form an executable program file, saved with the extension .sps (system default). Similar as Viewer, multiple Syntax Editors can be operated at the same time, but only one is designated. The SPSS process selected by the dialog box is only pasted in the currently designated Syntax Editor.

Why create the program file: When the large or complex data is processed, all the analysis processes can be collected in one program file to avoid repeated analysis processes due to small changes in the data. For some special or professional problems, the process cannot be implemented by menu or dialog box operation, but it can be implemented by the edited program file.

A1.2. Create and import data files

There are two sources of data files processed by SPSS, namely new data files created in the SPSS environment, and existing data files called from outside SPSS.

A1.2.1. *Menu File*

SPSS menu File (Figure A1.1), in addition to some basic operations same as general application software, has several special functions as follows:

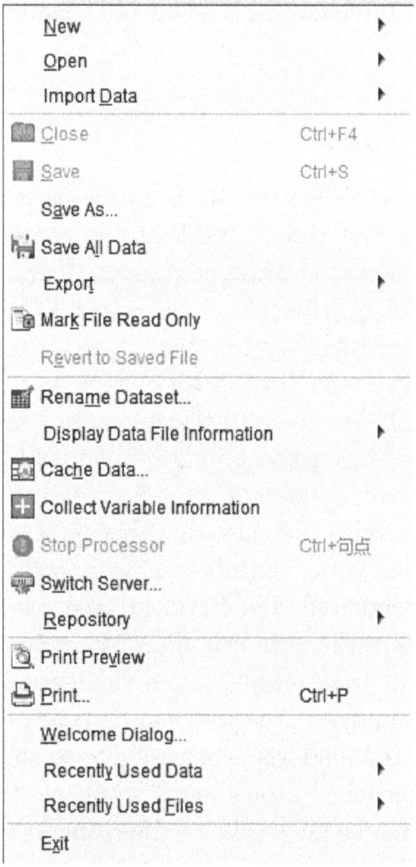

Figure A1.1 SPSS 25.0 menu File

1. Import Data: Click menu File/Import Data, and the options Database/Excel/CSV Data/Text Data/SAS.../Stata... pop up, which represent wizard import of database, Excel, CSV, text file, SAS file, and Stata file. This function is similar to that of File/Open/data.
2. Export: Opposite to Import Data, this function is to export the SPSS data to other formats, such as Excel and CSV, so it is the same as Save As.
3. Mark File Read Only: It locks the current data file in the read-only status. Click it to lock the data, and any editing is invalid.

The editing can be displayed in time, but it cannot be saved effectively. This function is important to protect the data file from being unintentionally modified or destroyed.

4. Rename Dataset: It changes the working name of the current file. Note that the working name is changed, not the file name of the data set.
5. Display Data File Information: Click it to display the details of the working file or external file.
6. Cache Data: Click it to avoid the process of reading data every time the program runs, which greatly speeds up the operation.
7. Collect Variable Information: Click it to search for variable information in some data files (e.g., SPSS file, SAS file, and Stata file) under the specific directory and display the variable information in the new data set. In some cases, if the data set file cannot be found, this function can be used to identify the name and position of the data set through variable information.
8. Stop Processor: Click it to stop the current SPSS operation command. If some parameters are found to have been incorrectly set in a complex analysis of a large data set, this command can be executed to stop the operation, but some commands involving data file modification (e.g., Compute Variable, Merge) cannot be stopped.

A1.2.2. *Create data file in the SPSS environment*

After SPSS is started, the system directly enters Data Editor, and data can be entered in Data Editor to form a data file. To clear the data in Data Editor, there is no need to exit the program. But click menu File/New/Data, and a new Data Editor is opened. Enter the data to form a new data file.

The data file is displayed in the two-dimensional format, in which each row represents a record or a case, while each column represents a variable. Different data types need to be processed by different statistical methods, and data files are expressed in different forms.

The first step to create a data file is to define variables. Activate Variable View in the lower left corner of Data Editor to define the following variables: Name, Type, Width, Decimals, Label, Values, Missing, Columns, Align, Measure, and Role.

The following principles should be followed to define variable names:

- The name should be no longer than 64 bytes (32 Chinese characters).
- The first character must be a letter or a Chinese character and the name cannot end with "_" or ".".
- There should be no spaces or special signs in the variable name, such as "!", "?", and "*".
- The variable name cannot be the same as the SPSS keyword, that is, ALL, AND, BY, EQ, GE, GT, LE, LT, NE, NOT, OR, TO, or WITH cannot be used as the variable name.
- There is no distinction of letter case of the variable name.
- There are nine types of variables for choice as follows:
- Numeric: Standard numeric variables.
- Comma: Comma numeric variables. Thousand bits are separated by commas, and decimals and integers are separated by dots.
- Dot: Dot numeric variables. Thousand bits are separated by dots, and decimals and integers are separated by commas.
- Scientific notation: Variables by scientific notation.
- Date: Date variables. The dialog box lists 27 date types, which can represent season, month, week, day, hour, minute, second, and percent second.
- Dollar: Numeric variables with a dollar sign.
- Custom currency: Custom variables.
- String: Character variables, which are used for identification rather than operation.
- Restricted Numeric (integer with leading zeros): Restricted numeric variables (integers with leading zeros).

In general, standard numeric variables, date variables, and character variables are most commonly used. System defaults are standard numeric variables.

Labels further explain variables. When a variable has complex meaning, it is more convenient to use the variable label. In Data Editor, when the cursor is moved to a variable name, the variable label is displayed.

Values label the value of a variable. If it is coded as "1=male, 2=female" and value labels are defined, the value "1" or "2" can be entered to display "male" or "female".

SPSS can define the missing value as a value (no more than three defined values), or an interval, or a value and an interval.

Column represents the column width of the display data, and the system default contains eight characters.

There are three types of data alignment, namely left alignment, center alignment, and right alignment.

Measure types classify variables into scale variables, ordinal variables, and nominal variables based on measure accuracy. This option is only used to distinguish between coordinate variables for statistical cartography and define the variables of SPSS decision tree module.

Role sets the variable relation for data mining and modeling. In default, SPSS assigns all variables as the role Input. In the existing versions of SPSS, there is less operation that needs to adjust the role of the variable, so general user can directly ignore this.

A1.2.3. *Call existing data file*

SPSS 25.0 can import SPSS (*.sav, *.zsav), Excel (*.xls, *.xlsx, *.xlsm), dBASE (*.dbf), ASCII (*.dat, *.txt, *.csv, *.tab), Access (*.mdb), Lotus (*.w*), and Foxpro (*.dbc) data files as well as various SAS data files.

1. Call SPSS data file (*.sav): Click menu File/Open/data, and the dialog box Open Data pops up and the file box displays SPSS data files with the extension ".sav" (system default). Select the object file and click Open, or double click the object file.
2. Import ASCII data file (text file, *.dat, *.txt, *.csv, *.tab): Click menu File/Import data/Text data or File/Open/data, the dialog box Open Data pops up. Select the file type Text, select a data file

and then click Open, and the dialog box Text Import Wizard pops up. Follow the prompts.

3. Import Excel file (*.xls, *.xlsx, *.xlsm): Click menu File/Import data/Excel or File/Open/Data, and the dialog box Open Data pops up. Select the file type *.xls, select a data file and then click Open, and the dialog box Opening Excel Data Source pops up. If there is an option ☑ Read variable names from the first row of data, the data of the first row is the variable name. If this option is not selected, the first raw is read as data, and the system automatically names variables as V1, V2, V3, ...
4. Import database file: Click menu File/Import Data/Database/ New Query, the dialog box Database Wizard pops up, which has three database types for choice. If other types of databases need to be imported, click Add ODBC Data Source, and the dialog box ODBC Data Source Manager pops up, which allows you to select the desired database type. This system supports more than 10 database types most commonly used. Follow the prompts to complete the import process step by step.

A1.2.4. *Data storage and file type*

SPSS 25.0 can also save data as data files, including SPSS (*.sav), Excel (*.xls), dBASE (*.dbf), and ASCII (*.dat, *.txt).

Major file types: Data files with the extension ".sav"; destination files with the extension ".spv"; program files with the extension ".sps".

Major button functions: OK: execute the selected operation; Paste: paste the statement command into the statement command window; Reset: reset the option; Cancel: cancel the option; Help: help.

A1.3. Process data file

Data is processed mainly through the menu Data and Transform as follows.

A1.3.1. *Data*

See Figure A1.2 for the menu Data. Its main functions meet the needs of various data sorting.

1. Define Variable Properties: It can define one variable or a set of variables and is more flexible than the variable definition window.

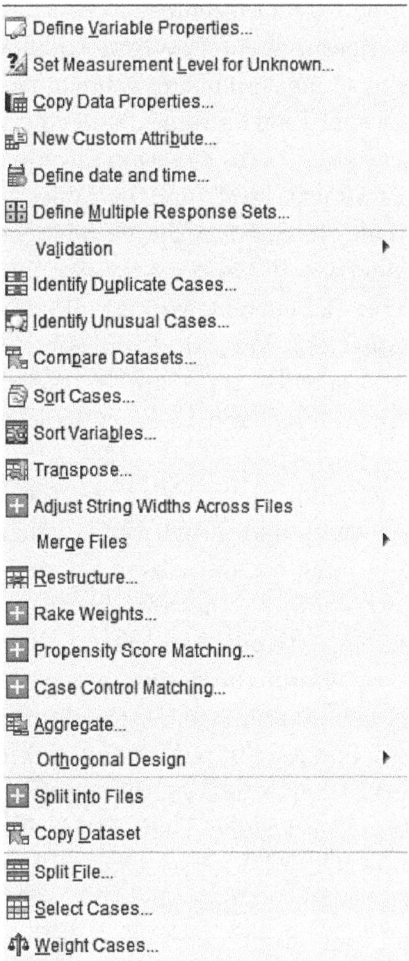

Figure A1.2 SPSS25.0 menu Data

Click menu Data/Define Variable Properties, and the dialog box Define Variable Properties pops up. Send the variables to be defined from the left view to the right and click Continue, and the dialog box pops up. Follow the prompts to define variables as required.

2. Set Measurement Level for Unknown: It is more convenient to set the variables with unknown measurement level in batches.
   Click menu Data/Set Measurement Level for Unknown, and the dialog box Set Measurement Level for Unknown pops up. Variables with unknown measurement level can be set in batches into nominal variables, ordinal variables, and continuous variables — namely scale variables. This function is only for variables with unknown measurement level, and variables with the measurement type set can be edited in the variable view.
3. Copy Data Properties: it can copy the variable characteristics of an external file or the current working file to a new file.
   Click menu Data/Copy Variable Properties, and the dialog box Copy Variable Properties pops up. It consists of five steps to copy variable properties, and there is a dialog box prompt for each step.
4. New Custom Attribute: According to the actual data, new attributes other than the 11 attributes provided by SPSS are generally used in large data management projects.
   Switch the data view to the variable view and click menu Data/New Custom Attribute, and the dialog box New Custom Attribute pops up. Enter the desired attribute name in the text box Attribute Name to create, enter the desired default attribute value in the text box Attribute Value, and select the variable to be set with default value into the list box Selected Variable on the upper right. Click Display Defined Attribute to view all the defined attributes. Click OK to see the new attribute on the right side of the variable view. Click the cell to edit it.
5. Define date and time: This process is mainly used for time series analysis. See the reference book.
6. Define Multiple Responses Sets: It redefines the variables that represent the multiple-choice answers to the survey questions

into a set for the next analysis. It should be noted that the set defined here is not available in Multiple Response Frequency and Multiple Response Crosstab and cannot be saved into the data set. Click menu Data/Defined Multiple Responses Sets, and the window Define Multiple Responses Sets pops up. Select the variable representing the multiple-choice answer into the list box Variables in Set right above.

Select "variable coding" method: Select "Dicho" or "category", set the count value, enter "set name" and "set label", click "Add (A)," and click OK for the next analysis.

7. Validation: Check the data in line with predefined rules or custom rules to determine whether the observation unit value is valid.
8. Identify Duplicate Cases: Click menu Data/Identify Duplicate Cases, and the dialog box of identifying duplicate observation units pops up. Select one or more variables into the check box, and the data file arranges the selected observation units with the same variable value. This function is useful for data validation.
9. Identify Unusual Cases: It identifies the observation units with unusual value based on the variable information.
10. Compare Datasets: It compares the variable information of two data sets.
11. Sort Cases: It sorts the observations of selected variables. Click menu Data/Sort Cases, and the dialog box Sort Cases pops up. Select the variables sorted by the observation into the column Sort By (select variables to be sorted). If more than two variables are selected, the sorting result is in the order in which they are selected into the column. There are two sorting methods for choice, Ascending and Descending.
12. Sort Variable: It sorts variables based on their attributes (e.g., variable name and type).
13. Transpose: It transposes the rows and columns of the original data so that the rows and columns of the new file are the columns and rows of the original file. Click menu Data/Transpose, and the dialog box Transpose pops up.
14. Adjust String Width Across File: Omitted.
15. Merge Files

(1) Add Cases: It adds the observation units of an external file into the current data file. The number of observation units of the new data file after the merger should be the sum of those of the two files. Click menu Data/Merge Files/Add Cases.
(2) Add Variables: It adds variables from an external file to the current data file. Click menu Data/ Merge Files/Add Variables to start this function.

16. Restructure: Click this option, and the dialog box Restructure pops up, which restructures data according to the required data structure to generate a new data file.
17. Rake Weights: Omitted.
18. Propensity Score Matching: This option achieves 1:1 propensity score matching, as described in the section on propensity score.
19. Case Control Match: It achieves 1:1 individual matching of case and control, as described in the relevant section.
20. Aggregate: In data processing, sometimes some intermediate variables, such as mean, standard deviation, minimum, and maximum need to be formed into a new data file, so the function Aggregate can be applied to this operation.
    In the new data file (aggregate file), each categorical variable level produces only one new aggregate observation, the name and characteristics of the categorical variable are the same as the source file, and the categorical variable can be a numeric variable or a character variable.
    In the aggregate data file, the old response variables are aggregated into a new variable, the default variable name is the old variable name plus underscore and function name, and the new variable name can be modified and tagged as well.
21. Orthogonal Design: Omitted
22. Split into Files: It splits the data file into several files according to the split sign (one or several categorical variables) and saves them in the relevant directory. This function is used for the separate analysis of certain subgroups of people.
23. Copy Dataset: It copies the data set being operated into a new work window.

24. Split Files: It splits the data file into several parts based on the split sign (one or several categorical variables), and each part has the same analysis process. Sometimes data processing requires a hierarchical analysis of certain categorical variables, also called fixed-level analysis. For example, the separate analysis of males and females requires a split file. Click menu Data/Split Files, and the dialog box Split Files pops up.
25. Select Cases: In data analysis, sometimes the analyzer may be only interested in several levels (groups) of a categorical variable; or in discriminant analysis, 90% of the observation units may be used to create the discriminant function, while the remaining 10% are used to evaluate the discriminant function; or the analyzer is only interested in the observation units in a certain period of time or a certain number range. In this case, click menu Data/Select Cases..., and the dialog box Select Cases pops up.
26. Weight Cases: In data analysis, there may be a lot of repeated observations in the observation units. In this case, this function can be used to define a variable as the frequency of the above observations with a view to easier subsequent analysis. It is usually used for counting frequency table data, such as contingency table, and frequency table of ranked data. This process defines a variable to describe it as a frequency rather than a certain value. Click menu Data/Weight Cases, and the dialog box Weight Cases (observation unit weights) pops up, and then the frequency variable can be selected.

A1.3.2. *Transform*

In many cases, the original data is difficult to meet all the requirements of data analysis, so it needs to be transformed as appropriate. SPSS has powerful functions of data transformation, which can not only implement simple variable transformation and re-create categorical variables but also implement complex statistical function and logic function operations.

Click the main menu Transform, and the submenu Transform pops up, as shown in Figure A1.3. Its major functions include

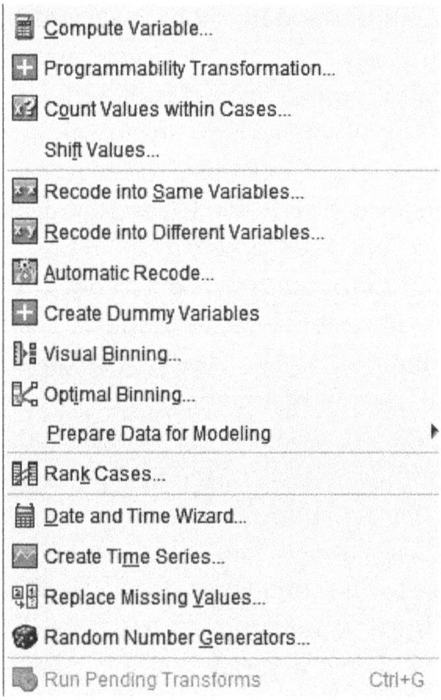

Figure A1.3 SPSS 25.0 menu Transform

Compute Variable..., Programmability Transformation, Count Values within Cases, Shift Values, Recode into Same Variables, Recode into Different Variables, Automatic Recode, Create Dummy Variables, Visual Binning, Optimal Binning, Prepare Data for Modeling, Rank Cases, Date and Time Wizard, Create Time Series, Replace Missing Values, and Random Number Generators.

1. Compute Variable...: It creates a new variable or replaces the old variable value after function compute according to the existing variable. Click menu Transform/Compute Variable..., and the dialog box Compute Variable pops up.

   The function can be entered into the expression view directly through the keyboard or the calculating board provided by the SPSS system or selected from the function box into the expression field. SPSS 25.0 provides about 180 functions, listed in

Functions and Special Variables. See the brief explanation of each function in the middle-lower box of the dialog box. The box Function Group displays function types, including arithmetic function, statistical function, distribution function, date function, random number function, logic function, missing value function, and character function. In the expression, character constants are enclosed in single or double quotes.
Function expressions and arithmetic expressions treat missing values in different ways, for example:

- For arithmetic expression $(x1 + x2 + x3)/3$
If at least one of the three variables is a missing value, the result of the expression is a missing value.
- For function expression MEAN (x1, x2, x3)
Only when all the three variables are missing values, the result of this expression is a missing value.
- For function expression MEAN.2 (x1, x2, x3)

As long as two or more variables are not missing values, the result of the expression is not a missing value.

2. Programmability Transformation: Omitted.
3. Count Values within Cases: This option is used to check whether the value of a variable has certain value(s), which can be a single value or a specified interval. A new binary variable is generated to indicate the number of occurrences of certain value(s) in the variable.
4. Shift Values: With the same function as function lag( ), this option moves variable values forward or backward and takes the front or rear value, which is often used in time series models.
5. Recode into Same Variables and Recode into Different Variables: Both options recode variables. For example, they reassign variables and transform continuous variables into discrete variables. Click menu Transform/Recode into Same Variables, and the dialog box Recode into Same Variables pops up. Select the variable into the box Variables, and the button Old and New Values is activated. Click this button, and the dialog box Old and New Values pops up. After reassignment, the new variable value replaces

the old variable value. Click Transform/Recode into Different Variables to retain the old variable, and a column of reassigned variables is generated. Other operations are completely the same as Recode into Same Variable.

6. Automatic Recode: It transforms a numeric variable value or a character variable value into a sequential integer starting from 1 and saves it as a new variable. Click menu Transform/Automatic Recode, and the dialog box Automatic Recode pops up. Select the old variable (e.g., "acc1") into the dialog box Variable→New Name and add a new variable name (e.g., "acc1a") in the text box New Name, and the button New Name is activated. Click the button, and the new variable is confirmed.
7. Create Dummy Variables: It automatically generates multiple dummy variables based on the category of variables, which is usually used in regression analysis. Click menu Transform/Create Dummy Variables, and the dialog box Create Dummy Variables pops up. Select the variable to be virtualized and name it, and then click OK to generate its dummy variable.
8. Visual Bining: It visually discretizes data and transforms continuous variables into categorical variables. This process can define the bining through the distribution of a visual variable, which is mainly used for bining continuous variables. Click menu Transform/Visual Bining, and the sub-dialog box Visual Bining pops up. Send the variables into the box Variables to Bin and click Continue, and the dialog box Visual Binning pops up. As soon as the variable in the box Variable is selected, its chart of frequency distribution (histogram) is displayed. Fill in the new variable name in the dialog box Binned Variable and click Make Cutpoints, and the dialog box Make Cutpoints pops up, which provides three options, namely Equal Width Intervals, Equal Percentiles Based on Scanned Cases, and Cutpoints at Mean and Selected Standard Deviations Based on Scanned Cases. After defining, click Apply to return to the previous dialog box, and the vertical line segment of each category boundary point is displayed on the histogram. Click the button Make Labels to automatically generate relevant value labels.

9. Optimal Bining: Some categorical variables act as "key indicator variables", so continuous variables are discretized into categorical variables in the principle of maximizing the differences in categorical variables, and then the discretized variables can be used for subsequent analysis. This function relates data modeling.
10. Prepare Data for Modeling: It is an intelligent preparation process of modeling data. Rank Cases: It ranks cases based on the observation of a variable in a certain order to generate a new variable representing its rank, without change in the order of the data itself. It differs from Sort Cases that reorders data based on the observation of a variable and generates no new variable. Click menu Transform/Rank Cases, and the dialog box Rank Cases pops up.
11. Date and Time Wizard: This function is highly flexible in the transformation between date variables and numeric and character variables as well as the calculation involving date and time, such as the transformation of a character variable containing date or time into a date variable and the transformation of a date variable into a numeric variable representing part date feature (year, month, day, week, etc.) that can be completed according to the prompts of the dialog interface.
12. Create Time Series: This dialog box allows the creation of a new variable based on the function of existing numeric time series variables, which is mainly used for time series analysis. See the reference book.
13. Replace Missing Values: Missing data is a problem frequently encountered in statistical analysis, such as the commonly used scale survey. Some SPSS statistical processes cannot be executed due to missing data, especially some time series data, so in order to make full use of the information of the original data and achieve effective statistical analysis, different processing methods can be selected to estimate and replace the missing value according to the research purpose and data distribution characteristics. Five alternative methods are listed to replace missing value as follows: replacing the missing value with the arithmetic mean of the variable, replacing the missing value with the arithmetic

mean of its neighbor points, replacing the missing value with the median of its neighbor points, estimating and replacing the missing value with the two valid observations before and after it based on the interpolation method (linear interpolation method), and estimating and replacing the missing value by linear regression (linear trend method).

Click menu Transform/Replace Missing Values, and the dialog box Replace Missing Values pops up.

14. Random Number Generators: Click menu Transform/Random Number Generators, and the dialog box Random Number Generators pops up. In the process of defining random number generators, the number of random seeds can be defined as well, such as fixed or not.

A1.4. Statistical analysis process

The main menu Analyze lists most contents of statistical analysis (Figure A1.4). The statistical analysis functions in the menu are briefly described as follows.

A1.4.1. *Reports*

Its major function is to summarize data, which can report and describe statistics in a self-defined format. In OLAP, it provides fast and flexible interactive modes so that the operator can freely select the report format and content of the form as required and the summarized results can be displayed in real time.

A1.4.2. *Descriptive Statistics*

The submenu Descriptive Statistics includes processes of Frequencies, Descriptives, Exploratory, Crosstabs, TURF, Ratio, PP diagram, and QQ diagram.

Frequencies: It describes data distribution characteristics mainly through frequency distribution table, bar graph, histogram, as well as various statistics of centralized tendency and dispersion tendency.

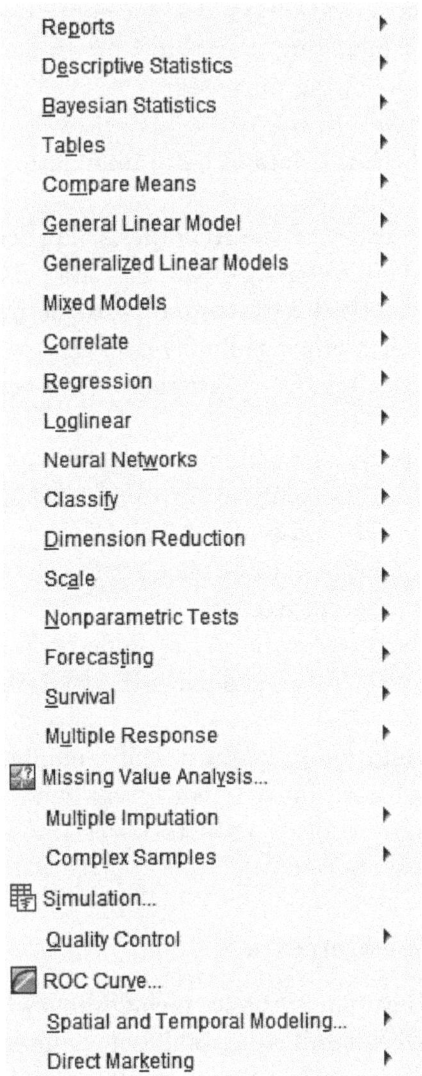

Figure A1.4 SPSS25.0 menu Analyze

Descriptives: It is mainly used to calculate various statistics describing centralized tendency and dispersion tendency. In addition, it has an important function to standardize variables, namely Z-transformation.

Explore: It can provide statistics, normality test, and descriptive statistical graphs, including stem-and-leaf display, histogram, and boxplot, with the following purposes:

- Preliminarily check the data to determine outliers and/or extreme values.
- Test the precondition of the hypothesis. For example, if normal distribution and homogeneity of variance are not satisfied, the data transformation method is prompted, and the parametric method or non-parametric method is finally decided.
- Identify the characteristics of differences between groups.

Crosstabs: It provides a number of methods of test and correlation measurement for the analysis of two-dimensional or multidimensional contingency data, especially $\chi 2$ test.

TURF: Short for Total Unduplicated Reach & Frequency, it is mainly used for marketing research.

Ratio: It analyzes the ratio of two quantitative variables, gives various statistics of the ratio, and saves the analysis results as a data file.

P-P diagram and Q-Q diagram: They mainly validate whether the distribution of a variable is consistent with the hypothesized distribution, which are often used to determine whether the data satisfies normal distribution.

A1.4.3. *Bayesian Statistics*

The sub-module Bayesian Statistics includes following processes, One Sample Normal, One Sample Binomial, One Sample Poisson, Related Sample Normal, Independent Samples, Pearson Correlation, Linear regression, One-way ANOVA, and Loglinear Models, to achieve relevant test methods in Bayesian Statistical Analysis.

A1.4.4. *Tables*

The SPSS process Tables is of great flexibility and convenience to categorize and summarize data with more categorical variables or deal with the questionnaire consisting of multiple responses. The process Crosstabs also lists categorical variables, but the process Tables has stronger list capabilities, greater flexibility, and more choices of output format. The menu Tables contains following options, Custom Tables, Multiple Response Sets, and Define Category Order.

A1.4.5. *Compare Means*

The submenu Compare Means includes the following five processes, Means, One-Sample t Test, Independent-Samples t Test, Paired-Samples t Test, and one-way ANOVA. The basic analysis process of quantitative data can be used for the calculation of 21 statistics as well as one-way ANOVA and linear tendency test. One-sample t Test is mainly used for the comparison between sample mean and population mean as well as the calculation of the descriptive statistic and the 95% confidence interval of the difference between sample mean and population mean. Independent-Samples t Test, also called Two-Sample t Test, is used to test the significant difference in the population mean of two independent samples. Paired-Samples t Test is used to compare paired measurement data and check the statistical significance of the difference between the D-value of population mean of paired samples and 0 as well as the correlation between paired samples. One-way ANOVA is used for the comparison of multiple sample means of completely random design data as well as multiple comparisons between sample means, which can also be used to compare multiple treatment groups with one control group.

A1.4.6. *General Linear Model*

The process General Linear Model of the main menu Analyze contains four sub-modules, namely Univariate, Repeated Measures, Multivariate, and Variance Components. The first two modules contain general ANOVA contents, such as one-way ANOVA, two-way ANOVA, Three-way ANOVA, factorial analysis, ANOVA for cross-over design, orthogonal design, split-plot design, and nested design, and ANOVA for the repeated measures. Not only can this process analyze the main effects of each factor on a response variable, but also it can analyze the interaction effects between factors; it can be used for both balanced and unbalanced design data as well as both complete and missing data; this process can also be used for regression analysis.

The module Multivariate is used for the comparison of multi-group means vectors, multivariate factor analysis, and multivariate regression analysis of experimental design in different forms. The module Variance Components provides four methods for variance component modeling.

A1.4.7. *Generalized Linear Models*

As an extension of General Linear Model, the module Generalized Linear Models consists of two processes, Generalized Linear Models and Generalized Estimating Equations (GEE). Generalized Linear Models allows abnormal distribution of the dependent variable. The dependent variable is linearly correlated to the factor and covariate through the specified contiguous function, which broadens the range of application of the traditional linear model, and the traditional linear model can be used as a special case of generalized linear models. GEE is mainly used for longitudinal data, repeated measurements, or aggregate data related to other dependent variables.

A1.4.8. *Mixed Models*

The module Mixed Models consists of Linear Mixed Models and Generalized Linear Mixed Models. Linear Mixed Models considers both fixed and random effects and can be used to analyze repeated measurements or highly aggregated data. Generalized Linear Mixed Models integrates Generalized Linear Models and Linear Mixed Models and analyzes the data with the dependent variable that does not satisfy the assumptions of independence and normality.

A1.4.9. *Correlate*

The module Correlate includes four processes: Bivariate, Partial, Distances, and Canonical Correlation. In the process Bivariate, the Pearson correlation coefficient can be selected for the data with bivariate normal distribution, while non-parametric methods, such as Spearman correlation coefficient or Kendall correlation coefficient, can be used for the data with bivariate abnormal distribution. In the process Partial, the partial correlation coefficient can be obtained, and the Pearson correlation coefficient can also be displayed. The process Distances can measure the spatial distance and similarities between observation units or variables. Canonical Correlation measures the correlation between two sets of variables.

A1.4.10. *Regression*

The module Regression contains different types of regression analysis, such as Automatic Linear Modeling, Linear, Curve Estimation, Partial Least Square Regression, Binary Logistic, Multinominal Logistic, Ordinal, Probit, Nonlinear Regression, Weighted Estimation, 2-stage Least Squares, and Optimal Scaling.

A1.4.11. *Loglinear*

The process General applies the method Generalized Linear Models to fit loglinear models or Logit models. It is mainly used for the confirmatory study, that is, it analyzes previously determined saturated or unsaturated, hierarchical or non-hierarchical loglinear models, gives the estimated values of these models and each parameter as well as the detailed results of relevant tests, and infers the correlation between categorical variables. In this process, categorical variables are not divided into dependent variables and independent variables. In addition, it is often used for the further analysis of selected optimal models.

The process Logit (Logit model or Logit analysis) refers to special loglinear models. Different from general loglinear models, their categorical variables are divided into dependent variables and independent variables. Logit model assumes that the observation frequency of different classification combinations of each independent variable obeys multinomial distribution, so it is also called multinomial distribution Logit model.

The module Model Selection is mainly applicable to exploratory research. This method requires that the candidate model be a hierarchical model. Categorical variables are not divided into dependent variables and independent variables. The selection process tends to solve three problems. First, the models with better and simpler fitting performance are selected from candidate Nested Models; second, the main effects and interaction effects included in the models are tested respectively; third, the parameters corresponding to the effects included in saturated models can be preliminary estimated and tested.

A1.4.12. *Neural Networks*

The module Neural Networks belongs to the category of machine learning. This module includes two methods, namely Multilayer Perception and Radial Basis Function, which can implement classification, forecast, and pattern recognition.

A1.4.13. *Classify*

The module Classify consists of the following seven processes: Two Step Cluster Analysis, K-Means Cluster Analysis, Hierarchical Cluster Analysis, Cluster Silhouettes Analysis, Decision Tree, Discriminant Analysis, and Nearest Neighbor Analysis.

Two Step Cluster Analysis is an exploratory sample clustering method with the precondition that variables are independent of each other and subject to a multivariate normal distribution (continuous variables) or joint multinomial-normal distribution (both categorical variables and continuous variables). It gives the optimal clustering solution according to the information criterion (Bayes or Ikeda information criterion) and works with graphic display.

As a sample clustering method, K-Means Cluster Analysis is effective for clustering large samples. It classifies n observation units into K classes, determines K initial class-centers, and then classifies the samples by the iterative method in the principle of minimum Euclidean distance of clustering center.

Hierarchical Cluster Analysis includes sample cluster and variable cluster. First, it considers n variables or samples as n classes, then merges the two classes with the closest property (or the largest similarity) into one new class, and divides it into $n-1$ classes. It then finds and merges the two closest classes and divides them into $n-2$ classes... until all the variables or samples are all clustered in one class. SPSS can output vertical icicle, horizontal icicle, or tree structure charts to indicate the classification result.

Decision Tree based on the idea of recursive partitioning uses some features (variable values) to decompose the study group into multiple subgroups with similar characteristics. Nearest Neighbor Analysis includes new observation cases into the class of the most similar cases.

Discriminant Analysis establishes a discriminant function group based on a batch of samples with known classes so that the function group can minimize the discriminant error of a sample when discriminating its class. This process can implement Fisher discriminant and canon discriminant.

A1.4.14. *Data Reduction*

The module Data Reduction includes three processes, namely Factor, Correspondence Analysis, and Optimal Scaling, all of which are used to the analysis of reduced variable dimensions.

A1.4.15. *Scale*

The module Scale includes Reliability Analysis and Multidimentional Scaling. Reliability Analysis is mainly used for internal consistency test, which generates Cronbach. α coefficient, split-half reliability coefficient, and intra-group correlation coefficient. Dimensional analysis includes three modules, namely Multidimentional Unfolding (PREFSCAL), Multidimensional Scaling (ALSCAL), and Multidimensional Scaling (PROXSCAL), applicable for multidimentional scaling in different scenarios.

A1.4.16. *Non-parametric Test*

The module Non-parametric Test includes three processes, namely One Sample, Independent Samples, and Related Samples, as well as Legacy Dialogs. The process can be selected according to the different data characteristics. Legacy Dialogs provides different non-parametric methods for choice, namely Chi-Square Test (checking whether the observed frequency matches the expected frequency), Binomial (comparison between sample rate and overall rate based on binomial distribution), Runs, One-Sample KS Test, two Independent Samples Tests, K Independent Samples Test, two Related Samples Test, and K Related Samples Test.

A1.4.17. *Forecasting*

The module Forecasting includes the following nine processes: Create Temporal Causal Models, Create Traditional Models, Apply Temporal Causal Models, Apply Traditional Models, Seasonal Decomposition, Spectral Analysis, Sequence Charts, Autocorrelations, and Cross-Correlations.

A1.4.18. *Survival*

The module Survival includes four processes, namely Life Tables, Kaplan-Meier, Cox Regression, and Cox w/Time-Dependent Covariate.

Survival is a statistical method used to process the data with survival time as response variables and with censored cases. Most survival time variables of such data hardly obey normal distribution. Different survival analysis methods can be applied according to different research purposes and data types. For example, Life Tables can be used for estimating the survival rate within a certain survival time, such as five-year survival rate after surgery; Kaplan-Meier can be used for estimating median survival time; both Life Tables and Kaplan-Meier can be used for comparing the survival time at different levels of a factor; and Cox Regression can be used for studying the effects of different factors on the survival time.

A1.4.19. *Multiple Response*

The response to the survey question is not merely the selected data, but a multiresponse analysis process can be used, which includes defining a data set and giving a crosstab of summary frequency table and contingency table.

A1.4.20. *Missing Value Analysis*

Missing Data Analysis is both different from and complementary to the process Replacing Missing Values in the main menu. Based on analysis, it provides EM algorithm and regression analysis to estimate the missing data.

A1.4.21. *Multiple Imputation*

Multiple Imputation uses the interpolation algorithm to generate a series of possible filling values for each missing value and thus generate a number of complete interpolation data sets, then analyzes each data set by the preset statistical method and synthesizes the series of results to form the final statistical inference. This module includes Analysis Patterns and Impute Missing Data Values.

A1.4.22. *Complex Samples*

As a new module added after SPSS 12.0, Complex Samples includes the processes including Select a Sample and Prepare for Analysis as well as a number of statistical analysis methods related to sampling. The process Select a Sample designs the sampling plan based on a sampling frame data file and forms a new data file. The process Prepare for Analysis develops a statistical analysis plan based on the new data file generated by the process Select a Sample. The statistical analysis methods listed in this module are all based on the new data file generated by sampling design, including statistical methods commonly used in observational studies such as basic statistical analysis, general linear model, and logistic regression.

A1.4.23. *Simulation*

This module uses Monte Carlo to evaluate the forecast model based on simulated sampling and calculate the model target. This process is repeated (usually tens of thousands or hundreds of thousands of times) to obtain the results of the target value distribution, which can also be used to answer questions about probabilistic characteristics.

A1.4.24. *Quality Control*

The module Quality Control includes Control Charts and Pareto Charts. With the basic principle that if a fluctuation is caused only by individual differences or random errors, the observation result obeys distribution with certain probability, such as the most common normal distribution, Control Charts can define whether the fluctuation of the observation is normal or abnormal, which is often used as a quality control tool. The main dialog box of Control Charts in SPSS provides four common quality control charts. Pareto Charts combines with bar graphs and line graphs, which uses the length of the straight bar to indicate the absolute number of each group and adds the curve of cumulative percentage of straight bars above the bar graph. Straight bars are arranged from low to high, and the gradual ascending trend of line segments indicates the increase in the cumulative percentage, which can intuitively identify the main cause of the problem. SPSS offers two types of Pareto Charts: Simple and Stacked.

A1.4.25. *ROC Curve*

ROC Curve is often used for evaluating the performance of medical diagnostic tests as well as the effects of forecast models. In the diagnostic test, the change in the critical value can generate multiple pairs of sensitivity and specificity values. The ROC Curve plotted with sensitivity as the ordinate and (1-specificity) as the abscissa can be used to calculate and compare the area under the ROC Curve (AUC value) to evaluate the effects of the diagnostic test. This module can be used for plotting ROC Curves and calculating AUC value.

A1.4.26. *Spatial and Temporal Modelling*

The geospatial modeling technology of this module is used to discover the mode in which the data contains geospatial (map) components. The geospatial modeling wizard provides a method to analyze geospatial data with or without time components.

A1.4.27. *Direct Marketing*

Direct Marketing provides a set of tools that are well designed to improve the effects of direct marketing activities, which can identify demographics, purchases, and other characteristics defining different consumer groups maximize positive responses for specific target groups.

References

[1] Wentong, Z, Chunwei, Q. *A Basic Course of SPSS.* 2nd ed. Higher Education Press; 2011.

[2] Wentong, Z, Wei, D. *An Advanced Course of SPSS.* 2nd ed. Higher Education Press; 2013.

[3] Chuanhua, Y. *SPSS and Statistical Analysis.* 2nd ed. Publishing House of Electronics Industry; 2014.

[4] SPSS Inc. *SPSS 25.0 Advanced Models.* Chicago: SPSS Inc.; 2018.

Jing Gu

APPENDIX A2

INTRODUCTION TO EXCEL FOR STATISTICS

The previous Excel book displayed 255 sheets, each consisting of 65,536 rows × 256 columns. Since the Excel is 2007 version, the capacity has been greatly expanded, and there is a table of 1,048,576 rows × 16,384 columns in each sheet (i.e., 1042^2 rows and 128^2 columns) (see Figure A2.1). Line numbers (e.g., 1, 2, 3, range: 1–1,048,576) and column labels (e.g., A, B, C, range: A–XFD) are, respectively, represented by numbers and letters. Each sheet can hold up to 1,048,576 observations and 16,384 variables.

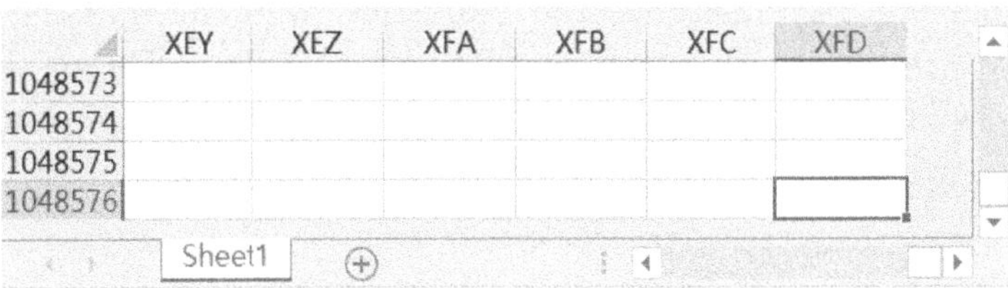

Figure A2.1 Excel interface

A2.1. Data editing and sorting function

Excel has excellent functions such as auto-filling, data editing, and data query. It can quickly create sub-lists of data for query results. R, SAS, SPSS, and other statistical software can easily read Excel file data, so for the studies that the sample size is not particularly large, Excel can be used as database-building software.

A2.2. Data analysis tool

Excel has an analysis tool called "Data Analysis." It is very useful for statisticians and other related people. After installing Microsoft Excel, you can't find "Data Analysis" in the Excel tools menu. You need to load "Add-Ins" to continue the installation.

Take Excel 2016 as an example. The way to install the Data Analysis tool is:

(1) Click File → Options → Add-Ins to bring up the add-ins interface.
(2) Select Analysis ToolPak on the right, click the Go button at the bottom of "Manage": Add-Ins, select Analysis Tool Library, Push Go... button, enter Add-Ins and select Analysis Tool Library, and click OK.

If the current Excel is not completely installed (it is recommended to install in a full installation format), you need to insert the same version of the Office software disk to install according to the installation prompt.

Once you have installed the "Add-Ins," you can find the Data Analysis option by opening the Data menu. Click "Data → Data Analysis" in the menu to pop up the data analysis menu interface (see Figure A2.2).

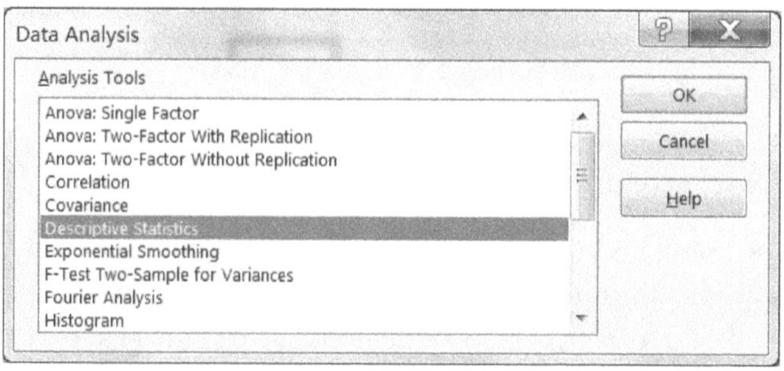

Figure A2.2 Excel "Data Analysis" dialog box

Using "Data Analysis" tools, you can easily perform common statistical analysis, such as statistical description of data, making histograms, performing t-tests, analysis of variance, correlation and regression analysis, and so on.

In addition, Excel's PivotTable can help us conduct exploratory analysis of statistical data. The calling method is as follows: Place the mouse in the data area, click "Insert→PivotTable" in the menu, and follow the prompts to complete the data sorting and analysis.

A2.3. Excel functions and formulas

There are nearly 400 built-in functions in Excel, including math and trigonometric functions, statistical functions, date and time functions, text functions, logic functions, query and reference functions, database functions, information functions, engineering functions, financial functions, user-defined functions, etc. The common statistical functions are shown in Table A2.1. Functions and operators [such as arithmetic operators (+, –, *, /, ^, %), comparison operators (=, >, <, >=, <=, <>), text operators (&) The reference operator (": (colon)," ", (comma)," "(space)")] can be used to create a variety of Excel formulas to complete a variety of complex statistical calculations.

In order to build a formula, you must first input "=". Inputting "=" is to indicate that the edit formula is about to begin.

Generally, the following steps can be used to build a formula:

(1) Select the cell in which you want to create a formula.
(2) Input "=". Generally, point the mouse pointer at the edit bar and click, then input "="; if you want to use the Excel function to create a formula, click the insert function "fx" button on the left side of the edit bar.
(3) Enter the contents of the formula, such as "=SUM(B4:G4)". If you enter a built-in function, such as the summation function SUM, Excel will automatically pop up the function's format text box, prompting the user for the correct function input format

Table A2.1 Common statistical functions

Number	Function	Example	Explanation (Result)
1	**AVERAGE** (**number1**,number2,...)	=AVERAGE (A2:A6)	Get the mean of a set of data (or cell references) Formula: $(\Sigma X)/n$
2	**BINOMDIST** (**number_s**, **trials**, **probability_s**, **cumulative**)	=BINOMDIST (6,10, 0.3, 0)	The probability of success is 6 times in 10 trials at an population rate of 0.3 (see Chapter 2); **Cumulative**=0 or FALSE calculates the probability density function; **Cumulative**=1 or TRUE calculates the cumulative distribution function
3	**CHIDIST** (**x**, **degrees_freedom**)	=CHIDIST (18.307, 10)	The P-value of the chi-squared value =18.307 in the chi-square distribution with a DF of 10 (0.05); see Chapter 7
4	**CHIINV** (**probability**, **degrees_freedom**)	=CHIINV (0.05,10)	The critical value of the test level=0.05 in the chi-square distribution with a DF= 10 (18.30703); see Chapter 7
5	**CONFIDENCE** (**alpha**, **standard_dev**, **size**)	=CONFIDENCE (0.05,2.5,50)	Half of the confidence interval width (0.693) from the $\alpha = 0.05$, $S = 2.5$, and $n = 50$ Formula: $Z_{\alpha/2}S/\sqrt{n}$; see Chapter 3
6	**CORREL**(**array1**,**array2**)	=CORREL(A2:A6,B2:B6)	Calculate the Pearson correlation coefficient between A2:A6 and B2:B6
7	**COUNT**(**value1**,value2,...)	=COUNT(A2:A8)	Count the number of numeric cells in the area (excluding blank cells, text, logical values)

(Continued)

Table A2.1 (*Continued*)

Number	Function	Example	Explanation (Result)
8	**COUNTIF(range,criteria)**	=COUNTIF (B2:B5,"> 55")	Calculate the number of cells in the range B2:B5 which values are greater than 55
9	**COVAR (array1,array2)**	=COVAR(A2:A6, B2:B6)	Calculate the covariance, which is the average of the sum of the products of the mean deviation of each pair of data points Formula: $[\Sigma(x-\bar{x})(y-\bar{y})]/n$
10	**DEVSQ (number1**,number2, ...)	=DEVSQ(A2:A8)	Calculate the sum of squares of mean deviation Formula: $\Sigma(x-\bar{x})^2$
11	**FDIST (x,degrees_freedom1, degrees_freedom2)**	=FDIST(15.21,6,4)	Calculate the $P-$value in the F =15.21 with DF1= 6 and DF2=4 (0.01); see Chapter 6
12	**FINV (probability, degrees_freedom1, degrees_freedom2)**	=FINV(0.01,6,4)	Obtain the critical value with the $\alpha = 0.01$ DF1= 6 and DF2= 4 (15.20675) and the inverse function of FDIST; see Chapter 6
13	**FISHER(x)**	=FISHER (0.75)	The normal transformation value of $r = 0.75$ (0.972955); the transformed value can be used to find the confidence interval of the correlation coefficient according to the normal method. Formula: Z =ATANH(r) =0.5ln[(1+r)/(1-r)]
14	**FISHERINV (y)**	=FISHERINV (0.972955)	The transformed value of Z =0.972955 to the correlation coefficient (0.75), The inverse function of FISHER; Formula: r =TANH(Z) = $(e^{2y}-1)/(e^{2y}+1)$

(*Continued*)

Table A2.1 (*Continued*)

Number	Function	Example	Explanation (Result)
15	**FREQUENCY (data_array, bins_array)**	=FREQUENCY (A2:A10,B2:B5)	Obtain a frequency table of continuous variables; A2: A10 is the original data, and B2:B5 is the upper limit of each group of the frequency table; see Chapter 1
16	**GEOMEAN (number1**,number2, . . .)	=GEOMEAN(4,5,8,7,11,4,3)	Calculate the geometric mean of the data (5.476987); see Chapter 1
17	**HARMEAN (number1**,number2, . . .)	=HARMEAN(A2:A8)	Calculates the harmonic mean of the data area A2:A8 (5.028376); see Chapter 1
18	**MAX(number1, number2**, . . .)	=MAX(A2:A6)	Find the maximum value in area A2:A6; see Chapter 1
19	**MEDIAN (number1**,number2, . . .)	=MEDIAN(A2:A7)	Find the median of data A2:A7, see Chapter 1
20	**MIN(number1**, number2, . . .)	=MIN(A2:A6)	Find the minimum value of data A2:A6; see Chapter 1
21	**MODE(number1**, number2, . . .)	=MODE(A2:A7)	Find the mode A9: the number of A7, that is, the most frequently occurring number
22	**NORMDIST** (**x, mean, standard_dev,cumulative**)	=NORMDIST(42,40, 1.5,TRUE)	Calculate the cumulative function of 42 in the normal distribution (40, 1.52) (0.908789); see Chapter 2; Cumulative= 0 or FALSE calculates the probability density function; Cumulative=1 or TRUE to calculate the cumulative distribution function

(*Continued*)

Table A2.1 (*Continued*)

Number	Function	Example	Explanation (Result)
23	**NORMINV (probability,mean,standard_dev)**	=NORMINV (0.908789,40,1.5)	Obtain the inverse function value (or quantile) of the normal distribution cumulative function (42); see Chapter 2
24	**NORMSDIST** (**z**)	=NORMSDIST (1.645)	Obtain a standard normal distribution cumulative function value of 1.645(0.95); see Chapter 2
25	**NORMSINV**(**probability**)	=NORMSINV(0.95)	Obtain the inverse function of NORMSDIST (the standard normal cumulative distribution function); obtain a critical value of P =0.05 (1.645); see Chapter 2
26	**PEARSON** (**array1**,**array2**)	=PEARSON(A2:A6, B2:B6)	Obtain the Pearson correlation coefficient, equal to the CORREL function
27	**PERCENTILE** (**array**, **k**)	=PERCENTILE(A2:A5,0.3)	Find the 30th percentile of the cell area A2:A5
28	**POISSON**(**x**, **mean**, **cumulative**)	=POISSON(2,5, TRUE)	Probability of occurrence of 2 times in a Poisson distribution with a mean of 5 (0.124652); Cumulative=0 or FALSE calculates the probability density function; Cumulative=1 or TRUE calculates the cumulative distribution function; See Chapter 2
29	**RSQ**(**known_y's**, **known_x's**)	=RSQ(A2:A8,B2:B8)	Calculate the determine the coefficient(R^2)

(*Continued*)

Table A2.1 (*Continued*)

Number	Function	Example	Explanation (Result)
30	**STANDARDIZE**(**x**, **mean**, **standard_dev**)	= STANDARDIZE(42, 40,1.5)	Converting the general normal distribution (μ, σ^2) to the standard normal distribution (0, 1^2), (1.333333) Formula: $z = (X - \overline{X})/S$
31	**STDEV**(**number1**, number2, ...)	=STDEV(A2:A11)	Unbiased estimation of the standard deviation of the data in the cell area A2:A11; see Chapter 1
32	**TDIST**(**x**, **degrees_freedom**, **tails**)	=TDIST(1.96,60,2)	Returns the two-sided P value of 1.96 in the t distribution with a degree of freedom of 60 (0.054644927); tails=2, two-sided; tails=1, one-sided; see chapter 5
33	**TINV**(**probability**, **degrees_freedom**)	=TINV(0.054645, 60)	Returns the critical value of $t$distribution with DF= 60 in the P =0.054645 two-sided value (1.959997462)
34	**VAR**(**number1**, number2, ...)	=VAR(A2:A11)	Estimate the variance of the sample of A2:A11 (i.e., the square of the standard deviation); see Chapter 1; Formula: $S^2 = \sum_{i=1}^{n} \frac{(X_i - \bar{X})^2}{n-1}$
35	**VARP**(**number1**, number2, ...)	=VARP(A2:A11)	Estimate the population variance of A2:A11; Formula: $\sigma^2 = \sum_{i=1}^{n} \frac{(X_i - \mu)^2}{n}$

(see Figure A2.3) (note that Excel 2002 or later only has this feature).

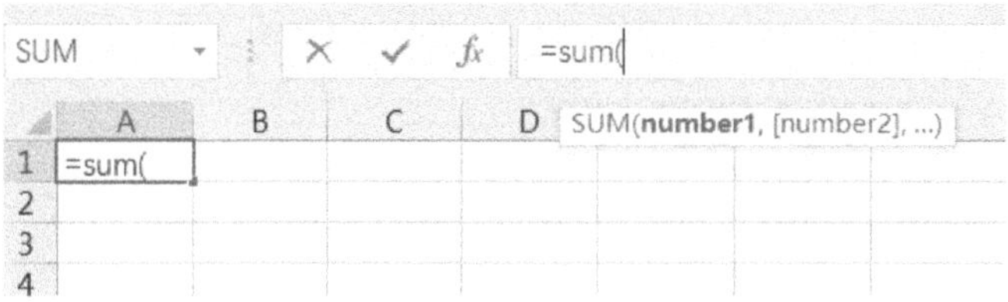

Figure A2.3 Edit bar input function icon

(4) In order to complete the editing of the formula, confirm the entered formula, press Enter or click the "√" button on the left side of the edit bar with the mouse; if you want to cancel the edited formula, click the "×" button in the edit bar.

In the matrix operation, you need to create a formula in multiple cells (that is, a cell area). In order to complete the formula editing, you must input Ctrl + Shift + Enter, instead of Enter.

A2.4. The principle of making computer experiments

Excel drawing function is very powerful, and the figure drawn by Excel after modification is very beautiful. There is a "linkage" relationship between cell data and excel analysis results. If one cell data is changed, the related Excel formula or chart changes accordingly, which has the effect of "change and see". This feature is conducive to making a vivid statistical computer experiment. Most of the computer experiments in this book are based on this principle.

The recent version of Excel "Developer" has been hidden. To make a scroll bar, you need to have "Developer". You can click File → Options → Customize Ribbon, find "Developer" in the lower middle part of the Main Tabs on the right (see Figure A2.4), and select "Developer" in the check box. In the future, it will be convenient to use "Developer" to make computer experiments. Click "Design Mode" in Figure A2.5 to enter the computer experiment program, then edit the computer experiment.

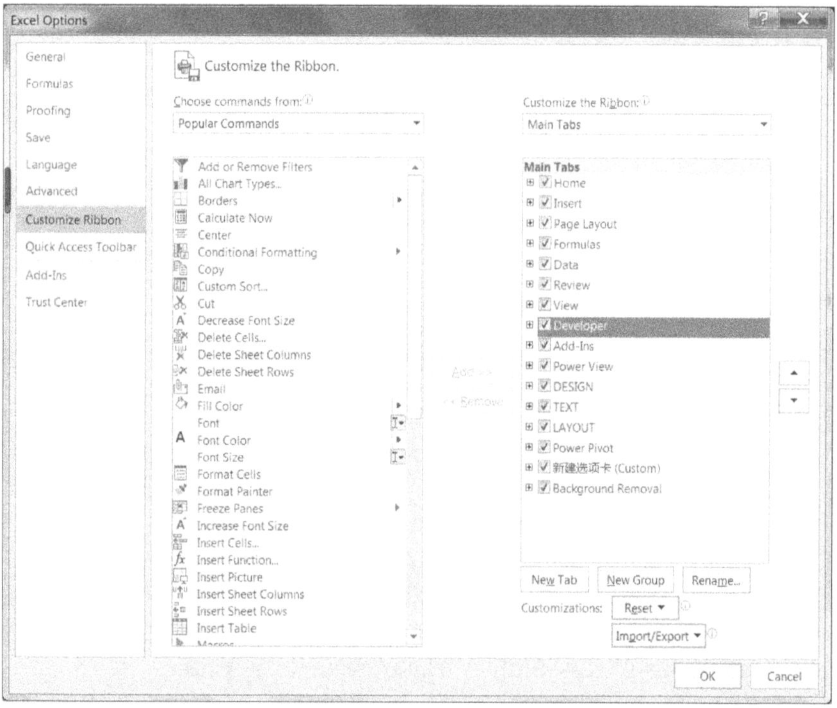

Figure A2.4 Add "Developer" in the main menu of Excel interface

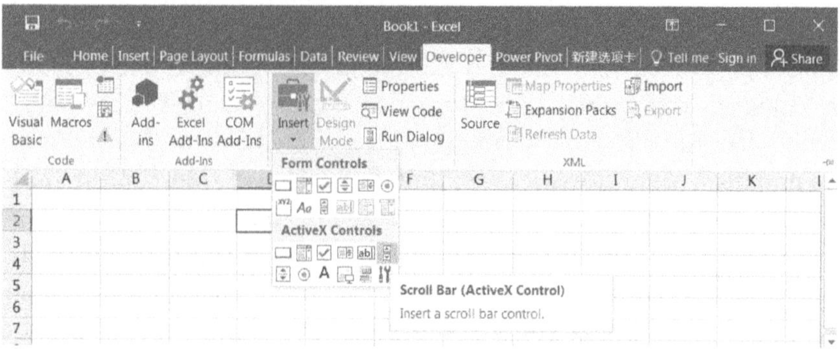

Figure A2.5 Insert such as Scroll Bar in Developer

Chuanhua Yu Yiran Cui

APPENDIX A3

INTRODUCTION TO R LANGUAGE

A3.1. R Introduction

A3.1.1. *What is R?*

R is a software system with the same statistical analysis and mapping functions as statistical software such as SAS and Stata. R is also a computer language that allows users to edit and use other editable tools. It was founded in the early 1990s by Ross Ihak and Robert Gentleman of the University of Auckland, New Zealand. It was derived from John Chambers in the 1970s; Chambers pioneered the development of the S language at Bell Labs. The R language is an interpreted language (sometimes called a scripting language), which means that the code does not need to be compiled before it runs. As a high-level language, R is designed to analyze data faster and more powerfully, and we don't need to know the details of how the code runs on the computer.

R provides a complete mathematical computing environment for data processing, calculation, and presentation, enabling any classic and modern statistical techniques to be flexibly applied. Some of these function codes have been embedded in the basic R language environment, and some of them are provided in the form of packages.

Even users can write their own functions to implement and extend. It is no exaggeration to say that the power of R is not impossible, but only unexpected.

A3.1.2. *R download and installation*

R is an open-source, completely free, and easy to install software that is compatible with different systems such as Windows, Linux, and Mac OS X. The latest version of R and R-based application packages can be downloaded from the official website of the R software (https://www.r-project.org).

After visiting the official website, in the Getting Started form on the home page, click the download R link (or click CRAN on the left). After selecting a recent mirroring, select a link compatible with your operating system in the Download and Install R form at the top of the page. If it's your first time installing R, then select base, then follow the instructions to select and start the download. After the download is complete, double-click the downloaded installation file and select the installation path to install.

A3.1.3. *The running platform of R*

After R is installed, using R under Windows or Mac OS X, a graphical user interface (R GUI) is available (or two, 32-bit or 64-bit, respectively). Double-click to open, you will get the GUI (Figure A3.1); through the R console code, you can run the code.

In addition to the code-running platform above that comes with R, R also has many running platforms, such as: Rstuido, RWinEdt, Rcommander, Tinn-R, etc., each integrated development environment (IDE) platform has its own style and characteristics; these platforms can generally give you a better experience than the platform that comes with R.

A3.1.4. *Getting to know R*

Start R's GUI. You can see the symbol ">" on the console as shown previously. After moving the cursor behind this, you can enter the

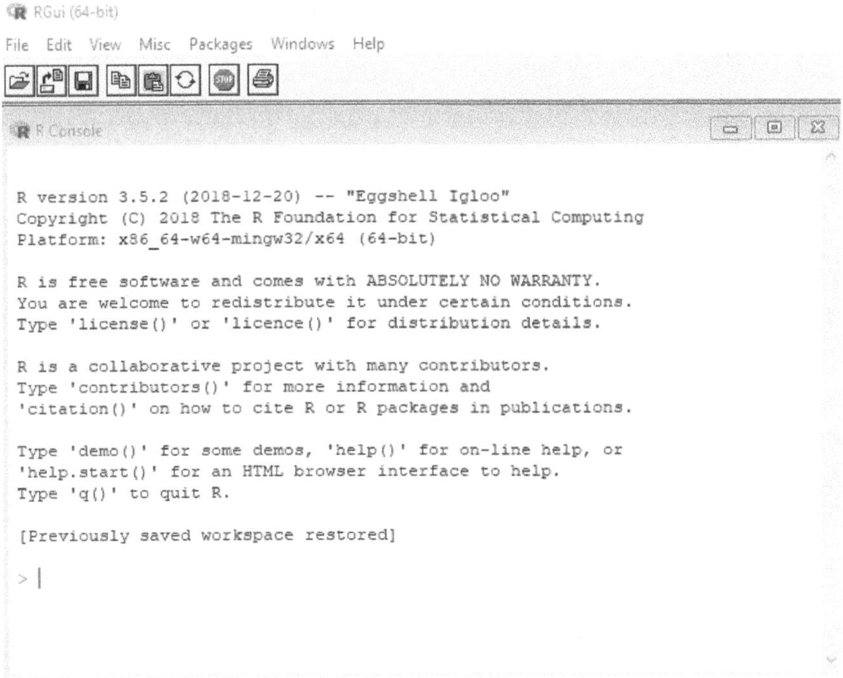

Figure A3.1 The R console Interface

code directly, such as entering $1 + 2$ after it:

```
> 1+2
```

After you press Enter, you can execute the code. Then immediately following the next line of the code, the following will appear:

```
[1] 3
```

This 3 is the result of running $1 + 2$, [1] will be seen in the next section, indicating the first position of the vector.

Through this simple example, you can see how the code of R is executed and easy to understand. The R language is an object-oriented interpretive programming language whose code is executed directly, step by step, without first forming a complete program form (such as SAS: data step and proc step).

The result of the above mentioned "1 + 2" operation can also be stored in:

```
> RES<-1+2
```

After executing the above code, nothing is displayed. The implication is that the operation "1 + 2" and the result is assigned to the object named "RES." Here "<−" is an assignment symbol, or it can be replaced with "=". But note that the assignment symbol in R is "<−", not "=", although most of the time they are equivalent.

The above code creates an object named "RES" and stores it in memory. To display the contents of the RES, enter the name of the object:

```
>RES

[1] 3
```

After pressing Enter, the contents of the RES can be displayed immediately. The function "print" is omitted here. The complete way of writing it should be:

```
>print(RES)

[1] 3
```

A3.1.5. *The object of R*

R is a language for object-oriented operations. There are many types of R objects, such as vectors, matrices, data frames, etc., which can store data, others objects include graphics, functions, environments, and so on. Objects can be purely the same element type, such as each element of the matrix is a numeric type; it can also be a composite image, such as a list object in R, each of which can also be a different type of object.

R objects have two basic properties: mode and length. The pattern categories of vectors are numerical, character, logical, and the like. As in the example below, where the first line of code, the colon function ":" indicates that a sequence of rules with a step size of 1 is generated. "<−" is said earlier, for the assignment of objects, you can also use the function assign; their specific usage can be seen in their help (see the next section). In addition, ";" in R is generally used to separate statements, indicating that there are two different complete statements before and after. The content after the "#" is not executed and is generally used to explain the previous code.

In the following, X and Y are object names. Object naming has the following rules: letters are case sensitive; object names can only be numbers, letters, "." and "_"; must start with a letter or "."; when the object begins with ".", the second character cannot be numbers.

```
>X<-2:5    # Build vector (2,3,4,5), and name it X

>X         # Print display X

[1] 2 3 4 5

>length(X)     # see the length of X

[1] 4

>Y<-X>3;Y      # create vector Y; and print Y

[1] FALSE FALSE  TRUE TRUE

>mode(Y)           # see the mode of Y

[1] "logical"
```

R also has a special type of NULL object, indicating that there is no value, similar to an empty set. In R objects, a class attribute can be used to support programming styles and operations for different types of objects. Some R functions will perform different operations depending on the category. For example, the plot() function may make different types of graphics for different categories of objects.

The currently defined object can also be viewed or deleted:

```
>objects()   #list all the current objects, you can also
               use ls()
```

```
[1] "X" "Y"
```

```
>rm(X)          #delete object X
```

```
>rm(list=ls())  #delete all current objects
```

A3.1.6. *Using help in R*

In learning R, one of the most important is to understand how to use help. There are several ways to use help. First, if you want to know the information of a function or data set, you can type "?" followed by the function name. If you want to find a function, enter two question marks (??) followed by the keywords associated with this function. Search for special characters, keywords, and multiple words requires single or double quotes, e.g:

```
>?lm    # Open the help page for the lm function
>??sum  # Search all subjects that contain " sum "
>?"if"  # Open the help page for if, for branch structure
```

The functions "help" and "help.search" are equivalent to ? and ??, respectively, but the arguments must be enclosed in quotes. The following commands are equivalent to the previous ones:

```
>help("lm")
>help.search("lm")
>help("if")
```

When you look at the help of a function, it will pop up the help page for that function, which details the usage, parameters, and results of the function. You can also use the example function to find related examples directly to better understand how they work:

```
>example(plot)
>demo() # list all displays
```

A3.1.7. *R package*

R packages are functions written for a particular task or a collection of these functions. There are two types of R packages. One is a series of default packages that come with them. This is included when installing the R software, and it is installed by default. If you want to view these packages, click on the RGUI window's package −> Load Packages to view them. It can also be viewed directly under the library folder of the R installation source file.

In addition, R also has a large number of non-self-contained packages; non-self-contained packages need to be manually downloaded and installed. There are many ways to install. The first one is to download the source file of this package and put it in the library folder. The download method is the same as the download of the R installer in A3.1.2 above. After the Download and Install R step, click package and find the package of the corresponding version to download. The second way is by clicking on the RGUI window in the package −> Install Package −> Recent Mirror −> the package you want to download. The third way can be installed directly via the install.packags function:

```
>install.packages(''ggplot2'') # download and install package
                                 ggplot2
```

The package call is also very simple; you can use the load package in the GUI window, or through the following code, checking the package upgrade is also the same:

```
>library(MASS)              # load package MASS
>help(package=MASS)         # check the functions in
                            package MASS by using help
>update.packages (mclust)   # upgrade package mclust
```

A3.1.8. *R working directory and space*

After R starts, it will set a path for the working directory on the local hard disk, through which you can search, read, or save files. By default, the working directory is the installation path for the R software. The getwd() function can be used to view the path of the current working directory. The format is as follows:

```
>getwd()
```

You can also change the current working directory settings

```
>setwd("D\\mydata") # Set the total directory to the D disk
                      mydata folder
```

Note that under the Windows operating system, the slash usage of the file path in R can be "\\" or "/", but not "\". Therefore, the setting of the above working directory is also equivalent to "setwd("D/mydata")." But you can't use "setwd("D/mydata")."

In the directory structure, simple names are usually used, you should avoid the directory name that contains some special characters, such as *, &, $, and so on.

To exit R, click close, or use the command:

```
>q( )
```

Before you exit, R will ask if you want to save the current workspace. If saved, the code currently on the R console will be saved to the current working directory. The next time you use it, you can load the workspace, for example, click File –> Load Workspace.

However, compared to saving the workspace, more often, we recommend saving the R code in a text editor, so as to avoid forgetting how to get different objects defined in the current workspace after a long time. For Text editor, you can click File –> New Program Script, then copy and paste the code, and save it.

A3.2. R data structure

Unlike SAS, etc., R can store data in different categories into the current memory, such as vectors, matrices, arrays, data frames, and so on. This section describes the creation, editing, and more of these different types of data structures.

A3.2.1. *Vector*

A vector is a sequence of elements of the same basic type. Common types are numeric vectors, character vectors, and logical vectors.

1. vector assignment

To create a vector in R, we usually use a connection function c (concatenate) to connect different components. For example, create a vector with the name X and the components are 1.4, –3.6, 0.5, –9.6, and 8.7; the code is:

```
>X<- c(1.4, -3.6, 0.5, -9.6, 8.7)
```

Or:

```
>assign("X", c(1.4, -3.6, 0.5, -9.6, 8.7))
```

You can also create character vectors in the same way:

```
>Y<- c("Cat", "Dog", "Pig", "Cow", "Sheep")
```

One of the great features of the R vector is the ability to name each element. In general, markup elements make the code more readable. You can use name = value to give it a name when you create a vector, or you can just name some elements in a vector and ignore other elements:

```
>names(X)<- Y # Name each component of vector X, corresponding
              to each component of Y
```

It can also be created directly by the vector name of each component when creating a vector:

```
>X<- c(Cat =1.4, Dog =-3.6, Pig =0.5, Cow =-9.6, Sheep =8.7)
```

2. Sequence of rules

As mentioned in Section 1.5, the colon function ":" is used to generate an equal sequence. For example, a:b means to generate a sequence of equalities up to "b" starting from "a" with an interval of 1 (or −1):

```
> 2.31 : 8.5

[1] 2.31 3.31 4.31 5.31 6.31 7.31 8.31

>8.2 : 2.3

[1] 8.2 7.2 6.2 5.2 4.2 3.2
```

In addition to this, there are several other functions that create a more general sequence. Among them, the seq function is the most common and can specify sequences in many different ways. The seq function is used as follows:

```
seq(from = 1, to = 1, by = ((to - from)/(length.out - 1)),
   length.out = NULL)
```

That is, a sequence from the "from" value to the "to" value; the interval step is "by" or the length is "length.out". The parameter values in the above parentheses are the default values:

```
> seq(from = 5, to = 9.4, by=0.5)

[1] 5.0 5.5 6.0 6.5 7.0 7.5 8.0 8.5 9.0

> seq(from = 5, by = 0.5, length.out=10)

[1] 5.0  5.5  6.0  6.5  7.0  7.5  8.0  8.5  9.0  9.5
```

Rep is a repeating function used to generate repeated sequences. The basic usage of the rep function is as follows:

$$\text{rep}(\text{x}, \text{times} = 1, \text{length.out} = \text{NA}, \text{each} = 1)$$

```
>  rep(2:4,times=3)

[1] 2 3 4 2 3 4 2 3 4

> rep(2:4,each=3)

[1] 2 2 2 3 3 3 4 4 4

>  rep(c(0,2),each=3,times=2)

[1] 0 0 0 2 2 2 0 0 0 2 2 2
```

3. Vector calculation

A numeric vector can perform basic operations of adding (+), subtracting (–), multiplying (*), dividing (/), and powering (ˆ), which means that each element of the vector is operated. Some commonly used arithmetic functions can be referred to as follows:

```
(1) Four arithmetic operations: +, -, *, /, ^, %%
    (modulo), %% (divisible)

(2) Rounding: ceiling, floor, round, signif, trunc
```

4. Vector index and subscript

For objects that contain multiple elements in R, such as vectors, matrices, arrays, and data frames, you can use subscripts to access some or all of the objects. This subscript operation is flexible and efficient. The general usage of subscript access is: X[subscript], where X is the object name and the subscript is enclosed in brackets [ ]. There are three types of subscripts: numeric, logical, and character.

The numeric subscript of a vector is the position corresponding to each element of the vector. The first element has a subscript of 1, and the subscript 0 is automatically ignored. The subscript vector of a positive integer value is selected, and the negative integer value is deleted.

```
> X<-rnorm(6);X # Generate 6 standard normal distribution random numbers and assign them to X; print X

[1]-0.7868257-0.4614661 0.1958343 0.1855816 0.1098954-1.5324978

>  X[2]        # Take the second element of X

[1] -0.4614661

>  X[c(2,4)]   # Take the second and fourth elements of X

[1] -0.4614661    0.1855816

>  X[-c(2,4)] # Delete the second and fourth elements of X

[1] -0.7868257 0.1958343 0.1098954 -1.5324978

>  X[2]<- 0 # Change the second element of X to 0

>X

[1] -0.7868257 0.0000000 0.1958343 0.1855816 0.1098954 -1.5324978
```

Logical subscripts are generally used to determine that certain conditions are met. For example, take all the elements of vector X that are greater than 0 in the above example:

```
> X>0

[1] FALSE FALSE TRUE TRUE TRUE FALSE

> X[X>0]

[1] 0.1958343  0.1855816  0.1098954
```

Character subscripts, generally related to the element name, must first define the name of the element, and then access its element or subset through the name of the vector.

A3.2.2. *Matrix and array*

Vectors are one-dimensional data structures, and sometimes you need to build multidimensional data structures. This is an array. A two-dimensional array is called a matrix.

1. Matrix assignment

Matrices are generally created using the matrix function, which has the general form:

```
matrix(data = NA, nrow = 1, ncol = 1, byrow = FALSE, dimnames = NULL))
```

where data is a data vector, nrow is the number of rows in the matrix, and ncol is the number of columns in the matrix. byrow refers to whether to place by row. The default value is FALSE, which is placed by column. dimnames is the name of the row and column of a two-dimensional matrix. For example, construct a 3*4 matrix:

```
>MAT<-matrix(1:12,nrow=3,ncol=4,byrow=T); MAT

        [,1]   [,2]  [,3]   [,4]

[1,]    1       2     3      4
[2,]    5       6     7      8
[3,]    9      10    11     12
```

Note that 1:12 above is the value of the parameter data, where the parameter name is omitted. The parameters of the function in R: when their corresponding parameter values are given in order, their parameter names can be omitted. byrow = T, where T is an abbreviation for TRUE. nrow = 3 and ncol = 4; these two parameters can also be omitted, because the length of data is 12. When the product of the nrow and ncol parameter values is not equal to the length of data, the previous part (less than the length of the data) is taken, or the loop starts from the first element (greater than the length of the data).

For matrices, the dim function returns a vector of integer values for its dimensions, similar to nrow and ncol:

```
> dim(MAT)

[1]  3  4
```

The rows and columns of the matrix also have row names and column names. For historical reasons, there is also a row.names function that works the same as the rownames function. But there is no corresponding col.names function. You can also use the dimnames function to view or define a row or column name directly in a list.

2. Array

A more general array can be defined by the array function, which has the general form of:

$$\text{array}(\text{x}, \text{dim} = \text{length}(\text{x}), \text{dimnames} = \text{NULL})$$

```
> A<-array(1:12,dim=c(2,4,3)); A

, , 1

     [,1] [,2] [,3] [,4]

[1,]    1    3    5    7

[2,]    2    4    6    8

, , 2

     [,1] [,2] [,3] [,4]

[1,]    9   11    1    3

[2,]   10   12    2    4
```

```
,,3

      [,1] [,2] [,3] [,4]

[1,]    5    7    9   11

[2,]    6    8   10   12
```

The above creates a three-dimensional array. When the dim argument is a vector of length 2, the array created at this time is a matrix. Arrays are the same as matrices and have different dimension names.

3. Subscripts of the matrix

Like the subscripts of vectors, matrices and arrays can also use subscripts to implement the selection of submatrices in matrix or modify matrix elements. The difference is that the subscript of the array is multidimensional; the subscript of the matrix is 2D; the first one is the row subscript and the second is the column subscript. The subscript index has the same numerical, logical, and direct use of the original name as the vector. It is perfectly fine to specify index subscripts in different ways in different dimensions. The subscripts for each dimension are separated by commas:

```
> M1<-matrix(round(rnorm(6),2),ncol=3); M1

      [,1]  [,2]  [,3]

[1,] -1.05  0.84  0.50

[2,]  0.23  0.29 -0.57


> M1[1,c(1,3)]

 [1] -1.05  0.50
```

```
> M1[ ,2]   # All elements of the second column
```

[1] 0.84 0.29

```
> M1[,-2]

      [,1] [,2]

[1,] -1.05 0.50

[2,] 0.23 -0.57
```

4. Straightening and splicing of the matrix

The matrix can also be directly converted into a vector, either using the as.vector function or directly using the c function:

```
> as.vector(M1)   # M1 is the matrix defined above

[1] -1.05 0.23 0.84 0.29 0.50 -0.57

> M2<-matrix(1:4,ncol=2)
> c(M1,M2)

2 [1] -1.05 0.23 0.84 0.29 0.50 -0.57 1.00 2.00 3.00 4.00
```

The cbind and rbind functions can be used for splicing different matrices, where the cbind function is spliced by columns, requiring the same number of rows in both matrices. The rbind function is spliced by lines, requiring the same number of columns in both matrices:

```
>   cbind(M1,M2)

      [,1] [,2]  [,3] [,4] [,5]

[1,] -1.05 0.84  0.50  1    3
```

```
[2,]  0.23 0.29 -0.57  2    4
```

```
> rbind(M1,M2)
```

```
Error in rbind(M1, M2) : The number of columns in the matrix
must match (see  arg2)
```

5. Matrix operations

Like the operations in the vector, the arithmetic operators (+, −, *, /) will process the matrix by element in the same way, that is, the arithmetic operations for the elements at the same position. Therefore, this requires that the two matrices of the operation have the same rank:

```
> M1+M2

Error in M1 + M2 : Non-integrated display

> M1[,-3]+M2

        [,1]  [,2]

[1,] -0.05  3.84

[2,]  2.23  4.29
```

The matrix can also do matrix multiplication: %*%, pay attention to the difference from the above arithmetic multiplication *, but also make sure they can operate.

```
>M2%*%M1

        [,1]  [,2]   [,3]

[1,] -0.36  1.71  -1.21

[2,] -1.18  2.84  -1.28
```

For other operations on the matrix, you can refer to the relevant papers, which will not be described in detail here.

A3.2.3. *Data frame*

Data frames are used to store spreadsheet-like data that is structured like a matrix. In R, the structure of the data frame storage data is also the data set most similar to other statistical software such as SAS, SPSS, etc. Each column can be regarded as a variable, and each row can be regarded as a sample.

The variable patterns in different columns of the data frame can be different. This is not the same as a matrix, where each column variable must be the same pattern class. Each column variable of the data frame can be a numeric, character, or logical vector, or a factor or other form.

The function data.frame is used to create a data frame:

```
>Mydata<-data.frame(Name=c("A","B","C"),
Sex=c("M","M","F"), Age=c(24,21,23))
> Mydata

  Name Sex Age 1 A M 24

2   B  M    21

3   C  F    23

> class(Mydata)

[1] "data.frame"
```

Note that in the above example, each line is automatically numbered from 1 to 3, where the number is actually the line name. If any vector entered has a name, the row name is taken from the first vector name. You can also specify a row name with the row.names parameter. Like a matrix, the name of a row can be retrieved or changed later by using the rownames function. Similarly, you can use the colnames and dimnames functions to get or set the names of columns and dimensions, respectively. In fact, almost all functions for matrices can be used on data frames.

The elements of the reference data frame are the same as the element methods of the reference matrix. You can use the subscript vector, you can also use the name vector, or you can use the dollar sign operator $. (The reference to the dollar sign can refer to the list or refer to the third section about the operation of the data frame.)

A3.2.4. *List*

1. List creation

A list is a special kind of data structure in R, which is a collection of different objects. Strictly speaking, a list is like a vector, except that the type of each element can be different. The list is created with the list function and can be specified like the c function in the following format:

$$\text{list}(\text{name1} = \text{object1}, \text{name2} = \text{object2}, ...)$$

Each element in the list, object1, object2, etc., can be any object in R, such as vectors, matrices, data frames, functions, and so on. Even, it can be the list itself. This type of data is called recursion, so it can be seen as a hierarchy. The list is created as follows:

```
> Scores<- data.frame(Math=c(85,90), English=c(75,70))
> Mylist<- list(Name="ZhangSan", Age=17,Scores= Scores)
> Mylist

$Name

  [1] "ZhangSan"

$Age

[1] 17

$Scores
```

```
Math English

1 85 75

2 90 70
```

A list has the same length as a vector, and its length is the number of top elements:

```
> length(Mylist)

[1] 3
```

Similar to a vector but different from a matrix, the list has no dimensions. Therefore, applying the dim, nrow, and ncol functions to the list returns NULL:

```
> dim(Mylist)

NULL
```

Unlike vectors, arithmetic operations have no effect on lists. Since the types of each element can be different, adding or multiplying two lists has no meaning. However, if the elements in the two lists are of the same type, they can be arithmetically operated. In this case, general arithmetic algorithms are applicable.

2. List references

The data reference of the list can be referenced in the format of "list name [[subscript]]," but the list is different from the vector, and only one element can be referenced at a time, such as the usage of [[1:2]] is wrong.

The subscripts of list elements are similar to vectors and are one-dimensional and can be accessed with brackets [ ]:

```
> Mylist [1:2]

$Name
```

```
[1] "ZhangSan"

$Age

[1] 17
```

The above reference is also equivalent to the code: Mylist [−3] or Mylist [c("Name", "Age")]. Note that the list is still a list by accessing the brackets [ ]:

```
> Mylist[3]

$Scores

    Math
   English
 1    85     75
 2    90     70

> class(Mylist[3])

[1] "list"
```

If you want to access the contents of a list element, you can use the double brackets [[ ]]. Here we must pay attention to the difference between single brackets and double brackets:

```
> Mylist[[3]]

    Math
   English
 1    85     75
 2    90     70

> identical(Mylist[3],Mylist[[3]])     # Determine
  if Mylist [3] and Mylist [[3]] are
```

```
  identical
[1] FALSE
```

You can also use the dollar sign $:

```
> Mylist$Scores

    Math
   English
 1   85     75
 2   90     70
```

A3.2.5. *Factor*

In addition to quantitative numerical variables, there are also qualitative categorical variables in the statistics. The categorical variables are divided into ordered and unordered. In R, such variables are uniformly represented by factors. The factor can be generated using the factor( ) function, which is generally used as:

factor(x = character(), levels, labels = levels, exclude = NA, ordered = is.ordered(x))

In the above function, x is generally a character vector; levels are the levels of the factor and can be specified by itself. When not specified, the different values of x are taken; labels are labels for each level; exclude means that a certain level is removed. By default, the missing value is removed; ordered means whether the parameter specified is in order and is generally unordered by default; you can also directly create an ordered factor of the specified order through the ordered function:

```
> Sex <- c("female", "male", "female",
   "male",
   "male", "female", "female", "male")
> Sexf <- factor(Sex)
```

[1] female male female male male female female male male female
Levels: female male

```
> levels(Sexf)   # view factor levels
```

```
[1] "female" "male"
```

```
> factor(Sex,labels=c("F","M"))
```

```
[1] F M  F  M  M  F

      F M Levels: F M
```

```
> factor(Sex,order=T)
```

```
[1] female male female male male female female male
Levels: female < male
```

The gl function makes it easier to generate factors regularly. Its general usage is:

$$\text{gl}(n, k, \text{length} = n^*k, \text{labels} = \text{seq\_len}(n), \text{ordered} = \text{FALSE})$$

In this function, n is the number of levels of the factor to be generated, k is the number of times each level needs to be repeated, "length" is the length of the factor, "labels" is the factor label, by default it is a natural sequence, and "ordered" is whether it is in order.

```
> gl(3,2)
```

```
[1] 1 1 2 2 3 3

Levels: 1 2 3
```

```
> gl(3,2,12)
```

```
 [1] 1 1 2 2 3 3 1 1 2 2 3 3

 Levels: 1 2 3

> gl(3, 2,labels=letters[1:3])

[1] a a b

b c c

Levels:

a b c
```

A3.3. Data operation

The previous section introduced the various data structures in R and how to create a data set. This section will introduce how to directly import data from different data sources and data formats in R and report the analysis results. In fact, R provides a wide range of data import tools, including text data, Excel data, Access data, SPSS data, SAS data, Stata data, web page data, and more. Like the input, R can also be saved as the corresponding various types of data.

A3.3.1. *Input and output of data*

1. Delimited plain text data

The read.table function in R can read and import text data with delimiters. This function reads a file in a tabular format and saves it as a data frame. Each row of the table appears in each row of the file. The syntax is as follows:

read.table(file, options)

In this syntax, "file" is the file name and "options" are options that control how the data is processed. Details can be seen in help.

Read in a text file called "student.txt" that contains basic information about the student's name, gender, and more. The file is opened in the computer. The first few lines are as Figure A3.2:

Name	Sex	Age	Height	Weight
Alice	F	13	56.5	84.0
Becka	F	13	65.3	98.0
Gail	F	14	64.3	90.0
Karen	F	12	56.3	77.0
Kathy	F	12	59.8	84.5

Figure A3.2 The student.txt file

This file can be read in with the following statement:

```
> setwd(''file path'')
> MyClass <- read.table ("student.txt", header=TRUE)
> is.data.frame(MyClass) # Determine if MyClass is a data
  frame

[1] TRUE

> head(MyClass) # Check the first 6 lines of MyClass

   Name  Sex Age Height Weight
1 Alice  F   13   56.5    84.0
2 Becka  F   13   65.3    98.0
3 Gail   F   14   64.3    90.0
4 Karen  F   12   56.3    77.0
5 Kathy  F   12   59.8    84.5
6 Mary   F   15   66.5   112.0
```

Note that you need to set the working directory before reading the file, or directly add the file path before the file name.

This parameter header indicates whether the first line of the file is used as the variable name. If there is no such "header = TRUE" parameter, the default is FALSE, and the first line of the file will be used as a sample.

The function saved as text corresponding to read.table is the write.table function, and its syntax is as follows:

$$\text{write.table(x, file, options)}$$

x is the name of the data variable that needs to be saved. File is the name of the file to save, and don't forget the suffix name. Options are options for some other control options. As with the function read.table, there are a number of additional options for tunable parameters. See help(read.table) for more details.

2. Excel data

The basic functions of R and the built-in package do not directly read the Excel data (suffixed with the name ".xls" or ".xlsx"). Therefore, if you need to directly read the imported Excel data, you need to use some non-self-contained packages, such as RODBC package, xlsx package, etc. For details, you can check its help.

Another way R can read an Excel file is to save the data in Excel as a tab-delimited file and then read it in other ways, such as the read.table function. The most common way to do this is to save the Excel file as a comma-delimited file (csv) and read it with the read.csv function. The basic syntax is as follows:

read.csv(file, header = TRUE, sep = ",", quote = "\"", ...)

Most of its parameters are the same as the read.table function, but note the difference between some of the default parameters between them, such as the read.csv function default header = TRUE. The corresponding function saved as a csv file is write.csv.

3. Other types of data

In addition to reading text data, R can also read data from other software, such as SPSS, SAS, Stata, etc. In the foreign package that comes with R, it contains functions for reading these data. You need to import the foreign package before using it:

```
> library(foreign)
```

Then, if you need to read spss data, you can call the function read.spss. For some other functions, directly view the help of the package.

In addition, R has many other packages that can read various types of data, such as xml data, ArcGIS spatial data, raster image data, or grab dynamic data. Readers can access relevant information as needed.

A3.3.2. *Management and operation of data*

After the function, as is described in the previous section, reads the data, most of it is stored in the form of a data frame. This section describes some simple, practical operations on these data.

1. Checking the data

After importing the data, you may first need to know what variables are in the data frame and what type of data they are. If the sample size is large or there are many variables, you cannot directly print this data by variable name to view it. The str() function can view all the variables and attributes in the data frame, such as the data imported in 3.1.1 MyClass:

```
> str(MyClass)    # View the data structure of MyClass

'data.frame':        15 obs. of     5 variables:

$Name   :Factor w/ 15 levels "Alfred","Alice",..: 2 3 5...

$Sex    :Factor w/ 2 levels "F","M": 1 1 1 1 1 1 1 2 ..

$Age    :int 13 13 14 12 12 15 14 14 14 15 ...

$Height:num 56.5 65.3 64.3 56.3 59.8 66.5 62.8 69 ...

$Weight:num 84 98 90 77 84.5 ...
```

The result shows that there are 15 rows of observations and 5 columns of variables in MyClass, and the types of each variable, as well as partial values, etc., are listed below. Sometimes you can also view some of the data through the head and tail functions:

```
> tail(MyClass,3) # View all data for the last 3 rows

      Name  Sex Age Height Weight

13   John    M  12  59.0    99.5
14 Robert    M  12  64.8   128.0
15 William   M  15  66.5   112.0
```

2. Reference and editing of data

Access to data can be done either by using subscript or by "$." In addition, each variable inside the data frame can be added to the search path of R through the attach function, so that each variable in the data frame can be directly accessed:

```
> Height

Error: object 'Height' not found

> attach(MyClass) # The search path of the connection object
  MyClass to R

> mean(Height) [1] 62.74

> detach(MyClass)
```

When you print Height directly, you will get an error and cannot find Height. But when the attach function adds the variable of the data frame Myclass to the search path of R, it can be found by printing Height. For example, to find the mean of Height, it is 62.74. Of course, before using the attach function, be sure to use a variable name that is unique. Finally, when the call is complete, use the detach function to remove it from the R search path.

In addition, R has a subset function that allows you to select variables and observations that meet different criteria from the data frame.

3. **Sort**

Sorting numeric data by size is often useful. The functions related to sorting in R are sort function, order function, and so on. The sort function syntax is as follows:

$$\text{sort}(x, \text{decreasing} = \text{FALSE}, ...)$$

The sort function returns the result of the x sort directly, and the decreasing parameter specifies whether to sort in ascending or descending order:

```
> sort(MyClass$Weight)

[1] 77.0 83.0 84.0 84.0 84.5 90.0 98.0 99.5 102.5

 [10] 102.5 112.0 112.0 112.5 128.0 133.0
```

If you sort the data box MyClass by weight, you can use the order function, which returns the sorted subscript:

```
> head(MyClass[order(MyClass$Weight),],5)

    Name     Sex   Age   Height    Weight

4   Karen     F    12     56.3      77.0
11  James     M    12     57.3      83.0
1   Alice     F    13     56.5      84.0
12  Jeffrey   M    13     62.5      84.0
5   Kathy     F    12     59.8      84.5
```

A3.4. R programming

A3.4.1. *Loop*

The loop structure repeatedly executes one or a series of statements until a condition is not true. There are three main types of loop structures in R: for, while, and repeat.

1. For loop

For is used to execute a statement repeatedly in a loop until the value of a variable is no longer included in the loop sequence seq. Its syntax is:

for (var in seq) statement

If you have a matrix and ask for the maximum value of each column, you can use a for loop:

```
> Mydata<-matrix(round(rnorm(30),3), ncol=6)
> Mydata

       [,1]   [,2]   [,3]   [,4]   [,5]   [,6]

[1,]  1.034 -0.764 -0.292 -0.935 -1.023  0.029

[2,] -1.684  0.895 -0.237  1.308 -0.007 -1.304

[3,]  0.461 -0.580  0.460 -0.732 -1.400  0.170

[4,] -0.656  1.542  0.666  0.223  0.783  0.765

[5,] -0.096 -0.147 -0.757  1.843  0.640 -1.104

> Colmax<-0
> for (i in 1:6) {Colmax[i]=max(Mydata[,i])}
> Colmax
[1] 1.034 1.542 0.666 1.843 0.783 0.765
```

In the above example for loop statement, the iterator variable i takes each value in 1, 2,..., 6 in order. Then, for each value, the statements in curly braces are executed in order.

It should be noted that when the amount of data is particularly large, the explicit loop for will slow down the running time of the program. In fact, the maximum value of each column of the above matrix can also be replaced by the apply function in R. In the apply family of R, including the functions tapply, sapply, etc., sometimes it is possible to perform some batch operations instead of loops:

```
> apply(Mydata,2,max)
[1] 1.034 1.542 0.666 1.843 0.783 0.765
```

2. While loop

The while loop executes a statement repeatedly until the condition is not true. The syntax is:

while (cond) statement

The while loop first checks the conditional cond of the loop inside the parenthesis. If the condition is true, the "statement" statement is executed; otherwise, the loop is terminated.

For example, generate a standard normal distribution random number such that the sum of its absolute values is less than 10:

```
> A<-0;i<-0
> while (sum(abs(A))<10){i=i+1;A[i]=rnorm(1)}
> round(A,3) # Preserve the 3-digit decimal of vector
    A and print
```

```
[1] -0.763 -0.836 -0.575 0.783 -0.168 -1.838 -2.976 -0.889

[9] 0.777 -0.093 1.209
```

3. Repeat loop

The repeat loop executes a statement repeatedly. In loop, break is usually used to jump out of the loop. Sometimes the next expression is used to enter the next loop in the middle. For details, please refer to other books.

A3.4.2. *Conditions*

In a conditional or branching structure, a statement or set of statements is executed only when a specified condition is met. Conditional execution structures include If or if-else, ifelse, and switch

1. if or if-else structure

The conditional structure if or if-else is the most important branch statement, and its syntax is:

if (*cond*) *statement 1*

if (*cond*) *statement 1* **else** *statement 2*

The above statement executes the statement 1 when the cond in the given parenthesis is true. The following statement states that when cond is true, the statement 1 is executed, otherwise statement 2 is executed.

2. ifelse structure

The cond in the above if-else structure is a scalar logical value. The ifelse structure is a vectorized version of the if-else structure. The syntax is:

ifelse(cond, statement1, statement2)

Cond is a logical vector value. When the "cond [i]" value in parentheses is true, statement 1 [i] is executed; when the "cond [i]" value is false, statement 2 [i] is executed.

3. Switch

In addition to the functions if and ifelse, there is switch function that can also execute select statements. Its syntax is:

switch(expr, ...)

where ... represents a statement that is bound to various possible output values of expr.

A3.4.3. *Function*

The R language itself provides a wealth of function code. In addition to this, R also allows users to construct their own functions, which is one of the biggest advantages of the R language. The code for the R constructor is a function whose general usage is:

```
functionname <-function(arg1, arg2, ...){
               statements
                   }
```

The so-called function, that is, given the input parameter value, the output value is obtained after a certain rule. In the above parentheses, arg1, arg2, etc. are the input parameter values. Through the statement, some values will be returned. These values can be any objects in R, such as vectors, lists, and so on. Functionname is the name of the function, and its reference is exactly the same as the general function. For example, to construct a function that finds the sum of the squares of two numbers and the square root, the code is as follows:

```
> myfunction <- function(x,y)

 {

 sqrt(x ^ 2 + y ^ 2)

 }

> myfunction (x=1,y=3)

[1] 10
```

Note that in general, objects defined inside a function can only be used inside the function. The data type of the returned object is arbitrary, from scalar to list. In fact, this variable is called a local variable. In addition to this, you can define a global variable that can be used outside of the function.

A3.5. R basic statistical method implementation

This section mainly introduces the implementation of the basic statistical methods in R. The specific statistical methods section can refer to the main article section of this book. Here is a brief introduction to the basic function code.

A3.5.1. *Descriptive statistics*

1. Simple statistics

The R language provides a number of functions that can directly calculate simple statistics such as mean, variance, and so on. Here are some common statistic functions:

(1) mean, variance and standard deviation: mean, var, sd;
(2) maximum, minimum and range: max, min, range;
(3) vector elements sum, product, accumulation and multiplication: sum, prod, cumsum, cumprod;
(4) medians, quantiles, and quartiles: meadian, quantile, IQR; and
(5) sort, rank: sort, order, rank (rank).

2. Distribution

The R language provides functions for implementing various distributions in probability theory. The corresponding R code representations and main parameters are as Table A3.1:

Table A3.1 The R code and main parameters for different distributions

Distribution name	R code	The main parameters	Distribution name	R code	The main parameters
Normal distribution	norm	mean,sd	Binomial distribution	binom	size, prob
Index distribution	exp	rate	Geometric distribution	geom	prob
Uniform distribution	unif	min,max	**Poisson distribution**	pois	lambda
Beta distribution	beta	shape1, shape2, ncp	Negative binomial distribution	Binomial	nbinom, size, prob
***t*-distribution**	t	t,df	Hyper geometric distribution	hyper	m,n,k
Chi-square distribution	Chisq	df	Gamma distribution	gamma	shape, scale
***F* distribution**	f	df1, df2	Cauchy distribution	cauchy	location, scale
Webb distribution	weibull	shape, scale	**Logistic distribution**	logis	location, scale
Lognormal	lnorm	meanlog, sdlog	**Wilcox distribution**	wilcox	m,n

By adding a different prefix to each distribution code, there are different functions corresponding to the distribution, each distribution corresponding to four functions:

d+ distribution: density function (density)
p+ distribution: probability distribution function (probability)
q+ distribution: quantile function (quantile)
r+ distribution: random number function (random)

For example:

```
> qt(p=1-0.05/2,df=10) #Find the critical value
  tα/2(10), α=0.05 [1] 2.228139
> runif(5,min=-1,max=1) # Generate 5 uniform random
  numbers between (-1,1)

[1] -0.06774079 0.61414148 0.14107337 -0.09538949 -0.44164047
```

3. Graphics

A major feature of the R language is its powerful graphics-making capabilities, which make it possible to quickly make a variety of visually beautiful graphics of data with simple functions. Currently, the R language mainly has four mature graphics systems, base, grid, lactice, and ggplot. The first three are included in the basic installation of R, but the grid and lactice packages need to be loaded, and ggplot is not included in the basic installation. In, you need to download and install it yourself. This section is a very simple introduction to the drawing in base, most of which are in the graphics package.

The most commonly used advanced drawing function is plot(), which is a generic function that accepts many different classes of objects as its drawing object parameters. Its usual usage is as follows:

$$\text{plot}(x, y = \text{NULL},\ \text{option})$$

x, y are the corresponding two axis variables. If x is a two-column matrix or data frame, then no more y is required, otherwise, both x and y must be numeric vectors. Options are graphical control parameters; see their help for details. For example, based on the data in the variable named MyClass data frame read in Section 3.1, the scatter plot code for height and weight is as Figure A3.3:

```
> attach(MyClass)
> plot(x=Height,y=Weight)
> detach(MyClass)
```

The result will be as follows:

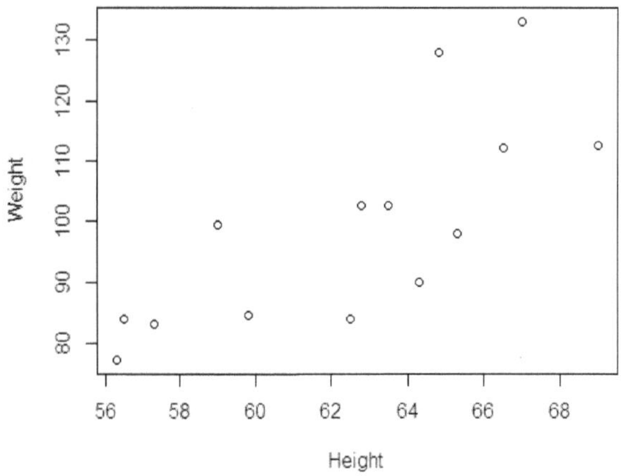

Figure A3.3 The scatter plot of Height and Weight

In addition to the plot function, R has a number of advanced drawing commands, such as:

(1) Histogram, bar chart, and pie chart: hist, barplot, pie
(2) Stem and leaf diagram, box line diagram and violin diagram: stem, boxplot, vioplot
(3) Scatter matrix, matrix and conditional map: pairs, matplot, coplot
(4) Unary function graph and 3D perspective: curve, persp
(5) qq diagram qqplot qqline qqnorm

In addition, R has many low-level mapping commands and graphical interaction functions such as points, lines, polygons, and so on.

A3.5.2. *Hypothesis test*

Hypothesis testing is a commonly used statistical method, and the R language provides a direct function of many different testing methods. A major feature of the R language about the validation function is that it basically contains the string "test." Therefore, we look for all functions that contain tests, and the results are as follows:

```
> apropos("test")
```

```
[1]".valueClassTest"        "ansari.test"            "bartlett.test"
[4]"binom.test"             "Box.test"               "chisq.test"
[7]"cor.test"               "file_test"              "fisher.test"
[10]"fligner.test"          "friedman.test"          "kruskal.test"
[13]"ks.test"               "mantelhaen.test"        "mauchly.test"
[16]"mcnemar.test"          "mood.test"              "oneway.test"
[19]"pairwise.prop.test"    "pairwise.t.test"        "pairwise.wilcox.test"
[22]"poisson.test"          "power.anova.test"       "power.prop.test"
[25]"power.t.test"          "PP.test"                "prop.test"
[28]"prop.trend.test"       "quade.test"             "shapiro.test"
[31]"t.test"                "testInheritedMethods"   "testPlatformEquivalence"
[34]"testVirtual"           "var.test"               "wilcox.test"
```

You can know what the test functions are by looking directly at the name. For example, "t.test" is used for t-test, and "chisq.test" is used for chi-square test. For different types of t-tests, such as single-sample, two-independent samples, etc., just adjust its corresponding parameters.

There is no function code provided directly in R for the normal distribution mean Z-test. The Z-test can be programmed manually or by downloading some other packages.

A3.5.3. *Linear model*

1. Analysis of variance

In the R software, the aov() function performs the calculation of the variance analysis. The basic usage is as follows: aov(formula, data = NULL, projections = FALSE, qr = TRUE, contrasts = NULL, ...); the formula is the model formula (see the next subsection); data is used to specify the variables in the formula; projections are to indicate whether to return the predicted value; qr are to indicate whether to return the QR decomposition; and contrasts are for the comparison of some factors.

For example, if you want to compare the height of students of different ages based on the data in the variable named MyClass data frame in Section 3.1, the code is as follows:

```
> MyClass$Age<-as.factor(MyClass$Age) #Transforming Age into factor
> Res.aov<-aov(Height~Age,data= MyClass)
> summary(Res.aov)
```

```
  Df Sum Sq Mean Sq F value Pr(>F)
Age 3 124.5 41.50 4.241 0.0321*
Residuals 11 107.6 9.78
---
Signif.codes: 0 ,,***" 0.001 ,,**" 0.01 ,,*" 0.05 ,,." 0.1,," 1
```

Among them, "Height∼Age" is a model formula. It should be noted that before the analysis of variance, it is necessary to ensure that the height is a quantitative numerical variable, and the age factor is a qualitative variable. In the original MyClass data frame, Age is a numerical variable, so before the analysis of variance, it is converted into a factor variable.

In addition, regarding the results of the analysis of variance, you can directly print the result "Res.aov" or the summary() function. However, the results of the directly printed analysis of variance do not include the p-value, while you can check the p-value in the summary() function. In the results of the variance analysis above, the p-value is 0.0321.

Multivariate analysis of variance is also an av() function. Now assume that the reaction variable is Y and there are two factors, denoted as F1 and F2, respectively, then:

(1) For formula parameters that have no interaction, they should be written as:

$$\text{formula} = Y \sim \text{F1} + \text{F2}$$

(2) For interacting formula parameters should be written:

$$\text{formula} = Y \sim \text{F1} + \text{F2} + \text{F1} : \text{F2}$$

or:

$$\text{formula} = Y \sim \text{F1} * \text{F2}$$

For the pairwise comparison, or the rank test of multiple sets of comparisons, see the test section in the previous section. For example, "pairwise.t.test" performs a pairwise comparison.

2. Regression analysis

The regression analysis in R uses the lm( ) function, and the generalized regression analysis uses the glm( ) function. The general usage of the lm() function is as follows:

lm (formula, data, options)

Formula is the same as the model formula, data is the sample data, and other parameters can refer to the help of lm. The formula is a formula object in R, which is generally expressed as the dependent variable on the left and the independent variable on the right, separated by "$\sim$" in the middle. Common simple regression formulas are expressed as follows:

(1) $Y \sim X$ or $Y \sim +X$: Represents a linear model, where *1* is the intercept term, or it can be omitted
(2) $Y \sim X_1 + X$: Binary linear model
(3) $Y \sim +X + IX^\wedge 2$ or $Y \sim$ poly $X2$: Quadratic polynomial model

For example, based on the data in the variable named MyClass data frame in Section 3.1, a simple linear regression of height and weight is given as follows:

```
> Res.lm<-lm(Height~Age,data = MyClass)
> summary(Res.lm)

Call:
lm(formula = Height ~ Weight, data = Data.ex1)

Residuals:
   Min      1Q      Median    3Q      Max
-3.6168 -2.2137  -0.0452  2.1603  3.9811

Coefficients:
            Estimate Std.  Error t  value   Pr(>|t|)
(Intercept) 44.23191     4.34547  10.179  1.46e-07***
```

```
Weight      0.18477      0.04282  4.315 0.000839***
---
Signif.codes: 0 ,,***" 0.001 ,,**" 0.01 ,,*" 0.05 ,,." 0.1 ,," 1

Residual standard error: 2.709 on 13 degrees of freedom
Multiple R-squared: 0.5889, Adjusted R-squared:
                    0.5573
F-statistic: 18.62 on 1 and 13 DF, p-value: 0.0008389
```

Through the above result, you can view the estimated value of the coefficient, check the p-value, and determine the coefficient and the model p-value and other information.

The result of regression in R, Res.lm, is essentially a list of lm values with class attribute values. The above results are extracted by the summary() function. In addition to this, there are some general functions that have special operations on lm class objects in order to extract relevant regression results, such as coef (fit coefficient), predict, and residuals.

References

[1] Zuur, AF, Ieno, EN, Meesters, EHWG. *A Beginner's Guide to R*. Springer; 2009.
[2] Cotton, R. *Learning R*. O'Reilly Media; 2013.
[3] Kabacoff, RI. *R in Action: Data Analysis and Graphics with R*. Manning Publications; 2015.

Songbo Hu

Appendix C

Statistical Tables

APPENDIX C1

FREQUENTLY USED TABLES

Table C1.1 Standard normal distribution

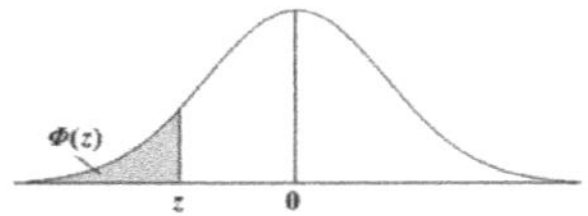

z	0.00	0.01	0.02	0.03	0.04	0.05	0.06	0.07	0.08	0.09
−3.0	0.00135	0.00131	0.00126	0.00122	0.00118	0.00114	0.00111	0.00107	0.00104	0.00100
−2.9	0.00187	0.00181	0.00175	0.00169	0.00164	0.00159	0.00154	0.00149	0.00144	0.00139
−2.8	0.00256	0.00248	0.00240	0.00233	0.00226	0.00219	0.00212	0.00205	0.00199	0.00193
−2.7	0.00347	0.00336	0.00326	0.00317	0.00307	0.00298	0.00289	0.00280	0.00272	0.00264
−2.6	0.00466	0.00453	0.00440	0.00427	0.00415	0.00402	0.00391	0.00379	0.00368	0.00357
−2.5	0.00621	0.00604	0.00587	0.00570	0.00554	0.00539	0.00523	0.00508	0.00494	0.00480
−2.4	0.00820	0.00798	0.00776	0.00755	0.00734	0.00714	0.00695	0.00676	0.00657	0.00639
−2.3	0.01072	0.01044	0.01017	0.00990	0.00964	0.00939	0.00914	0.00889	0.00866	0.00842
−2.2	0.01390	0.01355	0.01321	0.01287	0.01255	0.01222	0.01191	0.01160	0.01130	0.01101
−2.1	0.01786	0.01743	0.01700	0.01659	0.01618	0.01578	0.01539	0.01500	0.01463	0.01426
−2.0	0.02275	0.02222	0.02169	0.02118	0.02068	0.02018	0.01970	0.01923	0.01876	0.01831
−1.9	0.02872	0.02807	0.02743	0.02680	0.02619	0.02559	0.02500	0.02442	0.02385	0.02330
−1.8	0.03593	0.03515	0.03438	0.03362	0.03288	0.03216	0.03144	0.03074	0.03005	0.02938
−1.7	0.04457	0.04363	0.04272	0.04182	0.04093	0.04006	0.03920	0.03836	0.03754	0.03673
−1.6	0.05480	0.05370	0.05262	0.05155	0.05050	0.04947	0.04846	0.04746	0.04648	0.04551
−1.5	0.06681	0.06552	0.06426	0.06301	0.06178	0.06057	0.05938	0.05821	0.05705	0.05592

Table C1.1 (*Continued*)

z	0.00	0.01	0.02	0.03	0.04	0.05	0.06	0.07	0.08	0.09
−1.4	0.08076	0.07927	0.07780	0.07636	0.07493	0.07353	0.07215	0.07078	0.06944	0.06811
−1.3	0.09680	0.09510	0.09342	0.09176	0.09012	0.08851	0.08691	0.08534	0.08379	0.08226
−1.2	0.11507	0.11314	0.11123	0.10935	0.10749	0.10565	0.10383	0.10204	0.10027	0.09853
−1.1	0.13567	0.13350	0.13136	0.12924	0.12714	0.12507	0.12302	0.12100	0.11900	0.11702
−1.0	0.15866	0.15625	0.15386	0.15151	0.14917	0.14686	0.14457	0.14231	0.14007	0.13786
−0.9	0.18406	0.18141	0.17879	0.17619	0.17361	0.17106	0.16853	0.16602	0.16354	0.16109
−0.8	0.21186	0.20897	0.20611	0.20327	0.20045	0.19766	0.19489	0.19215	0.18943	0.18673
−0.7	0.24196	0.23885	0.23576	0.23270	0.22965	0.22663	0.22363	0.22065	0.21770	0.21476
−0.6	0.27425	0.27093	0.26763	0.26435	0.26109	0.25785	0.25463	0.25143	0.24825	0.24510
−0.5	0.30854	0.30503	0.30153	0.29806	0.29460	0.29116	0.28774	0.28434	0.28096	0.27760
−0.4	0.34458	0.34090	0.33724	0.33360	0.32997	0.32636	0.32276	0.31918	0.31561	0.31207
−0.3	0.38209	0.37828	0.37448	0.37070	0.36693	0.36317	0.35942	0.35569	0.35197	0.34827
−0.2	0.42074	0.41683	0.41294	0.40905	0.40517	0.40129	0.39743	0.39358	0.38974	0.38591
−0.1	0.46017	0.45620	0.45224	0.44828	0.44433	0.44038	0.43644	0.43251	0.42858	0.42465
0.0	0.50000	0.49601	0.49202	0.48803	0.48405	0.48006	0.47608	0.47210	0.46812	0.46414

Table C1.2 Critical values for the t-test

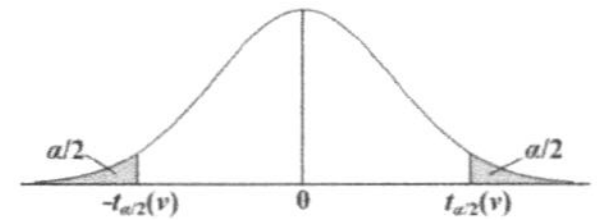

Degrees of freedom	α										
	One-tailed	0.25	0.20	0.10	0.05	0.025	0.010	0.005	0.0025	0.001	0.0005
ν	Two-tailed	0.50	0.40	0.20	0.10	0.050	0.020	0.010	0.0050	0.002	0.0010
1		1.00000	1.37638	3.07768	6.31375	12.70620	31.82052	63.65674	127.32134	318.30884	636.61925
2		0.81650	1.06066	1.88562	2.91999	4.30265	6.96456	9.92484	14.08905	22.32712	31.59905
3		0.76489	0.97847	1.63774	2.35336	3.18245	4.54070	5.84091	7.45332	10.21453	12.92398
4		0.74070	0.94096	1.53321	2.13185	2.77645	3.74695	4.60409	5.59757	7.17318	8.61030
5		0.72669	0.91954	1.47588	2.01505	2.57058	3.36493	4.03214	4.77334	5.89343	6.86883
6		0.71756	0.90570	1.43976	1.94318	2.44691	3.14267	3.70743	4.31683	5.20763	5.95882
7		0.71114	0.89603	1.41492	1.89458	2.36462	2.99795	3.49948	4.02934	4.78529	5.40788
8		0.70639	0.88889	1.39682	1.85955	2.30600	2.89646	3.35539	3.83252	4.50079	5.04131
9		0.70272	0.88340	1.38303	1.83311	2.26216	2.82144	3.24984	3.68966	4.29681	4.78091
10		0.69981	0.87906	1.37218	1.81246	2.22814	2.76377	3.16927	3.58141	4.14370	4.58689
11		0.69745	0.87553	1.36343	1.79588	2.20099	2.71808	3.10581	3.49661	4.02470	4.43698
12		0.69548	0.87261	1.35622	1.78229	2.17881	2.68100	3.05454	3.42844	3.92963	4.31779

Table C1.2 (*Continued*)

Degrees of freedom		α									
	One-tailed	0.25	0.20	0.10	0.05	0.025	0.010	0.005	0.0025	0.001	0.0005
ν	Two-tailed	0.50	0.40	0.20	0.10	0.050	0.020	0.010	0.0050	0.002	0.0010
13		0.69383	0.87015	1.35017	1.77093	2.16037	2.65031	3.01228	3.37247	3.85198	4.22083
14		0.69242	0.86805	1.34503	1.76131	2.14479	2.62449	2.97684	3.32570	3.78739	4.14045
15		0.69120	0.86624	1.34061	1.75305	2.13145	2.60248	2.94671	3.28604	3.73283	4.07277
16		0.69013	0.86467	1.33676	1.74588	2.11991	2.58349	2.92078	3.25199	3.68615	4.01500
17		0.68920	0.86328	1.33338	1.73961	2.10982	2.56693	2.89823	3.22245	3.64577	3.96513
18		0.68836	0.86205	1.33039	1.73406	2.10092	2.55238	2.87844	3.19657	3.61048	3.92165
19		0.68762	0.86095	1.32773	1.72913	2.09302	2.53948	2.86093	3.17372	3.57940	3.88341
20		0.68695	0.85996	1.32534	1.72472	2.08596	2.52798	2.84534	3.15340	3.55181	3.84952
21		0.68635	0.85907	1.32319	1.72074	2.07961	2.51765	2.83136	3.13521	3.52715	3.81928
22		0.68581	0.85827	1.32124	1.71714	2.07387	2.50832	2.81876	3.11882	3.50499	3.79213
23		0.68531	0.85753	1.31946	1.71387	2.06866	2.49987	2.80734	3.10400	3.48496	3.76763
24		0.68485	0.85686	1.31784	1.71088	2.06390	2.49216	2.79694	3.09051	3.46678	3.74540
25		0.68443	0.85624	1.31635	1.70814	2.05954	2.48511	2.78744	3.07820	3.45019	3.72514
26		0.68404	0.85567	1.31497	1.70562	2.05553	2.47863	2.77871	3.06691	3.43500	3.70661
27		0.68368	0.85514	1.31370	1.70329	2.05183	2.47266	2.77068	3.05652	3.42103	3.68959
28		0.68335	0.85465	1.31253	1.70113	2.04841	2.46714	2.76326	3.04693	3.40816	3.67391
29		0.68304	0.85419	1.31143	1.69913	2.04523	2.46202	2.75639	3.03805	3.39624	3.65941
30		0.68276	0.85377	1.31042	1.69726	2.04227	2.45726	2.75000	3.02980	3.38518	3.64596
31		0.68249	0.85337	1.30946	1.69552	2.03951	2.45282	2.74404	3.02212	3.37490	3.63346

(*Continued*)

Table C1.2 (*Continued*)

Degrees of freedom	α										
	One-tailed	0.25	0.20	0.10	0.05	0.025	0.010	0.005	0.0025	0.001	0.0005
ν	Two-tailed	0.50	0.40	0.20	0.10	0.050	0.020	0.010	0.0050	0.002	0.0010
32		0.68223	0.85300	1.30857	1.69389	2.03693	2.44868	2.73848	3.01495	3.36531	3.62180
33		0.68200	0.85265	1.30774	1.69236	2.03452	2.44479	2.73328	3.00824	3.35634	3.61091
34		0.68177	0.85232	1.30695	1.69092	2.03224	2.44115	2.72839	3.00195	3.34793	3.60072
35		0.68156	0.85201	1.30621	1.68957	2.03011	2.43772	2.72381	2.99605	3.34005	3.59115
36		0.68137	0.85172	1.30551	1.68830	2.02809	2.43449	2.71948	2.99049	3.33262	3.58215
37		0.68118	0.85144	1.30485	1.68709	2.02619	2.43145	2.71541	2.98524	3.32563	3.57367
38		0.68100	0.85118	1.30423	1.68595	2.02439	2.42857	2.71156	2.98029	3.31903	3.56568
39		0.68083	0.85094	1.30364	1.68488	2.02269	2.42584	2.70791	2.97561	3.31279	3.55812
40		0.68067	0.85070	1.30308	1.68385	2.02108	2.42326	2.70446	2.97117	3.30688	3.55097
41		0.68052	0.85048	1.30254	1.68288	2.01954	2.42080	2.70118	2.96696	3.30127	3.54418
42		0.68038	0.85026	1.30204	1.68195	2.01808	2.41847	2.69807	2.96296	3.29595	3.53775
43		0.68024	0.85006	1.30155	1.68107	2.01669	2.41625	2.69510	2.95916	3.29089	3.53163
44		0.68011	0.84987	1.30109	1.68023	2.01537	2.41413	2.69228	2.95553	3.28607	3.52580
45		0.67998	0.84968	1.30065	1.67943	2.01410	2.41212	2.68959	2.95208	3.28148	3.52025
46		0.67986	0.84951	1.30023	1.67866	2.01290	2.41019	2.68701	2.94878	3.27710	3.51496
47		0.67975	0.84934	1.29982	1.67793	2.01174	2.40835	2.68456	2.94563	3.27291	3.50990
48		0.67964	0.84917	1.29944	1.67722	2.01063	2.40658	2.68220	2.94262	3.26891	3.50507
49		0.67953	0.84902	1.29907	1.67655	2.00958	2.40489	2.67995	2.93973	3.26508	3.50044

Table C1.2 (Continued)

Degrees of freedom		α									
	One-tailed	0.25	0.20	0.10	0.05	0.025	0.010	0.005	0.0025	0.001	0.0005
ν	Two-tailed	0.50	0.40	0.20	0.10	0.050	0.020	0.010	0.0050	0.002	0.0010
50		0.67943	0.84887	1.29871	1.67591	2.00856	2.40327	2.67779	2.93696	3.26141	3.49601
60		0.67860	0.84765	1.29582	1.67065	2.00030	2.39012	2.66028	2.91455	3.23171	3.46020
70		0.67801	0.84679	1.29376	1.66691	1.99444	2.38081	2.64790	2.89873	3.21079	3.43501
80		0.67757	0.84614	1.29222	1.66412	1.99006	2.37387	2.63869	2.88697	3.19526	3.41634
90		0.67723	0.84563	1.29103	1.66196	1.98667	2.36850	2.63157	2.87788	3.18327	3.40194
100		0.67695	0.84523	1.29007	1.66023	1.98397	2.36422	2.62589	2.87065	3.17374	3.39049
120		0.67654	0.84463	1.28865	1.65765	1.97993	2.35782	2.61742	2.85986	3.15954	3.37345
140		0.67625	0.84420	1.28763	1.65581	1.97705	2.35328	2.61140	2.85221	3.14947	3.36138
160		0.67603	0.84387	1.28687	1.65443	1.97490	2.34988	2.60691	2.84649	3.14195	3.35237
180		0.67586	0.84362	1.28627	1.65336	1.97323	2.34724	2.60342	2.84205	3.13612	3.34540
200		0.67572	0.84342	1.28580	1.65251	1.97190	2.34514	2.60063	2.83851	3.13148	3.33984
220		0.67561	0.84326	1.28541	1.65181	1.97081	2.34342	2.59836	2.83562	3.12769	3.33530
240		0.67551	0.84312	1.28509	1.65123	1.96990	2.34199	2.59647	2.83322	3.12454	3.33152
260		0.67543	0.84301	1.28482	1.65074	1.96913	2.34078	2.59487	2.83119	3.12187	3.32834
280		0.67537	0.84291	1.28458	1.65031	1.96847	2.33974	2.59350	2.82945	3.11959	3.32561
300		0.67531	0.84282	1.28438	1.64995	1.96790	2.33884	2.59232	2.82795	3.11762	3.32325
500		0.67498	0.84234	1.28325	1.64791	1.96472	2.33383	2.58570	2.81955	3.10661	3.31009
1000		0.67474	0.84198	1.28240	1.64638	1.96234	2.33008	2.58075	2.81328	3.09840	3.30028
∞		0.67449	0.84163	1.28157	1.64488	1.96001	2.32642	2.57593	2.80716	3.09040	3.29072

Table C1.3 Confidence interval for the population proportion

Upperline: 95% CI Lower line: 99% CI

	x													
n	0	1	2	3	4	5	6	7	8	9	10	11	12	13
1	0–98													
	0–100													
2	0–84	1–99												
	0–93	0–100												
3	0–71	1–91	9–99											
	0–83	0–96	4–100											
4	0–60	1–81	7–93											
	0–73	0–89	3–97											
5	0–52	1–72	5–82	15–95										
	0–65	0–81	2–92	8–98										
6	0–46	0–64	4–78	12–88										
	0–59	0–75	2–86	7–93										
7	0–41	0–58	4–71	10–82	18–90									
	0–53	0–68	2–80	6–88	12–94									
8	0–37	0–53	3–65	9–76	16–84									
	0–48	0–63	1–74	5–83	10–90									
9	0–34	0–48	3–60	7–70	14–79	21–86								
	0–45	0–59	1–69	4–78	9–85	15–91								
10	0–31	0–45	3–56	7–65	12–74	19–81								
	0–41	0–54	1–65	4–74	8–81	13–87								
11	0–28	0–41	2–52	6–61	11–69	17–77	23–83							
	0–38	0–51	1–61	3–69	7–77	11–83	17–89							
12	0–26	0–38	2–48	5–57	10–65	15–72	21–79							
	0–36	0–48	1–57	3–66	6–73	10–79	15–85							

n	x = 0	1	2	3	4	5	6	7	8	9	10	11	12	13
13	0–25	0–36	2–45	5–54	9–61	14–68	19–75	25–81						
	0–34	0–45	1–54	3–62	6–69	9–76	14–81	19–86						
14	0–23	0–34	2–43	5–51	8–58	13–65	18–71	23–77						
	0–32	0–42	1–51	3–59	5–66	9–72	13–78	17–83						
15	0–22	0–32	2–41	4–48	8–55	12–62	16–68	21–73	27–79					
	0–30	0–40	1–49	2–56	5–63	8–69	12–74	16–79	21–84					
16	0–21	0–30	2–38	4–46	7–52	11–59	15–65	20–70	25–75					
	0–28	0–38	1–46	2–53	5–60	8–66	11–71	15–76	19–81					
17	0–20	0–29	2–36	4–43	7–50	10–56	14–62	18–67	23–72	28–77				
	0–27	0–36	1–44	2–51	4–57	7–63	10–69	14–74	18–78	22–82				
18	0–19	0–27	1–35	4–41	6–48	10–54	13–59	17–64	22–69	26–74				
	0–26	0–35	1–42	2–49	4–55	7–61	10–66	13–71	17–75	21–79				
19	0–18	0–26	1–33	3–40	6–46	9–51	13–57	16–62	20–67	24–71	29–76			
	0–24	0–33	1–40	2–47	4–53	6–58	9–63	12–68	16–73	19–77	23–81			
20	0–17	0–25	1–32	3–38	6–44	9–49	12–54	15–59	19–64	23–69	27–73			
	0–23	0–32	1–39	2–45	4–51	6–56	9–61	11–66	15–70	18–74	22–78			
21	0–16	0–24	1–30	3–36	5–42	8–47	11–52	15–57	18–62	22–66	26–70	30–74		
	0–22	0–30	1–37	2–43	3–49	6–54	8–59	11–63	14–68	17–71	21–76	24–80		
22	0–15	0–23	1–29	3–35	5–40	8–45	11–50	14–55	17–59	21–64	24–68	28–72		
	0–21	0–29	1–36	2–42	3–47	5–52	8–57	10–61	13–66	16–70	20–73	23–77		
23	0–15	0–22	1–28	3–34	5–39	8–44	10–48	13–53	16–57	20–62	23–66	27–69	31–73	
	0–21	0–28	1–35	2–40	3–45	5–50	7–55	10–59	13–63	15–67	19–71	22–75	25–78	
24	0–14	0–21	1–27	3–32	5–37	7–42	10–47	13–51	16–55	19–59	22–63	26–67	29–71	
	0–20	0–27	0–33	2–39	3–44	5–49	7–53	9–57	12–61	15–65	18–69	21–73	24–76	
25	0–14	0–20	1–26	3–31	5–36	7–41	9–45	12–49	15–54	18–58	21–61	24–65	28–69	31–72
	0–19	0–26	0–32	1–37	3–42	5–47	7–51	9–56	11–60	14–63	17–67	20–71	23–74	26–77

(*Continued*)

Table C1.3 (*Continued*)

	x													
n	0	1	2	3	4	5	6	7	8	9	10	11	12	13
26	0–13	0–20	1–25	2–30	4–35	7–39	9–44	12–48	14–52	17–56	20–60	23–63	27–67	30–70
	0–18	0–25	0–31	1–36	3–41	4–46	6–50	9–54	11–58	13–62	16–65	19–69	22–72	25–75
27	0–13	0–19	1–24	2–29	4–34	6–38	9–42	11–46	14–50	17–54	19–58	22–61	26–65	29–68
	0–18	0–25	0–30	1–35	3–40	4–44	6–48	8–52	10–56	13–60	15–63	18–67	21–70	24–73
28	0–12	0–18	1–24	2–28	4–33	6–37	8–41	11–45	13–49	16–52	19–56	22–59	25–63	28–66
	0–17	0–24	0–29	1–34	3–39	4–43	6–47	8–51	10–55	12–58	15–62	17–65	20–68	23–71
29	0–12	0–18	1–23	2–27	4–32	6–36	8–40	10–44	13–47	15–51	18–54	21–58	24–61	26–64
	0–17	0–23	0–28	1–33	2–37	4–42	6–46	8–49	10–53	12–57	14–60	17–63	19–66	22–70
30	0–12	0–17	1–22	2–27	4–31	6–35	8–39	10–42	12–46	15–49	17–53	20–56	23–59	26–63
	0–16	0–22	0–27	1–32	2–36	4–40	5–44	7–48	9–52	11–55	14–58	16–62	19–65	21–68
31	0–11	0–17	1–22	2–26	4–30	6–34	8–38	10–41	12–45	14–48	17–51	19–55	22–58	25–61
	0–16	0–22	0–27	1–31	2–35	4–39	5–43	7–47	9–50	11–54	13–57	16–60	18–63	20–66
32	0–11	0–16	1–21	2–25	4–29	5–33	7–36	9–40	12–43	14–47	16–50	19–53	21–56	24–59
	0–15	0–21	0–26	1–30	2–34	4–38	5–42	7–46	9–49	11–52	13–56	15–59	17–62	20–65
33	0–11	0–15	1–20	2–24	3–28	5–32	7–36	9–39	11–42	13–46	16–49	18–52	20–55	23–58
	0–15	0–20	0–25	1–30	2–34	3–37	5–41	7–44	8–48	10–51	12–54	14–57	17–60	19–63
34	0–10	0–15	1–19	2–23	3–28	5–31	7–35	9–38	11–41	13–44	15–48	17–51	20–54	22–56
	0–14	0–20	0–25	1–29	2–33	3–36	5–40	6–43	8–47	10–50	12–53	14–56	16–59	18–62
35	0–10	0–15	1–19	2–23	3–27	5–30	7–34	8–37	10–40	13–43	15–46	17–49	19–52	22–55
	0–14	0–20	0–24	1–28	2–32	3–35	5–39	6–42	8–45	10–49	12–52	14–55	16–57	18–60
36	0–10	0–15	1–18	2–22	3–26	5–29	6–33	8–36	10–39	12–42	14–45	16–48	19–51	21–54
	0–14	0–19	0–23	1–27	2–31	3–35	5–38	6–41	8–44	9–47	11–50	13–53	15–56	17–59
37	0–10	0–14	1–18	2–22	3–25	5–28	6–32	8–35	10–38	12–41	14–44	16–47	18–50	20–53
	0–13	0–18	0–23	1–27	2–30	3–34	4–37	6–40	7–43	9–46	11–49	13–52	15–55	17–58
38	0–10	0–14	1–18	2–21	3–25	5–28	6–32	8–34	10–37	11–40	13–43	15–46	18–49	20–51
	0–13	0–18	0–22	1–26	2–30	3–33	4–36	6–39	7–42	9–45	11–48	12–51	14–54	16–56

Table C1.3 (*Continued*)

	x													
n	0	1	2	3	4	5	6	7	8	9	10	11	12	13
39	0–9	0–14	1–17	2–21	3–24	4–27	6–31	8–33	9–36	11–39	13–42	15–45	17–48	19–50
	0–13	0–18	0–21	1–25	2–29	3–32	4–35	6–38	7–41	9–44	10–47	12–50	14–53	16–55
40	0–9	0–13	1–17	2–21	3–24	4–27	6–30	8–33	9–35	11–38	13–41	15–44	17–47	19–49
	0–12	0–17	0–21	1–25	2–28	3–32	4–35	5–38	7–40	9–43	10–46	12–49	13–52	15–54
41	0–9	0–13	1–17	2–20	3–23	4–26	6–29	7–32	9–35	11–37	12–40	14–43	16–46	18–48
	0–12	0–17	0–21	1–24	2–28	3–31	4–34	5–37	7–40	8–42	10–45	11–48	13–50	15–53
42	0–9	0–13	1–16	2–20	3–23	4–26	6–28	7–31	9–35	10–37	12–39	14–42	16–45	18–47
	0–12	0–17	0–20	1–24	2–27	3–30	4–33	5–36	7–39	8–42	9–44	11–47	13–49	15–52
43	0–9	0–12	1–16	2–19	3–23	4–25	5–28	7–31	8–33	10–36	12–39	14–41	15–44	17–45
	0–12	0–16	0–20	1–23	2–26	3–30	4–33	5–35	6–38	8–41	9–43	11–46	13–49	14–51
44	0–9	0–12	1–15	2–19	3–22	4–25	5–28	7–30	8–33	10–35	11–38	13–40	15–43	17–45
	0–11	0–16	0–19	1–23	2–26	3–29	4–32	5–35	6–37	8–40	9–42	11–45	12–47	14–50
45	0–8	0–12	1–15	2–18	3–21	4–24	5–27	7–30	8–32	9–34	11–37	13–39	15–42	16–44
	0–11	0–15	0–19	1–22	2–25	3–28	4–31	5–34	6–37	8–39	9–42	10–44	12–47	14–49
46	0–8	0–12	1–15	2–18	3–21	4–24	5–26	7–29	8–31	9–34	11–36	13–39	14–41	16–43
	0–11	0–15	0–19	1–22	2–25	3–28	4–31	5–33	6–36	7–39	9–41	10–43	12–46	13–48
47	0–8	0–12	1–15	2–17	3–20	4–23	6–26	6–28	8–31	9–34	11–36	12–38	14–40	16–43
	0–11	0–15	0–18	1–21	2–24	2–27	3–30	5–33	6–35	7–38	9–40	10–42	11–45	13–47
48	0–8	0–11	1–14	2–17	3–20	4–22	5–25	6–28	8–30	9–33	11–35	12–37	14–39	15–42
	0–10	0–14	0–18	1–21	2–24	2–27	3–29	5–32	6–35	7–37	8–40	10–42	11–44	13–47
49	0–8	0–11	1–14	2–17	2–20	4–22	5–25	6–27	7–30	9–32	10–35	12–37	13–39	15–41
	0–10	0–14	0–17	1–20	1–24	2–26	3–29	4–32	6–34	7–36	8–39	9–41	11–44	12–16
50	0–7	0–11	1–14	2–17	2–19	3–22	5–24	6–26	7–29	9–31	10–34	11–36	13–38	15–41
	0–10	0–14	0–17	1–20	1–23	2–26	3–28	4–31	5–33	7–36	8–38	9–40	11–43	12–45

(*Continued*)

Table C1.3 (*Continued*)

n	x: 14	15	16	17	18	19	20	21	22	23	24	25
27	32–71											
	27–76											
28	31–69											
	26–74											
29	30–68	33–71										
	25–72	28–75										
30	28–66	31–69										
	24–71	27–74										
31	27–64	30–67	33–70									
	23–69	26–72	28–75									
32	26–62	29–65	32–68									
	22–67	25–70	27–73									
33	26–61	28–64	31–67	34–69								
	21–66	24–69	26–71	29–74								
34	25–59	27–62	30–65	32–68								
	21–64	23–67	25–70	28–72								
35	24–58	26–61	29–63	31–66	34–69							
	20–63	22–66	24–68	27–71	29–73							
36	23–57	26–59	28–62	30–65	33–67							
	19–62	22–64	23–67	26–69	28–72							
37	23–55	25–58	27–61	30–63	32–66	34–68						
	19–60	21–63	23–65	25–68	28–70	30–73						
38	22–54	24–57	26–59	29–62	31–64	33–67						
	18–59	20–61	22–64	25–66	27–69	29–71						

Table C1.3 (*Continued*)

	x											
n	14	15	16	17	18	19	20	21	22	23	24	25
39	21–53	23–55	26–58	28–60	30–63	32–65	35–68					
	18–58	20–60	22–63	24–65	26–68	28–70	30–72					
41	21–52	23–54	25–57	27–59	29–62	32–64	34–66					
	17–57	19–59	21–61	23–64	25–66	27–68	30–71					
42	20–51	22–53	24–56	26–58	29–60	31–63	33–65	35–67				
	17–55	19–58	21–60	23–63	25–65	27–67	29–69	31–71				
42	20–50	22–52	24–54	26–57	28–59	30–61	32–64	34–66				
	16–54	18–57	20–59	22–61	24–64	26–66	28–67	30–70				
43	19–49	21–51	23–53	25–56	27–58	29–60	31–62	33–65	36–67			
	16–53	18–56	19–58	21–60	23–62	25–65	27–66	29–69	31–71			
44	19–48	21–50	22–52	24–55	26–57	28–59	30–61	33–63	35–65			
	15–52	17–55	19–57	21–59	23–61	25–63	26–65	28–68	30–70			
45	18–47	20–49	22–51	24–54	26–56	28–58	30–60	32–62	34–64	36–66		
	15–51	17–54	19–56	20–58	22–60	24–62	26–64	28–66	30–68	32–70		
46	18–46	20–48	21–50	23–53	25–55	27–57	29–59	31–61	33–63	35–65		
	15–50	16–53	18–55	20–57	22–59	23–61	25–63	27–65	29–67	31–69		
47	18–45	19–47	21–49	23–52	25–54	26–56	28–58	30–60	32–62	34–64	36–66	
	14–19	16–52	18–54	19–56	21–58	23–60	25–62	26–64	28–66	30–68	32–70	
48	17–44	19–46	21–48	22–51	24–53	26–53	28–57	30–59	31–61	33–63	35–65	
	14–49	16–51	17–53	19–55	21–27	22–59	24–61	26–63	28–65	29–67	31–69	
49	17–43	18–45	20–47	22–50	24–52	25–54	27–56	29–58	31–60	33–62	34–64	36–66
	14–48	15–50	17–52	19–54	20–56	22–58	23–60	25–62	27–64	29–66	31–68	32–70
50	16–43	18–45	20–47	21–49	23–51	25–53	26–55	28–57	30–59	32–61	34–63	36–65
	14–47	15–49	17–51	18–53	20–55	21–57	23–59	25–61	26–63	28–65	30–67	32–68

(Continued)

Table C1.3 (*Continued*)

	n							n				
x	50	60	70	80	90	100	x	60	70	80	90	100
1	0–11	0–9	0–8	0–7	0–6	0–5	26	31–57	26–49	22–44	20–39	18–36
	0–14	0–12	0–10	0–9	0–8	0–7		27–61	23–53	20–48	17–43	16–39
2	0–14	1–11	0–10	1–9	0–8	0–7	27	32–58	27–51	24–45	21–40	19–37
	0–17	0–14	0–13	0–11	0–10	0–9		29–62	24–55	21–49	18–44	16–40
3	1–17	1–14	1–12	1–11	1–10	1–8	28	34–60	29–52	25–46	22–42	20–38
	1–20	1–17	1–15	1–13	0–12	0–10		30–64	25–56	22–50	19–45	17–41
4	2–19	2–16	2–14	2–13	1–11	1–10	29	35–62	30–54	26–48	23–43	20–39
	1–23	1–20	1–17	1–15	1–14	1–12		32–65	27–57	23–51	20–46	18–42
5	3–22	3–18	3–16	2–14	2–13	2–11	30	37–63	31–55	27–49	24–44	21–40
	2–26	2–22	2–19	1–17	1–15	1–13		33–67	28–59	24–53	21–47	19–43
6	5–24	4–20	3–18	3–16	3–14	2–12	31		33–57	28–50	25–45	22–41
	3–29	3–24	2–21	2–19	2–17	2–14			29–60	25–45	22–49	20–44
7	6–27	5–23	4–20	4–17	3–15	3–14	32		34–58	29–51	26–46	23–42
	4–31	4–26	3–23	3–21	2–18	2–16			30–62	26–55	23–50	21–45
8	7–29	6–25	5–21	5–19	4–17	4–15	33		35–59	31–53	27–47	24–43
	6–33	4–29	4–25	3–22	3–20	3–17			32–63	27–56	24–51	21–46
9	9–31	7–26	6–23	5–20	5–18	4–16	34		36–61	32–54	28–48	25–44
	7–36	5–30	5–27	4–24	4–21	3–18			33–64	28–58	25–52	22–47
10	10–34	8–29	7–25	6–22	6–20	5–18	35		38–62	33–55	29–50	26–45
	8–38	7–32	6–28	5–25	4–22	4–19			34–66	30–59	26–53	23–48
11	12–36	10–30	8–26	7–23	6–21	5–19	36			34–56	30–51	27–46
	10–40	8–34	7–30	6–21	5–24	4–20				31–60	27–54	24–49
12	13–38	11–32	9–28	8–25	7–22	6–20	37			35–58	31–52	28–47
	11–43	9–36	7–32	6–28	6–25	5–21				32–61	28–55	25–50

Table C1.3 (*Continued*)

	n							n				
x	50	60	70	80	90	100	x	60	70	80	90	100
13	15–41	12–34	10–30	9–26	8–23	7–21	38			36–59	32–53	29–48
	12–45	10–38	8–33	7–30	6–27	6–23				33–62	29–56	26–51
14	16–43	13–36	11–31	10–27	9–25	8–22	39			37–60	33–54	29–49
	14–47	11–40	9–35	8–31	7–28	6–24				34–64	30–57	27–52
15	18–44	15–38	13–33	11–29	10–26	9–24	40			39–61	34–55	30–50
	15–49	12–42	10–37	9–33	8–30	7–26				35–65	31–59	28–53
16	20–46	16–40	14–34	12–30	11–27	9–25	41				35–56	31–51
	17–51	14–44	11–38	10–34	9–31	8–27					32–60	29–54
17	21–48	18–41	15–36	13–32	12–28	10–26	42				36–57	32–52
	18–53	15–46	12–40	11–35	10–32	9–29					33–61	30–55
18	23–50	19–43	16–37	14–33	12–30	11–27	43				37–59	33–53
	20–55	16–47	14–41	12–37	10–33	9–30					34–62	30–56
19	25–53	20–45	17–38	15–34	13–31	12–28	44				38–60	34–54
	21–57	17–49	15–43	13–38	11–35	10–31					35–63	31–57
20	27–55	22–47	18–40	16–36	14–32	13–29	45				39–61	35–55
	23–59	19–51	16–44	14–39	12–36	11–32					36–64	32–58
21	28–57	23–49	20–41	17–37	15–33	14–30	46					36–56
	24–61	20–52	17–46	15–41	13–37	12–33						33–59
22	30–59	25–50	21–43	18–39	16–35	14–31	47					37–57
	26–63	22–54	18–47	16–48	14–38	12–34						34–60
23	32–61	26–52	22–46	19–40	17–36	15–32	48					38–58
	28–65	23–56	19–49	17–44	15–39	13–35						35–61
24	34–63	28–53	23–46	20–41	18–37	16–33	49					39–59
	29–67	24–58	21–50	18–45	16–41	14–36						36–62
25	36–64	29–55	25–48	21–43	19–38	17–35	50					40–60
	31–69	26–59	22–52	19–46	17–42	15–38						37–63

Table C1.4 χ^2 distribution

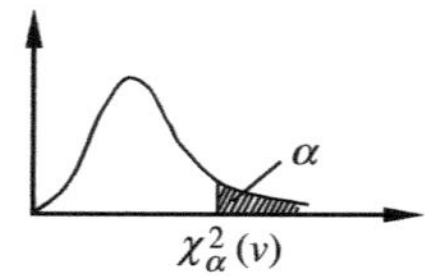

Degrees of freedom ν	α 0.995	0.990	0.975	0.950	0.900	0.750	0.500	0.250	0.100	0.050	0.025	0.010	0.005
1	0.000	0.000	0.001	0.004	0.016	0.102	0.455	1.323	2.706	3.841	5.024	6.635	7.879
2	0.010	0.020	0.051	0.103	0.211	0.575	1.386	2.773	4.605	5.991	7.378	9.210	10.597
3	0.072	0.115	0.216	0.352	0.584	1.213	2.366	4.108	6.251	7.815	9.348	11.345	12.838
4	0.207	0.297	0.484	0.711	1.064	1.923	3.357	5.385	7.779	9.488	11.143	13.277	14.860
5	0.412	0.554	0.831	1.145	1.610	2.675	4.351	6.626	9.236	11.070	12.833	15.086	16.750
6	0.676	0.872	1.237	1.635	2.204	3.455	5.348	7.841	10.645	12.592	14.449	16.812	18.548
7	0.989	1.239	1.690	2.167	2.833	4.255	6.346	9.037	12.017	14.067	16.013	18.475	20.278
8	1.344	1.646	2.180	2.733	3.490	5.071	7.344	10.219	13.362	15.507	17.535	20.090	21.955
9	1.735	2.088	2.700	3.325	4.168	5.899	8.343	11.389	14.684	16.919	19.023	21.666	23.589
10	2.156	2.558	3.247	3.940	4.865	6.737	9.342	12.549	15.987	18.307	20.483	23.209	25.188
11	2.603	3.053	3.816	4.575	5.578	7.584	10.341	13.701	17.275	19.675	21.920	24.725	26.757
12	3.074	3.571	4.404	5.226	6.304	8.438	11.340	14.845	18.549	21.026	23.337	26.217	28.300
13	3.565	4.107	5.009	5.892	7.042	9.299	12.340	15.984	19.812	22.362	24.736	27.688	29.819
14	4.075	4.660	5.629	6.571	7.790	10.165	13.339	17.117	21.064	23.685	26.119	29.141	31.319
15	4.601	5.229	6.262	7.261	8.547	11.037	14.339	18.245	22.307	24.996	27.488	30.578	32.801
16	5.142	5.812	6.908	7.962	9.312	11.912	15.338	19.369	23.542	26.296	28.845	32.000	34.267

Table C1.4 (*Continued*)

Degrees of freedom ν	α												
	0.995	0.990	0.975	0.950	0.900	0.750	0.500	0.250	0.100	0.050	0.025	0.010	0.005
17	5.697	6.408	7.564	8.672	10.085	12.792	16.338	20.489	24.769	27.587	30.191	33.409	35.718
18	6.265	7.015	8.231	9.390	10.865	13.675	17.338	21.605	25.989	28.869	31.526	34.805	37.156
19	6.844	7.633	8.907	10.117	11.651	14.562	18.338	22.718	27.204	30.144	32.852	36.191	38.582
20	7.434	8.260	9.591	10.851	12.443	15.452	19.337	23.828	28.412	31.410	34.170	37.566	39.997
21	8.034	8.897	10.283	11.591	13.240	16.344	20.337	24.935	29.615	32.671	35.479	38.932	41.401
22	8.643	9.542	10.982	12.338	14.041	17.240	21.337	26.039	30.813	33.924	36.781	40.289	42.796
23	9.260	10.196	11.689	13.091	14.848	18.137	22.337	27.141	32.007	35.172	38.076	41.638	44.181
24	9.886	10.856	12.401	13.848	15.659	19.037	23.337	28.241	33.196	36.415	39.364	42.980	45.559
25	10.520	11.524	13.120	14.611	16.473	19.939	24.337	29.339	34.382	37.652	40.646	44.314	46.928
26	11.160	12.198	13.844	15.379	17.292	20.843	25.336	30.435	35.563	38.885	41.923	45.642	48.290
27	11.808	12.879	14.573	16.151	18.114	21.749	26.336	31.528	36.741	40.113	43.195	46.963	49.645
28	12.461	13.565	15.308	16.928	18.939	22.657	27.336	32.620	37.916	41.337	44.461	48.278	50.993
29	13.121	14.256	16.047	17.708	19.768	23.567	28.336	33.711	39.087	42.557	45.722	49.588	52.336
30	13.787	14.953	16.791	18.493	20.599	24.478	29.336	34.800	40.256	43.773	46.979	50.892	53.672
31	14.458	15.655	17.539	19.281	21.434	25.390	30.336	35.887	41.422	44.985	48.232	52.191	55.003
32	15.134	16.362	18.291	20.072	22.271	26.304	31.336	36.973	42.585	46.194	49.480	53.486	56.328
33	15.815	17.074	19.047	20.867	23.110	27.219	32.336	38.058	43.745	47.400	50.725	54.776	57.648
34	16.501	17.789	19.806	21.664	23.952	28.136	33.336	39.141	44.903	48.602	51.966	56.061	58.964
35	17.192	18.509	20.569	22.465	24.797	29.054	34.336	40.223	46.059	49.802	53.203	57.342	60.275
36	17.887	19.233	21.336	23.269	25.643	29.973	35.336	41.304	47.212	50.998	54.437	58.619	61.581
37	18.586	19.960	22.106	24.075	26.492	30.893	36.336	42.383	48.363	52.192	55.668	59.893	62.883
38	19.289	20.691	22.878	24.884	27.343	31.815	37.335	43.462	49.513	53.384	56.896	61.162	64.181
39	19.996	21.426	23.654	25.695	28.196	32.737	38.335	44.539	50.660	54.572	58.120	62.428	65.476
40	20.707	22.164	24.433	26.509	29.051	33.660	39.335	45.616	51.805	55.758	59.342	63.691	66.766

(*Continued*)

Table C1.4 (*Continued*)

Degrees of freedom ν	α												
	0.995	0.990	0.975	0.950	0.900	0.750	0.500	0.250	0.100	0.050	0.025	0.010	0.005
41	21.421	22.906	25.215	27.326	29.907	34.585	40.335	46.692	52.949	56.942	60.561	64.950	68.053
42	22.138	23.650	25.999	28.144	30.765	35.510	41.335	47.766	54.090	58.124	61.777	66.206	69.336
43	22.859	24.398	26.785	28.965	31.625	36.436	42.335	48.840	55.230	59.304	62.990	67.459	70.616
44	23.584	25.148	27.575	29.787	32.487	37.363	43.335	49.913	56.369	60.481	64.201	68.710	71.893
45	24.311	25.901	28.366	30.612	33.350	38.291	44.335	50.985	57.505	61.656	65.410	69.957	73.166
46	25.041	26.657	29.160	31.439	34.215	39.220	45.335	52.056	58.641	62.830	66.617	71.201	74.437
47	25.775	27.416	29.956	32.268	35.081	40.149	46.335	53.127	59.774	64.001	67.821	72.443	75.704
48	26.511	28.177	30.755	33.098	35.949	41.079	47.335	54.196	60.907	65.171	69.023	73.683	76.969
49	27.249	28.941	31.555	33.930	36.818	42.010	48.335	55.265	62.038	66.339	70.222	74.919	78.231
50	27.991	29.707	32.357	34.764	37.689	42.942	49.335	56.334	63.167	67.505	71.420	76.154	79.490
51	28.735	30.475	33.162	35.600	38.560	43.874	50.335	57.401	64.295	68.669	72.616	77.386	80.747
52	29.481	31.246	33.968	36.437	39.433	44.808	51.335	58.468	65.422	69.832	73.810	78.616	82.001
53	30.230	32.018	34.776	37.276	40.308	45.741	52.335	59.534	66.548	70.993	75.002	79.843	83.253
54	30.981	32.793	35.586	38.116	41.183	46.676	53.335	60.600	67.673	72.153	76.192	81.069	84.502
55	31.735	33.570	36.398	38.958	42.060	47.610	54.335	61.665	68.796	73.311	77.380	82.292	85.749
56	32.490	34.350	37.212	39.801	42.937	48.546	55.335	62.729	69.919	74.468	78.567	83.513	86.994
57	33.248	35.131	38.027	40.646	43.816	49.482	56.335	63.793	71.040	75.624	79.752	84.733	88.236
58	34.008	35.913	38.844	41.492	44.696	50.419	57.335	64.857	72.160	76.778	80.936	85.950	89.477
59	34.770	36.698	39.662	42.339	45.577	51.356	58.335	65.919	73.279	77.931	82.117	87.166	90.715
60	35.534	37.485	40.482	43.188	46.459	52.294	59.335	66.981	74.397	79.082	83.298	88.379	91.952
61	36.301	38.273	41.303	44.038	47.342	53.232	60.335	68.043	75.514	80.232	84.476	89.591	93.186
62	37.068	39.063	42.126	44.889	48.226	54.171	61.335	69.104	76.630	81.381	85.654	90.802	94.419
63	37.838	39.855	42.950	45.741	49.111	55.110	62.335	70.165	77.745	82.529	86.830	92.010	95.649

Table C1.4 (*Continued*)

Degrees of freedom ν	α												
	0.995	0.990	0.975	0.950	0.900	0.750	0.500	0.250	0.100	0.050	0.025	0.010	0.005
64	38.610	40.649	43.776	46.595	49.996	56.050	63.335	71.225	78.860	83.675	88.004	93.217	96.878
65	39.383	41.444	44.603	47.450	50.883	56.990	64.335	72.285	79.973	84.821	89.177	94.422	98.105
66	40.158	42.240	45.431	48.305	51.770	57.931	65.335	73.344	81.085	85.965	90.349	95.626	99.330
67	40.935	43.038	46.261	49.162	52.659	58.872	66.335	74.403	82.197	87.108	91.519	96.828	100.554
68	41.713	43.838	47.092	50.020	53.548	59.814	67.335	75.461	83.308	88.250	92.689	98.028	101.776
69	42.494	44.639	47.924	50.879	54.438	60.756	68.334	76.519	84.418	89.391	93.856	99.228	102.996
70	43.275	45.442	48.758	51.739	55.329	61.698	69.334	77.577	85.527	90.531	95.023	100.425	104.215
71	44.058	46.246	49.592	52.600	56.221	62.641	70.334	78.634	86.635	91.670	96.189	101.621	105.432
72	44.843	47.051	50.428	53.462	57.113	63.585	71.334	79.690	87.743	92.808	97.353	102.816	106.648
73	45.629	47.858	51.265	54.325	58.006	64.528	72.334	80.747	88.850	93.945	98.516	104.010	107.862
74	46.417	48.666	52.103	55.189	58.900	65.472	73.334	81.803	89.956	95.081	99.678	105.202	109.074
75	47.206	49.475	52.942	56.054	59.795	66.417	74.334	82.858	91.061	96.217	100.839	106.393	110.286
76	47.997	50.286	53.782	56.920	60.690	67.362	75.334	83.913	92.166	97.351	101.999	107.583	111.495
77	48.788	51.097	54.623	57.786	61.586	68.307	76.334	84.968	93.270	98.484	103.158	108.771	112.704
78	49.582	51.910	55.466	58.654	62.483	69.252	77.334	86.022	94.374	99.617	104.316	109.958	113.911
79	50.376	52.725	56.309	59.522	63.380	70.198	78.334	87.077	95.476	100.749	105.473	111.144	115.117
80	51.172	53.540	57.153	60.391	64.278	71.145	79.334	88.130	96.578	101.879	106.629	112.329	116.321
81	51.969	54.357	57.998	61.261	65.176	72.091	80.334	89.184	97.680	103.010	107.783	113.512	117.524
82	52.767	55.174	58.845	62.132	66.076	73.038	81.334	90.237	98.780	104.139	108.937	114.695	118.726
83	53.567	55.993	59.692	63.004	66.976	73.985	82.334	91.289	99.880	105.267	110.090	115.876	119.927
84	54.368	56.813	60.540	63.876	67.876	74.933	83.334	92.342	100.980	106.395	111.242	117.057	121.126
85	55.170	57.634	61.389	64.749	68.777	75.881	84.334	93.394	102.079	107.522	112.393	118.236	122.325
86	55.973	58.456	62.239	65.623	69.679	76.829	85.334	94.446	103.177	108.648	113.544	119.414	123.522
87	56.777	59.279	63.089	66.498	70.581	77.777	86.334	95.497	104.275	109.773	114.693	120.591	124.718

(*Continued*)

Table C1.4 (*Continued*)

Degrees of freedom ν	α 0.995	0.990	0.975	0.950	0.900	0.750	0.500	0.250	0.100	0.050	0.025	0.010	0.005
88	57.582	60.103	63.941	67.373	71.484	78.726	87.334	96.548	105.372	110.898	115.841	121.767	125.913
89	58.389	60.928	64.793	68.249	72.387	79.675	88.334	97.599	106.469	112.022	116.989	122.942	127.106
90	59.196	61.754	65.647	69.126	73.291	80.625	89.334	98.650	107.565	113.145	118.136	124.116	128.299
91	60.005	62.581	66.501	70.003	74.196	81.574	90.334	99.700	108.661	114.268	119.282	125.289	129.491
92	60.815	63.409	67.356	70.882	75.100	82.524	91.334	100.750	109.756	115.390	120.427	126.462	130.681
93	61.625	64.238	68.211	71.760	76.006	83.474	92.334	101.800	110.850	116.511	121.571	127.633	131.871
94	62.437	65.068	69.068	72.640	76.912	84.425	93.334	102.850	111.944	117.632	122.715	128.803	133.059
95	63.250	65.898	69.925	73.520	77.818	85.376	94.334	103.899	113.038	118.752	123.858	129.973	134.247
96	64.063	66.730	70.783	74.401	78.725	86.327	95.334	104.948	114.131	119.871	125.000	131.141	135.433
97	64.878	67.562	71.642	75.282	79.633	87.278	96.334	105.997	115.223	120.990	126.141	132.309	136.619
98	65.694	68.396	72.501	76.164	80.541	88.229	97.334	107.045	116.315	122.108	127.282	133.476	137.803
99	66.510	69.230	73.361	77.046	81.449	89.181	98.334	108.093	117.407	123.225	128.422	134.642	138.987
100	67.328	70.065	74.222	77.929	82.358	90.133	99.334	109.141	118.498	124.342	129.561	135.807	140.169

Table C1.5-1 F-distribution

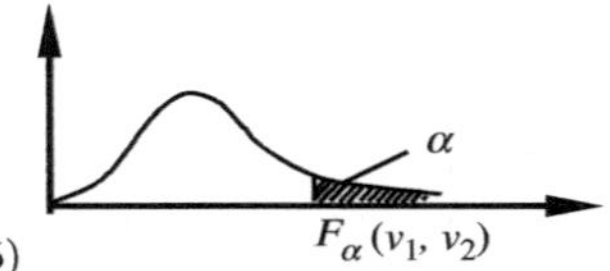

(analysis of variance, α for one-tailed, $\alpha = 0.05$)

Degrees of freedom denominator ν_2	Degrees of freedom, numerator ν_1											
	1	2	3	4	5	6	7	8	9	10	11	12
1	161.4476	199.5000	215.7073	224.5832	230.1619	233.9860	236.7684	238.8827	240.5433	241.8817	242.9835	243.9060
2	18.5128	19.0000	19.1643	19.2468	19.2964	19.3295	19.3532	19.3710	19.3848	19.3959	19.4050	19.4125
3	10.1280	9.5521	9.2766	9.1172	9.0135	8.9406	8.8867	8.8452	8.8123	8.7855	8.7633	8.7446
4	7.7086	6.9443	6.5914	6.3882	6.2561	6.1631	6.0942	6.0410	5.9988	5.9644	5.9358	5.9117
5	6.6079	5.7861	5.4095	5.1922	5.0503	4.9503	4.8759	4.8183	4.7725	4.7351	4.7040	4.6777
6	5.9874	5.1433	4.7571	4.5337	4.3874	4.2839	4.2067	4.1468	4.0990	4.0600	4.0274	3.9999
7	5.5914	4.7374	4.3468	4.1203	3.9715	3.8660	3.7870	3.7257	3.6767	3.6365	3.6030	3.5747
8	5.3177	4.4590	4.0662	3.8379	3.6875	3.5806	3.5005	3.4381	3.3881	3.3472	3.3130	3.2839
9	5.1174	4.2565	3.8625	3.6331	3.4817	3.3738	3.2927	3.2296	3.1789	3.1373	3.1025	3.0729
10	4.9646	4.1028	3.7083	3.4780	3.3258	3.2172	3.1355	3.0717	3.0204	2.9782	2.9430	2.9130
11	4.8443	3.9823	3.5874	3.3567	3.2039	3.0946	3.0123	2.9480	2.8962	2.8536	2.8179	2.7876
12	4.7472	3.8853	3.4903	3.2592	3.1059	2.9961	2.9134	2.8486	2.7964	2.7534	2.7173	2.6866
13	4.6672	3.8056	3.4105	3.1791	3.0254	2.9153	2.8321	2.7669	2.7144	2.6710	2.6347	2.6037
14	4.6001	3.7389	3.3439	3.1122	2.9582	2.8477	2.7642	2.6987	2.6458	2.6022	2.5655	2.5342
15	4.5431	3.6823	3.2874	3.0556	2.9013	2.7905	2.7066	2.6408	2.5876	2.5437	2.5068	2.4753
16	4.4940	3.6337	3.2389	3.0069	2.8524	2.7413	2.6572	2.5911	2.5377	2.4935	2.4564	2.4247
17	4.4513	3.5915	3.1968	2.9647	2.8100	2.6987	2.6143	2.5480	2.4943	2.4499	2.4126	2.3807
18	4.4139	3.5546	3.1599	2.9277	2.7729	2.6613	2.5767	2.5102	2.4563	2.4117	2.3742	2.3421
19	4.3807	3.5219	3.1274	2.8951	2.7401	2.6283	2.5435	2.4768	2.4227	2.3779	2.3402	2.3080
20	4.3512	3.4928	3.0984	2.8661	2.7109	2.5990	2.5140	2.4471	2.3928	2.3479	2.3100	2.2776

(*Continued*)

Table C1.5-1 (*Continued*)

Degrees of freedom denominator	Degrees of freedom, numerator ν_1											
ν_2	1	2	3	4	5	6	7	8	9	10	11	12
21	4.3248	3.4668	3.0725	2.8401	2.6848	2.5727	2.4876	2.4205	2.3660	2.3210	2.2829	2.2504
22	4.3009	3.4434	3.0491	2.8167	2.6613	2.5491	2.4638	2.3965	2.3419	2.2967	2.2585	2.2258
23	4.2793	3.4221	3.0280	2.7955	2.6400	2.5277	2.4422	2.3748	2.3201	2.2747	2.2364	2.2036
24	4.2597	3.4028	3.0088	2.7763	2.6207	2.5082	2.4226	2.3551	2.3002	2.2547	2.2163	2.1834
25	4.2417	3.3852	2.9912	2.7587	2.6030	2.4904	2.4047	2.3371	2.2821	2.2365	2.1979	2.1649
26	4.2252	3.3690	2.9752	2.7426	2.5868	2.4741	2.3883	2.3205	2.2655	2.2197	2.1811	2.1479
27	4.2100	3.3541	2.9604	2.7278	2.5719	2.4591	2.3732	2.3053	2.2501	2.2043	2.1655	2.1323
28	4.1960	3.3404	2.9467	2.7141	2.5581	2.4453	2.3593	2.2913	2.2360	2.1900	2.1512	2.1179
29	4.1830	3.3277	2.9340	2.7014	2.5454	2.4324	2.3463	2.2783	2.2229	2.1768	2.1379	2.1045
30	4.1709	3.3158	2.9223	2.6896	2.5336	2.4205	2.3343	2.2662	2.2107	2.1646	2.1256	2.0921
31	4.1596	3.3048	2.9113	2.6787	2.5225	2.4094	2.3232	2.2549	2.1994	2.1532	2.1141	2.0805
32	4.1491	3.2945	2.9011	2.6684	2.5123	2.3991	2.3127	2.2444	2.1888	2.1425	2.1033	2.0697
33	4.1393	3.2849	2.8916	2.6589	2.5026	2.3894	2.3030	2.2346	2.1789	2.1325	2.0933	2.0595
34	4.1300	3.2759	2.8826	2.6499	2.4936	2.3803	2.2938	2.2253	2.1696	2.1231	2.0838	2.0500
35	4.1213	3.2674	2.8742	2.6415	2.4851	2.3718	2.2852	2.2167	2.1608	2.1143	2.0750	2.0411
36	4.1132	3.2594	2.8663	2.6335	2.4772	2.3638	2.2771	2.2085	2.1526	2.1061	2.0666	2.0327
37	4.1055	3.2519	2.8588	2.6261	2.4696	2.3562	2.2695	2.2008	2.1449	2.0982	2.0587	2.0248
38	4.0982	3.2448	2.8517	2.6190	2.4625	2.3490	2.2623	2.1936	2.1375	2.0909	2.0513	2.0173
39	4.0913	3.2381	2.8451	2.6123	2.4558	2.3423	2.2555	2.1867	2.1306	2.0839	2.0443	2.0102
40	4.0847	3.2317	2.8387	2.6060	2.4495	2.3359	2.2490	2.1802	2.1240	2.0772	2.0376	2.0035
42	4.0727	3.2199	2.8270	2.5943	2.4377	2.3240	2.2371	2.1681	2.1119	2.0650	2.0252	1.9910
44	4.0617	3.2093	2.8165	2.5837	2.4270	2.3133	2.2263	2.1572	2.1009	2.0539	2.0140	1.9797
46	4.0517	3.1996	2.8068	2.5740	2.4174	2.3035	2.2164	2.1473	2.0909	2.0438	2.0039	1.9695
48	4.0427	3.1907	2.7981	2.5652	2.4085	2.2946	2.2074	2.1382	2.0817	2.0346	1.9946	1.9601
50	4.0343	3.1826	2.7900	2.5572	2.4004	2.2864	2.1992	2.1299	2.0734	2.0261	1.9861	1.9515

Table C1.5-1 (*Continued*)

Degrees of freedom denominator ν_2	Degrees of freedom, numerator ν_1											
	14	16	20	24	30	40	50	75	100	200	500	∞
1	245.3640	246.4639	248.0131	249.0518	250.0951	251.1432	251.7742	252.6180	253.0411	253.6770	254.0593	254.3132
2	19.4244	19.4333	19.4458	19.4541	19.4624	19.4707	19.4757	19.4824	19.4857	19.4907	19.4937	19.4957
3	8.7149	8.6923	8.6602	8.6385	8.6166	8.5944	8.5810	8.5630	8.5539	8.5402	8.5320	8.5265
4	5.8733	5.8441	5.8025	5.7744	5.7459	5.7170	5.6995	5.6759	5.6641	5.6461	5.6353	5.6281
5	4.6358	4.6038	4.5581	4.5272	4.4957	4.4638	4.4444	4.4183	4.4051	4.3851	4.3731	4.3650
6	3.9559	3.9223	3.8742	3.8415	3.8082	3.7743	3.7537	3.7258	3.7117	3.6904	3.6775	3.6689
7	3.5292	3.4944	3.4445	3.4105	3.3758	3.3404	3.3189	3.2897	3.2749	3.2525	3.2389	3.2298
8	3.2374	3.2016	3.1503	3.1152	3.0794	3.0428	3.0204	2.9901	2.9747	2.9513	2.9371	2.9276
9	3.0255	2.9890	2.9365	2.9005	2.8637	2.8259	2.8028	2.7715	2.7556	2.7313	2.7166	2.7067
10	2.8647	2.8276	2.7740	2.7372	2.6996	2.6609	2.6371	2.6048	2.5884	2.5634	2.5481	2.5379
11	2.7386	2.7009	2.6464	2.6090	2.5705	2.5309	2.5066	2.4734	2.4566	2.4308	2.4151	2.4045
12	2.6371	2.5989	2.5436	2.5055	2.4663	2.4259	2.4010	2.3671	2.3498	2.3233	2.3071	2.2963
13	2.5536	2.5149	2.4589	2.4202	2.3803	2.3392	2.3138	2.2791	2.2614	2.2343	2.2176	2.2065
14	2.4837	2.4446	2.3879	2.3487	2.3082	2.2664	2.2405	2.2051	2.1870	2.1592	2.1422	2.1308
15	2.4244	2.3849	2.3275	2.2878	2.2468	2.2043	2.1780	2.1419	2.1234	2.0950	2.0776	2.0659
16	2.3733	2.3335	2.2756	2.2354	2.1938	2.1507	2.1240	2.0873	2.0685	2.0395	2.0217	2.0097
17	2.3290	2.2888	2.2304	2.1898	2.1477	2.1040	2.0769	2.0396	2.0204	1.9909	1.9727	1.9604
18	2.2900	2.2496	2.1906	2.1497	2.1071	2.0629	2.0354	1.9975	1.9780	1.9479	1.9294	1.9169
19	2.2556	2.2149	2.1555	2.1141	2.0712	2.0264	1.9986	1.9601	1.9403	1.9097	1.8909	1.8781
20	2.2250	2.1840	2.1242	2.0825	2.0391	1.9938	1.9656	1.9267	1.9066	1.8755	1.8562	1.8432
21	2.1975	2.1563	2.0960	2.0540	2.0102	1.9645	1.9360	1.8965	1.8761	1.8446	1.8250	1.8118
22	2.1727	2.1313	2.0707	2.0283	1.9842	1.9380	1.9092	1.8692	1.8486	1.8165	1.7966	1.7832
23	2.1502	2.1086	2.0476	2.0050	1.9605	1.9139	1.8848	1.8444	1.8234	1.7909	1.7708	1.7571
24	2.1298	2.0880	2.0267	1.9838	1.9390	1.8920	1.8625	1.8217	1.8005	1.7675	1.7470	1.7331
25	2.1111	2.0691	2.0075	1.9643	1.9192	1.8718	1.8421	1.8008	1.7794	1.7460	1.7252	1.7111

(*Continued*)

Table C1.5-1 (*Continued*)

Degrees of freedom denominator	Degrees of freedom, numerator ν_1											
ν_2	14	16	20	24	30	40	50	75	100	200	500	∞
26	2.0939	2.0518	1.9898	1.9464	1.9010	1.8533	1.8233	1.7816	1.7599	1.7261	1.7050	1.6907
27	2.0781	2.0358	1.9736	1.9299	1.8842	1.8361	1.8059	1.7638	1.7419	1.7077	1.6863	1.6718
28	2.0635	2.0210	1.9586	1.9147	1.8687	1.8203	1.7898	1.7473	1.7251	1.6905	1.6689	1.6542
29	2.0500	2.0073	1.9446	1.9005	1.8543	1.8055	1.7748	1.7320	1.7096	1.6746	1.6527	1.6377
30	2.0374	1.9946	1.9317	1.8874	1.8409	1.7918	1.7609	1.7176	1.6950	1.6597	1.6375	1.6223
31	2.0257	1.9828	1.9196	1.8751	1.8283	1.7790	1.7478	1.7043	1.6814	1.6457	1.6233	1.6079
32	2.0147	1.9717	1.9083	1.8636	1.8166	1.7670	1.7356	1.6917	1.6687	1.6326	1.6099	1.5943
33	2.0045	1.9613	1.8977	1.8528	1.8056	1.7557	1.7241	1.6799	1.6567	1.6202	1.5973	1.5816
34	1.9949	1.9516	1.8877	1.8427	1.7953	1.7451	1.7134	1.6688	1.6454	1.6086	1.5854	1.5695
35	1.9858	1.9424	1.8784	1.8332	1.7856	1.7351	1.7032	1.6583	1.6347	1.5976	1.5742	1.5581
36	1.9773	1.9338	1.8696	1.8242	1.7764	1.7257	1.6936	1.6484	1.6246	1.5872	1.5635	1.5472
37	1.9692	1.9256	1.8612	1.8157	1.7678	1.7168	1.6845	1.6390	1.6151	1.5773	1.5534	1.5370
38	1.9616	1.9179	1.8534	1.8077	1.7596	1.7084	1.6759	1.6301	1.6060	1.5679	1.5438	1.5272
39	1.9545	1.9107	1.8459	1.8001	1.7518	1.7004	1.6678	1.6217	1.5974	1.5590	1.5347	1.5179
40	1.9476	1.9037	1.8389	1.7929	1.7444	1.6928	1.6600	1.6137	1.5892	1.5505	1.5260	1.5090
42	1.9350	1.8910	1.8258	1.7796	1.7308	1.6787	1.6456	1.5988	1.5740	1.5347	1.5097	1.4924
44	1.9236	1.8794	1.8139	1.7675	1.7184	1.6659	1.6325	1.5852	1.5601	1.5203	1.4948	1.4772
46	1.9132	1.8688	1.8031	1.7564	1.7070	1.6542	1.6206	1.5728	1.5474	1.5070	1.4812	1.4632
48	1.9037	1.8592	1.7932	1.7464	1.6967	1.6435	1.6096	1.5614	1.5357	1.4948	1.4686	1.4503
50	1.8949	1.8503	1.7841	1.7371	1.6872	1.6337	1.5995	1.5508	1.5249	1.4835	1.4569	1.4384

Table C1.5-1 (*Continued*)

Degrees of freedom denominator ν_2	Degrees of freedom, numerator ν_1											
	1	2	3	4	5	6	7	8	9	10	11	12
60	4.0012	3.1504	2.7581	2.5252	2.3683	2.2541	2.1665	2.0970	2.0401	1.9926	1.9522	1.9174
70	3.9778	3.1277	2.7355	2.5027	2.3456	2.2312	2.1435	2.0737	2.0166	1.9689	1.9283	1.8932
80	3.9604	3.1108	2.7188	2.4859	2.3287	2.2142	2.1263	2.0564	1.9991	1.9512	1.9105	1.8753
90	3.9469	3.0977	2.7058	2.4729	2.3157	2.2011	2.1131	2.0430	1.9856	1.9376	1.8967	1.8613
100	3.9361	3.0873	2.6955	2.4626	2.3053	2.1906	2.1025	2.0323	1.9748	1.9267	1.8857	1.8503
110	3.9274	3.0788	2.6871	2.4542	2.2969	2.1821	2.0939	2.0236	1.9661	1.9178	1.8767	1.8412
120	3.9201	3.0718	2.6802	2.4472	2.2899	2.1750	2.0868	2.0164	1.9588	1.9105	1.8693	1.8337
130	3.9140	3.0658	2.6743	2.4414	2.2839	2.1690	2.0807	2.0103	1.9526	1.9042	1.8630	1.8273
140	3.9087	3.0608	2.6693	2.4363	2.2789	2.1639	2.0756	2.0051	1.9473	1.8989	1.8576	1.8219
150	3.9042	3.0564	2.6649	2.4320	2.2745	2.1595	2.0711	2.0006	1.9428	1.8943	1.8530	1.8172
160	3.9002	3.0525	2.6611	2.4282	2.2707	2.1557	2.0672	1.9967	1.9388	1.8903	1.8489	1.8131
170	3.8967	3.0491	2.6578	2.4248	2.2673	2.1523	2.0638	1.9932	1.9353	1.8868	1.8453	1.8095
180	3.8936	3.0461	2.6548	2.4218	2.2643	2.1492	2.0608	1.9901	1.9322	1.8836	1.8422	1.8063
190	3.8909	3.0435	2.6521	2.4192	2.2616	2.1466	2.0580	1.9874	1.9294	1.8808	1.8393	1.8034
200	3.8884	3.0411	2.6498	2.4168	2.2592	2.1441	2.0556	1.9849	1.9269	1.8783	1.8368	1.8008
210	3.8861	3.0389	2.6476	2.4146	2.2571	2.1419	2.0534	1.9827	1.9247	1.8760	1.8345	1.7985
220	3.8841	3.0369	2.6456	2.4127	2.2551	2.1400	2.0514	1.9807	1.9226	1.8739	1.8324	1.7964
230	3.8822	3.0351	2.6438	2.4109	2.2533	2.1381	2.0495	1.9788	1.9207	1.8720	1.8304	1.7944
240	3.8805	3.0334	2.6422	2.4093	2.2516	2.1365	2.0479	1.9771	1.9190	1.8703	1.8287	1.7927
250	3.8789	3.0319	2.6407	2.4078	2.2501	2.1350	2.0463	1.9756	1.9174	1.8687	1.8271	1.7910
260	3.8775	3.0305	2.6393	2.4064	2.2487	2.1335	2.0449	1.9741	1.9160	1.8672	1.8256	1.7895
270	3.8761	3.0292	2.6380	2.4051	2.2474	2.1322	2.0436	1.9728	1.9146	1.8659	1.8242	1.7881
280	3.8749	3.0280	2.6368	2.4039	2.2462	2.1310	2.0424	1.9715	1.9134	1.8646	1.8229	1.7869
290	3.8737	3.0269	2.6357	2.4028	2.2451	2.1299	2.0412	1.9704	1.9122	1.8634	1.8218	1.7857
300	3.8726	3.0258	2.6347	2.4017	2.2441	2.1289	2.0402	1.9693	1.9112	1.8623	1.8206	1.7845

(*Continued*)

Table C1.5-1 (*Continued*)

Degrees of freedom denominator	Degrees of freedom, numerator ν_1											
ν_2	1	2	3	4	5	6	7	8	9	10	11	12
310	3.8716	3.0249	2.6337	2.4008	2.2431	2.1279	2.0392	1.9683	1.9101	1.8613	1.8196	1.7835
320	3.8707	3.0240	2.6328	2.3999	2.2422	2.1269	2.0382	1.9674	1.9092	1.8603	1.8186	1.7825
330	3.8698	3.0231	2.6320	2.3990	2.2413	2.1261	2.0374	1.9665	1.9083	1.8594	1.8177	1.7816
340	3.8690	3.0223	2.6312	2.3982	2.2405	2.1253	2.0365	1.9657	1.9075	1.8586	1.8169	1.7807
350	3.8682	3.0215	2.6304	2.3975	2.2398	2.1245	2.0358	1.9649	1.9067	1.8578	1.8161	1.7799
360	3.8674	3.0208	2.6297	2.3967	2.2391	2.1238	2.0350	1.9641	1.9059	1.8570	1.8153	1.7791
370	3.8667	3.0201	2.6290	2.3961	2.2384	2.1231	2.0343	1.9634	1.9052	1.8563	1.8146	1.7784
380	3.8660	3.0195	2.6284	2.3954	2.2377	2.1224	2.0337	1.9628	1.9045	1.8556	1.8139	1.7777
390	3.8654	3.0189	2.6278	2.3948	2.2371	2.1218	2.0331	1.9622	1.9039	1.8550	1.8132	1.7770
400	3.8648	3.0183	2.6272	2.3942	2.2366	2.1212	2.0325	1.9616	1.9033	1.8544	1.8126	1.7764
420	3.8637	3.0172	2.6261	2.3932	2.2355	2.1202	2.0314	1.9605	1.9022	1.8533	1.8115	1.7753
440	3.8627	3.0162	2.6252	2.3922	2.2345	2.1192	2.0304	1.9594	1.9012	1.8522	1.8104	1.7742
460	3.8618	3.0153	2.6243	2.3913	2.2336	2.1183	2.0295	1.9585	1.9002	1.8513	1.8095	1.7732
480	3.8609	3.0145	2.6235	2.3905	2.2328	2.1175	2.0286	1.9577	1.8994	1.8504	1.8086	1.7724
500	3.8601	3.0138	2.6227	2.3898	2.2320	2.1167	2.0279	1.9569	1.8986	1.8496	1.8078	1.7715
600	3.8570	3.0107	2.6198	2.3868	2.2290	2.1137	2.0248	1.9538	1.8955	1.8465	1.8046	1.7683
700	3.8548	3.0086	2.6176	2.3847	2.2269	2.1115	2.0226	1.9516	1.8932	1.8442	1.8023	1.7660
800	3.8531	3.0070	2.6160	2.3831	2.2253	2.1099	2.0210	1.9500	1.8916	1.8425	1.8006	1.7643
900	3.8518	3.0057	2.6148	2.3818	2.2240	2.1086	2.0197	1.9487	1.8903	1.8412	1.7993	1.7629
1000	3.8508	3.0047	2.6138	2.3808	2.2231	2.1076	2.0187	1.9476	1.8892	1.8402	1.7982	1.7618
∞	3.8416	2.9958	2.6050	2.3720	2.2142	2.0987	2.0097	1.9385	1.8800	1.8308	1.7887	1.7523

Table C1.5-1 (*Continued*)

Degrees of freedom denominator ν_2	Degrees of freedom, numerator ν_1											
	14	16	20	24	30	40	50	75	100	200	500	∞
60	1.8602	1.8151	1.7480	1.7001	1.6491	1.5943	1.5590	1.5085	1.4814	1.4377	1.4093	1.3894
70	1.8357	1.7902	1.7223	1.6738	1.6220	1.5661	1.5300	1.4779	1.4498	1.4042	1.3743	1.3530
80	1.8174	1.7716	1.7032	1.6542	1.6017	1.5449	1.5081	1.4548	1.4259	1.3786	1.3472	1.3248
90	1.8032	1.7571	1.6883	1.6389	1.5859	1.5284	1.4910	1.4366	1.4070	1.3582	1.3256	1.3021
100	1.7919	1.7456	1.6764	1.6267	1.5733	1.5151	1.4772	1.4220	1.3917	1.3416	1.3079	1.2833
110	1.7827	1.7363	1.6667	1.6167	1.5630	1.5043	1.4660	1.4099	1.3791	1.3279	1.2931	1.2675
120	1.7750	1.7285	1.6587	1.6084	1.5543	1.4952	1.4565	1.3998	1.3685	1.3162	1.2804	1.2540
130	1.7686	1.7219	1.6519	1.6014	1.5470	1.4875	1.4485	1.3912	1.3595	1.3062	1.2695	1.2422
140	1.7630	1.7162	1.6460	1.5954	1.5408	1.4809	1.4416	1.3838	1.3517	1.2975	1.2600	1.2319
150	1.7582	1.7113	1.6410	1.5902	1.5354	1.4752	1.4357	1.3773	1.3448	1.2899	1.2516	1.2227
160	1.7540	1.7071	1.6366	1.5856	1.5306	1.4702	1.4304	1.3716	1.3388	1.2832	1.2442	1.2145
170	1.7504	1.7033	1.6327	1.5816	1.5264	1.4657	1.4258	1.3666	1.3335	1.2772	1.2375	1.2071
180	1.7471	1.7000	1.6292	1.5780	1.5227	1.4618	1.4217	1.3621	1.3288	1.2718	1.2315	1.2004
190	1.7441	1.6970	1.6261	1.5748	1.5194	1.4583	1.4180	1.3581	1.3245	1.2670	1.2260	1.1943
200	1.7415	1.6943	1.6233	1.5720	1.5164	1.4551	1.4146	1.3545	1.3206	1.2626	1.2211	1.1887
210	1.7391	1.6919	1.6208	1.5694	1.5136	1.4522	1.4116	1.3512	1.3171	1.2586	1.2165	1.1835
220	1.7370	1.6897	1.6185	1.5670	1.5112	1.4496	1.4088	1.3482	1.3139	1.2549	1.2123	1.1787
230	1.7350	1.6876	1.6164	1.5648	1.5089	1.4472	1.4063	1.3454	1.3110	1.2515	1.2084	1.1743
240	1.7332	1.6858	1.6145	1.5628	1.5069	1.4450	1.4040	1.3429	1.3083	1.2484	1.2049	1.1701
250	1.7315	1.6841	1.6127	1.5610	1.5049	1.4430	1.4019	1.3405	1.3058	1.2456	1.2015	1.1663
260	1.7300	1.6825	1.6111	1.5593	1.5032	1.4411	1.3999	1.3384	1.3035	1.2429	1.1985	1.1627
270	1.7285	1.6811	1.6096	1.5578	1.5016	1.4394	1.3981	1.3364	1.3014	1.2404	1.1956	1.1593
280	1.7272	1.6797	1.6082	1.5563	1.5001	1.4378	1.3964	1.3345	1.2994	1.2381	1.1929	1.1561
290	1.7260	1.6785	1.6069	1.5550	1.4986	1.4363	1.3948	1.3328	1.2975	1.2359	1.1903	1.1530
300	1.7249	1.6773	1.6057	1.5537	1.4973	1.4349	1.3934	1.3312	1.2958	1.2339	1.1879	1.1502

(*Continued*)

Table C1.5-1 (*Continued*)

Degrees of freedom denominator ν_2	Degrees of freedom, numerator ν_1 14	16	20	24	30	40	50	75	100	200	500	∞
310	1.7238	1.6762	1.6045	1.5526	1.4961	1.4336	1.3920	1.3296	1.2942	1.2320	1.1857	1.1475
320	1.7228	1.6752	1.6035	1.5515	1.4949	1.4323	1.3907	1.3282	1.2926	1.2302	1.1835	1.1449
330	1.7218	1.6742	1.6025	1.5504	1.4939	1.4312	1.3895	1.3269	1.2912	1.2285	1.1815	1.1424
340	1.7209	1.6733	1.6015	1.5494	1.4928	1.4301	1.3883	1.3256	1.2898	1.2269	1.1796	1.1401
350	1.7201	1.6725	1.6006	1.5485	1.4919	1.4291	1.3873	1.3244	1.2885	1.2254	1.1778	1.1379
360	1.7193	1.6717	1.5998	1.5477	1.4910	1.4281	1.3862	1.3233	1.2873	1.2239	1.1761	1.1358
370	1.7186	1.6709	1.5990	1.5468	1.4901	1.4272	1.3853	1.3222	1.2862	1.2226	1.1745	1.1337
380	1.7179	1.6702	1.5983	1.5461	1.4893	1.4263	1.3844	1.3212	1.2851	1.2213	1.1729	1.1318
390	1.7172	1.6695	1.5976	1.5453	1.4885	1.4255	1.3835	1.3202	1.2840	1.2200	1.1714	1.1299
400	1.7166	1.6688	1.5969	1.5446	1.4878	1.4247	1.3827	1.3193	1.2831	1.2189	1.1700	1.1281
420	1.7154	1.6676	1.5956	1.5433	1.4864	1.4232	1.3811	1.3176	1.2812	1.2167	1.1673	1.1248
440	1.7143	1.6665	1.5945	1.5421	1.4852	1.4219	1.3797	1.3161	1.2796	1.2147	1.1649	1.1216
460	1.7133	1.6655	1.5934	1.5411	1.4841	1.4207	1.3784	1.3147	1.2780	1.2128	1.1627	1.1187
480	1.7124	1.6646	1.5925	1.5401	1.4830	1.4196	1.3773	1.3134	1.2766	1.2111	1.1606	1.1160
500	1.7116	1.6638	1.5916	1.5392	1.4821	1.4186	1.3762	1.3122	1.2753	1.2096	1.1587	1.1135
600	1.7083	1.6604	1.5881	1.5355	1.4782	1.4145	1.3719	1.3073	1.2701	1.2033	1.1508	1.1029
700	1.7059	1.6580	1.5856	1.5329	1.4755	1.4116	1.3688	1.3039	1.2664	1.1987	1.1450	1.0947
800	1.7041	1.6562	1.5837	1.5310	1.4735	1.4094	1.3665	1.3013	1.2635	1.1953	1.1406	1.0882
900	1.7028	1.6548	1.5822	1.5294	1.4719	1.4077	1.3647	1.2993	1.2613	1.1925	1.1371	1.0829
1000	1.7017	1.6536	1.5811	1.5282	1.4706	1.4063	1.3632	1.2976	1.2596	1.1903	1.1342	1.0784
∞	1.6919	1.6436	1.5706	1.5174	1.4592	1.3941	1.3502	1.2830	1.2436	1.1702	1.1066	1.0105

Table C1.5-2 *F*-distribution

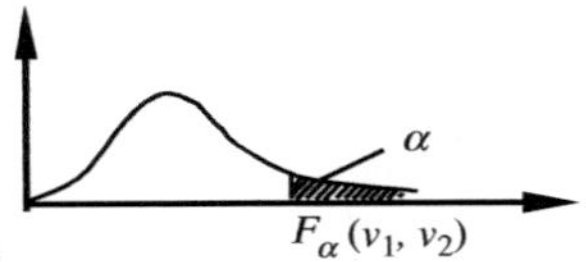

(analysis of variance, α for one-tailed, α = 0.01)

Degrees of freedom denominator	Degrees of freedom, numerator ν_1											
ν_2	1	2	3	4	5	6	7	8	9	10	11	12
1	4052.1807	4999.5000	5403.3520	5624.5833	5763.6496	5858.9861	5928.3557	5981.0703	6022.4732	6055.8467	6083.3168	6106.3207
2	98.5025	99.0000	99.1662	99.2494	99.2993	99.3326	99.3564	99.3742	99.3881	99.3992	99.4083	99.4159
3	34.1162	30.8165	29.4567	28.7099	28.2371	27.9107	27.6717	27.4892	27.3452	27.2287	27.1326	27.0518
4	21.1977	18.0000	16.6944	15.9770	15.5219	15.2069	14.9758	14.7989	14.6591	14.5459	14.4523	14.3736
5	16.2582	13.2739	12.0600	11.3919	10.9670	10.6723	10.4555	10.2893	10.1578	10.0510	9.9626	9.8883
6	13.7450	10.9248	9.7795	9.1483	8.7459	8.4661	8.2600	8.1017	7.9761	7.8741	7.7896	7.7183
7	12.2464	9.5466	8.4513	7.8466	7.4604	7.1914	6.9928	6.8400	6.7188	6.6201	6.5382	6.4691
8	11.2586	8.6491	7.5910	7.0061	6.6318	6.3707	6.1776	6.0289	5.9106	5.8143	5.7343	5.6667
9	10.5614	8.0215	6.9919	6.4221	6.0569	5.8018	5.6129	5.4671	5.3511	5.2565	5.1779	5.1114
10	10.0443	7.5594	6.5523	5.9943	5.6363	5.3858	5.2001	5.0567	4.9424	4.8491	4.7715	4.7059
11	9.6460	7.2057	6.2167	5.6683	5.3160	5.0692	4.8861	4.7445	4.6315	4.5393	4.4624	4.3974
12	9.3302	6.9266	5.9525	5.4120	5.0643	4.8206	4.6395	4.4994	4.3875	4.2961	4.2198	4.1553
13	9.0738	6.7010	5.7394	5.2053	4.8616	4.6204	4.4410	4.3021	4.1911	4.1003	4.0245	3.9603
14	8.8616	6.5149	5.5639	5.0354	4.6950	4.4558	4.2779	4.1399	4.0297	3.9394	3.8640	3.8001
15	8.6831	6.3589	5.4170	4.8932	4.5556	4.3183	4.1415	4.0045	3.8948	3.8049	3.7299	3.6662
16	8.5310	6.2262	5.2922	4.7726	4.4374	4.2016	4.0259	3.8896	3.7804	3.6909	3.6162	3.5527
17	8.3997	6.1121	5.1850	4.6690	4.3359	4.1015	3.9267	3.7910	3.6822	3.5931	3.5185	3.4552
18	8.2854	6.0129	5.0919	4.5790	4.2479	4.0146	3.8406	3.7054	3.5971	3.5082	3.4338	3.3706

(*Continued*)

Table C1.5-2 (*Continued*)

Degrees of freedom denominator	Degrees of freedom, numerator ν_1											
ν_2	1	2	3	4	5	6	7	8	9	10	11	12
19	8.1849	5.9259	5.0103	4.5003	4.1708	3.9386	3.7653	3.6305	3.5225	3.4338	3.3596	3.2965
20	8.0960	5.8489	4.9382	4.4307	4.1027	3.8714	3.6987	3.5644	3.4567	3.3682	3.2941	3.2311
21	8.0166	5.7804	4.8740	4.3688	4.0421	3.8117	3.6396	3.5056	3.3981	3.3098	3.2359	3.1730
22	7.9454	5.7190	4.8166	4.3134	3.9880	3.7583	3.5867	3.4530	3.3458	3.2576	3.1837	3.1209
23	7.8811	5.6637	4.7649	4.2636	3.9392	3.7102	3.5390	3.4057	3.2986	3.2106	3.1368	3.0740
24	7.8229	5.6136	4.7181	4.2184	3.8951	3.6667	3.4959	3.3629	3.2560	3.1681	3.0944	3.0316
25	7.7698	5.5680	4.6755	4.1774	3.8550	3.6272	3.4568	3.3239	3.2172	3.1294	3.0558	2.9931
26	7.7213	5.5263	4.6366	4.1400	3.8183	3.5911	3.4210	3.2884	3.1818	3.0941	3.0205	2.9578
27	7.6767	5.4881	4.6009	4.1056	3.7848	3.5580	3.3882	3.2558	3.1494	3.0618	2.9882	2.9256
28	7.6356	5.4529	4.5681	4.0740	3.7539	3.5276	3.3581	3.2259	3.1195	3.0320	2.9585	2.8959
29	7.5977	5.4204	4.5378	4.0449	3.7254	3.4995	3.3303	3.1982	3.0920	3.0045	2.9311	2.8685
30	7.5625	5.3903	4.5097	4.0179	3.6990	3.4735	3.3045	3.1726	3.0665	2.9791	2.9057	2.8431
31	7.5298	5.3624	4.4837	3.9928	3.6745	3.4493	3.2806	3.1489	3.0428	2.9555	2.8821	2.8195
32	7.4993	5.3363	4.4594	3.9695	3.6517	3.4269	3.2583	3.1267	3.0208	2.9335	2.8602	2.7976
33	7.4708	5.3120	4.4368	3.9477	3.6305	3.4059	3.2376	3.1061	3.0003	2.9130	2.8397	2.7771
34	7.4441	5.2893	4.4156	3.9273	3.6106	3.3863	3.2182	3.0868	2.9810	2.8938	2.8205	2.7580
35	7.4191	5.2679	4.3957	3.9082	3.5919	3.3679	3.2000	3.0687	2.9630	2.8758	2.8026	2.7400
36	7.3956	5.2479	4.3771	3.8903	3.5744	3.3507	3.1829	3.0517	2.9461	2.8589	2.7857	2.7232
37	7.3734	5.2290	4.3595	3.8734	3.5579	3.3344	3.1668	3.0357	2.9302	2.8431	2.7698	2.7073
38	7.3525	5.2112	4.3430	3.8575	3.5424	3.3191	3.1516	3.0207	2.9151	2.8281	2.7549	2.6923
39	7.3328	5.1944	4.3274	3.8425	3.5277	3.3047	3.1373	3.0064	2.9010	2.8139	2.7407	2.6782
40	7.3141	5.1785	4.3126	3.8283	3.5138	3.2910	3.1238	2.9930	2.8876	2.8005	2.7274	2.6648
42	7.2796	5.1491	4.2853	3.8021	3.4882	3.2658	3.0988	2.9681	2.8628	2.7758	2.7027	2.6402
44	7.2484	5.1226	4.2606	3.7784	3.4651	3.2430	3.0762	2.9457	2.8405	2.7536	2.6804	2.6179
46	7.2200	5.0986	4.2383	3.7570	3.4442	3.2224	3.0558	2.9254	2.8203	2.7334	2.6602	2.5977
48	7.1942	5.0767	4.2180	3.7374	3.4251	3.2036	3.0372	2.9069	2.8018	2.7150	2.6418	2.5793
50	7.1706	5.0566	4.1993	3.7195	3.4077	3.1864	3.0202	2.8900	2.7850	2.6981	2.6250	2.5625

Table C1.5-2 (*Continued*)

Degrees of freedom denominator	Degrees of freedom, numerator ν_1											
ν_2	14	16	20	24	30	40	50	75	100	200	500	∞
1	6142.6740	6170.1012	6208.7302	6234.6309	6260.6486	6286.7821	6302.5172	6323.5610	6334.1100	6349.9672	6359.5007	6365.8326
2	99.4278	99.4367	99.4492	99.4575	99.4658	99.4742	99.4792	99.4858	99.4892	99.4942	99.4972	99.4992
3	26.9238	26.8269	26.6898	26.5975	26.5045	26.4108	26.3542	26.2784	26.2402	26.1828	26.1483	26.1253
4	14.2486	14.1539	14.0196	13.9291	13.8377	13.7454	13.6896	13.6147	13.5770	13.5202	13.4859	13.4632
5	9.7700	9.6802	9.5526	9.4665	9.3793	9.2912	9.2378	9.1660	9.1299	9.0754	9.0424	9.0205
6	7.6049	7.5186	7.3958	7.3127	7.2285	7.1432	7.0915	7.0218	6.9867	6.9336	6.9015	6.8801
7	6.3590	6.2750	6.1554	6.0743	5.9920	5.9084	5.8577	5.7892	5.7547	5.7024	5.6707	5.6496
8	5.5589	5.4766	5.3591	5.2793	5.1981	5.1156	5.0654	4.9976	4.9633	4.9114	4.8799	4.8589
9	5.0052	4.9240	4.8080	4.7290	4.6486	4.5666	4.5167	4.4492	4.4150	4.3631	4.3317	4.3107
10	4.6008	4.5204	4.4054	4.3269	4.2469	4.1653	4.1155	4.0479	4.0137	3.9617	3.9302	3.9091
11	4.2932	4.2134	4.0990	4.0209	3.9411	3.8596	3.8097	3.7421	3.7077	3.6555	3.6238	3.6025
12	4.0518	3.9724	3.8584	3.7805	3.7008	3.6192	3.5692	3.5014	3.4668	3.4143	3.3823	3.3609
13	3.8573	3.7783	3.6646	3.5868	3.5070	3.4253	3.3752	3.3070	3.2723	3.2194	3.1871	3.1655
14	3.6975	3.6187	3.5052	3.4274	3.3476	3.2656	3.2153	3.1468	3.1118	3.0585	3.0260	3.0041
15	3.5639	3.4852	3.3719	3.2940	3.2141	3.1319	3.0814	3.0124	2.9772	2.9235	2.8906	2.8685
16	3.4506	3.3720	3.2587	3.1808	3.1007	3.0182	2.9675	2.8981	2.8627	2.8084	2.7752	2.7529
17	3.3533	3.2748	3.1615	3.0835	3.0032	2.9205	2.8694	2.7996	2.7639	2.7092	2.6757	2.6531
18	3.2689	3.1904	3.0771	2.9990	2.9185	2.8354	2.7841	2.7139	2.6779	2.6227	2.5889	2.5661
19	3.1949	3.1165	3.0031	2.9249	2.8442	2.7608	2.7093	2.6386	2.6023	2.5467	2.5124	2.4894
20	3.1296	3.0512	2.9377	2.8594	2.7785	2.6947	2.6430	2.5718	2.5353	2.4792	2.4446	2.4213
21	3.0715	2.9931	2.8796	2.8010	2.7200	2.6359	2.5838	2.5123	2.4755	2.4189	2.3840	2.3604
22	3.0195	2.9411	2.8274	2.7488	2.6675	2.5831	2.5308	2.4588	2.4217	2.3646	2.3294	2.3056
23	2.9727	2.8943	2.7805	2.7017	2.6202	2.5355	2.4829	2.4105	2.3732	2.3156	2.2800	2.2560
24	2.9303	2.8519	2.7380	2.6591	2.5773	2.4923	2.4395	2.3667	2.3291	2.2710	2.2351	2.2108
25	2.8917	2.8133	2.6993	2.6203	2.5383	2.4530	2.3999	2.3267	2.2888	2.2303	2.1941	2.1695
26	2.8566	2.7781	2.6640	2.5848	2.5026	2.4170	2.3637	2.2900	2.2519	2.1930	2.1564	2.1316
27	2.8243	2.7458	2.6316	2.5522	2.4699	2.3840	2.3304	2.2564	2.2180	2.1586	2.1217	2.0966

(*Continued*)

Table C1.5-2 (*Continued*)

Degrees of freedom denominator	Degrees of freedom, numerator ν_1											
ν_2	14	16	20	24	30	40	50	75	100	200	500	∞
28	2.7946	2.7160	2.6017	2.5223	2.4397	2.3535	2.2997	2.2253	2.1867	2.1268	2.0896	2.0643
29	2.7672	2.6886	2.5742	2.4946	2.4118	2.3253	2.2714	2.1965	2.1577	2.0974	2.0598	2.0343
30	2.7418	2.6632	2.5487	2.4689	2.3860	2.2992	2.2450	2.1698	2.1307	2.0700	2.0321	2.0064
31	2.7182	2.6396	2.5249	2.4451	2.3619	2.2749	2.2205	2.1449	2.1056	2.0444	2.0063	1.9803
32	2.6963	2.6176	2.5029	2.4229	2.3395	2.2523	2.1976	2.1217	2.0821	2.0206	1.9821	1.9559
33	2.6758	2.5971	2.4822	2.4021	2.3186	2.2311	2.1762	2.0999	2.0602	1.9982	1.9594	1.9330
34	2.6566	2.5779	2.4629	2.3827	2.2990	2.2112	2.1562	2.0795	2.0396	1.9772	1.9381	1.9114
35	2.6387	2.5599	2.4448	2.3645	2.2806	2.1926	2.1374	2.0604	2.0202	1.9574	1.9180	1.8911
36	2.6218	2.5430	2.4278	2.3473	2.2633	2.1751	2.1197	2.0423	2.0019	1.9387	1.8991	1.8720
37	2.6059	2.5270	2.4118	2.3312	2.2470	2.1585	2.1030	2.0253	1.9847	1.9211	1.8812	1.8538
38	2.5909	2.5120	2.3967	2.3160	2.2317	2.1430	2.0872	2.0092	1.9684	1.9045	1.8642	1.8366
39	2.5768	2.4978	2.3824	2.3016	2.2171	2.1282	2.0723	1.9940	1.9530	1.8887	1.8481	1.8203
40	2.5634	2.4844	2.3689	2.2880	2.2034	2.1142	2.0581	1.9795	1.9383	1.8737	1.8329	1.8048
42	2.5387	2.4596	2.3439	2.2629	2.1780	2.0884	2.0319	1.9528	1.9112	1.8458	1.8045	1.7760
44	2.5164	2.4373	2.3214	2.2401	2.1550	2.0650	2.0083	1.9285	1.8866	1.8205	1.7786	1.7498
46	2.4962	2.4170	2.3009	2.2195	2.1341	2.0438	1.9867	1.9065	1.8642	1.7974	1.7550	1.7258
48	2.4777	2.3985	2.2823	2.2007	2.1150	2.0244	1.9670	1.8862	1.8436	1.7762	1.7333	1.7037
50	2.4609	2.3816	2.2652	2.1835	2.0976	2.0066	1.9490	1.8677	1.8248	1.7567	1.7133	1.6833

Table C1.5-2 (*Continued*)

Degrees of freedom denominator ν_2	Degrees of freedom, numerator ν_1											
	1	2	3	4	5	6	7	8	9	10	11	12
60	7.0771	4.9774	4.1259	3.6490	3.3389	3.1187	2.9530	2.8233	2.7185	2.6318	2.5587	2.4961
70	7.0114	4.9219	4.0744	3.5996	3.2907	3.0712	2.9060	2.7765	2.6719	2.5852	2.5122	2.4496
80	6.9627	4.8807	4.0363	3.5631	3.2550	3.0361	2.8713	2.7420	2.6374	2.5508	2.4777	2.4151
90	6.9251	4.8491	4.0070	3.5350	3.2276	3.0091	2.8445	2.7154	2.6109	2.5243	2.4513	2.3886
100	6.8953	4.8239	3.9837	3.5127	3.2059	2.9877	2.8233	2.6943	2.5898	2.5033	2.4302	2.3676
110	6.8710	4.8035	3.9648	3.4946	3.1882	2.9703	2.8061	2.6771	2.5727	2.4862	2.4132	2.3505
120	6.8509	4.7865	3.9491	3.4795	3.1735	2.9559	2.7918	2.6629	2.5586	2.4721	2.3990	2.3363
130	6.8339	4.7722	3.9359	3.4669	3.1612	2.9437	2.7797	2.6509	2.5466	2.4602	2.3871	2.3244
140	6.8194	4.7600	3.9246	3.4561	3.1507	2.9333	2.7695	2.6407	2.5365	2.4500	2.3769	2.3142
150	6.8069	4.7495	3.9149	3.4467	3.1416	2.9244	2.7606	2.6319	2.5277	2.4412	2.3681	2.3053
160	6.7960	4.7403	3.9064	3.4386	3.1336	2.9166	2.7528	2.6242	2.5200	2.4335	2.3604	2.2977
170	6.7863	4.7322	3.8989	3.4314	3.1267	2.9097	2.7460	2.6174	2.5132	2.4268	2.3537	2.2909
180	6.7778	4.7250	3.8923	3.4251	3.1205	2.9036	2.7400	2.6114	2.5072	2.4208	2.3477	2.2849
190	6.7702	4.7186	3.8863	3.4194	3.1149	2.8982	2.7346	2.6061	2.5019	2.4154	2.3423	2.2795
200	6.7633	4.7129	3.8810	3.4143	3.1100	2.8933	2.7298	2.6012	2.4971	2.4106	2.3375	2.2747
210	6.7571	4.7077	3.8762	3.4097	3.1055	2.8888	2.7254	2.5969	2.4927	2.4063	2.3332	2.2704
220	6.7515	4.7029	3.8719	3.4055	3.1014	2.8848	2.7214	2.5929	2.4888	2.4023	2.3292	2.2664
230	6.7463	4.6986	3.8679	3.4017	3.0977	2.8812	2.7178	2.5893	2.4852	2.3988	2.3256	2.2628
240	6.7417	4.6947	3.8642	3.3982	3.0943	2.8778	2.7145	2.5860	2.4819	2.3955	2.3223	2.2595
250	6.7373	4.6911	3.8609	3.3950	3.0912	2.8748	2.7114	2.5830	2.4789	2.3925	2.3193	2.2565
270	6.7297	4.6846	3.8549	3.3893	3.0856	2.8693	2.7060	2.5776	2.4735	2.3871	2.3140	2.2511
280	6.7263	4.6817	3.8523	3.3868	3.0832	2.8669	2.7036	2.5752	2.4711	2.3847	2.3116	2.2487
290	6.7231	4.6791	3.8498	3.3845	3.0809	2.8646	2.7014	2.5730	2.4689	2.3825	2.3093	2.2465
300	6.7201	4.6766	3.8475	3.3823	3.0787	2.8625	2.6993	2.5709	2.4668	2.3804	2.3073	2.2444
260	6.7334	4.6877	3.8578	3.3921	3.0883	2.8719	2.7086	2.5802	2.4761	2.3897	2.3165	2.2537
310	6.7173	4.6743	3.8454	3.3802	3.0767	2.8605	2.6973	2.5690	2.4649	2.3785	2.3053	2.2425
320	6.7147	4.6721	3.8434	3.3783	3.0748	2.8587	2.6955	2.5671	2.4631	2.3766	2.3035	2.2407

(*Continued*)

Table C1.5-2 (*Continued*)

Degrees of freedom denominator	Degrees of freedom, numerator ν_1											
ν_2	1	2	3	4	5	6	7	8	9	10	11	12
330	6.7123	4.6700	3.8415	3.3765	3.0731	2.8569	2.6938	2.5654	2.4614	2.3749	2.3018	2.2389
340	6.7100	4.6681	3.8397	3.3748	3.0714	2.8553	2.6922	2.5638	2.4598	2.3733	2.3002	2.2373
350	6.7078	4.6663	3.8380	3.3732	3.0699	2.8538	2.6906	2.5623	2.4582	2.3718	2.2987	2.2358
360	6.7058	4.6646	3.8364	3.3716	3.0684	2.8523	2.6892	2.5609	2.4568	2.3704	2.2973	2.2344
370	6.7039	4.6630	3.8350	3.3702	3.0670	2.8509	2.6878	2.5595	2.4555	2.3690	2.2959	2.2330
380	6.7020	4.6614	3.8335	3.3689	3.0657	2.8496	2.6865	2.5582	2.4542	2.3678	2.2946	2.2318
390	6.7003	4.6600	3.8322	3.3676	3.0644	2.8484	2.6853	2.5570	2.4530	2.3666	2.2934	2.2305
400	6.6987	4.6586	3.8309	3.3664	3.0632	2.8472	2.6842	2.5559	2.4518	2.3654	2.2923	2.2294
420	6.6956	4.6560	3.8286	3.3641	3.0610	2.8451	2.6820	2.5537	2.4497	2.3633	2.2901	2.2272
440	6.6928	4.6537	3.8264	3.3620	3.0590	2.8431	2.6801	2.5518	2.4478	2.3613	2.2882	2.2253
460	6.6903	4.6516	3.8244	3.3602	3.0572	2.8413	2.6783	2.5500	2.4460	2.3596	2.2864	2.2235
480	6.6880	4.6496	3.8226	3.3584	3.0555	2.8396	2.6766	2.5484	2.4444	2.3579	2.2848	2.2219
500	6.6858	4.6478	3.8210	3.3569	3.0540	2.8381	2.6751	2.5469	2.4429	2.3565	2.2833	2.2204
600	6.6773	4.6407	3.8144	3.3505	3.0478	2.8321	2.6691	2.5409	2.4369	2.3505	2.2773	2.2144
700	6.6712	4.6356	3.8097	3.3460	3.0434	2.8277	2.6649	2.5367	2.4327	2.3463	2.2731	2.2102
800	6.6667	4.6318	3.8062	3.3427	3.0401	2.8245	2.6617	2.5335	2.4295	2.3431	2.2699	2.2070
900	6.6631	4.6288	3.8034	3.3400	3.0376	2.8220	2.6592	2.5310	2.4270	2.3406	2.2674	2.2045
1000	6.6603	4.6264	3.8012	3.3380	3.0355	2.8200	2.6572	2.5290	2.4250	2.3386	2.2655	2.2025
∞	6.6351	4.6054	3.7818	3.3194	3.0174	2.8022	2.6395	2.5115	2.4075	2.3211	2.2479	2.1849

Table C1.5-2 (*Continued*)

Degrees of freedom denominator	Degrees of freedom, numerator ν_1											
ν_2	14	16	20	24	30	40	50	75	100	200	500	∞
60	2.3943	2.3148	2.1978	2.1154	2.0285	1.9360	1.8772	1.7937	1.7493	1.6784	1.6327	1.6008
70	2.3477	2.2679	2.1504	2.0674	1.9797	1.8861	1.8263	1.7410	1.6954	1.6220	1.5743	1.5406
80	2.3131	2.2332	2.1153	2.0318	1.9435	1.8489	1.7883	1.7015	1.6548	1.5792	1.5296	1.4944
90	2.2865	2.2064	2.0882	2.0044	1.9155	1.8201	1.7588	1.6707	1.6231	1.5456	1.4943	1.4576
100	2.2654	2.1852	2.0666	1.9826	1.8933	1.7972	1.7353	1.6461	1.5977	1.5184	1.4656	1.4274
110	2.2482	2.1679	2.0491	1.9648	1.8751	1.7784	1.7160	1.6258	1.5767	1.4960	1.4417	1.4022
120	2.2339	2.1536	2.0346	1.9500	1.8600	1.7628	1.7000	1.6090	1.5592	1.4770	1.4215	1.3807
130	2.2219	2.1415	2.0223	1.9376	1.8473	1.7497	1.6865	1.5946	1.5443	1.4609	1.4041	1.3622
140	2.2117	2.1312	2.0119	1.9269	1.8364	1.7384	1.6748	1.5823	1.5315	1.4469	1.3890	1.3459
150	2.2028	2.1223	2.0028	1.9177	1.8270	1.7286	1.6648	1.5716	1.5204	1.4347	1.3757	1.3316
160	2.1951	2.1145	1.9949	1.9097	1.8187	1.7201	1.6559	1.5623	1.5106	1.4240	1.3640	1.3188
170	2.1883	2.1076	1.9879	1.9026	1.8115	1.7125	1.6482	1.5540	1.5020	1.4144	1.3535	1.3073
180	2.1823	2.1016	1.9818	1.8963	1.8050	1.7059	1.6413	1.5466	1.4942	1.4059	1.3440	1.2969
190	2.1769	2.0961	1.9763	1.8907	1.7993	1.6999	1.6351	1.5400	1.4873	1.3982	1.3355	1.2874
200	2.1721	2.0913	1.9713	1.8857	1.7941	1.6945	1.6295	1.5341	1.4811	1.3912	1.3277	1.2788
210	2.1677	2.0869	1.9668	1.8811	1.7894	1.6896	1.6244	1.5287	1.4754	1.3848	1.3206	1.2709
220	2.1637	2.0829	1.9628	1.8770	1.7851	1.6852	1.6199	1.5238	1.4702	1.3790	1.3141	1.2636
230	2.1601	2.0792	1.9590	1.8732	1.7813	1.6811	1.6157	1.5193	1.4655	1.3737	1.3081	1.2567
240	2.1568	2.0759	1.9556	1.8697	1.7777	1.6774	1.6118	1.5151	1.4611	1.3688	1.3026	1.2504
250	2.1537	2.0728	1.9525	1.8665	1.7744	1.6740	1.6083	1.5113	1.4571	1.3643	1.2974	1.2445
260	2.1509	2.0700	1.9496	1.8636	1.7714	1.6709	1.6050	1.5078	1.4534	1.3601	1.2926	1.2390
270	2.1483	2.0674	1.9470	1.8609	1.7686	1.6680	1.6020	1.5046	1.4500	1.3562	1.2882	1.2338
280	2.1459	2.0649	1.9445	1.8584	1.7660	1.6653	1.5992	1.5016	1.4468	1.3525	1.2840	1.2289
290	2.1437	2.0627	1.9422	1.8560	1.7636	1.6627	1.5966	1.4987	1.4438	1.3491	1.2801	1.2243
300	2.1416	2.0606	1.9401	1.8538	1.7614	1.6604	1.5942	1.4961	1.4410	1.3459	1.2764	1.2200
310	2.1396	2.0586	1.9380	1.8518	1.7593	1.6582	1.5919	1.4936	1.4384	1.3430	1.2729	1.2159
320	2.1378	2.0567	1.9362	1.8499	1.7573	1.6561	1.5897	1.4913	1.4360	1.3401	1.2697	1.2120

(*Continued*)

Table C1.5-2 (*Continued*)

Degrees of freedom denominator	Degrees of freedom, numerator ν_1											
ν_2	14	16	20	24	30	40	50	75	100	200	500	∞
330	2.1361	2.0550	1.9344	1.8481	1.7555	1.6542	1.5877	1.4892	1.4337	1.3375	1.2666	1.2083
340	2.1344	2.0534	1.9327	1.8464	1.7537	1.6524	1.5858	1.4871	1.4315	1.3350	1.2637	1.2048
350	2.1329	2.0518	1.9312	1.8448	1.7521	1.6507	1.5840	1.4852	1.4295	1.3326	1.2609	1.2014
360	2.1315	2.0504	1.9297	1.8433	1.7505	1.6490	1.5824	1.4834	1.4275	1.3304	1.2582	1.1982
370	2.1301	2.0490	1.9283	1.8419	1.7490	1.6475	1.5808	1.4816	1.4257	1.3283	1.2557	1.1952
380	2.1288	2.0477	1.9270	1.8405	1.7477	1.6461	1.5792	1.4800	1.4239	1.3262	1.2534	1.1923
390	2.1276	2.0465	1.9257	1.8392	1.7463	1.6447	1.5778	1.4784	1.4223	1.3243	1.2511	1.1895
400	2.1264	2.0453	1.9245	1.8380	1.7451	1.6434	1.5764	1.4770	1.4207	1.3225	1.2489	1.1868
420	2.1243	2.0431	1.9223	1.8358	1.7428	1.6409	1.5739	1.4742	1.4178	1.3191	1.2449	1.1817
440	2.1223	2.0412	1.9203	1.8337	1.7406	1.6387	1.5716	1.4717	1.4151	1.3160	1.2412	1.1770
460	2.1205	2.0394	1.9185	1.8318	1.7387	1.6367	1.5695	1.4694	1.4127	1.3131	1.2377	1.1727
480	2.1189	2.0377	1.9168	1.8301	1.7370	1.6349	1.5676	1.4673	1.4105	1.3105	1.2346	1.1687
500	2.1174	2.0362	1.9152	1.8285	1.7353	1.6332	1.5658	1.4654	1.4084	1.3081	1.2317	1.1649
600	2.1114	2.0301	1.9091	1.8222	1.7288	1.6263	1.5587	1.4577	1.4001	1.2983	1.2198	1.1491
700	2.1071	2.0258	1.9047	1.8177	1.7242	1.6215	1.5536	1.4521	1.3942	1.2913	1.2110	1.1370
800	2.1039	2.0226	1.9013	1.8144	1.7207	1.6178	1.5498	1.4480	1.3897	1.2860	1.2043	1.1274
900	2.1014	2.0201	1.8988	1.8117	1.7180	1.6150	1.5468	1.4447	1.3863	1.2818	1.1990	1.1196
1000	2.0994	2.0180	1.8967	1.8096	1.7158	1.6127	1.5445	1.4421	1.3835	1.2784	1.1947	1.1130
∞	2.0817	2.0002	1.8785	1.7910	1.6966	1.5925	1.5233	1.4188	1.3583	1.2475	1.1535	1.0148

Table C1.5-3 F-distribution

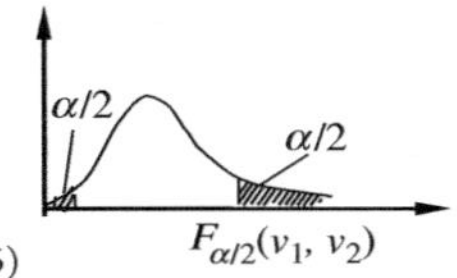

(homogeneity test of variance, α for two-tailed, $\alpha = 0.05$)

Degrees of freedom denominator	Degrees of freedom, numerator ν_1											
ν_2	1	2	3	4	5	6	7	8	9	10	11	12
1	161.4476	199.5000	215.7073	224.5832	230.1619	233.9860	236.7684	238.8827	240.5433	241.8817	242.9835	243.9060
2	18.5128	19.0000	19.1643	19.2468	19.2964	19.3295	19.3532	19.3710	19.3848	19.3959	19.4050	19.4125
3	10.1280	9.5521	9.2766	9.1172	9.0135	8.9406	8.8867	8.8452	8.8123	8.7855	8.7633	8.7446
4	7.7086	6.9443	6.5914	6.3882	6.2561	6.1631	6.0942	6.0410	5.9988	5.9644	5.9358	5.9117
5	6.6079	5.7861	5.4095	5.1922	5.0503	4.9503	4.8759	4.8183	4.7725	4.7351	4.7040	4.6777
6	5.9874	5.1433	4.7571	4.5337	4.3874	4.2839	4.2067	4.1468	4.0990	4.0600	4.0274	3.9999
7	5.5914	4.7374	4.3468	4.1203	3.9715	3.8660	3.7870	3.7257	3.6767	3.6365	3.6030	3.5747
8	5.3177	4.4590	4.0662	3.8379	3.6875	3.5806	3.5005	3.4381	3.3881	3.3472	3.3130	3.2839
9	5.1174	4.2565	3.8625	3.6331	3.4817	3.3738	3.2927	3.2296	3.1789	3.1373	3.1025	3.0729
10	4.9646	4.1028	3.7083	3.4780	3.3258	3.2172	3.1355	3.0717	3.0204	2.9782	2.9430	2.9130
11	4.8443	3.9823	3.5874	3.3567	3.2039	3.0946	3.0123	2.9480	2.8962	2.8536	2.8179	2.7876
12	4.7472	3.8853	3.4903	3.2592	3.1059	2.9961	2.9134	2.8486	2.7964	2.7534	2.7173	2.6866
13	4.6672	3.8056	3.4105	3.1791	3.0254	2.9153	2.8321	2.7669	2.7144	2.6710	2.6347	2.6037
14	4.6001	3.7389	3.3439	3.1122	2.9582	2.8477	2.7642	2.6987	2.6458	2.6022	2.5655	2.5342
15	4.5431	3.6823	3.2874	3.0556	2.9013	2.7905	2.7066	2.6408	2.5876	2.5437	2.5068	2.4753
16	4.4940	3.6337	3.2389	3.0069	2.8524	2.7413	2.6572	2.5911	2.5377	2.4935	2.4564	2.4247
17	4.4513	3.5915	3.1968	2.9647	2.8100	2.6987	2.6143	2.5480	2.4943	2.4499	2.4126	2.3807

(Continued)

Table C1.5-3 (*Continued*)

Degrees of freedom denominator	Degrees of freedom, numerator ν_1											
ν_2	1	2	3	4	5	6	7	8	9	10	11	12
18	4.4139	3.5546	3.1599	2.9277	2.7729	2.6613	2.5767	2.5102	2.4563	2.4117	2.3742	2.3421
19	4.3807	3.5219	3.1274	2.8951	2.7401	2.6283	2.5435	2.4768	2.4227	2.3779	2.3402	2.3080
20	4.3512	3.4928	3.0984	2.8661	2.7109	2.5990	2.5140	2.4471	2.3928	2.3479	2.3100	2.2776
21	4.3248	3.4668	3.0725	2.8401	2.6848	2.5727	2.4876	2.4205	2.3660	2.3210	2.2829	2.2504
22	4.3009	3.4434	3.0491	2.8167	2.6613	2.5491	2.4638	2.3965	2.3419	2.2967	2.2585	2.2258
23	4.2793	3.4221	3.0280	2.7955	2.6400	2.5277	2.4422	2.3748	2.3201	2.2747	2.2364	2.2036
24	4.2597	3.4028	3.0088	2.7763	2.6207	2.5082	2.4226	2.3551	2.3002	2.2547	2.2163	2.1834
25	4.2417	3.3852	2.9912	2.7587	2.6030	2.4904	2.4047	2.3371	2.2821	2.2365	2.1979	2.1649
26	4.2252	3.3690	2.9752	2.7426	2.5868	2.4741	2.3883	2.3205	2.2655	2.2197	2.1811	2.1479
27	4.2100	3.3541	2.9604	2.7278	2.5719	2.4591	2.3732	2.3053	2.2501	2.2043	2.1655	2.1323
28	4.1960	3.3404	2.9467	2.7141	2.5581	2.4453	2.3593	2.2913	2.2360	2.1900	2.1512	2.1179
29	4.1830	3.3277	2.9340	2.7014	2.5454	2.4324	2.3463	2.2783	2.2229	2.1768	2.1379	2.1045
30	4.1709	3.3158	2.9223	2.6896	2.5336	2.4205	2.3343	2.2662	2.2107	2.1646	2.1256	2.0921
31	4.1596	3.3048	2.9113	2.6787	2.5225	2.4094	2.3232	2.2549	2.1994	2.1532	2.1141	2.0805
32	4.1491	3.2945	2.9011	2.6684	2.5123	2.3991	2.3127	2.2444	2.1888	2.1425	2.1033	2.0697
33	4.1393	3.2849	2.8916	2.6589	2.5026	2.3894	2.3030	2.2346	2.1789	2.1325	2.0933	2.0595
34	4.1300	3.2759	2.8826	2.6499	2.4936	2.3803	2.2938	2.2253	2.1696	2.1231	2.0838	2.0500
35	4.1213	3.2674	2.8742	2.6415	2.4851	2.3718	2.2852	2.2167	2.1608	2.1143	2.0750	2.0411
36	4.1132	3.2594	2.8663	2.6335	2.4772	2.3638	2.2771	2.2085	2.1526	2.1061	2.0666	2.0327
37	4.1055	3.2519	2.8588	2.6261	2.4696	2.3562	2.2695	2.2008	2.1449	2.0982	2.0587	2.0248
38	4.0982	3.2448	2.8517	2.6190	2.4625	2.3490	2.2623	2.1936	2.1375	2.0909	2.0513	2.0173
39	4.0913	3.2381	2.8451	2.6123	2.4558	2.3423	2.2555	2.1867	2.1306	2.0839	2.0443	2.0102
40	4.0847	3.2317	2.8387	2.6060	2.4495	2.3359	2.2490	2.1802	2.1240	2.0772	2.0376	2.0035
42	4.0727	3.2199	2.8270	2.5943	2.4377	2.3240	2.2371	2.1681	2.1119	2.0650	2.0252	1.9910
44	4.0617	3.2093	2.8165	2.5837	2.4270	2.3133	2.2263	2.1572	2.1009	2.0539	2.0140	1.9797
46	4.0517	3.1996	2.8068	2.5740	2.4174	2.3035	2.2164	2.1473	2.0909	2.0438	2.0039	1.9695
48	4.0427	3.1907	2.7981	2.5652	2.4085	2.2946	2.2074	2.1382	2.0817	2.0346	1.9946	1.9601
50	4.0343	3.1826	2.7900	2.5572	2.4004	2.2864	2.1992	2.1299	2.0734	2.0261	1.9861	1.9515

Table C1.5-3 (*Continued*)

Degrees of freedom denominator ν_2	Degrees of freedom, numerator ν_1											
	14	16	20	24	30	40	50	75	100	200	500	∞
1	245.3640	246.4639	248.0131	249.0518	250.0951	251.1432	251.7742	252.6180	253.0411	253.6770	254.0593	254.3132
2	19.4244	19.4333	19.4458	19.4541	19.4624	19.4707	19.4757	19.4824	19.4857	19.4907	19.4937	19.4957
3	8.7149	8.6923	8.6602	8.6385	8.6166	8.5944	8.5810	8.5630	8.5539	8.5402	8.5320	8.5265
4	5.8733	5.8441	5.8025	5.7744	5.7459	5.7170	5.6995	5.6759	5.6641	5.6461	5.6353	5.6281
5	4.6358	4.6038	4.5581	4.5272	4.4957	4.4638	4.4444	4.4183	4.4051	4.3851	4.3731	4.3650
6	3.9559	3.9223	3.8742	3.8415	3.8082	3.7743	3.7537	3.7258	3.7117	3.6904	3.6775	3.6689
7	3.5292	3.4944	3.4445	3.4105	3.3758	3.3404	3.3189	3.2897	3.2749	3.2525	3.2389	3.2298
8	3.2374	3.2016	3.1503	3.1152	3.0794	3.0428	3.0204	2.9901	2.9747	2.9513	2.9371	2.9276
9	3.0255	2.9890	2.9365	2.9005	2.8637	2.8259	2.8028	2.7715	2.7556	2.7313	2.7166	2.7067
10	2.8647	2.8276	2.7740	2.7372	2.6996	2.6609	2.6371	2.6048	2.5884	2.5634	2.5481	2.5379
11	2.7386	2.7009	2.6464	2.6090	2.5705	2.5309	2.5066	2.4734	2.4566	2.4308	2.4151	2.4045
12	2.6371	2.5989	2.5436	2.5055	2.4663	2.4259	2.4010	2.3671	2.3498	2.3233	2.3071	2.2963
13	2.5536	2.5149	2.4589	2.4202	2.3803	2.3392	2.3138	2.2791	2.2614	2.2343	2.2176	2.2065
14	2.4837	2.4446	2.3879	2.3487	2.3082	2.2664	2.2405	2.2051	2.1870	2.1592	2.1422	2.1308
15	2.4244	2.3849	2.3275	2.2878	2.2468	2.2043	2.1780	2.1419	2.1234	2.0950	2.0776	2.0659
16	2.3733	2.3335	2.2756	2.2354	2.1938	2.1507	2.1240	2.0873	2.0685	2.0395	2.0217	2.0097
17	2.3290	2.2888	2.2304	2.1898	2.1477	2.1040	2.0769	2.0396	2.0204	1.9909	1.9727	1.9604
18	2.2900	2.2496	2.1906	2.1497	2.1071	2.0629	2.0354	1.9975	1.9780	1.9479	1.9294	1.9169
19	2.2556	2.2149	2.1555	2.1141	2.0712	2.0264	1.9986	1.9601	1.9403	1.9097	1.8909	1.8781
20	2.2250	2.1840	2.1242	2.0825	2.0391	1.9938	1.9656	1.9267	1.9066	1.8755	1.8562	1.8432
21	2.1975	2.1563	2.0960	2.0540	2.0102	1.9645	1.9360	1.8965	1.8761	1.8446	1.8250	1.8118
22	2.1727	2.1313	2.0707	2.0283	1.9842	1.9380	1.9092	1.8692	1.8486	1.8165	1.7966	1.7832
23	2.1502	2.1086	2.0476	2.0050	1.9605	1.9139	1.8848	1.8444	1.8234	1.7909	1.7708	1.7571
24	2.1298	2.0880	2.0267	1.9838	1.9390	1.8920	1.8625	1.8217	1.8005	1.7675	1.7470	1.7331
25	2.1111	2.0691	2.0075	1.9643	1.9192	1.8718	1.8421	1.8008	1.7794	1.7460	1.7252	1.7111

(*Continued*)

Table C1.5-3 (*Continued*)

Degrees of freedom denominator	Degrees of freedom, numerator ν_1											
ν_2	14	16	20	24	30	40	50	75	100	200	500	∞
26	2.0939	2.0518	1.9898	1.9464	1.9010	1.8533	1.8233	1.7816	1.7599	1.7261	1.7050	1.6907
27	2.0781	2.0358	1.9736	1.9299	1.8842	1.8361	1.8059	1.7638	1.7419	1.7077	1.6863	1.6718
28	2.0635	2.0210	1.9586	1.9147	1.8687	1.8203	1.7898	1.7473	1.7251	1.6905	1.6689	1.6542
29	2.0500	2.0073	1.9446	1.9005	1.8543	1.8055	1.7748	1.7320	1.7096	1.6746	1.6527	1.6377
30	2.0374	1.9946	1.9317	1.8874	1.8409	1.7918	1.7609	1.7176	1.6950	1.6597	1.6375	1.6223
31	2.0257	1.9828	1.9196	1.8751	1.8283	1.7790	1.7478	1.7043	1.6814	1.6457	1.6233	1.6079
32	2.0147	1.9717	1.9083	1.8636	1.8166	1.7670	1.7356	1.6917	1.6687	1.6326	1.6099	1.5943
33	2.0045	1.9613	1.8977	1.8528	1.8056	1.7557	1.7241	1.6799	1.6567	1.6202	1.5973	1.5816
34	1.9949	1.9516	1.8877	1.8427	1.7953	1.7451	1.7134	1.6688	1.6454	1.6086	1.5854	1.5695
35	1.9858	1.9424	1.8784	1.8332	1.7856	1.7351	1.7032	1.6583	1.6347	1.5976	1.5742	1.5581
36	1.9773	1.9338	1.8696	1.8242	1.7764	1.7257	1.6936	1.6484	1.6246	1.5872	1.5635	1.5472
37	1.9692	1.9256	1.8612	1.8157	1.7678	1.7168	1.6845	1.6390	1.6151	1.5773	1.5534	1.5370
38	1.9616	1.9179	1.8534	1.8077	1.7596	1.7084	1.6759	1.6301	1.6060	1.5679	1.5438	1.5272
39	1.9545	1.9107	1.8459	1.8001	1.7518	1.7004	1.6678	1.6217	1.5974	1.5590	1.5347	1.5179
40	1.9476	1.9037	1.8389	1.7929	1.7444	1.6928	1.6600	1.6137	1.5892	1.5505	1.5260	1.5090
42	1.9350	1.8910	1.8258	1.7796	1.7308	1.6787	1.6456	1.5988	1.5740	1.5347	1.5097	1.4924
44	1.9236	1.8794	1.8139	1.7675	1.7184	1.6659	1.6325	1.5852	1.5601	1.5203	1.4948	1.4772
46	1.9132	1.8688	1.8031	1.7564	1.7070	1.6542	1.6206	1.5728	1.5474	1.5070	1.4812	1.4632
48	1.9037	1.8592	1.7932	1.7464	1.6967	1.6435	1.6096	1.5614	1.5357	1.4948	1.4686	1.4503
50	1.8949	1.8503	1.7841	1.7371	1.6872	1.6337	1.5995	1.5508	1.5249	1.4835	1.4569	1.4384

Table C1.5-3 (*Continued*)

Degrees of freedom denominator	Degrees of freedom, numerator ν_1											
ν_2	1	2	3	4	5	6	7	8	9	10	11	12
60	4.0012	3.1504	2.7581	2.5252	2.3683	2.2541	2.1665	2.0970	2.0401	1.9926	1.9522	1.9174
70	3.9778	3.1277	2.7355	2.5027	2.3456	2.2312	2.1435	2.0737	2.0166	1.9689	1.9283	1.8932
80	3.9604	3.1108	2.7188	2.4859	2.3287	2.2142	2.1263	2.0564	1.9991	1.9512	1.9105	1.8753
90	3.9469	3.0977	2.7058	2.4729	2.3157	2.2011	2.1131	2.0430	1.9856	1.9376	1.8967	1.8613
100	3.9361	3.0873	2.6955	2.4626	2.3053	2.1906	2.1025	2.0323	1.9748	1.9267	1.8857	1.8503
110	3.9274	3.0788	2.6871	2.4542	2.2969	2.1821	2.0939	2.0236	1.9661	1.9178	1.8767	1.8412
120	3.9201	3.0718	2.6802	2.4472	2.2899	2.1750	2.0868	2.0164	1.9588	1.9105	1.8693	1.8337
130	3.9140	3.0658	2.6743	2.4414	2.2839	2.1690	2.0807	2.0103	1.9526	1.9042	1.8630	1.8273
140	3.9087	3.0608	2.6693	2.4363	2.2789	2.1639	2.0756	2.0051	1.9473	1.8989	1.8576	1.8219
150	3.9042	3.0564	2.6649	2.4320	2.2745	2.1595	2.0711	2.0006	1.9428	1.8943	1.8530	1.8172
160	3.9002	3.0525	2.6611	2.4282	2.2707	2.1557	2.0672	1.9967	1.9388	1.8903	1.8489	1.8131
170	3.8967	3.0491	2.6578	2.4248	2.2673	2.1523	2.0638	1.9932	1.9353	1.8868	1.8453	1.8095
180	3.8936	3.0461	2.6548	2.4218	2.2643	2.1492	2.0608	1.9901	1.9322	1.8836	1.8422	1.8063
190	3.8909	3.0435	2.6521	2.4192	2.2616	2.1466	2.0580	1.9874	1.9294	1.8808	1.8393	1.8034
200	3.8884	3.0411	2.6498	2.4168	2.2592	2.1441	2.0556	1.9849	1.9269	1.8783	1.8368	1.8008
210	3.8861	3.0389	2.6476	2.4146	2.2571	2.1419	2.0534	1.9827	1.9247	1.8760	1.8345	1.7985
220	3.8841	3.0369	2.6456	2.4127	2.2551	2.1400	2.0514	1.9807	1.9226	1.8739	1.8324	1.7964
230	3.8822	3.0351	2.6438	2.4109	2.2533	2.1381	2.0495	1.9788	1.9207	1.8720	1.8304	1.7944
240	3.8805	3.0334	2.6422	2.4093	2.2516	2.1365	2.0479	1.9771	1.9190	1.8703	1.8287	1.7927
250	3.8789	3.0319	2.6407	2.4078	2.2501	2.1350	2.0463	1.9756	1.9174	1.8687	1.8271	1.7910
260	3.8775	3.0305	2.6393	2.4064	2.2487	2.1335	2.0449	1.9741	1.9160	1.8672	1.8256	1.7895
270	3.8761	3.0292	2.6380	2.4051	2.2474	2.1322	2.0436	1.9728	1.9146	1.8659	1.8242	1.7881
280	3.8749	3.0280	2.6368	2.4039	2.2462	2.1310	2.0424	1.9715	1.9134	1.8646	1.8229	1.7869
290	3.8737	3.0269	2.6357	2.4028	2.2451	2.1299	2.0412	1.9704	1.9122	1.8634	1.8218	1.7857
300	3.8726	3.0258	2.6347	2.4017	2.2441	2.1289	2.0402	1.9693	1.9112	1.8623	1.8206	1.7845
310	3.8716	3.0249	2.6337	2.4008	2.2431	2.1279	2.0392	1.9683	1.9101	1.8613	1.8196	1.7835
320	3.8707	3.0240	2.6328	2.3999	2.2422	2.1269	2.0382	1.9674	1.9092	1.8603	1.8186	1.7825
330	3.8698	3.0231	2.6320	2.3990	2.2413	2.1261	2.0374	1.9665	1.9083	1.8594	1.8177	1.7816
340	3.8690	3.0223	2.6312	2.3982	2.2405	2.1253	2.0365	1.9657	1.9075	1.8586	1.8169	1.7807

(*Continued*)

Table C1.5-3 (*Continued*)

Degrees of freedom denominator	Degrees of freedom, numerator ν_1											
ν_2	1	2	3	4	5	6	7	8	9	10	11	12
350	3.8682	3.0215	2.6304	2.3975	2.2398	2.1245	2.0358	1.9649	1.9067	1.8578	1.8161	1.7799
360	3.8674	3.0208	2.6297	2.3967	2.2391	2.1238	2.0350	1.9641	1.9059	1.8570	1.8153	1.7791
370	3.8667	3.0201	2.6290	2.3961	2.2384	2.1231	2.0343	1.9634	1.9052	1.8563	1.8146	1.7784
380	3.8660	3.0195	2.6284	2.3954	2.2377	2.1224	2.0337	1.9628	1.9045	1.8556	1.8139	1.7777
390	3.8654	3.0189	2.6278	2.3948	2.2371	2.1218	2.0331	1.9622	1.9039	1.8550	1.8132	1.7770
400	3.8648	3.0183	2.6272	2.3942	2.2366	2.1212	2.0325	1.9616	1.9033	1.8544	1.8126	1.7764
420	3.8637	3.0172	2.6261	2.3932	2.2355	2.1202	2.0314	1.9605	1.9022	1.8533	1.8115	1.7753
440	3.8627	3.0162	2.6252	2.3922	2.2345	2.1192	2.0304	1.9594	1.9012	1.8522	1.8104	1.7742
460	3.8618	3.0153	2.6243	2.3913	2.2336	2.1183	2.0295	1.9585	1.9002	1.8513	1.8095	1.7732
480	3.8609	3.0145	2.6235	2.3905	2.2328	2.1175	2.0286	1.9577	1.8994	1.8504	1.8086	1.7724
500	3.8601	3.0138	2.6227	2.3898	2.2320	2.1167	2.0279	1.9569	1.8986	1.8496	1.8078	1.7715
600	3.8570	3.0107	2.6198	2.3868	2.2290	2.1137	2.0248	1.9538	1.8955	1.8465	1.8046	1.7683
700	3.8548	3.0086	2.6176	2.3847	2.2269	2.1115	2.0226	1.9516	1.8932	1.8442	1.8023	1.7660
800	3.8531	3.0070	2.6160	2.3831	2.2253	2.1099	2.0210	1.9500	1.8916	1.8425	1.8006	1.7643
900	3.8518	3.0057	2.6148	2.3818	2.2240	2.1086	2.0197	1.9487	1.8903	1.8412	1.7993	1.7629
1000	3.8508	3.0047	2.6138	2.3808	2.2231	2.1076	2.0187	1.9476	1.8892	1.8402	1.7982	1.7618
∞	3.8416	2.9958	2.6050	2.3720	2.2142	2.0987	2.0097	1.9385	1.8800	1.8308	1.7887	1.7523

Table C1.5-3 (*Continued*)

Degrees of freedom denominator	Degrees of freedom, numerator ν_1											
ν_2	14	16	20	24	30	40	50	75	100	200	500	∞
60	1.8602	1.8151	1.7480	1.7001	1.6491	1.5943	1.5590	1.5085	1.4814	1.4377	1.4093	1.3894
70	1.8357	1.7902	1.7223	1.6738	1.6220	1.5661	1.5300	1.4779	1.4498	1.4042	1.3743	1.3530
80	1.8174	1.7716	1.7032	1.6542	1.6017	1.5449	1.5081	1.4548	1.4259	1.3786	1.3472	1.3248
90	1.8032	1.7571	1.6883	1.6389	1.5859	1.5284	1.4910	1.4366	1.4070	1.3582	1.3256	1.3021
100	1.7919	1.7456	1.6764	1.6267	1.5733	1.5151	1.4772	1.4220	1.3917	1.3416	1.3079	1.2833
110	1.7827	1.7363	1.6667	1.6167	1.5630	1.5043	1.4660	1.4099	1.3791	1.3279	1.2931	1.2675
120	1.7750	1.7285	1.6587	1.6084	1.5543	1.4952	1.4565	1.3998	1.3685	1.3162	1.2804	1.2540
130	1.7686	1.7219	1.6519	1.6014	1.5470	1.4875	1.4485	1.3912	1.3595	1.3062	1.2695	1.2422
140	1.7630	1.7162	1.6460	1.5954	1.5408	1.4809	1.4416	1.3838	1.3517	1.2975	1.2600	1.2319
150	1.7582	1.7113	1.6410	1.5902	1.5354	1.4752	1.4357	1.3773	1.3448	1.2899	1.2516	1.2227
160	1.7540	1.7071	1.6366	1.5856	1.5306	1.4702	1.4304	1.3716	1.3388	1.2832	1.2442	1.2145
170	1.7504	1.7033	1.6327	1.5816	1.5264	1.4657	1.4258	1.3666	1.3335	1.2772	1.2375	1.2071
180	1.7471	1.7000	1.6292	1.5780	1.5227	1.4618	1.4217	1.3621	1.3288	1.2718	1.2315	1.2004
190	1.7441	1.6970	1.6261	1.5748	1.5194	1.4583	1.4180	1.3581	1.3245	1.2670	1.2260	1.1943
200	1.7415	1.6943	1.6233	1.5720	1.5164	1.4551	1.4146	1.3545	1.3206	1.2626	1.2211	1.1887
210	1.7391	1.6919	1.6208	1.5694	1.5136	1.4522	1.4116	1.3512	1.3171	1.2586	1.2165	1.1835
220	1.7370	1.6897	1.6185	1.5670	1.5112	1.4496	1.4088	1.3482	1.3139	1.2549	1.2123	1.1787
230	1.7350	1.6876	1.6164	1.5648	1.5089	1.4472	1.4063	1.3454	1.3110	1.2515	1.2084	1.1743
240	1.7332	1.6858	1.6145	1.5628	1.5069	1.4450	1.4040	1.3429	1.3083	1.2484	1.2049	1.1701
250	1.7315	1.6841	1.6127	1.5610	1.5049	1.4430	1.4019	1.3405	1.3058	1.2456	1.2015	1.1663
260	1.7300	1.6825	1.6111	1.5593	1.5032	1.4411	1.3999	1.3384	1.3035	1.2429	1.1985	1.1627
270	1.7285	1.6811	1.6096	1.5578	1.5016	1.4394	1.3981	1.3364	1.3014	1.2404	1.1956	1.1593
280	1.7272	1.6797	1.6082	1.5563	1.5001	1.4378	1.3964	1.3345	1.2994	1.2381	1.1929	1.1561
290	1.7260	1.6785	1.6069	1.5550	1.4986	1.4363	1.3948	1.3328	1.2975	1.2359	1.1903	1.1530
300	1.7249	1.6773	1.6057	1.5537	1.4973	1.4349	1.3934	1.3312	1.2958	1.2339	1.1879	1.1502

(*Continued*)

Table C1.5-3 (*Continued*)

Degrees of freedom denominator	Degrees of freedom, numerator ν_1											
ν_2	14	16	20	24	30	40	50	75	100	200	500	∞
310	1.7238	1.6762	1.6045	1.5526	1.4961	1.4336	1.3920	1.3296	1.2942	1.2320	1.1857	1.1475
320	1.7228	1.6752	1.6035	1.5515	1.4949	1.4323	1.3907	1.3282	1.2926	1.2302	1.1835	1.1449
330	1.7218	1.6742	1.6025	1.5504	1.4939	1.4312	1.3895	1.3269	1.2912	1.2285	1.1815	1.1424
340	1.7209	1.6733	1.6015	1.5494	1.4928	1.4301	1.3883	1.3256	1.2898	1.2269	1.1796	1.1401
350	1.7201	1.6725	1.6006	1.5485	1.4919	1.4291	1.3873	1.3244	1.2885	1.2254	1.1778	1.1379
360	1.7193	1.6717	1.5998	1.5477	1.4910	1.4281	1.3862	1.3233	1.2873	1.2239	1.1761	1.1358
370	1.7186	1.6709	1.5990	1.5468	1.4901	1.4272	1.3853	1.3222	1.2862	1.2226	1.1745	1.1337
380	1.7179	1.6702	1.5983	1.5461	1.4893	1.4263	1.3844	1.3212	1.2851	1.2213	1.1729	1.1318
390	1.7172	1.6695	1.5976	1.5453	1.4885	1.4255	1.3835	1.3202	1.2840	1.2200	1.1714	1.1299
400	1.7166	1.6688	1.5969	1.5446	1.4878	1.4247	1.3827	1.3193	1.2831	1.2189	1.1700	1.1281
420	1.7154	1.6676	1.5956	1.5433	1.4864	1.4232	1.3811	1.3176	1.2812	1.2167	1.1673	1.1248
440	1.7143	1.6665	1.5945	1.5421	1.4852	1.4219	1.3797	1.3161	1.2796	1.2147	1.1649	1.1216
460	1.7133	1.6655	1.5934	1.5411	1.4841	1.4207	1.3784	1.3147	1.2780	1.2128	1.1627	1.1187
480	1.7124	1.6646	1.5925	1.5401	1.4830	1.4196	1.3773	1.3134	1.2766	1.2111	1.1606	1.1160
500	1.7116	1.6638	1.5916	1.5392	1.4821	1.4186	1.3762	1.3122	1.2753	1.2096	1.1587	1.1135
600	1.7083	1.6604	1.5881	1.5355	1.4782	1.4145	1.3719	1.3073	1.2701	1.2033	1.1508	1.1029
700	1.7059	1.6580	1.5856	1.5329	1.4755	1.4116	1.3688	1.3039	1.2664	1.1987	1.1450	1.0947
800	1.7041	1.6562	1.5837	1.5310	1.4735	1.4094	1.3665	1.3013	1.2635	1.1953	1.1406	1.0882
900	1.7028	1.6548	1.5822	1.5294	1.4719	1.4077	1.3647	1.2993	1.2613	1.1925	1.1371	1.0829
1000	1.7017	1.6536	1.5811	1.5282	1.4706	1.4063	1.3632	1.2976	1.2596	1.1903	1.1342	1.0784
∞	1.6919	1.6436	1.5706	1.5174	1.4592	1.3941	1.3502	1.2830	1.2436	1.1702	1.1066	1.0105

Table C1.6 *H*-distribution Kruskal–Wallis *H*-test

				α				
N	n_1	n_2	n_3	0.10	0.05	0.025	0.01	0.001
7	3	2	2		4.71			
	3	3	1		5.14			
8	5	2	1	4.200	5.000			
	4	2	2	4.458	5.333	5.500		
	4	3	1	4.056	5.208	5.833		
	3	3	2	4.556	5.361	5.556		
9	7	1	1	4.267				
	6	2	1	4.200	4.822	5.600		
	5	2	2	4.373	5.160	6.000	6.533	
	5	3	1	4.018	4.960	6.044		
	4	3	2	4.511	5.444	6.000	6.444	
	4	4	1	4.167	4.967	6.167	6.667	
	3	3	3	4.622	5.600	5.956	7.200	
10	8	1	1	4.418				
	7	2	1	4.200	4.706	5.727		
	6	2	2	4.545	5.345	5.745	6.655	
	6	3	1	3.909	4.855	5.945	6.873	
	5	3	2	4.651	5.251	6.004	6.909	
	5	4	1	3.987	4.985	5.858	6.955	
	4	3	3	4.709	5.791	6.155	6.745	
	4	4	2	4.555	5.455	6.327	7.036	
11	8	2	1	4.011	4.909	5.420		
	7	2	2	4.526	5.143	5.818	7.000	
	7	3	1	4.173	4.952	5.758	7.030	
	6	3	2	4.682	5.348	6.136	6.970	
	6	4	1	4.038	4.947	5.856	7.106	
	5	3	3	4.533	5.648	6.315	7.079	8.727
	5	4	2	4.541	5.273	6.068	7.205	8.591
	5	5	1	4.109	5.127	6.000	7.309	
	4	4	3	4.545	5.598	6.394	7.144	8.909
12	8	2	2	4.587	5.356	5.817	6.663	
	8	3	1	4.010	4.881	6.064	6.804	
	7	3	2	4.582	5.357	6.201	6.839	8.654
	7	4	1	4.121	4.986	5.791	6.986	
	6	3	3	4.590	5.615	6.436	7.410	8.692
	6	4	2	4.494	5.340	6.186	7.340	8.827
	6	5	1	4.128	4.990	5.951	7.182	
	5	4	3	4.549	5.656	6.410	7.445	8.795
	5	5	2	4.623	5.338	6.346	7.338	8.938
	4	4	4	4.654	5.692	6.615	7.654	9.269

(Continued)

Table C1.6 (*Continued*)

				α				
N	n_1	n_2	n_3	0.10	0.05	0.025	0.01	0.001
13	8	3	2	4.451	5.316	6.195	7.022	8.791
	8	4	1	4.038	5.044	5.885	6.973	8.901
	7	3	3	4.603	5.620	6.449	7.228	9.262
	7	4	2	4.549	5.376	6.184	7.321	9.198
	7	5	1	4.035	5.064	5.953	7.061	9.178
	6	4	3	4.604	5.610	6.538	7.500	9.170
	6	5	2	4.596	5.338	6.196	7.376	9.189
	6	6	1	4.000	4.945	5.923	7.121	9.692
	5	4	4	4.668	5.657	6.673	7.760	9.168
	5	5	3	4.545	5.705	6.549	7.578	9.284
14	8	3	3	4.543	5.617	6.588	7.350	9.426
	8	4	2	4.500	5.393	6.193	7.350	9.293
	8	5	1	3.967	4.869	5.864	7.110	9.579
	7	4	3	4.527	5.623	6.578	7.550	9.670
	7	5	2	4.485	5.393	6.221	7.450	9.640
	7	6	1	4.033	5.067	6.067	7.254	9.747
	6	4	4	4.595	5.681	6.667	7.795	9.681
	6	5	3	4.535	5.602	6.667	7.590	9.669
	6	6	2	4.438	5.410	6.210	7.467	9.752
	5	5	4	4.523	5.666	6.760	7.823	9.606
15	8	4	3	4.529	5.623	6.562	7.585	9.742
	8	5	2	4.466	5.415	6.260	7.440	9.781
	8	6	1	4.015	5.015	5.933	7.256	9.840
	7	4	4	4.562	5.650	6.707	7.814	9.841
	7	5	3	4.535	5.607	6.627	7.697	9.874
	7	6	2	4.500	5.357	6.223	7.490	10.060
	7	7	1	3.986	4.986	6.057	7.157	9.871
	6	5	4	4.522	5.661	6.750	7.936	9.961
	6	6	3	4.558	5.625	6.725	7.725	10.150
	5	5	5	4.560	5.780	6.740	8.000	9.920
16	8	4	4	4.561	5.779	6.750	7.853	10.010
	8	5	3	4.514	5.614	6.614	7.706	10.040
	8	6	2	4.463	5.404	6.294	7.522	10.110
	8	7	1	4.045	5.041	6.047	7.308	10.030
	7	5	4	4.542	5.733	6.738	7.931	10.160
	7	6	3	4.550	5.689	6.694	7.756	10.260
	7	7	2	4.491	5.398	6.328	7.491	10.240
	6	5	5	4.547	5.729	6.788	8.028	10.290
	6	6	4	4.548	5.724	6.812	8.000	10.340

Table C1.6 (*Continued*)

N	n_1	n_2	n_3	α 0.10	0.05	0.025	0.01	0.001
17	8	5	4	4.549	5.718	6.782	7.992	10.290
	8	6	3	4.575	5.678	6.658	7.796	10.370
	8	7	2	4.451	5.403	6.339	7.571	10.360
	8	8	1	4.044	5.039	6.005	7.314	10.160
	7	5	5	4.571	5.708	6.835	8.108	10.450
	7	6	4	4.562	5.706	6.787	8.039	10.460
	7	7	3	4.613	5.688	6.708	7.810	10.450
	6	6	5	4.542	5.765	6.848	8.124	10.520
18	8	5	5	4.555	5.769	6.843	8.116	10.640
	8	6	4	4.563	5.743	6.795	8.045	10.630
	8	7	3	4.556	5.698	6.671	7.827	10.540
	8	8	2	4.509	5.408	6.351	7.654	10.460
	7	6	5	4.560	5.770	6.857	8.157	10.750
	7	7	4	4.563	5.766	6.788	8.142	10.690
	6	6	6	4.643	5.801	6.889	8.222	10.890
19	8	6	5	4.550	5.750	6.867	8.226	10.890
	8	7	4	4.548	5.759	6.837	8.118	10.840
	8	8	3	4.555	5.734	6.682	7.889	10.690
	7	6	6	4.530	5.730	6.897	8.257	11.000
	7	7	5	4.546	5.746	6.886	8.257	10.920
20	8	6	6	4.599	5.770	6.932	8.313	11.100
	8	7	5	4.551	5.782	6.884	8.242	11.030
	8	8	4	4.579	5.743	6.886	8.168	10.970
	7	7	6	4.568	5.793	6.927	8.345	11.130
21	8	7	6	4.553	5.781	6.917	8.333	11.280
	8	8	5	4.573	5.761	6.920	8.297	11.180
	7	7	7	4.594	5.818	6.954	8.378	11.320
22	8	7	7	4.585	5.802	6.980	8.363	11.420
	8	8	6	4.572	5.779	6.953	8.367	11.370
23	8	8	7	4.571	5.791	6.980	8.419	11.550
24	8	8	8	4.595	5.805	6.995	8.465	11.700
27	9	9	9	4.582	5.845	7.041	8.564	11.950
	∞	∞	∞	4.605	5.991	7.378	9.210	13.820

Table C1.7 *T*-critical values of the Wilcoxon singed-rank test

n	One-tailed: 0.05 Two-tailed: 0.10	0.025 0.05	0.01 0.02	0.005 0.010
5	0–15			
6	2–19	0–21		
7	3–25	2–26	0–28	
8	5–31	3–33	1–35	0–36
9	8–37	5–40	3–42	1–44
10	10–45	8–47	5–50	3–52
11	13–53	10–56	7–59	5–61
12	17–61	13–65	9–69	7–71
13	21–70	17–74	12–79	9–82
14	25–80	21–84	15–90	12–93
15	30–90	25–95	19–101	15–105
16	35–101	29–107	23–113	19–117
17	41–112	34–119	27–126	23–130
18	47–124	40–131	32–139	27–144
19	53–137	46–144	37–153	32–158
20	60–150	52–158	43–167	37–173
21	67–164	58–173	49–182	42–189
22	75–178	65–188	55–198	48–205
23	83–193	73–203	62–214	54–222
24	91–209	81–219	69–231	61–239
25	100–225	89–236	76–249	68–257
26	110–241	98–253	84–267	75–276
27	119–259	107–271	92–286	83–295
28	130–276	116–290	101–305	91–315
29	140–295	126–309	110–325	100–335
30	151–314	137–328	120–345	109–356
31	163–333	147–349	130–366	118–378
32	175–353	159–369	140–388	128–400
33	187–374	170–391	151–410	138–423
34	200–395	182–413	162–433	148–447
35	213–417	195–435	173–457	159–471
36	227–439	208–458	185–481	171–495
37	241–462	221–482	198–505	182–521
38	256–485	235–506	211–530	194–547
39	271–509	249–531	224–556	207–573
40	286–534	264–556	238–582	220–600
41	302–559	279–582	252–609	233–628
42	319–584	294–609	266–637	247–656
43	336–610	310–636	281–665	261–685
44	353–637	327–663	296–694	276–714
45	371–664	343–692	312–723	291–744
46	389–692	361–720	328–753	307–774
47	407–721	378–750	345–783	322–806
48	426–750	396–780	362–814	339–837
49	446–779	415–810	379–846	355–870
50	466–809	434–841	397–878	373–902

Table C1.8 ***T*-critical values of the Wilcoxon rank sum test**

	$P(1)$	$P(2)$
Line 1	0.05	0.1
Line 2	0.25	0.05
Line 3	0.01	0.02
Line 4	0.005	0.01

n_1 (smaller)	$n_2 - n_1$: 0	1	2	3	4	5	6	7	8	9	10
2				3–13	3–15	3–17	4–18	4–20	4–22	4–24	5–25
							3–19	8–21	3–23	3–25	4–26
3	6–15	6–18	7–20	8–22	8–25	9–27	10–29	10–32	11–34	11–37	12–39
			6–21	7–23	7–26	8–28	8–31	9–33	9–36	10–38	10–41
					6–27	6–30	7–32	7–35	7–38	8–40	8–42
							6–33	6–36	6–39	7–41	7–44
4	11–25	12–28	13–31	14–34	15–37	16–40	17–43	18–46	19–49	20–5	21–55
	10–26	11–29	12–32	13–35	14–38	14–42	15–45	16–48	17–51	18–54	19–57
		10–30	11–33	11–37	12–40	13–43	13–47	14–50	15–53	15–57	16–60
			10–34	10–38	11–41	11–45	12–48	12–52	13–55	13–59	14–62
5	19–36	20–40	21–44	23–47	24–51	26–54	27–58	28–62	30–65	31–69	33–72
	17–38	18–42	20–45	21–49	22–53	23–57	24–61	26–64	27–68	28–72	29–76
	16–39	17–43	18–47	19–51	20–55	21–59	22–63	23–67	24–71	25–75	26–79
	15–40	16–44	16–49	17–53	18–57	19–61	20–65	21–69	23–73	22–78	23–82
6	28–50	29–55	31–59	33–63	35–67	37–71	38–76	40–80	42–84	44–88	46–92

(Continued)

Table C1.8 (*Continued*)

n_1 (smaller)	$n_2 - n_1$										
	0	1	2	3	4	5	6	7	8	9	10
	26–52	27–57	29–61	31–65	32–70	34–74	35–79	37–83	38–88	40–92	42–96
	24–54	25–59	27–63	28–68	29–73	30–78	32–82	33–87	34–92	36–96	37–101
	23–55	24–60	25–65	26–70	27–75	28–80	30–84	31–89	32–94	33–99	34–104
7	39–66	41–71	43–76	45–81	47–86	49–91	52–95	54–100	56–105	58–110	61–114
	36–69	38–74	40–79	42–84	44–89	46–94	48–99	50–104	52–109	54–114	56–119
	34–71	35–77	37–82	39–87	40–93	42–98	41–103	45–109	47–114	49–119	51–124
	32–73	34–78	35–84	37–89	38–95	40–100	41–106	43–111	44–117	46–122	47–128
8	51–85	54–90	56–96	59–101	62–106	64–112	67–117	69–123	72–128	75–133	77–139
	49–87	51–93	53–99	55–105	58–110	60–116	62–122	65–127	67–133	70–138	72–144
	45–91	47–97	49–103	51–109	53–115	56–120	58–126	60–132	62–138	64–144	66–150
	43–93	45–99	47–105	49–111	51–117	53–123	54–130	56–136	58–142	60–148	62–165
9	66–105	69–111	72–117	75–123	78–129	81–135	84–141	87–147	90–153	93–159	96–165
	62–109	65–115	68–121	71–127	73–134	76–140	79–146	82–152	84–159	87–165	90–171
	59–112	61–119	63–126	66–132	68–139	71–145	73–152	76–158	78–165	81–171	83–178
	56–115	58–122	61–128	63–135	65–142	67–149	69–156	72–162	74–169	76–176	78–183
10	82–128	86–134	89–141	92–148	96–154	99–161	103–167	106–174	110–180	113–187	117–193
	78–132	81–139	84–146	88–152	91–159	94–166	97–173	100–180	103–187	107–193	110–200
	94–136	77–143	79–151	82–158	85–165	88–172	91–179	93–187	96–194	99–201	102–208
	71–139	73–147	76–154	79–161	81–169	84–176	86–184	89–191	92–198	94–206	97–213

Table C1.9 Critical values of the Spearman rank correlation coefficient r_s

	α			
n	0.10	0.05	0.02	0.01
4	1.000			
5	0.900	1.000	1.000	
6	0.829	0.886	0.943	1.000
7	0.714	0.786	0.893	0.929
8	0.643	0.738	0.833	0.881
9	0.600	0.700	0.783	0.833
10	0.564	0.648	0.745	0.794
11	0.536	0.618	0.709	0.755
12	0.503	0.587	0.678	0.727
13	0.484	0.560	0.648	0.703
14	0.464	0.538	0.626	0.679
15	0.446	0.521	0.604	0.654
16	0.429	0.503	0.582	0.635
17	0.414	0.485	0.566	0.615
18	0.401	0.472	0.550	0.600
19	0.391	0.460	0.535	0.584
20	0.380	0.447	0.520	0.570
25	0.337	0.398	0.466	0.511
30	0.306	0.362	0.425	0.467
35	0.283	0.335	0.394	0.433
40	0.264	0.313	0.368	0.405
45	0.248	0.294	0.347	0.382
50	0.235	0.279	0.329	0.363
60	0.214	0.255	0.300	0.331
70	0.198	0.235	0.278	0.307
80	0.185	0.200	0.260	0.287
90	0.174	0.207	0.245	0.271
100	0.165	0.197	0.233	0.257

Table C1.10 Sample size required for one group or pareddesigned t-test

	One-tailed: Two-tailed:	$\alpha = 0.005$ $\alpha = 0.01$				$\alpha = 0.01$ $\alpha = 0.02$					$\alpha = 0.025$ $\alpha = 0.05$					$\alpha = 0.05$ $\alpha = 0.1$				
δ/σ	$1-\beta = 0.99$	0.95	0.90	0.80	0.50	0.99	0.95	0.90	0.80	0.50	0.99	0.95	0.90	0.80	0.50	0.99	0.95	0.90	0.80	0.50
0.15																				122
0.20										139					99					70
0.25					110					90				128	64			139	101	45
0.30				134	78				115	63			119	90	45		122	97	71	32
0.35			125	99	58			109	85	47		109	88	67	34		90	72	52	24
0.40		115	97	77	45		101	85	66	37	117	84	68	51	26	101	70	55	40	19
0.45		92	77	62	37	110	81	68	53	30	93	67	54	41	21	80	55	44	33	15
0.50	100	75	63	51	30	90	66	55	43	25	76	54	44	34	18	65	45	36	27	13
0.55	83	63	53	42	26	75	55	46	36	21	63	45	37	28	15	54	38	30	22	11
0.60	71	53	45	36	22	63	47	39	31	18	53	38	32	24	13	46	32	26	19	9
0.65	61	46	39	31	20	55	41	34	27	16	46	33	27	21	12	39	28	22	17	8
0.70	53	40	34	28	17	47	35	30	24	14	40	29	24	19	10	34	24	19	15	8
0.75	47	36	30	25	16	42	31	27	21	13	35	26	21	16	9	30	21	17	13	7
0.80	41	32	27	22	14	37	28	24	19	12	31	22	19	15	9	27	19	15	12	6
0.85	37	29	24	20	13	33	25	21	17	11	28	21	17	13	8	24	17	14	11	6
0.90	34	26	22	18	12	29	23	19	16	10	25	19	16	12	7	21	15	13	10	5
0.95	31	24	20	17	11	27	21	18	14	9	23	17	14	11	7	19	14	11	9	5
1.0	28	22	19	16	10	25	19	16	13	9	21	16	13	10	6	18	13	11	8	5
1.1	24	19	16	14	9	21	16	14	12	8	18	13	11	9		15	11	9	7	
1.2	21	16	14	12	8	18	14	12	10	7	15	12	10	8	6	13	10	8	6	

Table C1.10 (*Continued*)

	One-tailed: / Two-tailed:	$\alpha = 0.005$ / $\alpha = 0.01$				$\alpha = 0.01$ / $\alpha = 0.02$					$\alpha = 0.025$ / $\alpha = 0.05$					$\alpha = 0.05$ / $\alpha = 0.1$				
δ/σ	$1-\beta = 0.99$	0.95	0.90	0.80	0.50	0.99	0.95	0.90	0.80	0.50	0.99	0.95	0.90	0.80	0.50	0.99	0.95	0.90	0.80	0.50
1.3	18	15	13	11	8	16	13	11	9	6	14	10	9	7	5	11	8	7	6	
1.4	16	13	12	10	7	14	11	10	9	6	12	9	8	7		10	8	7	5	
1.5	15	12	11	9	7	13	10	9	8	6	11	8	7	6		9	7	6		
1.6	13	11	10	8	6	12	10	9	7	5	10	8	7	6		8	6	6		
1.7	12	10	9	8	6	11	9	8	7		9	7	6	5		8	6	5		
1.8	12	10	9	8	6	10	8	7	7		8	7	6			7	6			
1.9	11	9	8	7	6	10	8	7	6		8	6	6			7	5			
2.0	10	8	8	7	5	9	7	7	6		7	6	5			6				
2.1	10	8	7	7		8	7	6	6	7	6					6				
2.2	9	8	7	6		8	7	6	5	7	6					6				
2.3	9	7	7	6		8	6	6			6	5				5				
2.4	8	7	7	6		7	6	6			6									
2.5	8	7	6	6		7	6	6			6									
3.0	7	6	6	5		6	5	5			5									
3.5	6	5	5			5														
4.0	6																			

Table C1.11 Sample size for t-test of comparing two means

	One-tailed: $\alpha = 0.005$ Two-tailed: $\alpha = 0.01$					One-tailed: $\alpha = 0.01$ Two-tailed: $\alpha = 0.02$				
δ/σ	$1-\beta = 0.99$	0.95	0.9	0.8	0.5	0.99	0.95	0.9	0.8	0.5
0.05										
0.10										
0.15										
0.20										
0.25										
0.30										123
0.35					110					90
0.40					85					70
0.45				118	68				101	55
0.50				96	55			106	82	45
0.55			101	79	46		106	88	68	38
0.60		101	85	67	39		90	74	58	32
0.65		87	73	57	34	104	77	64	49	27
0.70	100	75	63	50	29	90	66	55	43	24
0.75	88	66	55	44	26	79	58	48	38	21
0.80	77	58	49	39	23	70	51	43	33	19
0.85	69	51	43	35	21	62	46	38	30	17
0.90	62	46	39	31	19	55	41	34	27	15
0.95	55	42	35	28	17	50	37	31	24	14
1.00	50	38	32	26	15	45	33	28	22	13
1.1	42	32	27	22	13	38	28	23	19	11
1.2	36	27	23	18	11	32	24	20	16	9
1.3	31	23	20	16	10	28	21	17	14	8
1.4	27	20	17	14	9	24	18	15	12	8
1.5	24	18	15	13	8	21	16	14	11	7
1.6	21	16	14	11	7	19	14	12	10	6
1.7	19	15	13	10	7	17	13	11	9	6
1.8	17	13	11	10	6	15	12	10	8	5
1.9	16	12	11	9	6	14	11	9	8	5
2.0	14	11	10	8	6	13	10	9	7	5
2.1	13	10	9	8	5	12	9	8	7	5
2.2	12	10	8	7	5	11	9	7	6	4
2.3	11	9	8	7	5	10	8	7	6	4
2.4	11	9	8	6	5	10	8	7	6	4
2.5	10	8	7	6	4	9	7	6	5	4
3.0	8	6	6	5	4	7	6	5	4	3
3.5	6	5	5	4	3	6	5	4	4	
4.0	6	5	4	4		5	4	4	3	

Table C1.11 (*Continued*)

	One-tailed: $\alpha = 0.025$ Two-tailed: $\alpha = 0.05$					One-tailed: $\alpha = 0.05$ Two-tailed: $\alpha = 0.1$				
δ/σ	$1-\beta = 0.99$	0.95	0.9	0.8	0.5	0.99	0.95	0.9	0.8	0.5
0.05	—	—	—	—	—	—	—	—	—	—
0.10	—	—	—	—	—	—	—	—	—	—
0.15	—	—	—	—	—	—	—	—	—	—
0.20	—	—	—	—	—	—	—	—	—	137
0.25	—	—	—	—	124	—	—	—	—	88
0.30	—	—	—	—	87	—	—	—	—	61
0.35	—	—	—	—	64	—	—	—	102	45
0.40	—	—	—	100	50	—	—	108	78	35
0.45	—	—	105	79	39	—	108	86	62	28
0.50	—	106	86	64	32	—	88	70	51	23
0.55	—	87	71	53	27	112	73	58	42	19
0.60	104	74	60	45	23	89	61	49	36	16
0.65	88	63	51	39	20	76	52	42	30	14
0.70	76	55	44	34	17	66	45	36	26	12
0.75	67	48	39	29	15	57	40	32	23	11
0.80	59	42	34	26	14	50	35	28	21	10
0.85	52	37	31	23	12	45	31	25	18	9
0.90	47	34	27	21	11	40	28	22	16	8
0.95	42	30	25	19	10	36	25	20	15	7
1.00	38	27	23	17	9	33	23	18	14	7
1.1	32	23	19	14	8	27	19	15	12	6
1.2	27	20	16	12	7	23	16	13	10	5
1.3	23	17	14	11	6	20	14	11	9	5
1.4	20	15	12	10	6	17	12	10	8	4
1.5	18	13	11	9	5	15	11	9	7	4
1.6	16	12	10	8	5	14	10	8	6	4
1.7	14	11	9	7	4	12	9	7	6	3
1.8	13	10	8	6	4	11	8	7	5	—
1.9	12	9	7	6	4	10	7	6	5	—
2.0	11	8	7	6	4	9	7	6	4	—
2.1	10	8	6	5	3	8	6	5	4	—
2.2	9	7	6	5	—	8	6	5	4	—
2.3	9	7	6	5	—	7	5	5	4	—
2.4	8	6	5	4	—	7	5	4	4	—
2.5	8	6	5	4	—	6	5	4	3	—
3.0	6	5	4	4	—	5	4	3	—	—
3.5	5	4	4	3	—	4	3	—	—	—
4.0	4	4	3	—	—	4	—	—	—	—

Table C1.12 λ-value
(used in sample size calculation for comparison among multiple proportions)
($\alpha = 0.05$)

	β								
ν	0.9	0.8	0.7	0.6	0.5	0.4	0.3	0.2	0.1
1	0.43	1.24	2.06	2.91	3.84	4.90	6.17	7.85	10.51
2	0.62	1.73	2.78	3.83	4.96	6.21	7.70	9.63	12.65
3	0.78	2.10	3.30	4.50	5.76	7.15	8.79	10.90	14.17
4	0.91	2.40	3.74	5.05	6.42	7.92	9.68	11.94	15.41
5	1.03	2.67	4.12	5.53	6.99	8.59	10.45	12.83	16.47
6	1.13	2.91	4.46	5.96	7.50	9.19	11.14	13.62	17.42
7	1.23	3.13	4.77	6.35	7.97	9.73	11.77	14.35	18.28
8	1.32	3.33	5.06	6.71	8.40	10.24	12.35	15.02	19.08
9	1.40	3.53	5.33	7.05	8.81	10.71	12.89	15.65	19.83
10	1.49	3.71	5.59	7.37	9.19	11.15	13.40	16.24	20.53
11	1.56	3.88	5.83	7.68	9.56	11.57	13.89	16.80	21.20
12	1.64	4.05	6.06	7.97	9.90	11.98	14.35	17.34	21.83
13	1.71	4.20	6.29	8.25	10.23	12.36	14.80	17.85	22.44
14	1.77	4.36	6.50	8.52	10.55	12.73	15.22	18.34	23.02
15	1.84	4.50	6.71	8.78	10.86	13.09	15.63	18.81	23.58
16	1.90	4.65	6.91	9.03	11.16	13.43	16.03	19.27	24.13
17	1.97	4.78	7.10	9.27	11.45	13.77	16.41	19.71	24.65
18	2.03	4.92	7.29	9.50	11.73	14.09	16.78	20.14	25.16
19	2.08	5.05	7.47	9.73	12.00	14.41	17.14	20.56	25.65
20	2.14	5.18	7.65	9.96	12.26	14.71	17.50	20.96	26.13
21	2.20	5.30	7.83	10.17	12.52	15.01	17.84	21.36	26.60
22	2.25	5.42	8.00	10.38	12.77	15.30	18.17	21.74	27.06
23	2.30	5.54	8.16	10.59	13.02	15.59	18.50	22.12	27.50
24	2.36	5.66	8.33	10.79	13.26	15.87	18.82	22.49	27.94
25	2.41	5.77	8.48	10.99	13.49	16.14	19.13	22.85	28.37
26	2.46	5.88	8.64	11.19	13.72	16.41	19.44	23.20	28.78
27	2.51	5.99	8.79	11.38	13.95	16.67	19.74	23.55	29.19

Table C1.12 (*Continued*)

	β								
ν	0.9	0.8	0.7	0.6	0.5	0.4	0.3	0.2	0.1
28	2.56	6.10	8.94	11.57	14.17	16.93	20.04	23.89	29.60
29	2.60	6.20	9.09	11.75	14.39	17.18	20.33	24.22	29.99
30	2.65	6.31	9.24	11.93	14.60	17.43	20.61	24.55	30.38
31	2.69	6.41	9.38	12.11	14.82	17.67	20.89	24.87	30.76
32	2.74	6.51	9.52	12.28	15.02	17.91	21.17	25.19	31.13
33	2.78	6.61	9.66	12.45	15.23	18.15	21.44	25.50	31.50
34	2.83	6.70	9.79	12.62	15.43	18.38	21.70	25.80	31.87
35	2.87	6.80	9.93	12.79	15.63	18.61	21.97	26.11	32.23
36	2.91	6.89	10.06	12.96	15.82	18.84	22.23	26.41	32.58
37	2.96	6.99	10.19	13.12	16.01	19.06	22.48	26.70	32.93
38	3.00	7.08	10.32	13.28	16.20	19.28	22.73	26.99	33.27
39	3.04	7.17	10.45	13.44	16.39	19.50	22.98	27.27	33.61
40	3.08	7.26	10.57	13.59	16.58	19.71	23.23	27.56	33.94
50	3.46	8.10	11.75	15.06	18.31	21.72	25.53	30.20	37.07
60	3.80	8.86	12.81	16.38	19.88	23.53	27.61	32.59	39.89
70	4.12	9.56	13.79	17.60	21.32	25.20	29.52	34.79	42.48
80	4.41	10.21	14.70	18.74	22.67	26.75	31.29	36.83	44.89
90	4.69	10.83	15.56	19.80	23.93	28.21	32.96	38.74	47.16
100	4.95	11.41	16.37	20.81	25.12	29.59	34.54	40.56	49.29
110	5.20	11.96	17.14	21.77	26.25	30.90	36.04	42.28	51.33
120	5.44	12.49	17.88	22.68	27.34	32.15	37.47	43.92	53.27

Table C1.13 λ-value
(used in sample size calculation for comparison among multiple proportions)

$1-\beta$	$1-\beta = 0.80$		$1-\beta = 0.90$	
k	$\alpha = 0.01$	$\alpha = 0.05$	$\alpha = 0.01$	$\alpha = 0.05$
2	11.68	7.85	14.88	10.51
3	13.80	9.64	17.43	12.66
4	15.46	10.91	19.25	14.18
5	16.75	11.94	20.74	15.41
6	17.87	12.83	22.03	16.47
7	18.88	13.63	23.19	17.42
8	19.79	14.36	24.24	18.29
9	20.64	15.03	25.22	19.09
10	21.43	15.65	26.13	19.83
11	22.18	16.25	26.99	20.54
12	22.89	16.81	27.80	21.20
13	23.57	17.34	28.58	21.84
14	24.22	17.85	29.32	22.44
15	24.84	18.34	30.04	23.03
16	25.44	18.82	30.73	23.59
17	26.02	19.27	31.39	24.13
18	26.58	19.71	32.04	24.65
19	27.12	20.14	32.66	25.16
20	27.65	20.56	33.27	25.66

INDEX

Lightning Source UK Ltd.
Milton Keynes UK
UKHW021502180321
380529UK00003B/114

9 789811 228865

D BS

7/11/23